THE MANAGEMENT OF
DEPRESSION

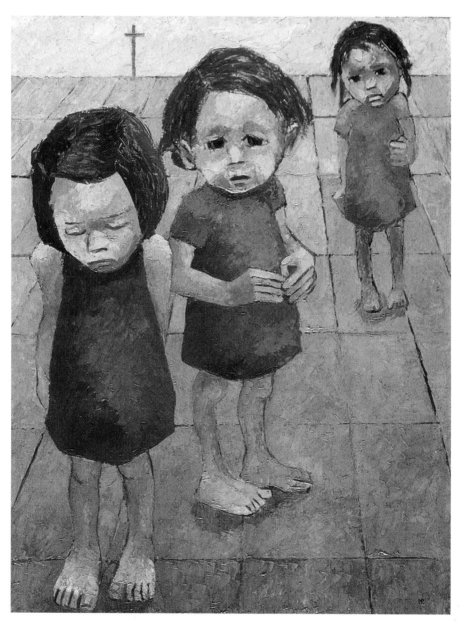

Frontispiece *The Cross* by Marion Patrick *c.* 1967; oil on hardboard. Reproduced with the kind permission of Bethlem Royal Hospital Archives and Museum, and the Ridehalgh family on behalf of the late Marion Patrick.

The Management of
DEPRESSION

EDITED BY
STUART CHECKLEY

BM, BCh FRCP, FRCPsych
Dean, Institute of Psychiatry,
Denmark Hill, London

Blackwell
Science

© 1998 by
Blackwell Science Ltd
Editorial Offices:
Osney Mead, Oxford OX2 0EL
25 John Street, London WC1N 2BL
23 Ainslie Place, Edinburgh EH3 6AJ
350 Main Street, Malden
  MA 02148 5018, USA
54 University Street, Carlton
  Victoria 3053, Australia
10 rue Casimir Delavigne
  75006 Paris, France

Other Editorial Offices:
Blackwell Wissenschafts-Verlag GmbH
Kurfürstendamm 57
10707 Berlin, Germany

Blackwell Science KK
MG Kodenmacho Building
7–10 Kodenmacho Nihombashi
Chuo-ku, Tokyo 104, Japan

First published 1998

Set by Setrite Typesetters, Hong Kong
Printed and bound in Great Britain
at the University Press, Cambridge

The Blackwell Science logo is a
trade mark of Blackwell Science Ltd,
registered at the United Kingdom
Trade Marks Registry

DISTRIBUTORS

  Marston Book Services Ltd
  PO Box 269
  Abingdon
  Oxon OX14 4YN
  (*Orders*: Tel: 01235 465500
         Fax: 01235 465555)
USA
  Blackwell Science, Inc.
  Commerce Place
  350 Main Street
  Malden, MA 02148 5018
  (*Orders*: Tel: 800 759 6102
         781 388 8250
        Fax: 781 388 8255)
Canada
  Copp Clark Professional
  200 Adelaide St, West, 3rd Floor
  Toronto, Ontario, M5H 1W7
  (*Orders*: Tel: 416 597-1616
        800 815-9417
        Fax: 416 597-1617)
Australia
  Blackwell Science Pty Ltd
  54 University Street
  Carlton, Victoria 3053
  (*Orders*: Tel: 3 9347 0300
        Fax: 3 9347 5001)

A catalogue record for this title
is available from the British Library

ISBN 0-86542-987-1

Library of Congress
Cataloging-in-publication Data

Management of depression / edited by Stuart
Checkley.
    p.   cm.
    Includes bibliographical references and
index.
    ISBN 0-86542-987-1
    1. Depression, Mental. I. Checkley, Stuart.
RC537.M34 1997
616.85'270651–dc21
                        97-6410
                        CIP

Contents

Contents

List of contributors

LUCY C. AITKEN MRCPsych, *Senior Registrar in Old Age Psychiatry, Withington Hospital, Nell Lane, Manchester M20 2LR*

ROBERT C. BALDWIN, DM, FRCP, FRCPsych, *Old Age Service, Psychiatry Directorate, Central Manchester Healthcare NHS Trust, York House, York Place, Oxford Road, Manchester M13 9WL*

PAUL BEBBINGTON, MA, PhD, FRCP, FRCPsych, *Professor of Social and Community Psychiatry and Behavioural Sciences, University College London, Archway Wing, Whittington Hospital, Highgate Hill, London N19 5NF*

KAMALDEEP BHUI MSc, MRCPsych, *Wellcome Research Fellow, Institute of Psychiatry, De Crespigny Park, Denmark Hill, London SE5 8AZ*

STUART CHECKLEY BM, BCh, FRCP, FRCPsych, *Dean and Professor of Psychoneuroendocrinology, Institute of Psychiatry, De Crespigny Park, Denmark Hill, London SE5 8AF*

JOHN COOKSON BM, DPhil, FRCP, FRCPsych, *Consultant and Honorary Senior Lecturer in Psychiatry, Royal London Hospital (St Clements), 2A Bow Road, London E3 4LL*

PHILIP J. COWEN MD, FRCPsych, *Professor of Psychopharmacology, Psychopharmacology Research Unit, Warneford Hospital, Headington, Oxford OX3 7JX*

ERIC FOMBONNE MD, MRCPysch, *Reader in Epidemiological Child Psychiatry and Honorary Consultant, Department of Child and Adolescent Psychiatry, Institute of Psychiatry, De Crespigny Park, Denmark Hill, London SE5 8AF*

DAVID GOLDBERG DM, FRCP, FRCPsych, *Professor of Psychiatry, Institute of Psychiatry, De Crespigny Park, Denmark Hill, London SE5 8AF*

GILLIAN E. HARDY MSc, *Clinical Research Fellow, Psychological Therapies Research Centre, University of Leeds, 17 Blenheim Terrace, Leeds LS2 9JT*

TIRRIL O. HARRIS MA, *Senior Research Fellow, Royal Holloway, University of London, 11 Bedford Square, London WC1D 3RA*

MATTHEW HOTOPF BSc, MBBS MRCPsych, MSc, *Clinical Research Fellow and Lecturer in Psychiatry, Department of Psychological Medicine, Institute of Psychiatry, De Crespigny Park, Denmark Hill, London SE5 8AZ*

R. CHANNI KUMAR MD, PhD, FRCPsych, *Professor of Perinatal Psychiatry, Department of Perinatal Psychiatry, Institute of Psychiatry, De Crespigny Park, Denmark Hill, London SE5 8AF*

MALCOLM H. LADER DSc, PhD, MD, FRCPsych, *Professor of Clinical Psychopharmacology, Institute of Psychiatry, De Crespigny Park, Denmark Hill, London SE5 8AF*

DOMINIC LAM PhD, *Senior Lecturer in Clinical Psychology, Department of Psychology, Institute of Psychiatry, De Crespigny Park, Denmark Hill, London SE5 8AF*

ANTHONY MANN MD, FRCP, FRCPsych, *Professor of Epidemiological Psychiatry, Institute of Psychiatry, De Crespigny Park, Denmark Hill, London SE5 8AF*

MAUREEN MARKS Dphil, *Senior Lecturer, Department of Perinatal Psychiatry, Institute of Psychiatry, De Crespigny Park, Denmark Hill, London SE5 8AF*

ALLAN I. F. SCOTT BSc, MPhil, MD, MBA, MRCPsych, *Consultant Psychiatrist, Andrew Duncan Clinic, Royal Edinburgh Hospital, Morningside Terrace, Edinburgh EH10 5HF*

DAVID A. SHAPIRO BA, MSc, PhD, FBPsS, *Professor of Clinical Psychology and Director, Psychological Therapies Research Centre, University of Leeds, 17 Blenheim Terrace, Leeds, LS2 9JT*

GERALDINE STRATHDEE MBBCh, MRCPsych, *Head of Service Development, Sainsbury's Centre for Mental Health, 134–138 Borough High Street, London SE1 1LB*

DAVID TAYLOR, BSc MSc, MRPharms, *Chief Pharmacist, Maudsley Hospital, Denmark Hill, London SE5 8AZ*

EDWARD WATKINS MSc, CPsychol, *Institute of Psychiatry, De Crespigny Park, Denmark Hill, London SE5 8AF*

SCOTT WEICH MRCPsych, MSc, *Senior Lecturer in Psychiatry, Academic Department of Psychiatry, Royal Free Hospital Medical School, Rowland Hill Street, London NW3 2PF*

SIMON WESSELY, MA, BM, BCh, MSc, MD, FRCP, MRCPsych, *Professor of Epidemiological and Liaison Psychiatry, King's College School of Medicine and Institute of Psychiatry, De Crespigny Park, Denmark Hill, London SE5 8AF*

RUTH WILLIAMS MA, CPsychol, *Senior Lecturer in Clinical Psychology, Institute of Psychiatry, De Crespigny Park, Denmark Hill, London SE5 8AF*

Introduction

The purpose of this book is to bring together from different disciplines what is known about the management of depression. A great deal has been learnt during the last 30 years concerning the effectiveness of the main physical and psychological treatments for depression. Important advances have also been made in understanding the biological and psychosocial causes of depression and the mechanisms by which physical and psychological treatments work. Yet most of these advances have been made in isolation from each other. There has been some integration between the psychological and social studies of depression but little between the psychosocial and biological. Most cases of depression in the community can be treated satisfactorily either with psychological or with physical treatment, yet little is known about interactions between the two, and in everyday practice most clinicians operate within an exclusively biological or psychosocial framework. The intention of this book is to bring these different approaches together whenever possible.

The first section of the book deals with epidemiology and aetiological models in so far as they relate to the treatment of depression. For a much fuller account of aetiology the reader is referred to Paykel (1992)[1] and more specialist reviews (Bloom & Kupfer 1995).[2] In order to discuss the management of depression in the different levels of care in which it presents, it is first necessary to have an understanding of the epidemiology of this extremely common disorder (Chapter 1), and second to understand how depression presents at different levels of care and, also, which filters regulate the movement of patients from one level of care (e.g. primary or secondary) to another (Chapter 2). The next four chapters summarize, from a clinical perspective, the biological, social and psychological models of depression. Genetic studies have defined both the environmental and genetic contribution as lifetime

---

[1]Paykel, E.S. (1992) *Handbook of Affective Disorders*, 2nd edn. Churchill Livingstone, Edinburgh.

[2]Bloom, F.E. & Kupfer, D.J. (1995) *Psychopharmacology: the Fourth Generation of Progress*. Raven Press, New York.

vulnerability to all forms of depression, and have clearly shown the different balance between the influence of nature (genetics) and nurture (environment) in different forms of depression (unipolar and bipolar). The psychosocial model described in Chapter 4 accounts for most of the variance in onset in the majority of episodes of unipolar depression, and for much of the variance in rates of recovery. The model is extremely well cross-referenced throughout the book and clearly provides one unifying theme. Another is provided by the cognitive model of depression (Chapter 5), which seeks to explain the mechanisms of action of cognitive therapy but also provides a good understanding of the psychological mediators between the effects of distal and proximal social processes on the onset of depression (Chapter 4). Another unifying theme is attachment (Chapter 6), which, as well as being central to any understanding of interpersonal psychotherapy, is also implicated in mechanisms of social support. Few links currently exist between these psychosocial models and the biology of depression, but a neuroendocrine mechanism which might underlie the psychosocial model is described in Chapter 3. Biological models come into their own in understanding the mechanisms of action of currently established antidepressant treatments and in suggesting new forms of treatment for the future (Chapter 3).

The second section of the book reviews what is known of the wanted and unwanted effects of the main antidepressant treatments. Few, if any, of these treatments produce a change in depression ratings which is greater than the standard deviation of the baseline score. For this reason it is necessary to be certain that all treatments are given in an optimal manner: where possible each chapter in this section indicates what is thought to be the optimal use of the treatment in question. Available information on the unwanted as well as the wanted effects of antidepressant treatment is reviewed particularly in the case of antidepressant medication (Chapter 11), for which most prescribing decisions within any class of drug are made on the basis of unwanted rather than wanted drug effects.

The final section of the book describes the management of depression in the very different settings and age groups at which it presents. Although there are some striking and unexplained differences (e.g., the fact that antidepressant drugs do not appear to be effective in childhood depression), the similarities between these final chapters are much greater than the differences: all adopt a multidisciplinary model; most refer to the psychosocial model mentioned in Chapter 4; most use cognitive models and/or cognitive therapy; and yet all have expertise in the appropriate use of physical treatments.

It is a pleasure to acknowledge the timely and excellent chapters which my colleagues have written for this book. Many of us have collaborated in clinical and academic matters over the years and it is hoped that this will be an advantage rather than a disadvantage to the overall aim of the book; which is to integrate different approaches to the treatment of depression. I would also like to acknowledge particularly the contribution made by Claire Daunton who provided editorial assistance in the preparation of the manuscripts.

Stuart Checkley

1 The assessment and epidemiology of affective disorder

PAUL BEBBINGTON

The aim of this chapter is to review the epidemiology of affective disorder in the light of constraints which arise from problems of measurement. The central problem is that epidemiology is essentially a medical discipline and therefore exploits the concept of disease. Diseases are primarily categories. While, for many diseases, what starts off as a categorical concept ends by revealing underlying continuities, the continuous distribution of depressive symptoms in the general population is obvious from the outset. There is little evidence for valid cut-points, and a disease-based approach must therefore be offset by a robust scepticism: the categories beloved of the epidemiologist should be treated as particularly tentative fictions. Such fictions may assist the progress of knowledge, but if we are to rely on them, they must be used consistently.

Modern psychiatric classifications and case definition

The purpose of any classification is to aid communication. In psychiatry we use mental phenomena (and sometimes physical correlates) as the basis of classification so that diagnostic classes and also series of exemplars of a given class can be compared. This is done in order to test ideas relating to the cause, outcome and treatment of the disorders that are represented by the class.

Diagnostic classes depend on two sets of definition: that relating to the class itself and that relating to the elements making up the criteria for class recognition. In psychiatry the first type of definition relates to the *syndromes* that form the basis of disorders, while the second relates to *clinical phenomena*, mainly symptoms. Symptoms are used according to given rules to construct syndromes. In recent years these rules have been set out explicitly in the Diagnostic Criteria for Research (DCR) attached to specific classifications such as DSM-III-R (American Psychiatric Association (APA), 1987), DSM-IV (APA, 1994) and ICD-10, so precisely that it is possible to incorporate them into computer algorithms such as CATEGO (Wing *et al.*, 1990) and OPCRIT (McGuffin *et al.*, 1991).

Once the presence of symptoms has been established, the information can be entered into the computer program in order to provide a diagnostic classification. Human idiosyncrasy can be reduced to an absolute minimum in this process. However, researchers must then decide how carefully the underlying symptoms should be identified. The choices include unstructured clinical assessment, responses to questionnaires, and semi-structured research interviews; each has its own problems.

1   Unstructured clinical judgement introduces variability into the process of case allocation, since researchers are relying merely on their devotion to a common educational tradition. The identification of clinical symptoms may consequently be biased by prior prejudices in favour of a particular diagnosis. This situation is even worse when the judgements of others (for example the treating physician) are used, as with the diagnostic information recorded in case registers or in national statistics.

2   In order to be practicable, questionnaires should comprise simple responses to unelaborated questions. However, symptoms are traditionally recognized through an assessment of mental experiences that demand quite elaborate enquiry. They are usually established by a process of clinical cross-examination. This process is rather complicated since it requires the questioner to frame further questions in a flexible way in the light of the answers given by the subject. While it might be possible to encapsulate this procedure in a branching algorithm, it would be exhaustive and exhausting. It might require paths comprising over a dozen questions just to establish the presence of depressed mood. In these circumstances there are clearly limits to the process of standardization, and we are probably better off relying on the shortcuts available from using the skills of trained clinicians. Since diagnosis is built around symptoms defined and elicited in this manner, redefinition in terms of answers to much more limited questions would involve changing the concept of diagnosis itself. No-one has seriously suggested that the conceptualization of psychiatric symptoms should be changed; therefore if a questionnaire is used, phenomena may be recorded as present when subsequent clinical enquiry might reveal otherwise, and vice versa. Nevertheless, structured questionnaires allow lay interviewers to be used, with considerable cost savings.

3   Semi-structured research interviews are costly in clinical time, and the way in which symptoms are established makes it impossible to standardize the procedure entirely (Robins, 1995). Because of the reliance on clinical judgement and the effect this has on the choice of follow-up questions, some variability will remain. This is the price paid for greater validity, that is, the closer approximation to the clinical consensus about the nature of given symptoms.

Classifications in psychiatry were originally developed on the basis of an informal process of abstraction, involving the exercise of considerable intellectual effort; revision of classificatory schemata in the early days relied almost wholly on clinical reflection. However, since the classifications are set up primarily for scientific purposes, they should be properly modified in the light of empirical research which permits definitive statements about their utility, and the standardized and operationalized classifications which are now available offer an opportunity for using research in this way. Unfortunately, much of the pressure for change has continued to originate from clinical and political demands. Revisions have sometimes had the appearance of tinkering in order to capture some imagined essence of the included disorders (Birley, 1990). What looks like fine-tuning can nevertheless make considerable differences to whether disorders meet criteria or not, and thus affects prevalence data disproportionately. Classifications should only be jettisoned on grounds of inadequate scientific utility and as seldom as possible, since too rapid revision defeats the objective of comparison. Moreover, classifications are created by committees, and the natural tendency to horse-trading between experts selected precisely because they are powerful and opinionated leads to an overelaborate structure, an excess of allowable classes and subclasses, and complicated defining criteria.

All these tendencies are apparent in the classification of affective disorders in DSM and ICD-10 (World Health Organization (WHO), 1992). Thus in DSM-III-R there are potentially 14 categories to consider before allocating someone with depressed mood, and in ICD-10 (WHO, 1992) there are 22 categories. It is the author's view that greater utility would accrue from limiting the primary categories to three (bipolar disorder, unipolar depressive psychosis and unipolar non-psychotic depression), and epidemiological research often uses these categories in any case.

However, DSM and ICD are clearly the major accepted classifications. What are their implications for case definition and identification? For the purpose of illustration, Table 1.1 compares the criteria relating to major depressive disorders (MDD) and depressive episode (DE). It will be seen that, although there is a welcome convergence between DSM and ICD, the categorization is far from identical. This has serious implications for studies of affective disorder, particularly those seeking to establish prevalence and comorbidity. The categories are far enough apart to cause discrepancies in identification, but probably too close together for empirical studies to establish their relative validity. Moreover, a few DSM and several ICD categories lack DCRs, and the existence of such rag-bag categories takes away from the comparability that the system as a whole strives for.

The disorders with explicit DCRs are the more severe ones. This is reflected in reported prevalences. Thus in the Epidemiologic Catchment Area (ECA) studies, despite anxieties that the instrument used (the Diagnostic Interview Schedule (DIS); Robins *et al.*, 1985) overestimated prevalence: the prevalence of MDD was only 1.7–3.1% (Robins & Regier, 1991). In its mild form, the ICD category DE has a slightly lower threshold than MDD, but the 1-month

Table 1.1 Criteria for depressive episode.

DSM-III-R/DSM-IV	ICD-10
Symptoms present nearly every day in the same 2-week period	Episode must have lasted at least 2 weeks with symptoms nearly every day
Change from normal functioning	Change from normal functioning
Key symptoms (n = 2) Depressed mood Anhedonia	*Key symptoms (n = 3)* Depressed mood Anhedonia Fatigue/loss of energy
Ancillary symptoms (n = 7) Fatigue/loss of energy Weight/appetite loss/gain Insomnia/hypersomnia Observed agitation/retardation Low self-esteem/guilt Impaired thinking/concentration Suicidal thoughts	*Ancillary symptoms (n = 7)* Weight and appetite change Sleep disturbance Subjective or objective agitation/retardation Low self-esteem/confidence Self reproach/guilt Impaired thinking/concentration Suicidal thoughts
Criteria: 1 key, 5 symptoms in total **Plus** significant distress **Or** social impairment	*Criteria:* Mild episode: 2 key, 4 symptoms in total Moderate episode: 2 key, 6 symptoms in total Severe episode: 3 key, 8 symptoms in total
Exclusions Not mixed episode Not substance related Not organic Not bereavement Not psychotic	*Exclusions* No history (ever) of manic symptoms Not substance related Not organic

prevalence of all forms of depressive episode reported in the current British National Survey of Psychiatric Morbidity is still only 2.1% (Jenkins *et al.*, 1997a, 1997b). 'Moderate' and 'severe' episodes are correspondingly rare. However, several community surveys have used the 9th edition of the Present-State Examination (PSE), which, in so far as it approximates to genuine diagnostic categories, deals with disorders of somewhat lower threshold (Bebbington, 1990). The disorders lying between the two thresholds would fall into other DSM and ICD categories. These include dysthymia (which demands a minimum course, albeit fluctuating, of 2 years) and in ICD, mixed anxiety/depression, which lacks DCRs. In the British National Survey, we followed the ICD suggestion and constructed our own criteria for this category. These comprised of a failure to meet criteria for other conditions, despite a score of 12 or more on the revised Clinical Interview Schedule (CIS-R) (Lewis *et al.*, 1992). So defined, the disorder had a nationwide prevalence of 7.7%, reflecting a threshold considerably lower than that for MDD or DE (Jenkins *et al.*, 1997b).

Clinical studies of depressive disorder are likely to concern cases that mainly meet criteria for MDD or DE. However, in the case of *community* and *primary care studies*, we are faced with a serious dilemma. It is clear the classificatory systems are failing in their primary objective of assisting research. Researchers will either use the categories of MDD and DE and accept that they will find relatively few cases to study at relatively high cost, or they will stick with the less severe conditions they have traditionally studied. If they choose the second course, many of the cases will fall into classes that do not have specific DCRs, and comparability will be lost.

It should be noted that the relatively high threshold of the core affective categories in DSM and ICD-10 also has consequences for the use of screening instruments. Thus data from the Camberwell Community Needs Survey (Bebbington *et al.*, 1997b) suggest that in relation to ICD-10 cases, the GHQ-28 had a sensitivity of 81%, a specificity of 65% and a positive predictive value of 32%. The last figure indicates a need to interview three community subjects who score above cut-off to identify one ICD-10 case. Thus screening instruments may require modification for use with the new classifications.

Measuring frequency

Frequency can be measured in a variety of ways: incidence; point, period and lifetime prevalence; and morbid risk. General population surveys commonly report period or lifetime prevalence, while investigations of clinical series often use first contact or admission as a proxy for incidence.

While community psychiatric surveys date back to Rosanoff's (1916) study in Nassau County, it is only recently that they have provided adequate diagnostic information based on standardized methods of assessment allowing the comparison of research from different locations (Dohrenwend & Dohrenwend, 1982). Two groups of studies are of particular value, those based on the PSE-ID-CATEGO system (Wing *et al.*, 1978), and those using DIS (Robins *et al.*, 1985) developed for the ECA surveys. The first group is linked to ICD-9 (WHO, 1978), the second to DSM-III (APA, 1980).

Studies using the 9th edition of the PSE and providing a breakdown of diagnostic categories are listed in Table 1.2. CATEGO depressive categories correspond to ICD-9 codes 296.2 (depressive psychosis) and 300.4 (neurotic depression). The data for the Camberwell Needs for Care Survey (Bebbington *et al.*, 1997a, 1997b) were derived from the 10th edition of the PSE, which is incorporated into an instrument called SCAN (WHO, 1992). There is downward compatibility, so these data were processed by the CATEGO-IV system to produce equivalent categories in the other studies. However, this procedure must be viewed with considerable reservation (P.E. Bebbington & L. Marsden, unpublished information).

Data on depression from the DIS surveys are given in Table 1.3. For dysthymia, only lifetime data are available. These have now been collated by the Cross-National Collaborative Group (1992; Weissman *et al.* 1996), with a

Table 1.2 Prevalence of CATEGO depressive classes (%).

Site	n	Male	Female	Total
Group 1				
Canberra (Henderson et al., 1979)*	756 (157)	2.6	6.7	4.8
Camberwell (Bebbington et al., 1981)*	800 (310)	4.8	9.0	7.0
Edinburgh (Surtees et al., 1983)	576	–	6.9	–
Nijmegen (Hodiamont et al., 1987)*	3232 (486)	–	–	5.5
Finland (Lehtinen et al., 1990)†	742	2.4	6.5	4.6
Camberwell (Bebbington & Marsden, 1997b)*	760 (408)	5.7	5.2	5.4
Group 2				
Athens (Mavreas et al., 1986)	489	4.3	10.1	7.4
Santander (Vazquez-Barquero et al., 1987)*	1223 (452)	4.5	7.8	6.2
Camberwell (Cypriot) (Mavreas & Bebbington, 1987)	307	4.2	7.1	5.6
Sardinia (Carta et al., 1991)	374	5.2	11.0	8.3
Group 3				
Uganda (Orley & Wing, 1979)	206	17.0	21.0	18.9
Palembang (Bahar, 1989)	839 (100)	–	–	6.5
Dubai (Ghubash et al., 1992)	300	–	13.7	–

* Two-stage survey—numbers given PSE at second stage in brackets. Prevalences weighted to represent original population.
† Age adjusted figures.
Studies that do not give a breakdown in terms of CATEGO classes are not included.

view to providing standard reporting of data. The range of prevalences given in Table 1.4 is difficult to explain, as it does not correspond to the obvious cultural differences between the locations of the surveys. There are, for example, very high rates in Europe compared with the USA, but the studies from Canada and New Zealand are also high. High rates in Beirut are perhaps understandable, and have similarities to the PSE data from another high-trauma site, the Uganda of the mid-1970s (Orley & Wing, 1979). The difficulties in the overall interpretation of these results suggest differences in the application of the interview.

Since these surveys were undertaken, data have been published from two large-scale investigations based on national probability samples, the American National Comorbidity Survey (NCS) (Kessler et al., 1993, 1994a,b) and the British National Survey of Psychiatric Morbidity (Meltzer et al., 1995; Jenkins et al., 1997b). They involved interviews with 8000 and 10000 subjects, respectively (see Table 1.5). Using the Composite International Diagnostic Interview (CIDI; Robins et al., 1988) in its University of Michigan variant, Kessler and colleagues (1993) obtained a noticeably high prevalence for DSM-III-R MDD—the NCS is one of the first based on CIDI, and the use of this instrument by lay interviewers may result in lower thresholds than its predecessors. The National Survey of Psychiatric Morbidity (Meltzer et al., 1995) also used lay interviewers. It was based on the revised version of the CIS-R (Lewis et al.,

Table 1.3 Six-month prevalence of major depressive episode (%).

Site	*n*	Male	Female	Total
ECA Studies				
Baltimore (Myers *et al.*, 1984)	3481	1.3	3.0	2.2
New Haven (Myers *et al.*, 1984)	3058	2.2	4.6	3.5
St Louis (Myers *et al.*, 1984)	3004	1.7	4.5	3.2
Piedmont (Blazer *et al.*, 1985)*	3921	–	–	1.7
Los Angeles (Burnham *et al.*, 1987)	3125	–	–	3.1
Other sites				
Puerto Rico (Canino, *et al.*, 1987)	1551	2.4	3.3	3.0
Edmonton (Bland *et al.*, 1988)	3258	2.5	3.9	3.2
Taiwan (Hwu *et al.*, 1989)†				
Taipei	5004	–	–	0.6
Small town	3005	–	–	1.1
Rural	2995	–	–	0.8
Christchurch (Oakley-Browne *et al.*, 1989)	1498	3.4	7.1	5.3
Munich (Wittchen *et al.*, 1992)‡	1366 (501)	–	–	3.0

* Weighted to take account of over-sampling of elderly.
† One-year prevalence.
‡ Two-stage survey—numbers given DIS at second stage in brackets. Prevalences weighted to represent original population.

Table 1.4 Recent surveys based on national probability samples.

Study	n	Location	Age range	Period	Disorder	Prevalence	
						Male	Female
National Comorbidity Study (Kessler et al., 1994a,b)	8098	48 contiguous United States	15–54	1 year	Major depressive disorder	7.7	12.9
National Survey of Psychiatric Morbidity (Jenkins et al., 1997b)	10 108	Great Britain (except Highlands and Islands)	18–64	1 week	Depressive episode	1.8	2.7

1992), a lay-administered interview that provides ICD-10 diagnoses (WHO, 1992). It can be seen from Table 1.4 that despite the similar procedure of the CIDI and the DIS, the prevalences in the ECA studies are closer to those in the British National Survey of Psychiatric Morbidity. These discrepancies require direct comparison of the instruments in a single sample before any idea of their clinical significance can be derived. Such a study is currently underway (T.S. Brugha, H.M. Sharp, S.A. Cooper *et al.*, unpublished information).

Depressive disorder has an ill-defined threshold and usually does not result in referral to specialist services, so there are particular difficulties in interpreting data based on referred series of patients (Bebbington, 1988). Nevertheless, provided we are cautious, such studies remain of value, especially if they corroborate and amplify community surveys.

Table 1.5 Incidence of depressive disorder based on rates of first admission to hospital.

Study	Place and date	Category	Male	Female	Total
			\multicolumn{3}{c}{Incidence per 10^5}		
Depressive psychosis, etc.					
Shepherd (1957)	Buckinghamshire 1945–7	Non-neurotic affective disorder	6.5	12.6	–
Norris (1959)	London 1947–9	Manic depressive psychosis	14.1	25.9	–
Jaco (1960)	Texas 1951–2	Affective psychosis	13.0	22.0	–
Sadoun *et al.* (1978)	France 1975	Manic depressive reaction	11.0	17.0	–
Joenson & Wang (1983)	Denmark 1970–9	Manic depressive psychosis	–	–	22.4
DHSS (1985)	England 1978–82	Affective psychosis	6.0	10.0	–
Finlay Jones (pers. comm., 1987)	Western Australia 1977–83	Depressive psychosis	11.6	15.5	–
Wells (pers. comm., 1987)	New Zealand 1980–3	Depressive psychosis	9.8	14.6	–
All depressions					
Joenson & Wang (1983)	Denmark 1970–9		–	–	55.6
DHSS (1985)	England 1978–82		32.0	54.0	–
Finlay Jones (pers. comm., 1987)	Western Australia 1977–83		28.9	39.2	–
Wells (pers. comm., 1987)	New Zealand 1980–3		27.9	47.2	–
O'Hare & Walsh (1985)	Ireland		52.3	87.9	70.0

Data on first admission rates from all over the developed world are presented in Table 1.5. It is, of course, dangerous to expect at the outset that very much weight can be placed on such data, due to the vagaries of diagnostic practice and admission policies. While both of these influences have changed over the years, this is particularly true of admission policies because of the recent acceleration in the drive to manage psychiatric disorders in the community, and the resulting reduction in bed availability. For this reason I have limited data to a 40-year period ending in the mid-1980s. During this period it is likely that most severe affective disorders led to admission to hospital, although one would expect more variation in the practice regarding milder conditions. Severity appears to be the main determinant of admission, overriding social influences (Hurry *et al.*, 1980).

The results in Table 1.5 are of some interest. The admission rates for severe types of affective disorder (obviously loosely defined) fall into a relatively restricted range: from 6 to 14 per 10^5 for men and from 10 to 26 per 10^5 for women. The sex ratio ranges from 1.3 to 1.9. Surprisingly, the rates for *all* depressive disorders are also fairly consistent, from 28 to 52 per 10^5 for males and from 39 to 88 per 10^5 for females. The implication is that the thresholds for admission to hospital were rather similar in the different locations quoted, otherwise the ratio of severe depressions to all depressions would have varied more. It is just possible, therefore, that the differences in the figures reflect real differences in susceptibility in the local populations, at least in some cases, for example the comparison between London and Buckinghamshire. It is also possible that the values for severe depression represent ballpark figures for the true incidence of the condition. However, before concluding this, we should see whether further illumination can be obtained from case register studies.

These provide data on incidence based on all contacts with services (Table 1.6). They avoid duplicate counts and probably use categories that are more consistently applied than routinely collected national data (Wing, 1972). They are restricted to relatively small geographical areas, but at least the social characteristics of the areas are known in detail. It might be hoped that register data would reveal a greater consistency, especially for severe depressions, as they would virtually all be referred for specialist treatment. The inconsistencies shown in Table 1.6 probably do reflect considerable variation in the register definitions of disorder. It is suspected from other sources that the categories of depressive psychosis in Salford and of manic depressive psychosis in Aarhus are broader than equivalent usages in the other sites. The differences between London and Aberdeen are likely to reflect a real difference in incidence between an inner city area and a predominantly rural one. Nevertheless, the values for severe depressions are around twice those obtained if first admission is used as a proxy for incidence, suggesting that even in this period only around half of severe depressions resulted in admission. It may perhaps be concluded that the incidence of severe depression is three or four times that of schizophrenia.

There are special difficulties in studying the epidemiology of bipolar affective disorder, centred around the fact that bipolarity can only be recognized at an unspecified time after the onset of first affective symptoms. I have discussed these at length elsewhere (Bebbington & Ramana, 1995). Moreover, surveys based on lay assessment are likely to over-recognize mania. For these reasons, community surveys provide poor data on prevalence; on balance the values for bipolar disorder in many studies are probably overestimates. Table 1.7 lists prevalence both for manic episode and for bipolar disorder from available studies.

Changes over time

The prevalence of depressive disorders is not guaranteed to be set for all time. In particular, several authors have raised the possibility that the frequency is increasing as the century proceeds (Klerman, 1978, 1988; Schwab *et al.*, 1979).

Table 1.6 Incidence of depression derived from inceptions on case registers.

Study	Place	Base population	Disorder type	Incidence per 10^5		
				Male	Female	Total
Depressive psychosis, etc.						
Adelstein et al. (1968)	Salford, England	>15 years	Depressive psychosis	65	123	97
Baldwin (1971)	NE Scotland	All	Manic depressive reactions	25	52	–
Pederson et al. (1972)	Monroe Co., N.Y.	>15 years	Psychotic depression	27	37	33
Weeke et al. (1975)	Aarhus Co., Denmark	All	Manic depressive psychosis	60	100	–
Der & Bebbington (1987)	Camberwell, England	>15 years	Severe depression	29	52	–
All depressions						
Baldwin (1971)	NE Scotland	All	All depressions	87	201	–
Weeke et al. (1975)	Aarhus Co., Denmark	All	All depressions	130	328	–
Der & Bebbington (1987)	Camberwell, England	>15 years	All depressions	144	270	–

Table 1.7 Six-month prevalence of mania and bipolar disorder based on community psychiatric surveys.

| Study | Location | Prevalence (%) | | |
		Manic episode	Bipolar I	Bipolar I and II
Faravelli *et al.* (1990)	Florence	–	1.7†	–
ECA studies				
(Robins & Regier, 1991;	New Haven	0.8	1.0	1.2
Myers *et al.*, 1984;	Baltimore	0.4	0.5	0.9
Burnham *et al.*, 1987)	St Louis	0.7	1.0	1.4
	Durham NC		0.3	0.6
	Los Angeles	0.2	0.4	0.7
Total		0.6	0.7	1.0
Other DIS studies				
Canino *et al.* (1987)	Puerto Rico	0.3	–	–
Bland *et al.* (1988)	Edmonton	0.1	–	–
Hwu *et al.* (1989)	Taiwan	0.1*†	–	–
Oakley-Brown *et al.* (1989)	Christchurch	0.1	–	–
Wittchen *et al.* (1992)	Munich	0.2	–	–
US National Comorbidity Survey				
Kessler *et al.* (1994a,b)	United States	1.4*	1.3*	1.3*

* One-year prevalence.
† Estimated from published data.

A distinction must be made between *age, period* and *cohort* effects, cohorts being groups defined by having birth dates occurring within a stipulated period. Subjects may be exposed to risk of disorder because they are passing through *an age of risk* (an age effect). This will be apparent in all cohorts that have passed that age. They may be exposed to disorder because they are passing through *a time of risk*. In this instance, different cohorts will suffer the disorder at different ages, corresponding to their age at the relevant date (a period effect). Finally, cohorts may exhibit differing lifetime risk because they are just different groups of people—the differences can be related neither to a given age nor to a given date, and there is a true *cohort effect*. It is very difficult to separate age, period and cohort effects statistically, because fixing any two of these factors constrains the third; it usually requires assumptions that go beyond what the data really allow (Wickramaratne *et al.*, 1989). An excellent account of the potential pitfalls in studies of this type is provided by Klerman & Weissman (1989).

There are a number of types of study that might reveal changing incidence and prevalence of disorder. The crudest indicator would be the finding that the mean rates from surveys within a geographical region were changing over time. However, little weight can be placed on such studies because of variation in methods, locations, and, in the case of referred series, referral practices.

In four instances, community surveys have been repeated in the same area after several years, using the same or translatable methods. These are the Midtown Manhattan Study (Srole *et al.*, 1962; Srole & Fischer, 1980), the Stirling County Study (Leighton *et al.*, 1963; Murphy, 1994), Lin and colleagues' (1989) study in Taiwan, and my own studies in Camberwell (Bebbington *et al.*, 1981, 1997b). If anything, the Manhattan study suggests that minor psychiatric disorders are becoming less prevalent, although once again it is impossible to distinguish period and cohort effects. The Stirling County study incorporates both a panel design based on repeated interviews with the same subjects, and repeated cross-sectional surveys of the study population in 1952, 1970 and 1992. Only results from the first two waves are so far available; depressive disorder was equally common at each date. Lin and colleagues (1989) surveyed general populations in Taiwan after a 15-year interval (1948–63), using the same methods on each occasion. They found a striking increase in neurotic disorders, but not in manic depressive psychosis.

The first Camberwell survey was carried out in 1978–9, the second in 1992–5. The first used the 9th edition of the PSE, the second, the 10th edition, which forms the core of the Schedules for Clinical Assessment in Neuropsychiatry (SCAN; Wing *et al.*, 1990; WHO, 1992). However, there is a translation programme which permits output equivalent to that for PSE–9. The 1-month prevalence of depressive disorders of all categories appears to have decreased in women but not in men, in whom it is very similar in the two studies (see Table 1.3). This is despite the considerable material deterioration of parts of the survey area in this period. However, as suggested above, problems in comparability of the instruments may have caused the later survey to give underestimates of prevalence. In the Lundby study, Hagnell and colleagues (1982, 1994) reinterviewed *the same population* after a number of years. Data collected in 1947, 1957 and 1972 in this Swedish rural community suggest that the incidence of severe depression is decreasing, but that depression of mild to moderate severity is increasing.

These results are obviously conflicting and this seems as likely to be due to their location and time as to methodological divergences. Recently, data from a range of studies have been used to analyse the age-specific incidence for successive cohorts of subjects (Klerman *et al.*, 1985; Gershon *et al.*, 1987; Lavori *et al.*, 1987; Joyce *et al.*, 1990; Lasch *et al.*, 1990; Burke *et al.*, 1991; Cross-National Collaborative Group, 1992; Kessler *et al.*, 1994b; Lewinsohn *et al.*, 1994), and these have been more consistent. It is possible to use *lifetime prevalence* (the proportion of the population that is suffering or has suffered from a given disease), as a first indication of changes in risk in succeeding cohorts. If there is no cohort effect, or there is a reduction in depressive experience with later birth date, cross-sectional surveys would be expected to show an increase in lifetime prevalence in older subjects, as they have had a longer life in which to become depressed.

In fact, there is a consistent *decline* in lifetime prevalence with age in a number of studies, including our own (Bebbington *et al.*, 1989). This suggests a cohort effect of increasing, and possibly earlier, incidence of depression in subjects with later birth dates. The direct examination of this possibility appears to confirm it. Klerman (1988) and, more recently, Wolk and Weissman (1995) have reviewed the available databases to illustrate that the relationship between age and incidence of depression has become steeper in sequential birth cohorts. In other words, as the twentieth century proceeds, the population is becoming increasingly prone to depression, and this emerges at a progressively younger age. It is of interest that very similar patterns are observed for bipolar disorder (Robins & Regier, 1991).

These illustrations are persuasive, but depend crucially on the subject's ability to remember past episodes. These are likely to be more remote and thus easier to forget in older subjects, and this may account for the findings described by Klerman (1988). Estimates of lifetime prevalence do seem to be of doubtful validity (Bromet *et al.*, 1986). Using a simulation of the effects of defective recall on the creation of apparent cohort effects, Giuffra and Risch (1994) have recently shown that really quite small (but constant) rates of forgetting produce curves strikingly similar to those that would be obtained if a genuine cohort effect existed without recall effects. The magnitude of recall effect required to mimic a true cohort effect is in line with what is known of test–retest studies of lifetime recall of depressive disorders. Hasin and Link (1988) also raised the possibility that older subjects are less able to recognize past disturbances in their functioning as psychological in nature—this would also be a cohort effect, but of a different type.

Despite this, the possibility of increasing proneness to depression in sequential birth cohorts clearly merits very serious attention. If the postulated cohort effects are genuine, they are very interesting. It would be difficult to argue that they arise from changes in gene frequency over so short a time, and the explanation must therefore be environmental, and probably social.

The social epidemiology of depressive disorder

One of the key objectives of epidemiology is the identification of sociodemographically defined high-risk groups. Although epidemiological study can, at best, only suggest the possible causal direction of observed associations, the results provide useful pointers for further research.

Social class

Social class, usually expressed as occupational class, is a measure of access to power, privilege and resources, and ought therefore to be inversely associated with vulnerability to depression. Twenty years ago, there were great hopes that the social origins of depression would be substantiated through studies of social class. There were certainly some grounds for these hopes (e.g. Dohrenwend & Dohrenwend, 1969; Warheit *et al.*, 1973; Uhlenhuth *et al.*, 1974; Comstock & Helsing, 1976; Brown & Harris, 1978; Surtees *et al.*, 1983). Many community surveys have reported a moderate predominance of minor affective disorder in the lower social classes, although the measurement of social class is far from consistent and the results are often dichotomized in a way to maximize the effect. Some large and well-conducted studies have recently failed to show much effect of social class. The ECA surveys report virtually no relationship betweeen affective disorder and social class (Robins & Regier, 1991), and the National Survey of Psychiatric Morbidity found only a reduced rate in Class I adults, with the prevalence of depression being essentially uniform in the remaining classes (Jenkins *et al.*, 1997b). The National Comorbidity Survey, on the other hand, did find significant associations with income and educational standing (Kessler *et al.*, 1994a,b). Over the years a number of other studies have failed to find associations between social class and depression (e.g. Taylor & Chave, 1964; Hare & Shaw, 1965; Blumenthal & Dielman, 1975; Brown *et al.*, 1977; Weissman & Myers, 1978; Bebbington *et al.*, 1981), nevertheless, there is still probably an overall consensus that the prevalence of disorder is indeed increased in those of lower social class, albeit much less so than some have claimed. This association seems likely to arise because of a direct effect of the disadvantages faced by those in the lower classes, rather than any downward drift exhibited by people afflicted by depression.

The association with social class is even less apparent for cases in contact with the psychiatric services (Birtchnell, 1971; Bagley, 1973; Der & Bebbington, 1987; Bebbington, 1988). Those of lower social class may be less able to access treatment and services, and severe disorders may, in any case, be less influenced by social adversity. In the study of Hurry *et al.* (1980), severity was the major determinant of referral, not social class, and this would tend to support the second interpretation. Thus the belief that social class reflects influences that may be causally related to the origins of depressive disorder has never been convincingly demonstrated.

There has been considerable argument over the social class distribution of bipolar disorder (Bebbington & Ramana, 1995). Clinical studies have suggested either no association with class or a tendency to cluster in higher classes. The ECA data, based on large community samples, suggest, on the contrary, that there is a consistent but small association with lower social class (Robins & Regier, 1991). It is unclear how any overidentification of bipolar cases would affect this finding.

Sex and depression

The data already presented emphasize that sex is one of the major determinants of frequency of depressive disorder. The female preponderance is extremely robust, and very few studies have failed to reflect it. Its causes are almost certainly multiple and complex (Bebbington *et al.* 1997a,b), but are illuminated by the identification of high-risk groups defined in other ways.

Marital status and child care

The most straightforward influence in the domestic arena is that of marital termination, for whatever reason. Early reports on marital status and depression relied on admission data (Ødegaard, 1953; Jaco, 1960), or case register information (Juel-Nielsen *et al.*, 1961; Adelstein *et al.*, 1968; Der & Bebbington, 1987), although these have now been supplemented by community surveys. The details vary (Bebbington, 1988), but the general finding of high rates in postmarital groups is robust. There are more women in postmarital groups because of an excess of widows and the longevity of divorced and separated women in relation to their ex-partners. Thus, postmarital status might account for some of the female excess of depression. Aseltine and Kessler (1993) have urged caution over findings from cross-sectional studies, emphasizing the problem of selection effects in studying the impact of marital breakdown on depression. They circumvented this by following up a general population sample for 3 years. Marital disruption was responsible for an increase in scores on a standard depression screening scale of one-third of a standard deviation. This was worse in women, but was less apparent where there had been long-term problems in the marriage.

However, in many studies women seem to cope better than men with the end of marriage (e.g. Aneshensel *et al.*, 1981). Moreover, age has a bearing on this issue. Depression in young women who are separated or divorced is compounded by the fact that they are often involved in childcare in disadvantageous circumstances. The high rates of depression in single mothers is confirmed in the recent British National Survey of Psychiatric Morbidity (Meltzer *et al.*, 1995). Kramer and his colleagues (1987) have pointed out that the increasing proportion of single mothers in western populations may have explosive consequences for mental health services (not to mention for the mothers themselves).

Some authors (Weissman & Klerman, 1977; Paykel & Rowan, 1979;

Weissman *et al.*, 1984) consider that being married connotes more stress for women than for men. Although not a universal finding (e.g. Ensel, 1982; Gebhardt & Klimitz, 1986), there is certainly good evidence that it is much less protective for women than for men (Bebbington *et al.*, 1981; Bebbington, 1987; Der & Bebbington, 1987; Bebbington & Tansella, 1989). Thus in one survey, single and divorced women had *lower* rates of minor affective disorder than their male counterparts, while wives had over five times the rate of husbands (Bebbington *et al.*, 1981). Many studies have found that young, married women looking after small children are particularly at risk (Baldwin, 1971; Richman, 1974, 1977; Grad de Alarcon *et al.*, 1975; Moss & Plewis, 1977; Brown & Harris, 1978; Bebbington *et al.*, 1981, 1984; Ensel, 1982).

However, marital status has different associations with affective disorder in different cultures. For instance, married women are at low risk of disorder in Mediterranean countries (Mavreas *et al.*, 1986; Vazquez-Barquero *et al.*, 1987), in rural New Zealand (Romans-Clarkson *et al.*, 1988) and in British orthodox Jews (Lowenthal *et al.*, 1995). These societies all accord a high value to the home-making role. This suggests not only that social variables are important in determining the sex ratio for depression, but that the association with relatively simple sociodemographic factors may itself be affected by more subtle sociocultural influences.

Employment status

There seems little doubt that becoming unemployed increases the risk of affective disorder (e.g. Finlay-Jones & Eckhardt, 1981; Kessler *et al.*, 1987; Eales, 1988; Meltzer *et al.*, 1995), although most resulting cases are minor (Warr, 1984). A longitudinal study of young people demonstrated that unemployment has ill-effects on mental health which are reversed when work is obtained (Banks & Jackson, 1982; Jackson *et al.*, 1982). Jenkins and colleagues (1982) found similar effects when employees were threatened with redundancy, effects that were neutralized if the threat was removed.

The benefits of employment are complex. Krause and Geyer-Pestello (1985) distinguished four aspects of work: job satisfaction; whether work is full- or part-time; pay satisfaction; and commitment to the work role. Surprisingly, they found that only the last two were related to depressive symptoms. Many workers in the field of unemployment research have been influenced by Jahoda's (1982) emphasis on the 'latent functions' of employment. She lists six such functions: time structure; social contact; activity; status; purposefulness; and sense of control. These aspects of employment are plainly important, and the effects of unemployment must include consequences related to them. So, for instance, Bolton and Oatley (1987) and Eales (1988) argue that when social support continues to be available, the impact of becoming unemployed is lessened. However, unemployment itself usually causes changes in the individual's social network (Jackson, 1988).

Kessler and colleagues (1987) studied three possible sources of strain: financial, marital, and that due to constriction of 'affiliative interaction'. Their longitudinal study suggested that the most important and direct consequence was financial, and that financial hardship increased the impact of any supervening misfortunes. The importance of money problems also emerged from the study of Frese and Mohr (1987).

In most countries women are less likely to be in paid employment than men, particularly if they are involved in home-making and child care. Moreover, if they do work, they may still retain arduous responsibilities at home. Overall, employment appears to have beneficial effects on psychological health, although this may be reduced or reversed if it gives rise to competing pressures and obligations. Leeflang *et al.* (1992) showed that the impact of short- and long-term unemployment did not differ between men and women.

For women, work has a particular set of meanings that lie behind the general association with reduced levels of psychiatric disorder. Rosenfield (1989) reviewed the value of employment in buffering women from the tendency to become depressed, and interpreted findings from community surveys in terms of power and personal control. The extent of any financial difficulty and of other commitments and burdens, and the availability of social support are crucial, as are interest and involvement. Warr and Parry (1982) concluded that most evidence pointed to a protective effect of employment in working class but not in middle class women. Parry (1986; Parry & Shapiro, 1986) has suggested that the important factor is whether work provides extra social support. If it does not, it may actually increase the burdens on women.

The benefits of employment are weaker in married women (Roberts & O'Keefe, 1981; Roberts *et al.*, 1982; Warr & Parry, 1982), still more so if they have children (McGee *et al.*, 1983; Parry, 1986). Full-time employment is particularly demanding (Cleary & Mechanic, 1983; Elliott & Huppert, 1991). Haw (1995) reports results of a community survey suggesting that the beneficial effects of employment are reduced in women with preschool children, but not in those whose children are at school. The most likely explanation for these findings is role conflict and overload. Thus, part of the excess of depressive disorders in women may be related both to their reduced involvement in employment and to the particular strains they are exposed to if they do work. Unfortunately, the economic circumstances in most Western countries are inducing more women to work, and for longer hours.

The effect of constraining social factors on sex differences in the frequency of depression

A number of authors have obtained interesting results from populations in which social differences between the sexes are artificially constrained. Thus Stangler and Printz (1980) found similar rates of depression in male and female university students, as did Jenkins (1985) in employed civil servants. Maffeo *et al.* (1990) found no sex differences in employed men and women once employment attributes were controlled. Levav *et al.* (1991) argued that there was more social equality for women living in a kibbutz, and thus if social factors were important determinants of depression the sex ratio should also be more equal. However, in their study, the sex discrepancy was maintained. Finally, Wilhelm and Parker (1989) reported that men and women matched for the putative social causes of depression showed no sex differences, even at 5-year follow-up. Neither did they show differences in attitudinal measures nor the experience of life events. Despite the attraction of this type of study, their results are ambiguous, as they cannot take account of the possibility of biased female representation due to selection effects.

Sex and bipolar disorder

In general, the sex difference seen in unpolar depression is not apparent in bipolar disorder (Bebbington & Ramana, 1995), and this is one of the major discriminating features of the two disorders. However, it is of interest that among subjects with bipolar disorder, women tend to have more depressive episodes (see, e.g., Angst, 1986). It is also of interest that there is no sex-related variation in the association of bipolar disorder with marital status: low rates are particular to married subjects of both sexes.

Age, sex and depressive disorders

Age has an important effect on the sex ratio seen in depressive disorders. However, there are methodological problems. Estimates of depressive disorders in childhood and adolescence are hampered by the relatively recent development of standardized methods of identifying and assessing these conditions in age groups where its expression differs from that in adulthood. Nevertheless, there is a clear increase in rates as the form of depressive disorder moves in adolescence towards that recognizable in adults.

In prepubertal children there is, if anything, a male predominance in depressive symptoms and disorders (Anderson *et al.*, 1987; Kashani & Carlson, 1987; Fleming & Offord, 1990), while during adolescence the F:M ratio approaches the 2:1-value seen in adults (Cohen *et al.*, 1993). Moreover, in a large, clinical sample this change in ratio was seen only in depression, not in conduct disorder or anxiety (Rutter, 1991; Angold & Rutter, 1992). Community surveys confirm that the adult sex ratio has fully developed by the age of 14–15 (Rutter *et al.*, 1976; McGee *et al.*, 1992).

In adulthood, the incidence of severe depressive disorder is generally found to increase with age in both sexes, while the sex ratio tends to decline (Bebbington, 1988). Milder conditions show a peak in early adult life; as this peak is relatively greater in women, this is also the stage at which the sex ratio is greatest. This age relationship can be contrasted with that for mania (Table 1.8).

Table 1.8 Age and the incidence of affective disorders (adapted from Der & Bebbington, 1987).

Disorder type	Sex	Age						
		15–24	25–34	35–44	45–54	55–64	65–74	75+
Mania and hypomania	Male	7.3	7.2	5.2	3.4	2.3	5.7	10.6
	Female	9.4	5.8	5.7	6.2	3.1	3.9	4.2
Severe affective disorder	Male	15.3	31.2	37.2	46.8	39.2	59.8	34.2
	Female	44.6	70.0	72.3	70.6	52.6	71.5	46.6
All depressions	Male	154.8	216.7	210.0	185.5	140.0	157.9	113.5
	Female	422.0	505.1	373.5	259.1	179.6	184.7	123.7

Findings based on prevalence are more ambiguous. In the ECA studies (Weissman *et al.*, 1988), the sex ratio for 1 year prevalence of MDD for the age groups 18–44, 45–64 and 65 and over was 3.0, 2.2 and 3.5, respectively. In the National Comorbidity Survey (Kessler *et al.*, 1993), the sex ratio was maintained to age 55, the age limit of the sample. Results from 2000 first-degree relatives assessed in the course of the NIMH Collaborative Study on the Psychobiology of Depression confirm that the discrepancy between the rate of major depressive disorder in men and women peaks between adolescence and early adulthood (Leon *et al.*, 1993).

The recent British National Survey of Psychiatric Morbidity (Meltzer *et al.*, 1995) suggests that after the age of 55, the sex ratio changes, both for depressive episodes and for mixed anxiety/depression, such that males predominate. This is due not to a rise in male rates but to a fall in female rates, and appears to be independent of changes in marital status, child-care arrangements and employment (Bebbington *et al.* 1997b). Fifty-five years is of interest because by then women have passed through the menopause, and in the past this was seen as a time of increased vulnerability for women, because of both social and hormonal changes.

Jorm (1987) carried out a meta-analysis of studies of depression over the age range, analysing separately those based on diagnosed cases of depression and those using continuous measures of depressive symptoms. The scatter of results indicated a non-linear relationship, and was best accounted for by a quadratic curve which cut the zero sex difference line at just over 10 and just under 80 years. The equation accounted for 27% of the variance. Thus the sex ratio was much reduced at the ends of the lifespan, but was maintained for some time after the menopausal years. Both men and women peaked in their early twenties, but the female peak was higher and declined more quickly.

While the timing of the development of a sex differential is clearly related to the timing of puberty, it is not clear whether it is more strongly related to the social or the biological consequences of that change. Since puberty starts at various ages, one way of assessing the impact of hormonal changes is to use age as a control variable. A number of authors (Brooks-Gunn & Warren, 1989; Paikoff *et al.*, 1991; Angold & Rutter, 1992) have found that controlling for age eliminated the contribution of pubertal stage to the adolescent increase of rates of depressive disorders in girls, although one well-conducted longitudinal community survey found that time since menarche was the determinant of high levels of depression in girls, rather than age itself (Patton *et al.*, 1995). We conclude that most evidence favours the importance of being in a pubertal cohort over the personal experience of puberty; this is easier to explain in social terms. The adolescent rise in rates of depressive disorder in females cannot, however, be accounted for in unidimensional terms, and originates from the complex interplay of bodily changes, individual and societal reactions to them, and the other things that tend to be happening in girls' lives at this time (Alsaker, 1994).

The inconsistent relationship between the sex ratio and the menopause make it hard to argue strongly that the ratio arises from high rates of depression during women's reproductive lives. This, in turn, weakens the argument for explanations in terms of gonadal hormones, and in any case the hormone system most clearly (and probably causally) related to depression is the corticoid response to stress, which does not vary between the sexes (Checkley, 1996). However, the strongest argument against a hormonal aetiology for the sex difference is the lack of a genetic contribution (Merikangas *et al.*, 1985). It is difficult to imagine a biological cause that does not show individual variability from genetic causes. This opens the door for non-biological explanations, of which, in my view, the most plausible relates to the disadvantages almost universally experienced by women. These are reflected in the burdens and conflicts of the roles open to them and, consequently, in the sociodemographic groupings characterized by high risk of depression.

Conclusions

Epidemiology is endlessly capable of generating hypotheses that can be tested in more refined and focused studies. This chapter attempts to give a flavour of the particular difficulties faced by epidemiologists when they study affective disorder, but at the same time to use epidemiological techniques to provide insights into the likely causes of individual variations in susceptibility.

References

Adelstein, A.M, Downham, D.Y, Stein, Z. & Susser, M.W. (1968) The epidemiology of mental illness in an English City. *Social Psychiatry*, **3**, 47–59.

Alsaker, F.D. (1994) Timing of puberty and reactions to pubertal changes. In: *Psychosocial Disturbances in Young People: Challenges for Prevention* (ed. M. Rutter), pp. 37–82. Cambridge University Press, Cambridge.

American Psychiatric Association (1980) *Diagnostic and Statistical Manual of Mental Disorders*, 3rd edn. American Psychiatric Association, Washington, DC.

American Psychiatric Association (1987) *Diagnostic and Statistical Manual of Mental Disorders*, revised 3rd edn. American Psychiatric Association, Washington, DC.

American Psychiatric Association (1994) *Diagnostic and Statistical Manual of Mental Disorders*, 4th edn. American Psychiatric Association, Washington, DC.

Anderson, J.C., Williams, S. & McGee, R. *et al.* (1987) DSM-III disorders in preadolescent children. *Archives of General Psychiatry*, **44**, 69–76.

Aneshensel, C.S., Frerichs, R.R. & Clark, V.A. (1981) Family roles and sex differences in depression. *Journal of Health and Social Behaviour*, **22**, 379–393.

Angold, A. & Rutter, M. (1992) Effects of age and pubertal status on depression in a large clinical sample. *Developmental Psychopathology*, **4**, 5–28.

Angst, J. (1986) The course of affective disorders. *Psychopathology*, **19** (Suppl. 2), 47–52.

Aseltine, R.H. Jr & Kessler, R.C. (1993) Marital disruption and depression in a community sample. *Journal of Health and Social Behaviour*, **34**, 237–251.

Bagley, C. (1973) Occupational class and symptoms of depression. *Social Science and Medicine*, **7**, 327–339.

Bahar, E. (1989) *Development and Mental Health. A psychiatric Epidemiological study in Developing Country: An Enquiry in Palembang, Indonesia*. PhD thesis. The Australian National University.

Baldwin, J.A. (1971) *Five year incidence of reported psychiatric disorder. Aspects of the Epidemiology of Mental Illness: Studies in Record Linkage*. Little, Brown & Co., Boston.

Banks, M.H. & Jackson, P.R. (1982) Unemployment and risk of minor psychiatric disorders in young people: cross-sectional and longitudinal evidence. *Psychological Medicine*, **12**, 789–798.

Bebbington, P.E. (1987) Life events and schizophrenia: The WHO collaborative study. *Social Psychiatry*, **22**, 179–180.

Bebbington, P.E. (1988) The social epidemiology of clinical depression. In: *Handbook of Studies in Social Psychiatry* (eds A. S. Henderson & G. Burrows), pp. 88–102. Elsevier, Amsterdam.

Bebbington, P.E. (1990) Population surveys of psychiatric disorder and the need for treatment. *Social Psychiatry and Psychiatric Epidemiology*, **25**, 33–40.

Bebbington, P.E. & Ramana, R. (1995) The epidemiology of bipolar affective disorder. *Social Psychiatry and Psychiatric Epidemiology*, **30**, 279–292.

Bebbington, P.E. & Tansella, M. (1989) Gender, marital status and treated affective disorders in South Verona: a case-register study. *Journal of Affective Disorders*, **17**, 83–91.

Bebbington, P.E., Hurry, J., Tennant, C., Sturt, E. & Wing, J.K. (1981) The epidemiology of mental disorders in Camberwell. *Psychological Medicine*, **11**, 561–580.

Bebbington, P.E., Sturt, E., Tennant, C. & Hurry, J. (1984) Misfortune and resilience: a community study of women. *Psychological Medicine*, **14**, 347–364.

Bebbington, P.E., Katz, R., McGuffin, P., Tennant, C. & Hurry, J. (1989) The risk of minor depression before age 65: results from a community survey. *Psychological Medicine*, **19**, 393–340.

Bebbington, P.E., Marsden, L., Brewin, C. & Lesage, A. (1996a) Measuring the need for psychiatric treatment in the general population: the Community Version of the MRC Needs for Care

Assessment. *Psychological Medicine*, **26**, 229–236.

Bebbington, P.E., Marsden, L. & Brewin, C. (1997) The needs for psychiatric treatment in the general population: the Camberwell Needs for Care Survey. *Psychological Medicine*, **27**, 821–834

Birley, J.L.T. (1990) DSM-III: From left to right or from right to left? *British Journal of Psychiatry*, **157**, 116–118.

Birtchnell, J. (1971) Social class, parental social class and social mobility in psychiatric patients and general population controls. *Psychological Medicine*, **1**, 209–221.

Bland, R.C., Newman, S.C. & Orn, H. (1988). Epidemiology of psychiatric disorders in Edmonton. *Acta Psychiatrica Scandinavica*, **77**, Supplementum 338.

Blazer, D., George, L.K. & Landerman R. *et al.* (1985). Psychiatric disoders: a rural/urban comparison. *Archives of General Psychiatry*, **42**, 651–656.

Blumenthal, M.D. & Dielman, T.E. (1975) Depressive symptomatology and role function in a general population. *Archives of General Psychiatry*, **32**, 985–991.

Bolton, W. & Oatley, K. (1987) A longitudinal study of social support and depression in unemployed men. *Psychological Medicine*, **17**, 453–460.

Bromet, E.J., Dunn, L.O., Connell, M.O., Dew, M.A. & Schulberg, H.C. (1986) Long-term reliability of diagnosing lifetime major depression in a community sample. *Archives of General Psychiatry*, **43**, 435–440.

Brooks-Gunn, J. & Warren, M.P. (1989) Biological and social contributions to negative affect in young adolescent girls. *Child Development*, **60**, 40–55.

Brown, G.W. & Harris, T.O. (1978) *Social Origins of Depression: A Study of Psychiatric Disorder in Women*. Tavistock, London.

Brown, G.W., Davidson, S., Harris, T., Maclean, U., Pollock, S. & Prudo, R. (1977) Psychiatric disorder in London and North Uist. *Social Science and Medicine*, **11**, 367–377.

Burnham, M.A., Hough, R.L., Escobar, J.I. *et al.* (1987) Six month prevalence of specific psychiatric disorders among Mexican Americans and non-Hispanic whites in Los Angeles. *Archives of General Psychiatry*, **44**, 687–694.

Burke, K.C., Burke, J.D., Rae, D.S. & Regier, D.A. (1991) Comparing age at onset of major depression and other psychiatric disorders by birth cohorts in five US community populations. *Archives of General Psychiatry*, **48**, 789–795.

Canino, G.J., Bird, H.R., Shrout, P.E. *et al.* (1987) The prevalence of specific psychiatric disorders in Puerto Rico. *Archives of General Psychiatry*, **44**, 727–735.

Carta, M.G., Carpiniello, B., Morosini, P.L. & Rudas, N. (1991). Prevalence of mental disorders in Sardinia: a community study in an inland mining district. *Psychological Medicine*, **21**, 1061–1071.

Checkley, S.A. (1996) The neuroendocrinology of depression and of chronic stress. *British Medical Bulletin*, **52**, 397–417.

Cleary, P.D. & Mechanic, D. (1983) Sex differences in psychological distress among married people. *Journal of Health and Social Behaviour*, **6**, 64–78.

Cohen, P., Cohen, J. & Brook., J. (1993) An epidemiological study of disorders in late childhood and adolescence. II. Persistence of disorders. *Journal of Child Psychology and Psychiatry*, **34**, 869–877.

Comstock, G.W. & Helsing, K.J. (1976) Symptoms of depression in two communities. *Psychological Medicine*, **6**, 551–563.

Cross-National Collaborative Group (1992) The changing rate of major depression. *Journal of the American Medical Association*, **268**, 3098–3105.

Der, G. & Bebbington, P.E. (1987) Depression in inner London: a register study. *Social Psychiatry*, **22**, 73–84.

DHSS (1985). In-patient Statistics from the Mental Health Enquiry, 1982, London, HMSO.

Dohrenwend, B.P. & Dohrenwend, B.S. (1969) *Social Status and Psychological Disorder: A Causal Inquiry*. John Wiley & Sons, New York.

Dohrenwend, B.P. & Dohrenwend, B.S. (1982) Perspectives on the past and future of psychiatric epidemiology. *American Journal of Public Health*, **72**, 1271–1279.

Eales, M.J. (1988) Depression and anxiety in unemployed men. *Psychological Medicine*, **18**, 935–945.

Elliott, J. & Huppert, F.A. (1991) In sickness and in health: associations between physical and mental well-being, employment and parental status in a British Nationwide sample of married women. *Psychological Medicine*, **21**, 515–524.

Ensel, W.M. (1982) The role of age in the relationship of gender and marital status to depression. *Journal of Nervous and Mental Disease*, **170**, 536–543.

Faravelli, C. Guerrini-Degl'Innocenti, B., Aiazzi, L., Incerpi, G. & Pallanti, S. (1990). Epidemiology of mood disorders: a community survey in Florence. *Journal of Affective Disorders*, **20**, 135–41.

Finlay-Jones, R. & Eckhardt, B. (1981) Psychiatric disorder among the young unemployed. *Australian and New Zealand Journal of Psychiatry*, **15**, 265–270.

Fleming, J.E. & Offord, D.R. (1990) Epidemiology of childhood depressive disorders: a critical review. *Journal of the American Academy of Child* and Adolescent Psychiatry, **29**, 571–580.

Frese, M. & Mohr, G. (1987) Prolonged unemployment and depression in older workers: a longitudinal study of intervening variables. *Social Science and Medicine*, **25**, 173–178.

Gebhardt, R. & Klimitz, H. (1986) Depressive Störungen, Geschlect und Zivilstand. *Zeitschrift für Klinische Psychologie*, **15**, 3–20.

Gershon, E., Hamovit, J.H., Guroff, J.J. & Nurnberger, J.I. (1987) Birth cohort changes in manic and depressive disorders in relatives of bipolar and schizoaffective patients. *Archives of General Psychiatry*, **44**, 314–319.

Ghubash, R. (1992), Hamde, E. & Bebbington, P.E. The Dubai Community Psychiatric Survey: Prevelence and sociodemographic correlates. *Social Psychiatry and Psychiatric Epidemiology*, **27**, 53–61.

Giuffra, L.A. & Risch, N. (1994) Diminished recall and the cohort effect of major depression: a simulation study. *Psychological Medicine*, **24**, 375–383.

Grad de Alarcon, J., Sainsbury, P. & Costain, W.R. (1975) Incidence of referred mental illness in Chichester and Salisbury. *Psychological Medicine*, **5**, 32–54.

Hagnell, O., Lanke, J., Rorsman, B. & Ojesjo, L. (1982) Are we entering an age of melancholy? Depressive illness in a prospective epidemiological study over 25 years: the Lundby Study, Sweden. *Psychological Medicine*, **12**, 279–289.

Hagnell, O., Ojesjo, L., Otterbeck, L. & Rorsman, B. (1994) Prevalence of mental disorders, personality traits and mental complaints in the Lundby Study. A point prevalence study of the 1957 Lundby cohort of 2,612 inhabitants of a geographically defined area who were re-examined in 1972 regardless of domicile. *Scandinavian Journal of Social Medicine*, **50**, 1–77.

Hare, E.H. & Shaw, G.K. (1965) *Mental Health on a New Housing Estate: A Comparative Study of Health in two Districts in Croydon.* Maudsley Monograph No. 12. Oxford University Press, Oxford.

Hasin, D. & Link, B. (1988) Age and recognition of depression: Implications for a cohort effect in major depression. *Psychological Medicine*, **18**, 683–688.

Haw, C.E. (1995) The family life cycle: a forgotten variable in the study of women's employment and wellbeing. *Psychological Medicine*, **25**, 727–738.

Henderson, S., Duncan-Jones, P., Byrne, D.G., Scott, R. & Adcock, S. (1979). Psychiatric disorders in Canberra: a standardised study of prevalence. *Acta Psychiatrica Scandinavica*, **60**, 355–374.

Hodiamant, P., Peer, N. & Syben, N. (1986). Epidemiological aspects of psychiatric disorder in a Dutch Health Area. *Psychological Medicine*, **16**: 495–506.

Hurry, J., Tennant, C. & Bebbington, P.E. (1980) Selective factors leading to psychiatric referral. *Acta Psychiatrica, Supplementum*, **285**, 315–323.

Hwu, H.-G., Yeh, E.-K. & Chang, L.-Y. (1989). Prevalence of psychiatric disorders in Taiwan defined by the Chinese Diagnostic Interview Schedule. *Acta Psychiatrica Scandinavica*, **79**, 136–147.

Jackson, P.R. (1988) Personal networks, support mobilization and employment. *Psychological Medicine*, **18**, 397–404.

Jackson, P.R., Stafford, E.M., Banks, M.H. & Warr, P.B. (1982) *Work involvement and employment status as influences on mental health: a test of an inter-actional model.* SAPU Memo 404. University of Sheffield.

Jaco, E.G. (1960) *The Social Epidemiology of Mental Disorders.* Russell Sage Foundation, New York.

Jahoda, M. (1982) *Employment and Unemployment.* Cambridge University Press, Cambridge.

Jenkins, R. (1985) Sex differences in minor psychiatric morbidity. *Psychological Medicine* (Suppl. 7).

Jenkins, R., MacDonald, A., Murray, J. & Strathdee, G. (1982) Minor psychiatric morbidity and the threat of redundancy in a professional group. *Psychological Medicine*, **12**, 799–807.

Jenkins, R., Bebbington, P., Brugha, T. *et al.* (1997a) The National Psychiatric Morbidity Surveys of Great Britain—an Overview. *Psychological Medicine*, **27**, 765–774.

Jenkins, R., Lewis, G., Bebbington, P. *et al.* (1997b) The National Psychiatric Morbidity Surveys of Great Britain—Initial findings from the Household Survey. *Psychological Medicine*, **27**, 775–791.

Joenson, S. & Wang, A.G. (1983). First admissions for psychiatric disorders: a comparison between the Faroe Islands and Denmark. *Acta Psychiatrica Scandinavica*, **68**: 66–71.

Jorm, A.F. (1987) Sex and age differences in depression: a quantitative synthesis of published research. *Australian and New Zealand Journal of Psychiatry*, **21**, 46–53.

Joyce, P.R., Oakley-Browne, M.A., Wells, J.E., Bushnell, J.A. & Hornblow, A.R. (1990) Birth cohort trends in major depression: increasing rates and earlier onset in New Zealand. *Journal of Affective Disorders*, **18**, 83–89.

Juel-Nielson, N., Bille, M., Flygenring, J. & Helgason, T. (1961) Frequency of depressive states within geographically delimited population groups. 3. Incidence (the Aarhus County Investigation). *Acta Psychiatrica Scandinavica*, (Suppl.) **162**, 69–80.

Kashani, J.H. & Carlson, G.A. (1987) Seriously depressed preschoolers. *American Journal of*

Psychiatry, **144**, 348–350.

Kessler, R.C., Turner, J.B. & House, J.S. (1987) Intervening processes in the relationship between unemployment and health. *Psychological Medicine*, **17**, 949–962.

Kessler, R.C., McGonagle, K.A. & Swartz, M. *et al.* (1993) Sex and depression in the National Comorbidity Survey. I: Lifetime prevalence, chronicity and recurrence. *Journal of Affective Disorders*, **29**, 85–96.

Kessler, R.C.McGonagle, K.A. & Zhao, S. *et al.* (1994a) Lifetime and 12-month prevalence of DSM-III-R psychiatric disorders in the United States: results from the National Comorbidity Study. *Archives of General Psychiatry*, **51**, 8–19.

Kessler, R.C. & McGonagle, K.A.Nelson, C.B. *et al.* (1994b) Sex and depression in the National Comorbidity Survey. II: Cohort effects. *Journal of Affective Disorders*, **30**, 15–26.

Klerman, G.L. (1978) Affective disorders. In: *The Harvard Guide to Modern Psychiatry* (eds M. Armand & M. D. Nicholi). Belknap Press, Cambridge, MA.

Klerman, G.L. (1988) The current age of youthful melancholia: evidence for increase in depression among adolescents and young adults. *British Journal of Psychiatry*, **152**, 4–14.

Klerman, G.L. & Weissman, M.M. (1989) Increasing rates of depression. *Journal of the American Medical Association*, **261**, 2229–2235.

Klerman, G.L., Lavori, P.W., Rice, J., Reich, T., Endicott, J. & Andreason, N.C. (1985) Birth-cohort trends in rates of major depressive disorder among relatives of patients with affective disorder. *Archives of General Psychiatry*, **421**, 689–693.

Kramer, M., Brown, H., Skinner, A., Anthony, J. & German, P. (1987) Changing living arrangements in the population and their potential effect on the prevalence of mental disorder: findings of the East Baltimore Mental Health Survey. In: *Psychiatric Epidemiology* (ed. B. Cooper), pp. 3–26. Croom Helm, London.

Krause, N. & Geyer-Pestello, H.F. (1985) Depressive symptoms among women employed outside the home. *American Journal of Community Psychology*, **13**, 49–67.

Lasch, K., Weissman, M., Wickramaratne, P. & Bruce, M.L. (1990) Birth-cohort changes in the rates of mania. *Psychiatry Research*, **33**, 31–37.

Lavori, P.W., Klerman, G.L., Keller, M.B., Reich, T., Rice, J. & Endicott, J. (1987) Age-period-cohort analysis of secular trends in onset of major depression: Findings in siblings of patients with major affective disorder. *Journal of Psychiatric Research*, **21**, 23–35.

Leeflang, R.L., Klein-Hesselink, D.J. & Spruit, I.P. (1992) Health effects of unemployment. II: Men and women. *Social Science and Medicine*, **34**, 351–363.

Lehtinen, V., Lindholm, T., Veijola, J. & Vaisanen, E. (1990). The prevalence of PSECATEGO disorders in a Finnish adult population cohort. *Social Psychiatry and Psychiatric Epidemiology*, **25**, 187–192.

Leighton, D.C., Harding, J.S., Macklin, D.B., MacMillan, A.M. & Leighton, A.H. (1963) *The Character of Danger Stirling County Study*. Vol. 3. Basic Books, New York.

Leon, A.D., Klerman, G.L. & Wickramaratne, P. (1993) Continuing female predominance in depressive illness. *American Journal of Public Health*, **83**, 754–757.

Levav, I., Gilboa, S. & Ruiz, R. (1991) Demoralization and gender differences in a kibbutz. *Psychological Medicine*, **21**, 1019–1028.

Lewinsohn, P.M., Clarke, G.N., Seeley, J.R. & Rohde, P. (1994) Major depression in community adolescents: age at onset, episode duration, and time to recurrence. *Journal of the American Academy of Child and Adolescent Psychiatry*, **33**.

Lewis, G., Pelosi, A.J., Araya, R.C. & Dunn, G. (1992) Measuring psychiatric disorder in the community: a standardized assessment for use by lay-interviewers. *Psychological Medicine*, **22**, 465–486.

Lin, T.Y., Chu, H.M., Rin, H., Hsu, C.C., Yeh, E.K. & Chen, C.C. (1989) Effects of social change on mental disorders in Taiwan: observations based on a 15 year follow-up survey of general populations in 3 communities. *Acta Psychiatrica Scandinavica*, (Suppl.) **348**, 11–33.

Lowenthal, K., Goldblatt, V., Gorton, T. *et al.* (1995) Gender and depression in Anglo-Jewry. *Psychological Medicine*, **25**, 1051–1064.

Maffeo, P.A., Ford, T.W. & Lavin, P.F. (1990) Gender differences in depression in an employment setting. *Journal of Personality Assessment*, **55**, 249–262.

Mavreas, V. & Bebbington, P.E. (1987). Psychiatric morbidity in London's Greek Cypriot community. I. Association with sociodemographic variables. *Social Psychiatry*, **22**, 150–159.

Mavreas, V.G., Beis, A., Mouyias, A., Rigoni, F. & Lyketsos, G.C. (1986) Prevalence of psychiatric disorder in Athens: a community study. *Social Psychiatry*, **21**, 172–181.

McGee, R., Williams, S., Kashani, J. & Silva, P. (1983) Prevalence of self reported depressive symptoms and associated factors in mothers in Dunedin. *British Journal of Psychiatry*, **143**, 473–479.

McGee, R., Feehan, M., Williams, S. & Anderson, J. (1992) DSM-III disorders from age 11 to age 15 years. *Journal of the American Academy of Child and Adolescent Psychiatry*, **31**, 50–59.

McGuffin, P., Farmer, A. & Harvey, I. (1991) A polydiagnostic application criteria in studies of psychotic illness. Development and reliability of the OPCRIT system [news]. *Archives of General Psychiatry*, **48**, 764–770.

Meltzer, H., Gill, B., Petticrew, M. & Hinds, K. (1995) *The prevalence of psychiatric morbidity among adults living in private households. OPCS Survey of Psychiatric Morbidity in Great Britain.* Report 1. HMSO, London.

Merikangas, K.R., Weissman, M.M. & Pauls, D.L. (1985) Genetic factors in the sex ratio of major depression. *Psychological Medicine*, **15**, 63–69.

Moss, P. & Plewis, I. (1977) Mental distress in mothers of pre-school children in Inner London. *Psychological Medicine*, **7**, 641–652.

Murphy, J.M. (1994) The Stirling County study: then and now. *International Review of Psychiatry*, **6**, 329–348.

Myers. J.K., Weissman, M.M. & Tischler, G.L. (1984). Six month prevalence of psychiatric disorders in three communities: 1980–1982. *Archives of General Psychiatry*, **41**, 959–67.

Norris, V. (1959). *Mental Illness in London*, Maudsley Monograph **No. 6**. London, OUP.

Oakley-Browne, M.A., Joyce, P.R., Wells, J.E., Bushnell, J.A. & Hornblow, A.R. (1989). Christchurch Psychiatric Epidemiology Study, Part I: Six month and other period prevalences of specific psychiatric disorders. *Australian and New Zealand Journal of Psychiatry*, **23**, 327–340.

Ødegaard, Ø. (1953) New data on marriage and mental disease: the incidence of psychosis in the widowed and the divorced. *Journal of Mental Disease*, **99**, 778–785.

O'Hare & Walsh (1985). *Activities of Irish Psychiatric Hospitals and Units.* Medico-Social Research Board, Dublin.

Orley, J. & Wing, J.K. (1979) Psychiatric disorders in two African villages. *Archives of General Psychiatry*, **36**, 513–520.

Paikoff, R.L., Brooks-Gunn, J. & Worren, M.P. (1991) Effects of girls' hormonal status on depressive and aggressive symptoms over the course of one year. *Journal of Youth and Adolescence*, **20**, 191–215.

Parry, G. (1986) Paid employment, life events, social support and mental health in working class mothers. *Journal of Health and Social Behaviour*, **27**, 193–208.

Parry, G. & Shapiro, D.A. (1986) Social support and life events in working class women. *Archives of General Psychiatry*, **43**, 315–323.

Patton, G.C., Hibbert, M. & Bowes, G. (1995) *Common psychiatric symptoms and health risk behaviours*

through the teens: a multiwave prospective study. Poster presented at WPA Section of Epidemiology and Community Psychiatry Conference New York, 15–17 May.

Paykel, E.S. & Rowan, P. (1979) Recent advances in research on affective disorders. In: *Recent Advances in Clinical Psychiatry.* (ed K. Grenville-Grossman), pp. 37–90. Churchill Livingstone, Edinburgh.

Pederson, A.M., Barry, D.J. & Babigian, H.M. (1972). Epidemiological considerations of psychotic depression. *Archives of General Psychiatry*, 27, 193–197.

Richman, N. (1974) The effect of housing on pre-school children and their mothers. *Developmental Medicine and Child Neurology*, **16**, 53–58.

Richman, N. (1977) Behaviour problems in preschool children: family and social factors. *British Journal of Psychiatry*, **131**, 523–527.

Roberts, C.R., Roberts, R.E. & Stevenson, J.M. (1982) Women, work, social support and psychiatric morbidity. *Social Psychiatry*, **17**, 167–173.

Roberts, R.E. & O'Keefe, S.J. (1981) Sex differences in depression re-examined. *Journal of Health and Social Behaviour*, **22**, 394–400.

Robins, L.N. (1995) How to choose among the riches: Selecting a diagnostic instrument. In: *Textbook in Psychiatric Epidemiology* (eds M. T. Tsuang, M. Tohen & G. E. P. Zahner), pp. 243–252. Wiley-Liss, New York.

Robins, L.N. & Regier, D.A. (1991) *Psychiatric Disorders in America: The Epidemiological Catchment Area Study.* Free Press, New York.

Robins, L.N., Helzer, J.E., Orvaschel, H. *et al.* (1985) The Diagnostic Interview Schedule. In: *Epidemiologic Field Methods in Psychiatry: The NIMH Epidemiologic Catchment Area Program* (eds W. W. Eaton & L. G. Kessler), pp. 143–170. Academic Press, Orlando.

Robins, L.N., Wing, J.K., Wittchen, H.U. *et al.* (1988) The Composite International Diagnostic Interview. *Archives of General Psychiatry*, **45**, 1069–1077.

Romans-Clarkson, S.E., Walton, V.A., Herbison, G.P. & Mullen, P.E. (1988) Marriage, motherhood and psychiatric morbidity in New Zealand. *Psychological Medicine*, **18**, 983–990.

Rosanoff, A.J. (1916) Survey of mental disorders in Nassau County, New York. *Psychiatric Bulletin*, **2**, 109–231.

Rosenfield, S. (1989) The effects of women's employment: personal control and sex differences in mental health. *Journal of Health and Social Behaviour*, **30**, 77–91.

Rutter, M. (1991) Age changes in depressive disorders: Some developmental considerations. In: *The Development of Emotion Regulation and*

Dysregulation (eds J. Garber & K. A. Dodge), pp. 273–300. Cambridge University Press, Cambridge.

Rutter, M., Tizard, J., Yule, W., Graham, P. & Whitmore, K. (1976) Research report: Isle of Wight studies, 1964–1974. *Psychological Medicine*, **6**, 313–332.

Sadoun, R., Quemada, N. & Chassague, M.M. (1978). *Statistiques Medicales des Etablissements Psychiatriques*, Paris, Editions INSERM.

Schwab, J.J., Bell, R.A., Warheit, G.J. & Schwab, R.B. (1979) *Social Order and Mental Health: The Florida Health Study*. Brunner/Mazel, New York.

Shepherd, M. (1957) *A Study of the Major Psychoses in an English County*, Maudsley Monograph **No. 3**. London, OUP.

Srole, L. & Fischer, A.K. (1980) The Midtown Manhattan longitudinal study vs. the 'Mental Paradise Lost' doctrine: a controversy joined. *Archives of General Psychiatry*, **37**, 209–221.

Srole, L., Langner, T.S., Michael, S.T., Opler, M.K. & Rennie, T.A.C. (1962) *Mental Health in the Metropolis*. Vol. 1: *The Mid-Town Manhattan Study*. McGraw-Hill, New York.

Stangler, R.S. & Printz, A.M. (1980) DSM-III: psychiatric diagnosis in a university population. *American Journal of Psychiatry*, **137**, 937–940.

Surtees, P.G., Dean, C., Ingham, J.G., Kreitman, N.B., Miller, P.McC. & Sashidharan, S.P. (1983) Psychiatric disorder in women from an Edinburgh community: associations with demographic factors. *British Journal of Psychiatry*, **142**, 238–246.

Taylor, Lord & Chave, S. (1964) *Mental Health and Environment*. Longman Green, London.

Uhlenhuth, E.H., Lipmann, R.S., Balter, M.B. & Stern, M. (1974) Symptom intensity and life stress in the city. *Archives of General Psychiatry*, **31**, 759–764.

Vazquez-Barquero, J.L., Diez-Manrique, J.F., Pena, C., Aldana, J., Samaniego-Rodriguez, C. & Menendez-Arango, J. (1987) A community mental health survey in Cantabria: a general description of morbidity. *Psychological Medicine*, **17**, 227–242.

Warheit, G.J., Holzer, C.E. & Schwab, J.J. (1973) An analysis of social class and racial differences in depressive symptomatology: a community study. *Journal of Health and Social Behaviour*, **14**, 291–295.

Warr, P.B. (1984) Economic recession and mental health: a review of research. *Tijdschrift voor Sociale Gesondheidszorg*, **62**, 298–308.

Warr, P. & Parry, G. (1982) Paid employment and women's psychological well-being. *Psychological Bulletin*, **91**, 498–516.

Weeke, A., Bille, M., Videbeck, T., Dupont, A. & Juel-Nielsen, N. (1975). Incidence of depressive syndromes in a Danish county. *Acta Psychiatrica Scandinavica*, **51**, 28–41.

Weissman, M.M. & Klerman, G.L. (1977) Sex differences and the epidemiology of depression. *Archives of General Psychiatry*, **3**, 98–112.

Weissman, M.M. & Myers, J. (1978) Rates and risks of depressive symptoms in a United States urban community. *Acta Psychiatrica Scandinavica*, **57**, 219–231.

Weissman, M.M., Bland, R.C. & Canino, G.J. *et al.* (1996). Cross-national epidemiology of major depression and bipolar disorder. *Journal of the American Medical Association*, **276**, 293–299.

Weissman, M.M., Leaf, P.J., Holzer, C.E., Myers, J.K. & Tischler, G.L. (1984) The epidemiology of depression: an update on sex differences in rates. *Journal of Affective Disorders*, **7**, 179–188.

Weissman, M.M., Leaf, P.J., Tischler, G.L. *et al.* (1988) Affective disorders in five United States communities. *Psychological Medicine*, **18**, 141–154.

Wickramaratne, P.J., Weissman, M.M., Leaf, P.J. & Holford, T.R. (1989) Age, period and cohort effects on the risk of major depression: results from five United States communities. *Journal of Clinical Epidemiology*, **42**, 333–343.

Wilhelm, K. & Parker, G. (1989) Is sex necessarily a risk factor to depression? *Psychological Medicine*, **19**, 401–413.

Wing, J.K. (1972) Principles of evaluation. In: *Evaluating a Community Psychiatric Service: The Camberwell Register, 1967–71* (eds J. K. Wing & A. M. Hailey). Oxford University Press, Oxford.

Wing, J.K., Mann, S.A., Leff, J.P. & Nixon, J.M. (1978) The concept of a 'case' in psychiatric population surveys. *Psychological Medicine*, **8**, 203–217.

Wing, J., Wing, J.K., Babor, T., Brugha, T., Burke, J. & Cooper, J.E. (1990) SCAN: Schedules for Clinical Assessment in Neuropsychiatry. *Archives of General Psychiatry*, **47**, 589–593.

Wittchen H.U., Esau C.A., von Zerssen D., Kreig J.C. & Zaudig M. (1992). Lifetime and six-month prevalence of mental disorders: the Munich follow-up study. *European Archives of Psychiatry and Clinical Neuroscience*, **241**, 247–258.

Wolk, S.I. & Weissman, M.M. (1995) Women and depression. In: *Review of Psychiatry* Vol. 14, (eds J. M. Oldham & M. B. Riba), pp. 227–259. American Psychiatric Press, Washington, DC.

World Health Organization (1978) *Mental Disorders: Glossary and Guide to their Classification in accordance with the Ninth Revision of the International Classification of Diseases*. WHO, Geneva.

World Health Organization (1992) *Tenth Revision of the International Classification of Diseases*. WHO, Geneva.

2 Depression presenting at different levels of care

DAVID GOLDBERG

Goldberg and Huxley (1992) have suggested a framework for understanding the pathway by which individuals become defined as mentally ill and eventually reach mental illness services. This framework serves to organize epidemiological data about mental illness into groupings which depend upon how far along this pathway individuals have reached, and draws attention to the 'filters' through which patients must pass in order to receive specialized treatments.

In many countries most patients are referred to the mental illness services by other professionals, so that one can postulate a filter between the community and the referring professional, as well as between that professional and the mental illness service. The framework consists of five levels at which survey data could be considered, each one corresponding to a stage on the pathway to psychiatric care. A set of four filters are postulated between these five levels, and these are shown in Table 2.1.

Table 2.1 Five levels and four filters [from Goldberg & Huxley, 1992].

Level	Description	Filter
1 The community	All adults who experience an episode of mental disorder in the course of 1 year	1 Illness behaviour
2 Primary care attenders (total)	All adults who experience an episode of mental disorder and seek help from a primary care physician	2 Ability to detect disorder
3 Primary care attenders (PCP) (detected)	All adults who are considered mentally disordered by their PCP: *whether or not they satisfy research criteria*	3 Referral to mental illness services
4 Mental illness services (total)	All adults treated by the mental illness services during the course of a year	4 Admission to psychiatric beds
5 Mental illness services (hospitalized)		

Table 2.2 Figures for the annual period prevalence for all mental disorders and for depression, England and Wales.

Level	All mental disorders	Depression only
1 The community	250–315	130*
2 GP attenders	230	80†
3 Conspicuous psychiatric morbidity	101.5	30.6‡
4 Mental illness services: all	20.8	6.82§
5 Mental illness services: in-patients	3.4	1.2¶

*Figures from OPCS 1995 inflated by 33% for annual inceptions.
†Figures from Blacker & Clare, 1987 (confirmed Nielsen & Williams, 1980), decreased by 0.80, to account for consultation rate.
‡,§,¶ From Goldberg & Huxley, 1992 (p. 47); see Goldberg & Huxley, 1992 (p. 29) for all mental disorders, and for corrections to notes * and †.

Recent estimates for all mental disorders for England and Wales are shown in Table 2.2. The figure for the community is obtained by averaging results from various surveys (which produce point prevalence data), and then inflating them to take account of inceptions that occur for each disorder during a calendar year. It can be seen that there are many more disorders in the community than are treated by primary care services, and that more disorders are treated in primary care than by specialist care. However, the various filters are selectively permeable to disorders of greater severity: so that severe mental disorders account only for about 4.5% of total disorders in the community, yet they account for 50% of those seen at level 5. The same effect is seen for severity within a particular disorder: so that many depressive illnesses seen in community settings are self-limiting disorders that will remit without specialist treatment, whereas those referred through to the specialist services are more likely to have a previous episode of illness, a family history of that illness, and abnormal personalities.

Depression is the commonest mental disorder seen in community settings, and estimates for its prevalence at all levels can also be found in Table 2.2.

Characteristics of depression in the community (level 1)

Depressive disorders encountered in community surveys are most likely to be accompanied by symptoms of anxiety, and least likely to be seen in subjects with abnormal personalities. Among women in Britain, the weekly period prevalence of mixed anxiety/depression is 99/1000 at risk, and the weekly prevalence of pure depressive episode is 25/1000 at risk. The corresponding figures for men are 54 and 17/1000. There are interesting ethnic differences, with Asian and Oriental women having particularly high rates for mixed anxiety/depression, although there are no clear effects for males (see Table 2.3). The sex ratio is greatest in community settings, and becomes less at level 4, since the 3rd filter (general practitioner (GP) referral) is selectively permeable to males (Goldberg & Huxley, 1992).

Table 2.3 Weekly period prevalence per 1000 population at risk for mixed anxiety/depression and depressive episode, by ethnic group (OPCS, 1995).

Disorder	White		West Indies or Africa		Asian or Oriental	
	Men	Women	Men	Women	Men	Women
Mixed anxiety/depression	54	96	58	136	68	160
Depressive episode	17	24	21	18	19	51

Table 2.4 Odds ratios for social and demographic characteristics with significant odds ratios for either mixed anxiety/depression or depressive episode (from OPCS, 1995).

Odds ratios	Mixed anxiety/depression	Depressive episode
Female gender	1.73**	1.47 NS
Lone parents	1.48**	2.60**
Living alone	1.47**	2.32**
Unemployed	1.73**	2.66**
Economically inactive	1.19 NS	2.87**
Urban life	1.30 NS	1.38**

** significant $P < 0.01$.

It can be seen from Table 2.4 that loneliness and unemployment are shared factors between the two conditions: there is a preponderance of females only for mixed anxiety/depression, and urban living, economic inactivity and having no qualifications (not shown, but odds ratio = 1.67**) for depressive episode. In a study of 100 couples who had experienced at least one depressogenic life event, it was shown (Nazroo *et al.*, 1996) that women were at greater risk of depression than men. This greater risk was restricted to those events involving children, housing or reproductive problems, and was only seen in those couples with clear gender differences in roles, with the woman viewing herself as being more responsible for these functions. In couples without these role differences, there was no gender difference in risk.

Many of these individuals do not see themselves as ill, despite possessing sufficient symptoms for a diagnosis of a mental disorder. They may see their state as being in an understandable relationship to some life situation, or they may seek help only for somatic symptoms which often accompany these states.

Effects of treatment in community cases

While nothing can really be said about the response to treatment in people who have not sought medical care, there was an advertisement in local newspapers for people with symptoms of depression (Lipman *et al.*, 1986) who were not in psychiatric treatment but who were prepared to take part in a 10-week research project with drugs. The 'symptomatic volunteers' (SVs) needed to be two standard deviations above the mean for depressive symptoms, and were given a range of depression scales (Hamilton Depression Scale, Raskin Depression Screen and Research Diagnostic Criteria for Depression). The SVs were each given a 2-week placebo washout period, and it was necessary for them still to be depressed at the end of this period. They were then assigned randomly to imipramine, chlordiazepoxide or placebo, and treatment was continued for 8 weeks with regular clinic visits. Differences at the end of the first week generally favoured chlordiazepoxide but these early advantages were soon lost, apart from subjects on this drug reporting generally better sleep. By the end of the trial most effects favoured imipramine, and these effects were seen both for anxiety and depression. However, it should be noted that the effects of imipramine were only 13% better than placebo (65% vs. 52% for global improvement, patient self-rated).

Depression at level 2

Many patients attend their GP with somatic symptoms that are accompanying states of depression and anxiety. They often do not see themselves as psychologically ill, but seek either an explanation for their symptoms or treatment which will relieve these symptoms. The WHO study of mental disorders in general health care (Ustun & Sartorius, 1995) confirmed previous British studies (for example, Bridges & Goldberg, 1985), by demonstrating that mental disorders usually present to primary care physicians with physical symptoms. In Manchester 76% presented in this way; across the world 69% did so. Across all centres the most common main complaint of patients with mental disorders was pain (29%), fatigue or poor sleep (7%), and other assorted somatic complaints (33%); only 5% presented with psychological symptoms. Some of these illnesses (47% in Manchester), are accompanying physical illnesses known to their doctors, but others are presenting with unexplained somatic symptoms. Thus, the old 'either/or' dichotomy, whereby patients were to be thought of as having either a physical illness or a mental one, is inappropriate: and this was true in all centres.

Across the world, some 7.1% of male, and 12.5% of female, consecutive attenders at GP surgeries have major depression according to the primary care version of the Composite International Diagnostic Interview (CIDI-PC).

This gender difference is statistically significant (see Table 2.5). However, there is considerable divergence between centres, and even the odds ratios need to be interpreted with caution: for example, the odds ratios are very different for Rio and Manchester, but this is produced by a great difference in the male rates for depression; the female rates are nearly identical. In Nagasaki rates are low for each sex, while in Ibadan the male rate is (non-significantly) higher than the female rate.

Table 2.5 Rates for current depression according to the CIDI-PC by gender for six selected centres from the WHO Study of Mental Disorders in General Medical Settings, showing odds ratios (Goldberg & LeCrubier, 1995).

Centre in WHO Study	Current depression	CIDI (primary care)	Odds ratio
	Men	Women	
Santiago de Chile	11.2	36.8	4.73
Rio de Janeiro	5.8	19.6	3.95
Manchester	13.9	18.3	1.40 NS
Bangalore	4.8	13.3	3.05
Ibadan	5.3	3.8	0.70 NS
Nagasaki	2.3	2.8	1.28 NS
All 15 centres	7.1	12.5	1.89

Detection of these depressive episodes by the primary care physicians was comparable with previous reports. Across the world, about 54% were diagnosed, but there were great variations between centres, with physicians in Verona, Manchester and Santiago detecting about 70%, while their colleagues in Nagasaki, Athens and Shanghai detected only about 20%. Depression was associated with high rates of self-reported disability.

The only demographic variable shown to be associated with depression in this study was poor educational level, but it should be noted that this was the only variable recorded in this particular study that reflected social disadvantage. Physical ill-health, as assessed by the primary care physicians, was not significantly related to depression in this study, nor were parous women at greater risk (Usrun & Sartorius, 1995, p. 330). The depressive syndrome observed varied from centre to centre, despite the constraints imposed by the DSM-III-R definition. Thus fatigue, often accompanied by insomnia and depressive thoughts, was common in Athens, Berlin, Groningen, Ibadan, Manchester, Paris and Verona: all European centres, with the exception of Ibadan. In Nagasaki, fatigue and depressive thoughts are accompanied by worthlessness and weight loss. In Bangalore there appeared to be a specific pattern, with thoughts of death and worthlessness being relatively common, while in the three American centres depressive thoughts and insomnia were common, often accompanied by weight gain (Goldberg & LeCrubier, 1995).

Ormel *et al.* (1993) have examined the long-term outcome of depressions and anxiety states encountered in primary care settings, using cases confirmed by two-stage screening. They found that pure depressions had a better outcome than either anxiety states or mixed anxiety/depressions at 3.5-year follow-up, but that partial remission, rather than full recovery, was the rule.

Would detection of these disorders help the patient?

In centres with high rates for detection, it is doubtful whether detection of these extra cases would bestow much more than marginal benefit on the patients; probably in the shape of a shorter duration of episode. Secondary analyses of data collected in surveys by Bridges and Goldberg, Kisely and Goldberg, and Creed and Ronalds indicate that in Manchester the undetected depressions are milder than the detected ones, and have a similar good outcome at follow-up to those depressions detected and treated by the primary care physicians (unpublished data). Simon and VonKorff (1995) have produced similar data in Seattle: 64% of their cases of major depression detected at second stage of the WHO study were recognized as depressed by the family physician, and 56% of these were prescribed and took antidepressant medication. The recognized cases were more severe than the unrecognized cases (GHQ-28 scores: 15.3 vs. 11.1, $P = 0.006$), but the outcomes were similar. The authors argue that in centres such as theirs treatment resources should be focused on more intensive follow-up and relapse prevention, rather than on better detection. In other centres, with low rates of detection, more might be gained by increasing detection rates in terms of better patient outcomes.

Depressions at level three: those detected by the general practitioner (conspicuous psychiatric morbidity)

Depressive illnesses at this level are necessarily a mixed bag, as many of these patients are not found to have illnesses at second-stage examination, but to have other mental illnesses, or no illnesses at all. Freeling and colleagues (1985) studied 143 patients identified as depressed by their GPs and treated with antidepressants; of these only 43% conformed with diagnostic criteria for either probable or definite depression. With modern aids to diagnosis, such as the primary care version of the ICD-10 (ICD-10-PC, Ustun *et al.*, 1995), both diagnosis and management of depressive disorders are likely to improve in the future. Schulberg and colleagues (1995) have carried out a feasibility study of pharmacological treatments for depression in primary care, following guidelines suggested by a national body; they found that only 33% of patients initially assigned to receive medication actually completed it, and that the guidelines were 'feasible but complex'.

What treatments are of benefit to depressions recognized by GPs?

A number of studies have randomized depressed patients to an active antidepressant drug or to a placebo, and failed to show a difference in outcome (see, for example Porter, 1970; Blashki *et al.*, 1971; Hazell *et al.*, 1995). However, Hazell's study relates to depressed adolescents, while earlier studies might have contained heterogeneous populations. Tan *et al.* (1994) randomized depressed, elderly patients to lofepramine or placebo, and found that both improved by a similar amount during the trial. Lofepramine tended to be more effective than placebo in those patients who were more depressed. On the other hand, subjects who were less depressed improved more on placebo than on lofepramine. Brown and colleagues (1988) point out that placebos are especially effective in those who are less depressed (shorter duration or fewer symptoms), and may be as high as 70%, rather greater than the figures likely to respond to antidepressants among more depressed patients.

Katon *et al.* (1995) randomized depressed patients to 'usual care' or enhanced or 'multifaceted care' (MC). The last consisted of greater frequency of visits, two with a psychiatrist. In those with major depression, MC produced greater compliance, greater satisfaction with treatment, and patients rated antidepressants as more helpful and had greater symptom reduction. However, in minor depression, MC produced better compliance but not better outcomes or satisfaction.

Banerji *et al.* (1989) found no differences in outcome between depressed primary care patients randomized to alprazolam or amitriptyline, although there was a more rapid response in those receiving the antidepressant. This finding is consistent with that described by the Depression Guideline Panel (1993), which reports differences between the responses to active drug and placebo which are as great for alprazolam and buspirone as those for conventional antidepressants (meta-analysis of eight studies for the former, 76 studies for the latter). In 1985 the National Institute of Mental Health (NIMH) Consensus Development Panel (NIMH, 1985) counselled against generalizing from one field to another, but 8 years later this valuable lesson did not appear to have influenced the Depression Guideline Panel, which produced evidence for the efficacy of antidepressants almost entirely from samples treated by specialist mental health services (Depression Guideline Panel, 1993). Table 6 of that report claims to cover primary care studies, but only two of the quoted studies are placebo controlled, and one of these (Rickels *et al.*, 1987) should have been included with the mental health studies. Paykel *et al.* (1988) carried out one of the best studies in British general practice, and this showed that confirmed depressives with Hamilton depression scores greater than 15 (approximately comparable to ICD-10 major depression) did indeed benefit from amitriptyline rather than placebo medication.

Part of the problem is that without quality control of the patients being diagnosed, the placebo response is often as great as the antidepressant response. Quitkin *et al.* (1993) studied a group of atypical depressives with reactive mood and hyperphagia, hypersomnolence and rejection sensitivity. These were randomized to imipramine, phenelzine and placebo. Phenelzine was consistently found to be superior to imipramine.

Effectiveness of psychotherapies in general practice

Thomas (1987) showed the importance of 'being positive' in his management of emotional distress. Sixty-four per cent of patients randomized to a 'positive' consultation improved, as compared with 39% of those receiving a 'negative' consultation. In the positive consultation the patient was given a firm diagnosis and told confidently that he/she would be better in a few days, while in the negative consultation the patient was told, 'I cannot be certain what the matter is with you.' Prescription of a placebo made no difference to outcome in this study. Brown (1994) argues that if the drug-placebo is given in a way which produces hope and an expectancy of improvement, then it is likely to do so.

Elkin *et al.* (1989) claim that the placebo response is often as high as 50%, and argue that no psychotherapeutic treatment for depression can better the effects of a properly administered drug-placebo. Robinson *et al.* (1990) argue that the advantage of psychotherapies over pill-placebo are an effect size of only 0.28 (NS), to be compared with an advantage over waiting list control with an effect size of 0.84. Four studies are usually quoted in support of cognitive behaviour therapy in general practice (Blackburn *et al.*, 1981; Teasdale *et al.*, 1984; Ross & Scott, 1985; Miranda & Munoz, 1994), but none of these assessed the psychotherapy against a drug–placebo; the control conditions were active drugs, treatment as usual and waiting list. Robinson *et al.* (1995) examine the extent to which cognitive behavioural techniques are being used by primary care physicians in their treatments of depression. Sixty-one per cent of patients in their survey say that physicians advise them to identify activities that they are already undertaking which help to make them feel better. These suggestions are associated with a greater use of such strategies, and with better compliance with medication during treatment.

Mynors-Wallace *et al.* (1995) have overcome Elkin and colleagues' objections, by showing that a method of psychotherapy (problem-solving) was as effective as an antidepressant in the treatment of major depression, and that both active treatments were more effective than a drug-placebo. Sixty per cent of those patients given problem-solving improved, to be compared with only 27% given the placebo.

In summary, before rushing into antidepressant treatment the wise doctor will carry out a careful diagnostic evaluation. Antidepressant medication should be reserved for those with severe depressive illnesses, those with suicidal thoughts, and those with well-established, previously untreated illnesses. Others might benefit from an expectant treatment, with hypnotics used to secure sleep, and a return visit after a short time. The importance of a positive attitude, restoring hope and the expectation of improvement cannot be overemphasized. Whether the doctor uses a placebo is a matter of professional preference; what is important is that potentially dangerous drugs are not used for what is, in fact, a placebo response. Of the psychotherapeutic possibilities only problem-solving seems better than a drug–placebo, but the use of cognitive techniques may enhance the quality of care and possibly reduce the risk of relapse.

Depression in mental health care (level 4)

It will be recalled from Table 2.2 that we are now dealing with a small subset of depressive illnesses. In countries where GPs act as gatekeepers to the specialist services, the ready availability of psychotropics in primary care and the delays often associated with secondary referral mean that placebo responders have been, to some degree, removed. Patients coming to mental health specialists are more likely to have a positive family history, and to have had previous episodes of mental illness than those seen in primary care. On average, the illnesses seen by mental health specialists are more severe in the sense of patients having higher mean symptom counts (Goldberg & Huxley, 1992), although it should be appreciated that owing to the greater size of the population in primary care, it is likely that in absolute numbers there are more severe illnesses in that location. Because assessments by mental health professionals typically take much longer than the 10 minutes or so available in primary care, it is likely that the diagnostic assessment will be more thorough, and antidepressants will only be offered to those satisfying diagnostic criteria for depressive illnesses.

Piccinelli and Wilkinson (1994) have shown that depressive illnesses at this level have only a 25% chance of recovering from the episode and then staying well for 10 years. Twenty-five per cent relapse within 1 year, and 75% within 10 years; 12% never recover.

Response to treatment in specialist care

Drugs

It would be tedious to rehearse the evidence that antidepressants do indeed have a significant effect on these illnesses; the interested reader is referred to the meta-analyses of treatment trials published by the Depression Guideline

Panel (1993, see pp. 47–54). It is worth recording that drugs with very different pharmacological actions appear to be effective, and that no drug is known which is effective for all patients. Rational choice is often governed by acceptable side-effects: amitriptyline, doxepin, trimipramine, maprotiline and trazodone are sedating, amoxapine and the selective serotonin re-uptake inhibitors (SSRIs) are alerting. SSRIs are free from anticholinergic effects and do not cause orthostatic hypotension, cardiac arrythmias or weight gain and so on. Tricyclics (TCAs) have therapeutic effects in about 51% of patients, SSRIs for 54%, monoamine oxidase inhibitors (MAOIs) for 57%, and heterocyclics for 62%. The size of the active drug–placebo difference is 16.5% for the heterocyclics, 20.1% for the SSRIs, 21.3% for the TCAs, and 30.9% for the MAOIs. As previously mentioned, among 'anxiolytics' alprazolam and buspirone have effects comparable to tricyclics, but chlordiazepoxide and diazepam have little antidepressant effect. Katona *et al.* (1995) have carried out a placebo-controlled trial of lithium augmentation of therapy by either fluoxetine (an SSRI) or lofepramine (a TCA); both of these drugs were equally effective, but the patients who had treatment supplemented by lithium had a greater response to treatment, but it was necessary to ensure a lithium level of at least 0.4 mmol L^{-1} to achieve this advantage.

Psychotherapy

The Depression Guideline Panel (1993) carried out a meta-analysis of 12 randomised controlled trials (RCTs) of cognitive behaviour therapy and found it to be effective in 46.6% of cases, with a therapy vs. drug-placebo advantage of only 8.3% (one study only), but an advantage over waiting list of 30.1%, and over active drug therapy of 15.3% (three studies). Interpersonal psychotherapy, on the other hand, was effective with 52.3% of patients, with an advantage over drug-placebo of 22.6% (also only one study), and an advantage over active drug therapy of 12.3%. The advantage of behaviour therapy over drug–placebo is unknown; but it is effective in 55.3% of patients, with an advantage over active drugs of 23.9% (two studies only), and over waiting list of 17%. Brief, dynamic therapy is effective in only 34.8% of patients, with an advantage over active drugs of 8.4% (two studies only).

Depressions among the physically ill, seen in hospital settings

Patients with physical disease may become depressed for a number of reasons including: the disease process itself, treatment received or a psychological reaction to finding oneself with a serious illness. It is also possible for depressive states to antedate the onset of physical disease. Treatment of depressive states will improve the quality of life remaining to the patient, and may, in some cases, even prolong survival. Patients with cancer have attracted particular attention since they have a serious life-threatening disease which may require special psychological counselling, and various measures of immune function can be readily made. It is necessary to modify the diagnostic criteria used for depression when it occurs among the physically ill, since several depressive symptoms can equally be produced by physical disease processes. Cohen-Cole *et al.* (1993) eliminate fatigue and anorexia, and require four of the remaining symptoms for a diagnosis. McDaniel *et al.* (1995) review 18 studies of depression among cancer patients, with rates varying between a high of 50% depression for carcinoma of the pancreas, and a low of 30% depression for leukaemias.

Sapolsky and Donnelly (1985) showed stress-induced hyperactivity of the hypothalamo-pituitary axis was associated with increased tumour growth. Levy and colleagues (1987, 1990) studied psychological factors which influence outcome in breast cancer, and showed these to be adjustment level, lack of social support, fatigue and depressive symptoms. Together, they accounted for 30% of the variance of natural killer cell activity (NKA): metastatic nodes were associated with depressive features and decreased NKA. Higher NKA can be consistently predicted by high quality, emotional support from spouse or intimate other, perceived social support from physician and process of actively seeking social support as coping strategy.

Treatment for the depressed physically-ill

Drugs

Costa *et al.* (1985) show reduced depressive symptoms and improved quality of life (QOL) in an RCT of mianserin vs. placebo in depressed women with cancer, and Evans *et al.* (1988) showed a relief of depressive symptoms and increased QOL in women with gynaecological cancer treated with imipramine. Since these early studies, because of their relative freedom from side-effects, SSRIs have proved suitable for patients with cancer.

Psychotherapy

Both Spiegel *et al.* (1989) and Fawzy *et al.* (1993) show that group psychotherapy prolongs survival time in patients with metastatic breast cancer and malignant melanoma, respectively. An earlier paper by Fawzy and colleagues (1990) showed that those receiving group psychotherapy had increases in large granular lymphocytes and natural killer (NK) cells, as well as higher NKA. Richardson *et al.* (1990) showed that patients with lymphomas and leukaemias receiving educational in-home supportive interventions had significantly longer survival times than controls, and Gruber *et al.* (1993) showed those receiving relaxation, guided imagery and biofeedback training had higher NKA and lymphocyte mitogen response compared with controls.

Greer *et al.* (1992) studied the effect of 'adjuvant psychological therapy'— a brief, problem-focused, cognitive-behavioural treatment programme, specifically designed for the needs of individuals—on the QOL of patients with cancer. The new treatment produced higher scores on scales measuring fighting spirit and psychosocial adjustment to illness, and lower scores on helplessness. At 4-month follow-up, differences between index and control patients were more marked for anxiety than for depression.

Depressions admitted to hospital (level 5)

Patients who are admitted to in-patient beds are more severely depressed than those treated in ambulant settings; they have higher mean symptom counts, are more likely to have psychotic phenomena and more likely to be seriously suicidal. It follows that placebo responses are less of a problem in this setting, and it becomes more reasonable to compare one drug with another, without including a placebo arm. Considering the greater severity of these illnesses, it is of interest that the results of treatment are comparable with those at level 4: the proportion responding to antidepressants is between 50 and 55% for all drug groups, and the drug-placebo differences are MAOIs 18.4%, TCAs 25.1%, SSRIs 25.5% and heterocyclics 39.3%. Raskin *et al.* (1978) carried out a multicentre study with 360 depressed in-patients, randomized to imipramine, chlorpromazine or placebo. There were no significant differences between the effects of imipramine and chlorpromazine, but both were more effective than the placebo. Patients receiving imipramine for more than 6 months had fewer relapses, while those responding positively to the placebo initially had the poorest outcome at 1 year: 57% had 'ups and downs' with marked fluctuations in course.

Electroconvulsive treatment (ECT) produces better short-term results for patients with retardation or depressive delusions, but the results at 6 months are no different from simulated ECT. For those without these features, real ECT confers no additional benefits over simulated ECT (Buchan *et al.*, 1992). Bilateral, brief-pulse ECT is just as efficacious as traditional ECT with constant-voltage modified sine-wave stimuli (Scott *et al.*, 1992).

As at level 4, lithium augmentation has a place in the treatment of drug-resistant depressions, and recurrent depression.

Conclusions

In summary, the depressive illnesses that are seen in the community are unlike those seen by mental health professionals, in that they are more likely to remit spontaneously, so that the performance of a drug-placebo is very good. Improvement with a placebo is associated with a short illness, a precipitating event and a good response to previous antidepressant treatment (Brown *et al.*, 1992). The enthusiastic claims for the efficacy of non-drug treatments for depressive illness seen in community settings must be considered with this in mind. However, severe depressive illnesses and those accompanied by ideas of suicide, should continue to attract pharmacological interventions. Depressions seen in association with serious physical illness merit energetic treatment, since not only will quality of life be improved, but the course of the associated physical illness may also be favourably influenced.

References

Banerji, J.R., Brantingham, P., McEwan, G.D. *et al.* (1989) A comparison of alprazolam and amitriptyline in the treatment of patients with neurotic or reactive depression. *Irish Journal of Medical Science*, **158**, 110–113.

Blackburn, I., Bishop, S. & Glen, A. (1981) The efficacy of cognitive therapy in depression. *British Journal of Psychiatry*, **139**, 181–189.

Blacker, C.V.R. & Clare, A.W. (1987) Depressive disorders in primary care. *British Journal of Psychiatry*, **150**, 737–751.

Blashki, T.G., Mowbray, R. & Davies, B. (1971) Controlled trial of amitriptyline in general practice. *British Medical Journal*, i, 133–138.

Bridges, K. & Goldberg, D.P. (1985) Somatic presentation of psychiatric diseases in primary care. *Journal of Psychosomatic Research*, **29**, 563–569.

Brown, W.A. (1994) Placebo as a treatment for depression. *Neuropsychopharmacology*, **10**, 265–269.

Brown, W.A., Dornseif, B.E. & Wernicke, J.F. (1988) Placebo response in depression: a search for predictors. *Psychiatry Research*, **26**, 259–264.

Brown, W.A., Johnson, M.F. & Chen, M.G. (1992) Clinical features of depressed patients who do and do not improve with PBO. *Psychiatry Research*, **41**, 203–214.

Buchan, H., Johnstone, E., McPherson, K., Palmer, R.L., Crow, T.J. & Brandon, S. (1992) Who benefits from electroconvulsive therapy? Combined results of the Leicester and Northwick Park trials. *British Journal of Psychiatry*, **160**, 355–359.

Cohen-Cole, S.A., Brown, F.W. & McDaniel, S.J. (1993) Diagnostic assessment of depression in the medically ill. In: *Psychiatric Care of the Medical Patient* (eds A. Stoudemire & B. Fogel), pp. 53–70. Oxford University Press, New York.

Costa, D., Mogos, I. & Toma, T. (1985) Efficacy and safety of Mianserin in the treatment of women with cancer. *Acta Psychiatrica Scandinavica*, **320**, 85–92.

Depression Guideline Panel (1993) *Depression in Primary Care. Vol. 2: Treatment of Major Depression*. US Dept of Health and Human Services, Washington, DC.

Elkin, I., Shea, M.T., Watkins, J.T. *et al.* (1989) NIMH treatment of depression collaborative treatment programme: general effectiveness of treatment. *Archives of General Psychiatry*, **46**, 971–982.

Evans, D.L., McCartney, C.F. & Haggerty, J.J. (1988) Treatment of depression in cancer patients is associated with better life adaptation: a pilot study. *Psychosomatic Medicine*, **50**, 72–76.

Fawzy, F.I., Kemeny, M.L., Fawzy, N.W. *et al.* (1990) A structured psychiatric intervention for cancer patients. II: Changes over time in immunological measures *Archives of General Psychiatry*, **47**, 729–735.

Fawzy, F.I., Fawzy, N.W., Hyun, C. *et al.* (1993) Malignant melanoma: effects of an early structured intervention coping, and affective state on recurrence and survival 6 years later. *Archives of General Psychiatry*, **50**, 681–689.

Freeling, P., Rao, B.M., Paykel, E.S., Sireling, L. & Burton, R. (1985) Unrecognised depression in general practice. *British Medical Journal*, **190**, 1880–1883.

Goldberg, D.P. & Huxley, P. (1992) *Common Mental Disorders: A Biosocial Model*. Routledge, London.

Goldberg, D.P. & LeCrubier, Y. (1995) Form and frequency of mental disorders across centres. In: *Mental Disorders in General Medical Settings* (eds V. Ustun & N. Sartorius), p. 398. John Wiley & Sons, Chichester.

Greer, S., Moorey, S., Baruch, J.D. *et al.* (1992) Adjuvant psychological therapy for patients with cancer: a prospective randomised trial. *British Medical Journal,* **304**, 675–680.

Gruber, B.L., Hersh, S.P., Hall, N.R. *et al.* (1993) Immunological responses of breast cancer patients to behavioural interventions. *Biofeedback Self Regulation,* **18**, 1–22.

Hazell, P., O'Connell, D., Heathcote, D. & Robertson, I. (1995) Efficacy of tricyclic drugs in treating child and adolescent depression: a meta-analysis. *British Medical Journal,* **310**, 897–890.

Katon, W., VonKorff, M., Lin, E. *et al.* (1995) Collaborative management to achieve treatment guidelines: impact of depression in primary care. *Journal of the American Medical Association,* **273**, 1026–1031.

Katona, C., Abou-Saleh, M.T., Harrison, D.A. *et al.* (1995) Placebo controlled trial of lithium augmentation of fluoxetine and lofepramine. *British Journal of Psychiatry,* **166**, 80–86.

Levy, S.M., Herbermann, R.B., Lippman, M. & d'Angelo, T. (1987) Correlation of stress factors with sustained depression of natural killer cell activity and predicted prognosis in patients with breast cancer. *Journal of Clinical Oncology,* **5**, 348–353.

Levy, S.M., Herbermann, R.B., Whiteside, T., Sanzo, K., Lee, J. & Kirkwood, J. (1990) Perceived social support and tumour oestrogen/ progesterone receptor status as predictors of NK activity in breast cancer patients. *Psychosomatic Medicine,* **52**, 73–85.

Lipman, R.S., Covi, L., Rickels, K. *et al.* (1986) Imipramine and chlordiazepoxide in depression and anxiety disorders. *Archives of General Psychiatry,* **43**, 68–86.

McDaniel, J.S., Musselman, D.L., Porter, M.R., Reed, D.A. & Nemeroff, C.B. (1995) Depression in Patients with cancer. *Archives of General Psychiatry,* **52**, 89–99.

Miranda, J. & Munoz, R. (1994) Intervention for minor depression in primary care patients. *Psychosomatic Medicine,* **56**, 136–141.

Mynors-Wallace, L., Gath, D., Lloyd Thomas, A. & Tomlinson, D. (1995) RCT comparing problem solving treatment with amitriptyline and placebo for major depression in primary care. *British Medical Journal,* **310**, 441–445.

Nazroo, J.Y., Edwards, A.C. & Brown, G.W. (1996) Gender differences in the onset of depression following a shared life event: a study of couples. *Psychological Medicine* **27**, 9–19.

Nielsen, A.C. & Williams, T. (1980) Depression in ambulatory medical patients. *Archives of General Psychiatry,* **37**, 999–1004.

(NIMH) National Institutes of Mental Health (1985) Consensus Development Panel-Mood Disorders: Pharmacologic prevention of recurrences. *American Journal of Psychiatry,* **142**, 469–476.

(OPCS) Office of Populations Censuses and Surveys (1995) *Morbidity in Great Britain, Report no. 1. The prevalence of psychiatric morbidity among adults living in private households.* HMSO, London.

Ormel, J., Oldehinkel, T., Brilman, E. & VandenBrink, W. (1993) Outcome of depression and anxiety in primary care. *Archives of General Psychiatry,* **50**, 759–766.

Paykel, E.S., Hollyman, J. & Freeling, P. (1988) Predictors of therapeutic benefit from amitriptyline in mild depression: a general practice placebo controlled trial. *Journal of Affective Disorders,* **14**, 83–95.

Piccinelli, M. & Wilkinson, G. (1994) Outcomes of depression in psychiatric settings. *British Journal of Psychiatry,* **164**, 297–304.

Porter, A.M.W. (1970) Depressive illness in general practice. A demographic study and a controlled trial of imipramine. *British Medical Journal,* **i**, 773–778.

Quitkin, F.M., Stewart, J.W., McGrath, P.J. *et al.* (1993) Columbia atypical depression: a subgroup of depressives with better response to MAOI than to tricyclic antidepressants or placebo. *British Journal of Psychiatry,* **21**, (Suppl.), 30–34.

Raskin, A., Boothe, H., Reatig, N. & Schulterbrand, J.R. (1978) Initial response to drugs in depressive illness and psychiatric and community adjustment a year later. *Psychological Medicine,* **8**, 71–80.

Richardson, J., Sheldon, D., Krailo, M. & Levine, A. (1990) The effect of compliance with treatment on survival among patients with haematologic malignancies. *Journal of Clinical Oncology* **8**, 356–364.

Rickels, K., Chung, H.R., Csanalosi, I.B. *et al.* (1987) Alprazolam, diazepam, imipramine and placebo in out-patients with major depression. *Archives of General Psychiatry,* **44**, 862–866.

Robinson, L.A., Berman, J.S. & Neimeyer, R.A. (1990) Psychotherapy for the treatment of depression: a comprehensive review of controlled outcome research. *Psychological Bulletin,* **108**, 30–49.

Robinson, P., Bush, T., VonKorff, M. *et al.* (1995) Primary care physician use of cognitive behavioural techniques with depressed patients. *Family Practice,* **40**, 352–357.

Ross, S. & Scott, M. (1985) An evaluation of the effectiveness of individual and group cognitive therapy in the treatment of depressed patients in an inner city health centre. *Journal of the Royal College of General Practitioners,* **35,** 239–242.

Sapolsky, R.M. & Donnelly, T.M. (1985) Vulnerability to stress-induced tumour growth increases with age: role of glucocorticoids. *Endocrinology,* **117,** 662–666.

Schulberg, H.C., Block, M.R., Madonia, M.J., Rodriguez, E., Scott, C.P. & Lave, J. (1995) Applicability of clinical pharmacology guidelines for major depression in primary care settings. *Archives of Family Medicine,* **4,** 106–112.

Scott, A.I., Rodger, C.R., Stocks, R.H. & Shering, A.P. (1992) Is old-fashioned electroconvulsive therapy more efficacious? A randomised comparative study of bilateral brief-pulse and bilateral sine-wave treatments. *British Journal of Psychiatry,* **160,** 360–364.

Simon, G. & Von Korff, M. (1995) Recognition, management and outcomes of depression in primary care. *Archives of Family Medicine,* **4,** 99–105.

Spiegel, D., Bloom, J.R., Kraemer, H.C. & Gottheil, E. (1989) Effect of psychosocial intervention on survival of patients with metastatic breast cancer. *Lancet,* **ii,** 888–891.

Tan, R.S., Barlow, R.J., Abel, C. *et al.* (1994) The effect of low dose lofepramine in depressed elderly patients in general medical wards. *British Journal of Clinical Pharmacology,* **37,** 321–324.

Teasdale, J., Fennell, M. & Hibbert, G. (1984) Cognitive therapy for major depression in primary care. *British Journal of Psychiatry,* **144,** 400–406.

Thomas, K.B. (1987) General practice consultations: is there any point in being positive? *British Medical Journal,* **294,** 1200–1202.

Ustun, B. & Sartorius, N. (1995) *Mental Disorders in General Medical Settings.* John Wiley & Sons, Chichester.

Ustun, B., Goldberg, D., Cooper, J., Simon, G.E. & Sartorius, N. (1995) New classification for mental disorders with management guidelines for use in primary care: ICD-10 PHC, Chapter 5. *British Journal of General Practice,* **45,** 211–215.

3 Biological models of depression and response to antidepressant treatments

STUART CHECKLEY

The purpose of this chapter is to review those advances in biological psychiatry which are of theoretical or practical relevance to the clinician who is assessing and treating depressed patients. The subject matter falls naturally into three sections. The first concerns aetiology: the biological causes of depression. The second concerns pathogenesis: the biological mediators of depression. The third concerns the biological mechanisms by which physical treatments exert a therapeutic effect.

Aetiology

What is genetic and what is environmental?

Depression runs in families and so the first question to address is whether the depressed members of a given family share their depression because of their shared genes or because of their shared environment. Monozygous (MZ) twins have 100% of their genes in common whereas dizygous (DZ) twins have 50% of their genes in common, and so by comparing the concordance rates of MZ with DZ twins it is possible to estimate the heritability of a disorder, or the proportion of the variation in phenotype that is accounted for by genetic factors. Nurnberger and Gershon (1992) have reviewed eight twin studies of major depression in which the overall concordance rates of MZ and DZ twins were 59.6% and 13.7%. They cited 59% as a typical estimate of the heritability of major depression on the basis of their review. In the case of bipolar affective illness the genetic influence is greater and concordance rates of 67% and 20% have been reported in MZ and DZ twins, respectively (Bertelsen *et al.*, 1977). On the basis of Bertelsen's study, McGuffin and Katz (1989) have estimated the heritability of bipolar affective disorder to be ~80%. There are many environmental factors, including pregnancy, psychotropic medication, sleep deprivation and expressed emotion in the social environment which influence the onset of illness in an individual who has a genetic predisposition for depressive illness.

The heritability of unipolar depression is lower than that of bipolar and, depending on the assumptions made in the calculations, was between 48% and 75% for the unipolar depressives in the Maudsley Twin Register (McGuffin *et al.*, 1996). When depression was identified in a community-based volunteer twin register then an even lower heritability was found, but a genetic influence could still be detected (Kendler *et al.*, 1992).

Genetic relationship between unipolar depression, anxiety and neuroticism

It is possible to determine from twin studies whether or not there is genetic covariation or shared heritability for different disorders. Several twin studies have reported genetic covariation for anxiety and depression including one which was appropriately entitled 'Major depression and generalized anxiety disorder: same genes and (partly) different environments' (Kendler *et al.*, 1992). Environmental studies reviewed elsewhere in this book suggest that the environmental difference between the triggers for anxiety and depression are that the life events which trigger anxiety involve threat, whereas the life events which trigger depression involve loss, humiliation and entrapment. Twin studies have also shown that approximately half of the association between the personality trait of neuroticism and lifetime risk of depression is due to genetics (Kendler *et al.*, 1993). The same group has also shown a common genetic liability to phobia, panic disorder and bulimia (Kendler *et al.*, 1995), which are genetically unrelated to the liability to depression, anxiety and neuroticism.

Genetic mechanisms

The method of linkage analysis has been outstandingly successful in the case of early onset familial Alzheimer's disease for which linkage has been established with loci on chromosomes 21 and 14 on which chromosomal mutations have been demonstrated subsequently (Sham, 1996). Comparable genome-wide searches for linkage have been conducted in multiple affected bipolar families with sufficient rigour for it to be possible to exclude the possibility that a single locus explains the inheritance of bipolar affective illness (Berretini, 1996). Attempts to fit epidemiological and genetic data to mathematical models have also argued against the notion that bipolar affective illness is due to a single gene of major effect (Craddock *et al.*, 1995). At least three, and possibly more, genes are likely to be involved. Although the findings of many linkage studies in affective illness have never been replicated, two findings have been. As much as 25% of bipolar illness in multiply affected families may be linked to a locus near the centromere on chromosome 18 and as much as 20% to a locus on chromosome 21q22.3

43

(Berretini, 1996). A candidate gene approach may be employed in conjunction with or instead of linkage analysis as in the recent identification of the serotonin transporter as a candidate gene in unipolar depression (Heils *et al.*, 1996; Ogilvie *et al.*, 1996; Collier *et al.*, 1997).

In the case of the related dimensions of depression, anxiety and neuroticism the search for genes of major effect is even less likely to be productive than in bipolar affective disorder. Many genes of small effect are likely to influence dimensions such as neuroticism, as has been demonstrated recently for fearfulness in the mouse (Flint *et al.*, 1995).

The biological basis of the main environmental causes of depression

The environmental causes of depression are reviewed in Chapter 4 and the main influences are summarized here in Fig. 3.1. These are known to explain

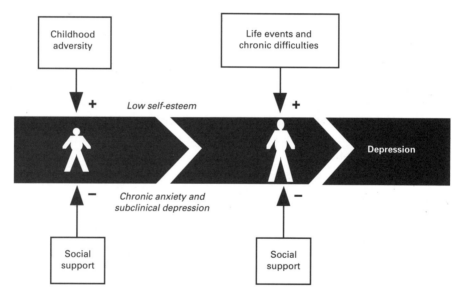

Fig. 3.1 A schematic summary of the psychosocial causes of depression as described in Chapter 4.

most of the variance in onset and much of the variance in offset of depression as studied in community samples. What might be the biological basis for this environmental influence? The main biological response to environmental stress is activation of the adrenal medulla and cortex which results in increased secretion of adrenaline and corticosteroid hormones (predominantly cortisol in man and corticosterone in the rat). Of these two adrenal products cortisol is much more important in depression. Corticosteroid hormones act at corticosteroid receptors in the brain (particularly the hippocampus) and mediate the influence of environmental stress on the development of several animal models of depression including learned helplessness (Papolos *et al.*, 1993) and immobility in the forced swim test (de Kloet *et al.*, 1988). In man, also, the central actions of cortisol can cause depression, as in Cushing's syndrome (Jeffcoate *et al.*, 1979; Kelly *et al.*, 1983). It may also be possible to treat depression by inhibiting the synthesis of cortisol (Murphy-Pearson *et al.*, 1991; O'Dwyer *et al.*, 1995). For all of these reasons, the corticosteroid response to environmental stress is a relevant biological measure for studies into the biological basis of the environmental causes of depression.

Most of the environmental influences on depression can be modelled in experimental animals and, in most cases, activation of the hypothalamic pituitary adrenal (HPA axis) results. Thus life at the bottom of the baboon social hierarchy involves limited access to food and mates and the intermittent receipt of displaced hostility from frustrated baboons higher up the hierarchy. This situation (which would be rated by social scientists as a 'chronic difficulty') is associated with increased activation of the HPA axis (Sapolsky, 1989). So, too, is the loss of social rank (Sapolsky, 1990; Jones *et al.*, 1995), which in man would be categorized as a life event with severe long-term consequences for the individual. In social psychiatry, vulnerability factors are psychosocial influences which increase the likelihood that an event or difficulty will be followed by depression. Childhood adversity is such a vulnerability factor, and in many animal studies environmental stress *in utero* or in neonatal life results in enhanced responsiveness of the HPA axis throughout adult life (Plotsky & Meaney, 1993). Conversely, increased maternal attention (produced experimentally by a procedure termed 'handling') results in reduced corticosteroid responses to stress throughout life (Meaney *et al.*, 1989).

In humans, social support is a protective factor which reduces the likelihood that a given event or difficulty will be followed by depression. In the experimental animal, social support (provided by the presence of members of the social group) reduces the size of the corticosteroid response to stress (Lyons & Levine, 1994). Human studies of the effects upon cortisol of social adversity have been less detailed than the animal studies but the results are broadly consistent. The secretion of cortisol is increased by life events (Willis *et al.*, 1987), particularly in the presence of depression (Calloway & Dolan, 1989). Social support buffers the cortisol response to stress, at least in children (Gunnar *et al.*, 1992), and sexual abuse (a powerful vulnerability factor for subsequent depression) results in lasting neuroendocrine changes which are similar to those seen in depression (de Bellis *et al.*, 1994).

For all these reasons the corticosteroid response to environmental stress is a convenient biological model of the environmental causes of depression (Fig. 3.2). It is a simplified model, and even within the corticosteroid system there are other steroids, the secretion of which is influenced by stress such as

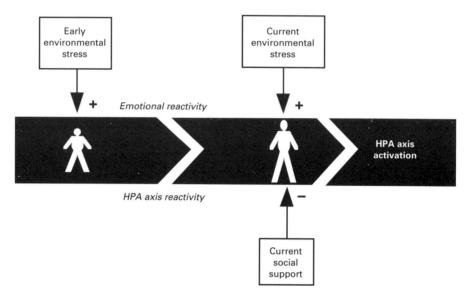

Fig. 3.2 A schematic summary of the effects of psychosocial stress upon the secretion of corticosteroid hormones.

dihydroepiandosterone, which have an antiglucocorticoid action. There are also many neurotransmitter systems such as noradrenaline (NA) and 5-hydroxytryptamine (5-HT) which adapt to acute and chronic stress (Abercrombie & Zigmond, 1995) but which are less accessible to human investigation at present. The model described in Fig. 3.2 should therefore be thought of as one aspect of the biological basis of the environmental causes of depression: the corticosteroid response to stress is an excellent 'marker' of the main environmental causes of depression, it may in some cases 'mediate' the environmental influence (O'Dwyer *et al.*, 1995) but it is not the whole story.

Less common environmental causes of depression

Childbirth is a very powerful environmental trigger for the onset of bipolar illness, with relapse rates of 30–50% in the first 6 weeks after childbirth (Dean *et al.*, 1989). The withdrawal of oestrogen and/or progesterone may be the cause, although so far it has not proved possible to prevent such relapses with oestrogen treatment. However, unipolar depression following childbirth can be treated with oestrogen, suggesting that oestrogen withdrawal may be the cause (Gregoire *et al.*, 1996). Cushing's syndrome is a rare endocrine disorder which is commonly associated with depression (Kelly *et al.*, 1983). Myxoedema is much commoner and is also associated with depression (Cleare *et al.*, 1996). Hypercalcaemia is another rare metabolic disorder which can be associated with depression. Although few depressive illnesses are triggered by such endocrine disturbances they are of theoretical importance and, in the case of resistant depression, can become practically important (see Chapter 20).

Biological changes in depression

These fall into three main groups:
1 changes in limbic forebrain function;
2 changes in cortical activity;
3 neurochemical studies.
There is, at present, no unitary hypothesis which satisfactorily links 1–3 and so in this chapter detail will only be given where this is of some clinical relevance.

Changes in limbic forebrain function

Neuroendocrine changes in depression

These are reviewed elsewhere (Checkley, 1992; Holsboer, 1995) and so only the most general statements will be reviewed here.
1 Depression is associated with more widespread and more severe neuroendocrine disturbances than any other psychiatric disorder, implying a greater disturbance of limbic and hypothalamic function in depression than in other cases.
2 Increased activation of the HPA axis leading to a sustained increase in cortisol secretion is the most common abnormality, being present in: 80% of the most severely depressed (i.e. psychotic) patients; 50% of in-patients with melancholia; and in less than 50% in mildly depressed out-patients. The causes of HPA axis activation in depression are multiple and probably include an increased central drive of the axis mediated by: increased production of the hypothalamic hormones arginine vasopressin and corticotropin-releasing hormone (Raadsheer *et al.*, 1994); impaired negative feedback control of the axis by cortisol (Carroll *et al.*, 1981; Young *et al.*, 1991); and hypertrophy of the adrenal gland (Rubin *et al.*, 1995) (Fig. 3.3).
3 Reduced secretion of thyroid-stimulating hormone (TSH) (Rubin *et al.*, 1987) with consequent blunting of the TSH response to thyrotropin releasing hormone (TRH) (Loosen *et al.*, 1987) is only slightly less common. There are other changes in the thyroid axis, including subclinical hypothyroidism (Rupprecht *et al.*, 1989) and an increased incidence of antithyroid antibodies (Nemeroff *et al.*, 1985).
4 Growth hormone (GH) responses to most stimuli are impaired in depression, particularly those which involve the alpha$_2$ adrenoceptor influence on GH secretion. (for review, see Checkley, 1992).

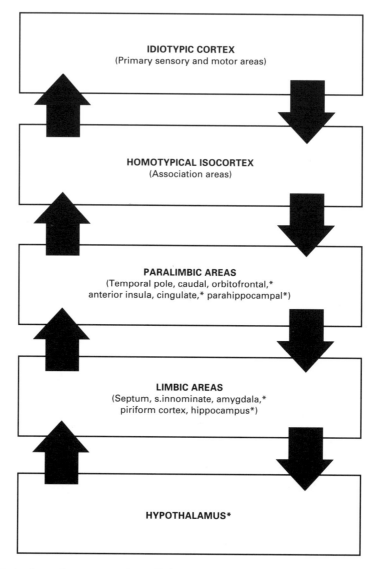

Fig. 3.3 A schematic representation of behavioural specialization and neural connectivity in the cerebral cortex and related limbic structures (adapted from Mesulam, 1985). Regions implicated in the pathogenesis of depression by studies cited in this chapter are indicated by asterisks.

5 Prolactin responses to indirectly acting 5-HT agonists such as fenfluramine and tryptophan are impaired in depression (Siever *et al.*, 1984; Cowen & Charig, 1987; O'Keane & Dinan, 1991).

6 Most neuroendocrine changes in depression can be seen to be either the consequence of chronic stress ((**2**) above) or of monoaminergic dysfunction ((**4**) and (**5**) above) or possibly of both.

7 Not only is depression uniquely capable of altering neuroendocrine function but it is also uniquely sensitive to changes in that function. Depression is the only psychiatric disorder which is causally related both to Cushing's syndrome (Jeffcoate *et al.*, 1979; Kelly *et al.*, 1983) and to myxoedema (Cleare *et al.*, 1996). Also in the postnatal period, it can be treated by oestrogen (Gregoire *et al.*, 1996) and the therapeutic response to standard treatment can be enhanced by additional treatment with thyroid hormones (Goodwin *et al.*, 1982).

8 The neuroanatomical location of the processes described in (2–7) include hypothalamic nuclei such as the ventromedial nuclei, where hypothalamic hormones are synthesized and the amygdala, which is involved in the activation of the stress response, and the hippocampus, which is involved in its termination. The hippocampus is uniquely endowed with corticosteroid receptors, which are known to mediate the influence of corticosteroid hormones on the development of several animal models of depression (de Kloet *et al.*, 1988; Papolos *et al.*, 1993). The hippocampus may therefore be involved in the pathogenesis of depression in Cushing's syndrome. The hippocampus and related limbic structures are also richly endowed with thyroid and oestrogen receptors which may mediate the effect of oestrogen and thyroxine on depression.

Sleep and depression

There is also a unique biological relationship between sleep and depression. Sleep disturbance in depression has been characterized by Kupfer (1995) as:

1 a decrease in sleep continuity and duration in unipolar depression;

2 an increased continuity and duration of sleep;

3 changes in rapid-eye-movement (REM) sleep in unipolar depression including reduced REM latency, increased first REM period and shift in distribution of REM sleep toward the first half of the night;

4 reduced slow-wave sleep, particularly during the first non-REM sleep period;

5 increased electroencephalogram power in higher wave bands.

Some of these changes are seen in disorders such as obsessive compulsive disorder, which is associated with depression, but all are more frequent in depression than in other psychiatric disorders. The two-way relationship between sleep and depression is demonstrated by the observation that among psychiatric disorders depression is uniquely amenable to treatment with sleep deprivation. Total sleep deprivation for one night results in a transient but significant reduction in the severity of depression in about 60% of all cases (Wu & Bunney, 1990). This effect develops progressively over the period of sleep deprivation and then is lost as soon as the patient falls asleep, even for a brief nap (Wu & Bunney, 1990). The involvement of the limbic system in the action of sleep deprivation in man has been suggested by a positron emission tomography (PET) study in which antidepressant response to total sleep deprivation was accompanied by a reduction in glucose metabolism in limbic regions (Wu *et al.*, 1992).

Biological rhythms and depression

Depression is a periodic disorder with tendencies both to relapse and remission. When the periodicity is regular then the question arises as to whether it is driven by an endogenous biological rhythm or clock, or whether the timing is derived from external stimuli which themselves are periodic. The only way to resolve the matter is to study the periodic phenomena in isolation from external cues to time.

One patient with a 48-hour bipolar illness has been studied in such conditions in complete sensory isolation and the periodicity of this illness was preserved. Under the conditions of complete sensory deprivation his sleep–wake cycle shortened to 19.5 h so that every 19.5 h he woke up at what he thought was the start of a new day: his bipolar illness, however, maintained a strict 48-hour periodicity showing that it was driven by a truly endogenous biological clock (Dirlich *et al.*, 1981). There is also some evidence that diurnal variation of depressed mood maintains its timing in the absence of clues to real clock time. It remains controversial as to whether the circadian system is altered in depression (Wirz-Justice, 1995) and the authors' data suggest that it is not (Thompson *et al.*, 1988; Checkley *et al.*, 1993). However, there is no controversy about the periodic nature of depression and the fact that in some cases this is driven by a truly endogenous biological clock (Dirlich *et al.*, 1981). Such regular periodicity is not seen for other psychiatric disorders and so suggests a unique relationship between depression and biological clocks. Animal studies indicate that the suprachiasmatic nucleus in the hypothalamus is the site of the 'master clock' (Moore, 1995; Ralph & Hurd, 1995), and so the evidence that depression is uniquely sensitive to biological rhythms is further evidence that the hypothalamus is involved in the pathogenesis of depression.

Changes in cortical activity in depression

The neuroendocrine and other physiological changes which I have reviewed thus far point to a dysfunction in hypothalamic and related subcortical limbic system regions in depressive illness. The following section will give an overview of recent advances in the functional neuroimaging of depression. It will show that changes in cerebral blood flow are best described in those cortical regions (orbitofrontal and cingulate) with reciprocal connections to the limbic system. Before changes in brain function can be studied by neuroimaging it must first be determined whether or not there are abnormalities in brain structure. Enlarged lateral ventricals in elderly depressed patients were first reported by Jacoby and Levy (1980) using computed tomography. More recent studies using magnetic resonance imaging (MRI) have confirmed these findings and have shown that they are associated with widening of the cerebral sulci (Tanaka *et al.*, 1982; Rabins *et al.*, 1991) particularly in the frontal and temporal lobes (Dolan *et al.*, 1986). These changes have been reported in elderly depressives but in younger depressives abnormalities in structure have not been consistently detected thus far (Pearlson & Schlaepfer, 1995). Elderly depressives have also been found to have areas of increased MRI signal density (termed hyperintensities) in subcortical regions such as the basal ganglia and thalamus: the significance of these hyperintensities is not known (Rabins *et al.*, 1991). Similar subcortical white matter lesions have also been reported in younger patients with bipolar affective disorder (Dupont *et al.*, 1990; Swayze *et al.*, 1990).

Functional neuroimaging in depression

Since neuronal activity is dependent on the supply of glucose from the blood, whenever there is an increase in the neuronal activity of a circumscribed brain region there will be an accompanying increase in the regional cerebral blood flow (rCBF) to that part of the brain. This can be measured in man either by functional MRI (which detects changes in the oxygenation of haemoglobin) or by PET or single photon emission tomography (SPET), in both of which a radioactive tracer is used (Goodwin, 1996).

State-dependent changes in cortical activity have attracted particular interest because they control for any abnormality in structure of the brain. Most reports to date have described state-dependent changes in depression in those parts of the cerebral cortex with the strongest connections to the limbic system. The limbic association cortex includes the orbitofrontal cortex, the cingulate gyrus and the parahippocampal cortex, and changes have consistently been reported in orbitofrontal cortex and anterior cingulate gyrus as patients have recovered from depression. In one PET (Bench *et al.*, 1995) and one SPET (Goodwin *et al.*, 1993) study drug status was well controlled between the depressed and recovered state, and in both experiments rCBF was reduced in orbitofrontal cortex and anterior cingulate gyrus in the depressed state and increased with clinical recovery. Changes in rCBF in the same areas but in the opposite direction have been reported following electroconvulsive therapy (ECT; Lerer *et al.*, 1994), total sleep deprivation (Ebert *et al.*, 1994; Wu *et al.*, 1992) and following drug treatment (Drevets *et al.*, 1992), but in none of these studies were the treatment conditions of the depressed and recovered patients well matched. Further studies are needed, but at present it would appear that activity in some limbic association areas is altered in depression and changed by a variety of antidepressant treatments.

Comparisons between depressed and control subjects, although not controlling for any structural change in depression, do reveal broadly similar findings as has been reviewed recently by Goodwin (1996). Reduced cerebral blood flow in anterior brain structures, particularly the inferomedial frontal cortex and anterior cingulate gyrus, have been reported in many studies, and reductions in parietal and temporal brain regions have also been frequently reported.

The induction of sad mood by the recollection of sad life events has been shown to activate the medial prefrontal cortex in studies using PET (Pardo *et al.*, 1993; George *et al.*, 1995) and magnetic resonance imaging (MRI) (S. Baker, unpublished data). The generation of depressing plans (preparing to attend one's mother's funeral) similarly activates the medial prefrontal cortex, whereas the generation of relatively emotionally neutral plans (preparing for one's mother coming to dinner) does not (Partiot *et al.*, 1995). One common feature of these two activation procedures is the activation of depressogenic schemata as described in Chapter 5. For this reason it has been argued that depressogenic schemata are 'stored' in the medial prefrontal cortex. Since the operation of stereotactic subcaudate tractotomy (SST), which is used for resistant depression (Poynton *et al.*, 1995), isolates the medial prefrontal cortex and reduces oxygen metabolism therein (Biver *et al.*, 1995) it is reasonable to suggest that SST disrupts the storage or processing of depressogenic schemata.

The neuroendocrine effects of depression mostly point to a disturbance of brain function at hypothalamic or higher levels. The effects of hormones (corticosteroid, oestrogen and thyroxine) on depression must be mediated by their receptors which are mostly localized in subcortical limbic forebrain structures, such as the hippocampus, amygdala and hypothalamus. In animal studies, hippocampal glucocorticoid receptors are clearly involved in animal models of depression. The first generation of functional neuroimaging studies have shown that the brain regions which show state-dependent changes in depression are mostly within the limbic association cortex. The functional relationship between these different areas has been described by Mesulam (1985) as described in Fig. 3.3.

Neurochemical studies

It is not possible to review in a short chapter the very large number of studies which have been conducted into the neurochemistry of depression over the last 30 years. Detailed reviews are available elsewhere of the many changes in 5-hydroxytryptamine (5-HT; Maes & Meltzer, 1995) and the fewer but still important changes in noradrenaline (NA; Schatzberg & Schildkraut, 1995) as well as the good reasons for implicating dopamine (Willner, 1995), acetyl choline (Janowsky & Overstreet, 1995) and neuropeptides (Holsboer, 1995; Plotsky *et al.*, 1995) in the pathogenesis of depression. For none of these neuro-transmitters is there a single hypothesis that explains satisfactorily the pathogenesis of depression. In the case of the monoamines NA and 5-HT there is now good evidence that depletion of NA and 5-HT, respectively, does not result in depression (Delgado *et al.*, 1991; Miller *et al.*, 1996a). How-ever, as will be reviewed in the next section, both procedures do reverse the therapeutic action of antidepressant drugs which are thought to act by increasing NA and 5-HT neurotransmission.

Mechanisms of action of antidepressant drugs

This section will give a simplified account of current understanding of the mechanisms of action of antidepressant drugs such as is needed by a clinician who prescribes such drugs, and needs to know the scientific basis for their actions and interactions. Thirty years ago when tricyclic antidepressants (TCAs) and monoamine oxidase inhibitors (MAOIs) were introduced into clini-cal practice, it was thought that they alleviated depression by increasing monoamine availability as a result of uptake inhibition and monoamine oxidase inhibition, respectively. However, it was soon appreciated that there is a discrepancy between the time course of drug action upon monoamines (which is immediate) and upon mood (which is delayed by 3–6 weeks). Fifteen years later it was discovered that adaptive changes at monoamine receptors were seen following chronic antidepressant treatment, and so it was proposed that these effects might explain the delayed onset of antidepressant action. The down-regulation of beta adrenoceptors (together with uncoupling from its second messenger) was the first adaptive change to be reported fol-lowing treatment with MAOIs, TCAs and ECT, and so this was proposed as the common mechanism of action of antidepressant drugs (Sulser, 1984). Over the ensuing years many more receptors have been described, many more drug effects upon them have been reported and attempts have been made, both in preclinical and clinical studies, to describe the net effect upon monoaminergic neurotransmission of the multiple effects of antidepressant drugs upon monoaminergic receptors. The wheel has now come full circle and once again it is thought that antidepressant drugs work by increasing monoaminergic neurotransmission. Adaptive changes at several receptors play an important part in this effect, and so an understanding of how at least some of these receptors function is needed by any clinician who is trying to understand how antidepressant medication works. For everyday purposes a working un-derstanding of the serotonergic and noradrenergic systems suffices, and so this chapter will focus almost exclusively on the effects of antidepressant drugs upon transmitter systems for 5-HT and NA.

Effect of antidepressant treatments upon 5-HT

5-Hydroxytryptamine (5-HT) and 5-HT receptors

The cell bodies of 5-HT neurones are located in the raphe nuclei of the hind brain from where projections arise to all brain regions. There are at least 14 receptor subtypes (Watson & Girdlestone, 1996) but so far a role in human psychopharmacology has only been established in four cases. These receptors fall within three families of receptors: 5-HT_1, 5-HT_2 and 5-HT_3. Members of the 5-HT_1 family of receptors have in common coupling of the receptor to the enzyme adenylate cyclase; the consequence of this is that the stimulation of 5-HT_1 receptors results in inhibition of adenylate cyclase activity, with a subsequent fall in intracellular concentrations of the second messenger cyclic AMP. The 5-HT_2 family of receptors are coupled to the phosphoinositide cycle. The consequence is that stimulation of the 5-HT_2 receptors results in increased intracellular concentrations of the second messengers diacylglycerol and inositol triphosphate. 5-HT_3 receptors are linked to the fast cation channel in the cell membrane. Stimulation of 5-HT_3 results in a rapid change in intracellular calcium and potassium concentrations.

Of the 5-HT_1 family of receptors 5-HT_{1A} receptors are of particular relevance to human psychopharmacology. They bind anxiolytic drugs such as buspirone, gepirone and ipsapirone as well as the beta antagonist pindolol, all of which can be given to human subjects. 5-HT_{1A} receptors are located postsynaptically and are abundant in the hippocampus. Receptors are also located in the cell bodies and dendrites of the 5-HT neurones in the raphe nucleus as somatodendritic receptors. The stimulation of somatodendritic 5-HT_{1A} receptors results in inhibition of 5-HT cell firing and consequent 5-HT release. In this way the 5-HT_{1A} somatodendritic receptor maintains a negative feedback control over 5-HT release. The presynaptic 5-HT_1-like receptor which is found on 5-HT axon terminals is the 5-HT_{1B} receptor in the rat and the 5-HT_{1D} receptor in humans; in human psychopharmacology the 5-HT_{1D} agonist sumatriptan is effective in the relief of migraine through its action at vascular 5-HT_{1D} receptors.

The 5-HT behavioural syndrome refers to a pattern of motor behaviour which is seen in experimental animals following maximal stimulation of the 5-HT system with drug combinations such as the 5-HT precursor tryptophan and a MAOI. The syndrome, which includes hyperactivity, tremor and stereotyped motor behaviours (Straub tail, forepaw treading, hind limb abduction, lateral head shakes), involves activation of 5-HT_{1A} receptors since it is reversed by 5-HT$_{1A}$ antagonists (Deakin & Green, 1978). The term '5-HT syndrome' is applied in clinical practice to somewhat comparable behaviours which are seen following excessive stimulation of the 5-HT system in man including confusion, agitation, myoclonus, hyper-reflexia, diaphoresis, shivering, tremor, diarrhoea, incoordination and fever (Sternbach, 1991). Again 5-HT$_{1A}$ receptors may be involved since some of these effects have been reversed by treatment with 5-HT$_{1A}$ antagonists (Guze & Baxter, 1986; Sandyk, 1986).

Of the 5-HT$_2$-like receptors, 5-HT$_{2A}$ receptors have a high affinity for ketanserin, spireprone and some TCAs. 5-HT$_{2A}$ receptors are located postsynaptically in the cerebral cortex where they can be visualized using PET and SPET ligands such as ketanserin and ritanserin. Increased numbers of 5-HT$_{2A}$ receptors have been found in the frontal cortex of some, but not all, depressed suicides (Arora & Meltzer, 1989; Arango *et al.*, 1992) and studies of living patients are being conducted at present.

5-HT$_3$ receptors are located in the peripheral nervous system and sensory afferents, and in hind brain regions such as the area postrema which is involved in the control of emesis. The 5-HT$_3$ antagonist ondansetron is a potent anti-emetic (Kenny *et al.*, 1992) and since the gastrointestinal side-effects of serotonin re-uptake inhibitors (SSRIs) can be inhibited by ondansetron, it is likely that they involve the stimulation of 5-HT$_3$ receptors.

Finally, mention should be made of the 5-hydroxytryptamine transporter (5-HTT), which is the site of selective and active re-uptake of 5-HT from the synapse. SSRIs and tricyclic antidepressant drug (TADs) bind to the 5-HTT and thereby inhibit the re-uptake of 5-HT. 5-HTTs are expressed in platelets as well as in the brain and in most (though not all) studies reduced numbers of platelet 5-HTTs have been repeated in depressed patients (Maes & Meltzer, 1995). More recently, genetic variations of the 5-HTT gene have been shown to be associated with genetic vulnerability towards depression.

Effects of antidepressant drugs upon the 5-HT system in experimental animals

All antidepressant treatments which affect 5-HT cause an immediate increase in the availability of 5-HT (Adell & Artigas, 1991; Sharp *et al.*, 1991). TADs and SSRIs achieve this by inhibiting 5-HT uptake, ECT and lithium do so by increasing 5-HT release and MAOIs by inhibiting metabolism. In all cases an increased availability of 5-HT results in the stimulation of the 5-HT$_{1A}$ somatodendritic receptors which exert a negative feedback control by 5-HT over the firing rate of 5-HT neurones (Chaput *et al.*, 1986; Blier *et al.*, 1990). This means that the initial consequence of increased 5-HT availability within the synapse is inhibition of 5-HT cell firing and therefore of 5-HT release.

However, with chronic antidepressant treatment an adaptive downregulation of the somatodendritic 5-HT$_{1A}$ receptor takes place and has the effect of overcoming this initial negative feedback. As a result, 5-HT cell firing and 5-HT release return to pretreatment values; the effect of uptake blockade by SSRIs is then to increase 5-HT neurotransmission (Blier *et al.*, 1988). After chronic TAD treatment an increased responsiveness of postsynaptic 5-HT$_{1A}$ receptors is seen (Blier *et al.*, 1986, 1987, 1990) together with downregulation of 5-HT$_{2A}$ receptors (Goodwin *et al.*, 1984). Since these changes occur in the absence of change in 5-HT cell firing, the net effect is an increase in 5-HT neurotransmission through postsynaptic 5-HT$_{1A}$ receptors. An enhanced responsiveness of postsynaptic 5-HT$_{2A}$ receptors is also seen after chronic electroconvulsive shock (ECS) (Keller *et al.*, 1981, Biegon & Israel, 1987; Burnet *et al.*, 1995), which also results in increased 5-HT neurotransmission since 5-HT cell firing and 5-HT release is unchanged following chronic ECS (Blier & Bouchard, 1992). A net increase in 5-HT neurotransmission is also seen following treatment with MAOIs as a result of downregulation of 5-HT$_{1A}$ somatodendritic receptors, and also of the alpha$_2$ adrenoceptor which is located on 5-HT terminals and which inhibits 5-HT release (Mongeau *et al.*, 1994). Although these different treatments have different acute and chronic effects upon 5-HT, in all cases, the net effect of chronic treatment is an increase in 5-HT neurotransmission in experimental animals.

Effects upon 5-HT of lithium given in combination with antidepressant drugs.

Lithium inhibits the functioning of the second messenger systems adenylate cyclase and phosphatidyl inositol turnover and as a result has many effects upon neuroreceptor function, including increased responsiveness of postsynaptic 5-HT$_{1A}$ receptors (Goodwin *et al.*, 1986; Blier *et al.*, 1987). Lithium also increases 5-HT release following acute treatment (Sharp *et al.*, 1991). The combination of lithium with antidepressant drugs results in greater increase in 5-HT release than is seen with either treatment alone and this may explain the basis of augmentation by lithium of antidepressant drug treatment (see below).

Interactions between 5-HT$_{1A}$ antagonists and antidepressant drug treatment

The ability of SSRI treatment to reduce cell firing in the raphe nucleus can be reduced by the selective blockade of 5-HT$_{1A}$ receptors (Arborelius *et al.*, 1995; Gartside *et al.*, 1995), which suggests that the effect of SSRIs on 5-HT function can be increased by concurrent autoreceptor blockade (see below).

Effects of 5-HT$_{1A}$ agonists on 5-HT

5-HT$_{1A}$ agonists such as gepirone and buspirone are effective as anxiolytics (Robinson *et al.*, 1990) and possibly as antidepressants (Jenkins *et al.*, 1990). They have the same effect on 5-HT cell firing as SSRIs and MAOIs. With acute treatment, cell firing is inhibited and with chronic treatment cell firing returns to baseline value as a result of downregulation of the 5-HT$_{1A}$ somatodendritic autoreceptors (Blier & de Montigny, 1990). The net effect is an increase in 5-HT neurotransmission.

Effects of antidepressant treatment on 5-HT function in man

Models have been developed for the clinical investigation of the above pharmacological mechanisms and many have been demonstrated to occur in man. Neuronal 5-HT uptake is conveniently modelled in platelets and platelet 5-HT content is reduced following the chronic administration of the SSRI fluvoxamine (Celada *et al.*, 1992). The hypothermic response to 5-HT$_{1A}$ agonists, which is thought to be a measure of 5-HT$_{1A}$ autoreceptor function, is reduced following chronic treatment with a number of antidepressant drugs (Lesch *et al.*, 1990, 1991). Neuroendocrine responses to 5-HT$_{1A}$ receptors are thought to involve postsynaptic 5-HT$_{1A}$ receptors and some but not all of these responses have been seen to be reduced in depression (Lesch, 1992; Moeller *et al.*, 1994) and following antidepressant drug treatment (Lesch *et al.*, 1991).

Effects of antidepressant treatment on neuroendocrine measures of
5-HT neurotransmission in man

The prolactin response to the 5-HT precursor tryptophan has been generally found to be reduced in depression and increased by chronic depressant treatment (Charney *et al.*, 1984; Price *et al.*, 1985, 1989; Cowen *et al.*, 1990). The prolactin response to the indirect 5-HT agonists fenfluramine and d-fenfluramine have also been reported to be reduced in many, though not all, studies of depressed patients. Both responses are increased following chronic treatment with TCAs and ECT (Upadhyaya *et al.*, 1991; Charney & Delgado, 1992; O'Keane *et al.*, 1992; Shapira *et al.*, 1992a,b). On balance the evidence suggests that, at least in neuroendocrine systems, 5-HT neurotransmission is increased in humans treated clinically with TCAs, SSRIs and probably also MAOIs.

Relationship between drug effects upon 5-HT and antidepressant response

There is good evidence that interfering with antidepressant effects upon

5-HT interferes with antidepressant response. This was first demonstrated when the antidepressant effect of imipramine was reversed by treatment with the 5-HT depleting agent parachlorophenylalanine (Shopsin *et al.*, 1975, 1976). More recently, a more acceptable form of 5-HT depletion has been produced by the administration of drinks rich in amino acids with and without tryptophan—the 5-HT precursor. The amino acid load stimulates the synthesis of protein which requires the essential amino acid tryptophan. When tryptophan is supplied in the drink the tryptophan is available, but in the tryptophan-free condition the tryptophan is withdrawn from the body's tryptophan stores and since these are needed for the synthesis of 5-HT, 5-HT synthesis is reduced. Animal studies have demonstrated falls in brain concentrations of tryptophan and 5-HT, and the 5-HT metabolite 5-hydroxyindoleacetic acid in rats treated with tryptophan-free diets (Young *et al.*, 1989). Comparable falls in plasma tryptophan have been reported in human subjects given the tryptophan-free amino acid drinks (Delgado *et al.*, 1990).

Depressed patients who have responded to antidepressant treatment relapse temporarily within a few hours of ingesting tryptophan-free amino acid-rich drinks (Delgado *et al.*, 1990). This effect has been demonstrated for all classes of antidepressant drugs with selective action upon 5-HT uptake (i.e. TCAs, SSRIs and MAOIs), but interestingly not for selective inhibitors of noradrenaline uptake such as desipramine and lofepramine (Heninger, 1995). Furthermore, when tryptophan-free drinks are given to untreated, depressed patients, no deterioration of their depression results (Delgado *et al.*, 1991); this means that 5-HT depletion as produced by typtophan-free drinks is not a sufficient cause of depression. However, the studies that have been reviewed provide good evidence that the antidepressant effects of TCAs, SSRIs and MAOIs involve an increase in 5-HT neurotransmission.

Further evidence for a causal link between antidepressant response and enhanced 5-HT neurotransmission comes from reports that the antidepressant response to a drug that enhances 5-HT neurotransmission can be increased by enhancing the drug effect upon 5-HT. This was first shown by enhancing the antidepressant response to the MAOI, tranylcypromine, with the tryptophan (Pare, 1963; Glassman & Platman, 1969). The tryptophan–MAOI combination, which in animals is a potent stimulus to the 5-HT syndrome, is a more potent antidepressant treatment than MAOI alone. More recent indirect evidence suggests that the augmentation of the antidepressant effect of antidepressant drugs by lithium may depend on enhanced 5-HT neurotransmission (Cowen *et al.*, 1991). Finally, there are suggestions that pindolol may accelerate the antidepressant response to SSRIs by removing 5-HT_{1A} autoreceptor-mediated negative feedback inhibition of the 5-HT neurone (Artigas *et al.*, 1994). The present state of knowledge suggests that enhance-

ment of 5-HT release is a common action of TCAs, SSRIs and MAOIs and
a sufficient cause of antidepressant response. However, it is not a necessary
component of the response because antidepressant effects can also be obtained
by selective inhibition of uptake.

Effects of antidepressant drugs on noradrenaline

Noradrenaline and its receptors

The noradrenergic system is similar in many respects to the serotonergic and
so will be described in less detail. Noradrenergic projections to the cerebral
cortex and limbic forebrain structures arise from cell bodies in the locus
coeruleus in the hind brain. The system that is activated in response to the
arousal is thought to be involved in psychological processes such as the mediation of anxiety, selective attention, learning and reinforcement (Robbins &
Everitt, 1995). The receptors at which NA (and adrenaline) exerts its physiological effects are termed adrenoreceptors. Their subdivision into alpha and
beta adrenoceptors was proposed on the basis of the opposing actions of the
chemically related compounds adrenaline and NA on the same physiological
processes (Ahlquist, 1948). Subsequently, alpha$_2$ adrenoceptors were distinguished from alpha$_1$ adrenoceptors on the basis of the presynaptic location of alpha$_2$ adrenoceptors, although it was later recognized that alpha$_2$
adrenoceptors are located both pre- and postsynaptically (Fillenz, 1990).
Clonidine is a clinically useful drug which can be used to probe the function of the alpha$_2$ adrenoceptors in depressed patients (see below). The subdivision of beta adrenoceptors was made on the basis of the preferential
activity of different beta adrenoceptor antagonists for cardiac and vascular
tissue (Lands *et al.*, 1967). Now that the genes for each of these adrenoceptors
have been identified, it is possible to study their structure and molecular
biology.

More recently a new class of receptor—the imidazoline receptor—has been
described, which also regulates the release of NA. Imidazoline receptors have
high affinity for imidazoline, clonidine and also for the alpha$_2$ antagonist
yohimbine, and a recently described endogenous ligand agmatine (Li *et al.*,
1994). Imidazoline receptors have been subcategorized into I$_1$ and I$_2$ receptors
on the basis of their preferential affinity for clonidine and imidazoline,
respectively (Michel & Eisberg, 1992). I$_1$ and I$_2$ receptors inhibit NA release
at NA terminals. The noradrenergic system has receptors located on
glia; both are present on human platelets and so are available for clinical
research.

Effects of antidepressant drugs upon the NA system in experimental animals

The net effects of antidepressant drugs upon NA and 5-HT neurones are surprisingly similar. For both neurotransmitters (see Table 3.1) the immediate
consequence of uptake inhibition is increased transmitter availability, and
in both cases this results in stimulation of somatodendritic autoreceptors
(alpha$_2$ adrenoceptors at NA neurones and 5-HT$_{1A}$ autoreceptors on 5-HT neurones), which results in reduced rates of cell firing and reduced transmitter
release. With both types of somatodendritic receptor downregulation occurs
following long-term treatment with selective re-uptake inhibitors, as a result
of which cell firing returns towards pretreatment values. The main differences between the adaptive responses of the NA and 5-HT systems concern
changes in postsynaptic receptor function. Concerning the noradrenergic system, downregulation of postsynaptic beta$_1$ adrenoceptors and/or uncoupling
of beta$_1$ adrenoceptors from the second messenger system is seen following
chronic treatment with almost all antidepressant treatments including ECT
(Sulser, 1984). Although studied in less detail, downregulation of both
pre- and postsynaptic alpha$_2$ adrenoceptors has been found following chronic
antidepressant treatments, as has upregulation of postsynaptic alpha$_1$
adrenoceptors (Heninger & Charney, 1987). Alpha$_2$ and imidazoline I$_2$ receptors
on NA terminals are both downregulated by chronic antidepressant treatment (Garcia-Sevilla *et al.*, 1996).

Effects of antidepressant drugs upon NA in man

In general, the effects of antidepressant drugs upon NA in man are equivalent
to those that are seen in animals. Various measures of the metabolism of NA
can be made in depressed patients treated with antidepressant drugs and these
indicate a reduction in the metabolic turnover of NA in man (Golden *et al.*,
1988; Sharma *et al.*, 1990). The alpha$_2$ and imidazoline I$_1$ receptor agonist
clonidine has measurable effects upon blood pressure, sedation, temperature
and the secretion of GH. The effects of antidepressant drugs upon these
alpha$_2$ adrenoceptor and/or imidazoline I$_1$ receptor-mediated responses are
similar in animals and man, suggesting that chronic treatment with antidepressant drugs downregulates alpha$_2$ adrenoceptors in experimental animals,
healthy human volunteers and depressed patients (Checkley *et al.*, 1986).
Downregulation of alpha$_2$ adrenoceptors and imidazoline I$_1$ receptors has been
demonstrated in the platelets of depressed patients (Garcia-Sevilla *et al.*, 1986,
1996) and in brain regions such as the frontal cortex (Garcia-Sevilla *et al.*, 1996),
hippocampus (Gonzalez *et al.*, 1994) and locus coeruleus (Ordway *et al.*, 1994).
From a clinical perspective the most important question is the determina-
tion of the net effect of antidepressant drug treatment on noradrenergic

Table 3.1 This table shows the acute (minutes) and chronic (7–14 days) effects of selective serotonin re-uptake inhibitors (SSRIs) and selective noradrenaline re-uptake inhibitors (SNRIs) on 5-HT and NA cell bodies in the raphe nuclei and locus coeruleus, respectively. (For the effects of SSRIS and TADs on pre- and post-synaptic receptors, please see text.)

	5-HT	NA
Acute effects of SSRIs and SNRIs, respectively, on 5-HT and NA neurones	(i) increased 5-HT availability (ii) stimulation of 5-HT$_{1A}$ somatodendritic receptors (iii) reduced 5-HT cell firing and reduced 5-HT release (iv) 5-HT availability returns to baseline value	(i) increased NA availability (ii) stimulation of alpha$_2$ somatodendritic receptors (iii) reduced NA cell firing and reduced NA release (iv) NA availability returns to baseline value
Chronic effects of SSRIs and SNRIs, respectively, on 5-HT and NA neurones	(i) downregulation of 5-HT$_{1A}$ somato-dendritic receptors (ii) cell firing and 5-HT release return to pretreatment values (iii) 5-HT uptake is still inhibited (iv) 5-HT availability is therefore increased	(i) downregulation of alpha$_2$ somatodendritic receptors (ii) cell firing and NA release return to pretreatment value (iii) NA uptake is still inhibited (iv) NA availability is therefore increased

neurotransmission. Some of the adaptive changes seen in animals will result in increased noradrenergic neurotransmission (downregulation of alpha$_2$ autoreceptors and upregulation of postsynaptic alpha$_1$ adrenoceptors), but others will have the effect of reduced noradrenergic neurotransmission (downregulation of postsynaptic beta$_1$ and alpha$_2$ adrenoceptors). How can the net effect of antidepressant drug treatment on noradrenergic neuro-transmission be determined in man?

The secretion of the pineal hormone melatonin is appropriate for this purpose, since the pineal gland is innervated by noradrenergic fibres which are endowed with prejunctional alpha$_2$ adrenoceptors and postjunctional alpha$_1$ and beta$_1$ adrenoceptors. Each of these receptors has been shown to influence the secretion of melatonin in animals and in man (Checkley & Palazidou, 1988). The secretion of melatonin is therefore controlled by the output of a typical noradrenergic system. The critical question is whether this is increased or reduced by chronic antidepressant treatment in man. Most studies have reported an increase (Checkley, 1991). One particularly informative experiment involved healthy volunteers receiving two stereoisomers of the highly selective noradrenaline uptake inhibitor oxaprotiline. The isomers differ mainly in their ability to inhibit noradrenaline uptake. The isomer that inhibited NA increased the secretion of melatonin after acute and chronic treatment, whereas the isomer with no effect on NA uptake had no effect on melatonin. Similar effects upon melatonin (and so presumably upon NA) have been found in healthy volunteers (Thompson *et al.*, 1985) and depressed patients (Sack & Lewy, 1986; Palazidou *et al.*, 1992) treated with the selective NA uptake inhibitor desipramine or with other antidepressant drugs (Murphy *et al.*, 1986).

Is the effect of antidepressant drugs on NA causally related to antidepressant response?

It will be recalled that whereas tryptophan depletion reverses the antidepressant effect of SSRIs, tryptophan depletion has no effect on the antidepressant effect of relatively selective NA uptake inhibitors (Delgado *et al.*, 1990). There is one report that the antidepressant effect of desipramine can be inhibited by inhibiting the synthesis of NA with alpha-methyl-para-tyrosine (AMPT; Delgado *et al.*, 1993), which suggests that the antidepressant response to desipramine depends on its ability to increase noradrenergic neurotransmission. AMPT given alone had no effect on drug-free depressed patients (Miller *et al.*, 1996a, 1996b). To date there is no evidence that increasing the effect of antidepressant drugs on noradrenergic transmission increases antidepressant response. At present it can be concluded that chronic treatment with selective NA uptake inhibitors results in a sustained increase in noradrenergic neurotransmission in man, and that this effect may be causally related to the mechanism of antidepressant action. As is the case for 5-HT, there is no evidence that an NA deficiency causes depression, even though there is evidence from neuroendocrine and other studies of NA changes in depression.

Effects of antidepressant drugs upon other receptor systems

For the purposes of the everyday treatment of depressed patients it is not necessary to review the many other neurochemical effects of antidepressant drugs. However, one which is of interest and has relevance to other parts of this chapter is the recent finding that antidepressant drug treatment increases the number of corticosteroid receptors in brain regions, particularly the hippocampus (Seckl & Fink, 1992). As a result of corticosteroid receptors in the hippocampus being involved in several animal models of depression (de Kloet *et al.*, 1988; Papolos *et al.*, 1993), the effects of antidepressants on these receptors may be relevant to the mode of action of antidepressant drugs. Corticosteroid receptors modulate 5-HT and NA neurotransmission through the hippocampus, and antidepressant drug effects on corticosteroid receptors require the presence of intact 5-HT pathways to the hippocampus. The view that antidepressant drugs may work via their effects on corticosteroid receptors is therefore not incompatible with the view that antidepressant effects are mediated through their effect on 5-HT and NA. However, from the perspective of the psychiatrist who is trying to augment the therapeutic response to a standard antidepressant drug, the view that antidepressant drugs work by enhancing 5-HT neurotransmission is currently of the greatest practical importance.

References

Abercrombie, E.D. & Zigmond, M.J. (1995) Modification of central catecholaminergic systems by stress and injury. In: *Psychopharmacology: The Fourth Generation of Progress* (eds F. E. Bloom & D. J. Kupfer), pp. 351–361. Raven Press: New York.

Adell, A. & Artigas, F. (1991) Differential effects of clomipramine given locally or systemically on extracellular 5-hydroxytryptamine in raphe nuclei and frontal cortex. An *in vivo* brain microdialysis study. *Naunyn Schmiedeberg's Archives of Pharmacology*, **343**, 237–244.

Ahlquist, R.P. (1948) A study of the adrenotropic receptor. *American Journal of Physiology*, **153**, 586–600.

Arango, V., Underwood, M.D. & Mann, J.J. (1992) Alterations in monoamine receptors in the brain of suicide victims. *Journal of Clinical Psychopharmacology*, **12**, 8–12.

Arborelius, L., Nomikos, G.G., Gultner, P. *et al.* (1995) *Naunyn Schmiedeberg's Archives of Pharmacology*, **352**, 157–165.

Arora, R.C. & Meltzer, H.Y. (1989) Increased serotonin 2 (5-HT2) receptor binding as measured by 3H-lysergic acid diethylamide (3H-LSD) in the blood platelets of depressed patients. *Life Science*, **44**, 725–734.

Artigas, F., Perez, V. & Alvarez, E. (1994) Pindolol induces a rapid improvement of depressed patients treated with serotonin reuptake inhibitors. *Archives of General Psychiatry*, **51**, 248–251.

de Bellis, M.D., Chrousos, G.P., Dorn, L.D. *et al.* (1994) Hypothalamic pituitary adrenal axis dysregulation in sexually abused girls with histories of abuse. *Journal of Clinical Endocrinology and Metabolism*, **78**, 249–250.

Bench, C.H., Friston, K.J. & Brown, R.G. *et al.* (1993) Regional cerebral blood flow in depression measured by positron emission tomography: the relationship with clinical dimensions. *Psychological Medicine*, **23**, 579–590.

Berretini, W. (1996) Genetic studies of bipolar disorders: new and recurrent findings. *Molecular Psychiatry*, **1**, 172–173.

Bertelsen, A., Harvald, B. & Gauge, M. (1977) A Danish twin study of manic-depressive disorders. *British Journal of Psychiatry*, **130**, 330–351.

Biegon, A. & Israel, M. (1987) Quantitative autoradiographic analysis of the effects of electroconvulsive shock on serotonin-2 receptors in male and female rats. *Journal of Neurochemistry*, **48**, 1386–1391.

Biver, F., Goldman, S., Francois, A. *et al.* (1995) Changes in metabolism of cerebral glucose after stereotactic leucotomy for refractory obsessive–compulsive disorder: a case report. *Journal of Neurology, Neurosurgery and Psychiatry*, **58**, 502–505.

Blier, P. & Bouchard, C. (1992) Effect of repeated electroconvulsive shocks on serotonergic neurons. *European Journal of Pharmacology*, **211**, 365–373.

Blier, P. & de Montigny, C. (1990) Differential effect of gepirone on presynaptic and postsynaptic serotonin receptors: single cell recording studies. *Journal of Clinical Psychopharmacology*, **10** (Suppl. 3), 13S–20S.

Blier, P., de Montigny, C. & Azzaro, A.J. (1986) Modification of serotonergic and noradrenergic neurotransmission by repeated administration of monoamine oxidase inhibitors: electrophysiological studies in threat. *Journal of Pharmacology and Experimental Therapeutics*, **237**, 987–994.

Blier, P., de Montigny, C. & Tardif, D. (1987) Short-term lithium treatment enhances responsiveness of postsynaptic 5-HT$_{1A}$ receptors without altering 5-HT autoreceptor sensitivity: an electrophysiological study in the rat brain. *Synapse*, **1**, 225–232.

Blier, P., Chaput, Y. & de Montigny, C. (1988) Long-term 5-HT reuptake blockade, but not monoamine oxidase inhibition, decreases the function of terminal 5-HT autoreceptors: an electrophysiological study in the rat brain.

Naunyn Schmiedeberg's Archives of Pharmacology, **337**, 246–254.

Blier, P., de Montigny, C. & Chaput, Y. (1990) A role for the serotonin system in the mechanism of action of antidepressant treatment: preclinical evidence. *Journal of Clinical Psychiatry,* **51**, (Suppl. 4), 14–20.

Bridges, P. (1992) Resistant depression and psychosurgery. In: *Handbook of Affective Disorders* (ed. E. S. Paykel), pp. 437–452. Churchill Livingstone, Edinburgh.

Brugha, T.S. & Bebbington P., McCarthy, P. *et al.* (1987) Social networks social support and the type of depressive illness. *Acta Psychiatrica Scandinavica,* **76**, 664–673.

Burnet P.W.J., Mead, A. & Eastwood, S.L. *et al.* (1995) Repeated ECS differentially effects rat brain 5HT$_{1A}$ and 5HT$_{2A}$ receptor expression. *NeuroReport,* **6**, 901–904.

Calloway, P. & Dolan, R. (1989) Endocrine changes and clinical profiles in depression. In: *Life Events and Illness* (eds G. W. Brown & T. O. Harris), pp. 139–160. Unwin Hyman, London.

Carroll, B.J., Feinberg, M., Greden, J.F. *et al.* (1981) A specific laboratory test for the diagnosis of melancholia. *Archives of General Psychiatry,* **38**, 15–22.

Celada, P., Dolan, M., Alvarez, E. *et al.* (1992) Effects of acute and chronic treatment with fluvoxamine on extracellular and platelet serotonin in the blood of major depressive patients. Relationships to clinical improvement. *Journal of Affective Disorders,* **25**, 243–250.

Chaput, Y. & de Montigny, C. (1991) Presynaptic and postsynaptic modifications of the serotonin system by long-term administration of antidepressant treatments: an *in vivo* electrophysiologic study in the rat. *Neuropsychopharmacology,* **5**, 219–229.

Chaput, Y., de Montigny, C. & Blier, P. (1986) Effects of a selective 5-HT reuptake blocker, citalopram, on the sensitivity of 5-HT autoreceptors: electrophysiological studies in the rat. *Naunyn Schmeideberg's Archives of Pharmacology,* **333**, 342–345.

Charney, D.S. & Delgado, P.L. (1992) Current concepts of the role of serotonin function in depression and anxiety. In: *Serotonin Receptor Subtypes: Pharmacological Significance and Clinical Implication* (eds S. Z. Langer, N. Brunello, G. Racagni, J. Mendlewicz), pp. 89–104. Karger, Basel.

Charney, D.S., Heninger, G.R. & Sternberg, D.E. (1984) Serotonin function and the mechanism of action of antidepressant treatment: effects of amitriptyline and desipramine. *Archives of General Psychiatry,* **41**, 359–365.

Checkley SA (1991) Neuroendocrine effects of psychotropic drugs. *Clinical Endocrinology and Metabolism,* **5**, 15–33.

Checkley, S.A. (1992) Neuroendocrinology. In: *Handbook of Affective Disorders* (ed. E. S. Paykel), pp. 255–266. Churchill Livingstone, London.

Checkley, S.A. (1998) The management of resistant depression. In: *The Management of Depression* (ed. S.A. Checkley), pp. 430–457. Blackwell Science, Oxford.

Checkley, S.A. & Palazidou, E. (1988) Melatonin and antidepressant drugs: clinical pharmacology. In: *Melatonin: Clinical Perspectives* (eds A. Miles, D. R. S. Philbrick, C. Thompson), pp. 190–204. Oxford University Press, Oxford.

Checkley, S.A., Corn, T.H., Glass, I.B. *et al.* (1986) Neuroendocrine and other studies of the mechanism of action of desipramine. In: *Antidepressants and their Receptor Function* (eds R. Porter, G. Bock, S. Clark), *CIBA Foundation Symposium,* **123**, 126–147. CIBA Foundation, London.

Cleare, A.J., McGregor, A., Chambers, S.M. *et al.* (1996) Thyroxine replacement increases central 5-hydroxytryptamine activity and reduces depressive symptoms in hypothyroidism. *Neuroendocrinology,* **64**, 65–69.

Collier, D.A., Stober, G., Li, T. *et al.* (1997) Susceptibility to bipolar affective disorder and unipolar depression is influenced by allelic variation of functional serotonin transporter expression. *Molecular Psychiatry* (in press).

Cowen, P.J. & Charig, E.M. (1987) Neuroendocrine responses to intravenous tryptophan in major depression. *Archives of General Psychiatry,* **44**, 958–966.

Cowen, P.J., McCance, S.L., Gelder, M.G. *et al.* (1990) The effect of amitriptyline on endocrine responses to intravenous L-tryptophan. *Psychiatry Research,* **31**, 201–208.

Cowen, P.J., McCance, S.L., Ware, C.J. *et al.* (1991) Lithium in tricyclic resistant depression: correlation of increased brain 5-HT function with clinical outcome. *British Journal of Psychiatry,* **159**, 341–346.

Craddock, N., Khodel, V., Van Eerdewegh, P. & Reich, T. (1995) Mathematical limits of multilocus models: the genetic transmission of bipolar disorder. *American Journal of Human Genetics,* **57**, 690–702.

Deakin, J.F.W. & Green, A.R. (1978) The effects of putative 5-hydroxytryptamine antagonists on the behaviour produced by administration of tranylcypromine and L-tryptophan or tranylcypromine and L-dopa to rats. *British Journal of Pharmacology,* **64**, 201–209.

Dean, C., Williams, R.J. & Brockington, I.F. (1989)

Is puerperal psychosis the same as bipolar manic depressive disorder? A family study. *Psychological Medicine,* **19**, 637–647.

Delgado, P.L., Charney, D.S. & Price, L.H. *et al.* (1990) Serotonin function and the mechanism of antidepressant action: reversal of antidepressant induced remission by rapid depletion of plasma tryptophan. *Archives of General Psychiatry,* **47**, 411–418.

Delgado, P.L., Price, L.H. & Miller, H.L. *et al.* (1991) Rapid serotonin depletion as a provocation challenge test for patients with major depression: relevance to antidepressant action and the neurobiology of depression. *Psychopharmacology Bulletin,* **27**, 321–330.

Delgado, P.L., Miller, H.L. & Salomon, R.M. *et al.* (1993) Monoamines and the mechanism of antidepressant action: effects of catecholamine depletion on mood of patients treated with antidepressant. *Psychopharmacology Bulletin,* **3**, 389–395.

Dirlich, G., Kammerloher, A. & Schulz, H. *et al.* (1981) Temporal co-ordination of rest–activity cycle. Body temperature, urinary free cortisol and mood in a patient with 48-hour unipolar depressive cycles in clinical and time-cue-free environments. *Biological Psychiatry,* **16**, 163–179.

Dolan, R.J., Calloway, S.P., Thacker, P.F. & Mann, A.H. (1986) The cerebral cortical appearance in depressed subjects. *Psychological Medicine,* **16**, 775–779.

Drevets, W.C., Videen, T.O. & Price, J.L. *et al.* (1992) A functional anatomical study of unipolar depression. *Journal of Neuroscience,* **12**, 3628–3641.

Dupont, R.M., Jernigan, T.L. & Butter, N. *et al.* (1990) Subcortical abnormalities detected in bipolar affective disorder using magnetic resonance imaging. *Archives of General Psychiatry,* **47**, 55–59.

Ebert, D., Feistel, H. & Kaschka, W. *et al.* (1994) Single photon emission computerized tomography assessment of cerebral dopamine D2 receptor blockade in depression before and after sleep deprivation: preliminary results. *Biological Psychiatry,* **35**, 880–885.

Fillenz, M. (1990) *Noradrenergic Neurones.* Cambridge University Press, Cambridge.

Flint, J., Corley, R., De Fries, J.C. *et al.* (1995) A simple genetic basis for a complex psychological trait in laboratory mice. *Science,* **269**, 1432–1435.

Garcia-Sevilla, J.A., Guimon, J., Garcia-Vallejo, P. & Fuster, M.J. (1986) Biochemical and functional evidence of supersensitive platelet α_2 adrenoreceptors in major affective disorder: effect of long-term lithium carbonate treatment. *Archives of General Psychiatry,* **43**, 51–57.

Garcia-Sevilla, J.A., Escriba, P.V., Sastre, M. *et al.* (1996) Immunodetection and quantitation of imidazoline receptor proteins in platelets of patients with major depression and in brains of suicide victims. *Archives of General Psychiatry,* **53**, 803–810.

Gartside, S.E., Umbers, V., Hajos, M. & Sharp, T. (1995) Interaction between a selective 5-HT$_{1A}$ receptor antagonist and an SSRI *in vivo*: effects on 5-HT cell firing and extracellular 5-HT. *British Journal of Pharmacology,* **115**, 1064–1070.

George, M.S., Ketter, T. & Parekh, P. *et al.* (1995) Brain activity during transient sadness and happiness in healthy women. *American Journal of Psychiatry,* **152**, 341–351.

Glassman, A.H. & Platman, S.R. (1969) Potentiation of monoamine oxidase inhibitor by tryptophan. *Journal of Psychiatric Research,* **7**, 83–88.

Golden, R.N., Markey, S.P. & Risbey, E.D. *et al.* (1988) Antidepressants reduce whole blood norepinephrine turnover while enhancing 6-hydroxymelatonin output. *Archives of General Psychiatry,* **45**, 150–154.

Gonzalez, A.M., Pascual, J., Meana, J.J. *et al.* (1994) Autoradiographic demonstration of increased α-2 adrenoreceptor agonist binding sites in the hippocampus and the frontal cortex of depressed suicide victims. *Journal of Neurochemistry,* **63**, 256–265.

Goodwin, F.K., Prange, A.J. & Post, R.M. *et al.* (1982) Potentiation of antidepressant effects by L-triiodothyronine in tricyclic non-responders. *American Journal of Psychiatry,* **139**, 34–38.

Goodwin, G.M. (1996) Functional imaging, affective disorder and dementia. *British Medical Bulletin,* **52**, 495–512.

Goodwin, G.M., Green, A.R. & Johnson, P. (1984) 5-HT$_2$ receptor characteristics in frontal cortex and 5-HT$_2$ receptor-mediated head-twitch behaviour following antidepressant treatment in mice. *British Journal of Pharmacology,* **83**, 235–242.

Goodwin, G.M., de Souza, R.J. & Wood, A.J. *et al.* (1986) The enhancement by lithium of the 5-HT$_{1A}$ mediated serotonin syndrome in the rat: evidence for a post-synaptic mechanism. *Psychopharmacology,* **90**, 488–493.

Goodwin, G.M., Austin, M.-P. & Dougall, N. *et al.* (1993) State changes in brain activity shown by the uptake of ^{99m}Tc-exametazine with single photon emission tomography in major depression before and after treatment. *Journal of Affective Disorders,* **29**, 243–253.

Gregoire, A.J.P., Kumar, R. & Everitt, B. *et al.* (1996) Transdermal oestrogen for severe postnatal depression. *Lancet,* **347**, 930–933.

Gunnar, M.R., Larson, M.C. & Hertsgaard, L. *et al.* (1992) The stressfulness of separation among nine-month-old infants: effects of social context variables and infant temperament. *Child Development*, **63**, 290–303.

Guze, B.H. & Baxter, L.R., Jr (1986) The serotonin syndrome: case responsive to propranolol (letter). *Journal of Clinical Psychopharmacology*, **6**, 119–120.

Heils, A., Teufel, A., Petri, S. *et al.* (1996) Allelic variation of human serotonin transporter gene expression. *Journal of Neurochemistry* (in press).

Heninger, G.R. (1995) Indoleamines: the role of serotonin in clinical disorders. In: *Psychopharmacology: The Fourth Generation of Progress* (eds F. E. Bloom & D. J. Kupfer), pp. 471–482. Raven Press, New York.

Heninger, G.R. & Charney, D.S. (1987) Mechanism of action of antidepressant treatments: implications for the etiology and treatment of depressive disorders. In: *Psychopharmacology: The Third Generation of Progress* (ed. H. Y. Meltzer), pp. 535–544. Raven Press, New York.

Holsboer, F. (1995) Neuroendocrinology of mood disorders. In: *Psychopharmacology: The Fourth Generation of Progress* (eds F. E. Bloom & D. J. Kupfer), pp. 957–970. Raven Press, New York.

Jacoby, R.J. & Levy, R. (1980) Computed tomography in the elderly. 3: Affective disorder. *British Journal of Psychiatry*, **136**, 270–275.

Janowsky, D.S. & Overstreet, D.H. (1995) The role of acetylcholine mechanisms in mood disorders. In: *Psychopharmacology: The Fourth Generation of Progress* (eds F. E. Bloom & D. J. Kupfer), pp. 945–956. Raven Press, New York.

Jeffcoate, W.J., Silverstone, J.T., Edwards, C.R.W. *et al.* (1979) Psychiatric manifestations of Cushing's Syndrome: response to lowering of plasma cortisol. *Quarterly Journal of Medicine*, **48**, 465–472.

Jenkins, S.W. *et al.* (1990) Gepirone in the treatment of major depression. *Journal of Clinical Psychopharmacology*, **10**, (Suppl. 3), 77S–85S.

Jones, I.H., Stoddart, D.M. & Mallick, J. (1995) Towards a sociobiological model of depression. *British Journal of Psychiatry*, **166**, 475–479.

Keller, K.J., Cascio, C.S. & Butler, J.A. *et al.* (1981) Differential effects of electroconvulsive shock and antidepressant drugs on serotonin-2 receptors in rat brain. *European Journal of Pharmacology*, **69**, 515–518.

Kelly, W.F., Checkley, S.A., Bender, D.A. *et al.* (1983) Cushing's Syndrome and depression: a prospective study of 26 patients. *British Journal of Psychiatry*, **142**, 16–19.

Kendler, K.S., Neale, M.C., Kessler, R.C. *et al.* (1992) Major depression and generalized anxiety disorder: same genes (partly) different environments? *Archives of General Psychiatry*, **49**, 716–722.

Kendler, K.S., Neale, M.C., Kessler, R.C. *et al.* (1993) A longitudinal twin study of personality and major depression in women. *Archives of General Psychiatry*, **50**, 853–862.

Kendler, K.S., Walters, E.E., Neale, M.C. *et al.* (1995) The structure of the genetic and environmental risk factors for six major psychiatric disorders in women. *Archives of General Psychiatry*, **52**, 374–383.

Kenny, G.N., Oates, J.L., Lesser, J. *et al.* (1992) Efficacy of orally administered ondansetron in the prevention of postoperative nausea and vomiting: a dose ranging study. *British Journal of Anaesthetics*, **68**, 466–470.

de Kloet, E.R., de Kloet, S., Schild, V. *et al.* (1988) Antiglucocorticoid RU 38486 attenuates retention of a behaviour and disinhibits the hypothalamic pituitary adrenal axis at different brain sites. *Neuroendocrinology*, **47**, 109–115.

Kupfer, D.J. (1995) Sleep research in depressive illness: clinical implications: a tasting menu. *Biological Psychiatry*, **38**, 391–403.

Lands, A.M., Arnold, A., McAuliff, J.P., Luduena, F.P. & Brown, T.G. (1967) Differentiation of receptor systems activated by sympathomimetic amines. *Nature*, **214**, 597–598.

Lerer, B. (1989) Neurochemical and other neurobiological consequences of ECT: implications for the pathogenesis and treatment of affective disorders. In: *Psychopharmacology: The Third Generation of Progress* (ed. H. Y. Meltzer), pp. 577–588. Raven Press, New York.

Lerer, B., Krausz, Y., Bonne, O. *et al.* (1994) ECT, antidepressant response and cerebral blood flow in patients with major depression. *Neuropsychopharmacology*, **10**, 568S.

Lesch, K.P. (1992) 5-HT$_{1A}$ receptor responsivity in anxiety disorders and depression. *Progress in Neuropsychopharmacology and Biological Psychiatry*, **15**, 723–733.

Lesch, K.P., Disselkamp-Tietze, J., Hoh, A. *et al.* (1990) 5-HT$_{1A}$ receptor function in unipolar depression: effect of chronic amitriptyline treatment. *Journal of Neural Transplantation*, **180**, 157–161.

Lesch, K.P., Hoh, A.H., Schulte, H.M. *et al.* (1991) Long-term fluoxetine treatment decreases 5-HT$_{1A}$ receptor responsivity in obsessive-compulsive disorder. *Psychopharmacology*, **105**, 410–420.

Li, G., Regunathan, S., Barrow, C.J., Eshraghi, J., Cooper, R. & Reis, D.J. (1994) Agmatine: an endogenous clonidine-displacing substance in the brain. *Science*, **263**, 966–969.

Loosen, P.T., Garbutt, J.C. & Prange, A. (1987) Evaluation of the diagnostic utility of the TRH-induced response in psychiatric disorders. *Pharmacopsychiatry*, **20**, 90–95.

Lyons, D.M. & Levine, S. (1994) Socioregulatory effects on squirrel monkey pituitary-adrenal activity: a longitudinal analysis of cortisol and ACTH. *Psychoneuroendocrinology*, **19**, 283–291.

Maes, M. & Meltzer, H.Y. (1995) The serotonin hypothesis of major depression. In: *Psychopharmacology: The Fourth Generation of Progress* (eds F. E. Bloom & D. J. Kupfer), pp. 933–944. Raven Press, New York.

McGuffin, P. & Katz, R. (1989) The genetics of depression and manic depressive illness. *British Journal of Psychiatry*, **155**, 294–304.

McGuffin, P., Katz, R. & Watkins, S. (1996) A hospital based twin register of the heritability of DSM-IV unipolar depression. *Archives of General Psychiatry*, **53**, 129–136.

Meaney, A.J., Aitkin, D.H., Viau, V. *et al.* (1989) Neonatal handling alters adrenocortical negative feedback sensitivity and hippocampal type II glucocorticoid receptor binding in the rat. *Neuroendocrinology*, **50**, 597–604.

Mesulam, M.-M. (1985) Patterns in behavioral neuroanatomy: associative areas, the limbic systema and hemispheric specialisation. In: *Principles of Behavioral Neurology* (ed. M.-M. Mesulam), pp. 1–70. Davis, Philadelphia.

Michel, M.C. & Eisberg, P. (1992) Keeping an eye on the I site: imidazoline-preferring receptors. *Trends in Pharmaceutical Sciences*, **113**, 369–370.

Miller, H.L., Delgado, P.L., Salomon, R.M. *et al.* (1996a) Clinical and biochemical effects of catecholamine depletion on antidepressant-induced remission of depression. *Archives of General Psychiatry*, **53**, 117–128.

Miller, H.L., Delgado, P.L., Salomon, R.M. *et al.* (1996b) Effects of a α-methyl-para-tyrosine (AMPT) in drug free depressed patients. *Neuropsychopharmacology*, **14**, 151–157.

Moeller, F.G., Steinberg, J.L., Fulton, M. *et al.* (1994) A preliminary neuroendocrine study with buspirone in major depression. *Neuropsychopharmacology*, **10**, 75–83.

Mongeau, R., de Montigny, C. & Blier, P. (1994) Electrophysiologic evidence for desensitization of alpha 2-adrenoceptors on serotonin terminals following long-term treatment with drugs increasing norepinephrine synaptic concentration. *Neuropsychopharmacology*, **10**, 41–51.

Murphy, D.L., Tamarkin, L., Sunderland, T. *et al.* (1986) Human plasma melatonin is elevated during treatment with monoamine oxidase inhibitors clorgyline and tranylcypromine but not deprenyl. *Psychiatry Research*, **17**, 119–127.

Murphy-Pearson, B., E., Dhar, V., Ghadirian, A.M. *et al.* (1991) Response to steroid hypertension in major depression resistant to antidepressant therapy. *Journal of Clinical Psychopharmacology*, **11**, 121–126.

Nemeroff, C.B., Simon, J.S., Haggerty, J.J., Jr *et al.* (1985) Antithyroid antibodies in depressed patients. *American Journal of Psychiatry*, **142**, 840–843.

Nurnberger, J.I., Gershon, E.S. (1992) Genetics. In: *Handbook of Affective Disorders* (ed E.S. Paykel), pp. 131–148. Churchill Livingstone, Edinburgh.

O'Dwyer, A.M., Lightman, S.A., Marks, M.N. *et al.* (1995) Treatment of major depression with metyrapone and hydrocortisone. *Journal of Affective Disorders*, **33**, 123–128.

Ogilvie, A.D., Battersby, S., Bubb, V.J. *et al.* (1996) Polymorphism in serotonin transporter gene associated with susceptibility to major depression. *Lancet*, **347**, 731–733.

O'Keane, V. & Dinan, T.G. (1991) Prolactin and cortisol responses to d-fenfluramine in major depression: evidence for diminished responsivity of central serotonergic function. *American Journal of Psychiatry*, **148**, 1009–1015.

O'Keane, V., McLoughlin, D. & Dinan, T.G. (1992) D-fenfluramine-induced prolactin and cortisol release in major depression: response to treatment. *Journal of Affective Disorders*, **26**, 143-150.

Ordway, G.A., Widdowson, P.S., Smith, K.S. & Halaris, A.E. (1994) Agonist binding to α2-adrenoreceptors is elevated in the locus coeruleus from suicide victims. *Journal of Neurochemistry*, **63**, 617–624.

Palazidou, E., Papadopoulos, A., Ratcliff, H. *et al.* (1992) Noradrenaline uptake inhibition increases melatonin secretion, a measure of noradrenergic neurotransmission in depressed patients. *Psychological Medicine*, **22**, 309–315.

Papolos, D.F., Edwards, E., Marmur, R. *et al.* (1993) Effects of the antiglucocorticoid RU 38486 on the induction of learned helplessness in Sprague-Dawley rats. *Brain Research*, **615**, 304–309.

Pardo, J.V., Pardo, P. & Raichle, M. (1993) Neural correlates of self-induced dysphoria. *American Journal of Psychiatry*, **150**, 713–719.

Pare, C.M.B. (1963) Potentiation of monoamine oxidase inhibitors by tryptophan. *Lancet*, **ii**: 527–528.

Partiot, A., Grafman, J., Sadato, N. *et al.* (1995) Brain activation during the generation of non-emotional and emotional plans. *NeuroReport, 6,* 1269–1272.

Pearlson, G.D. & Schlaepfer, T.E. (1995) Brain imaging in mood disorders: In: *Psychopharmacology the Fourth Generation of Progress* (eds F.E. Bloom & D.J. Kupfer), pp. 1019–1028. Raven Press, New York.

Plotsky, P.M. & Meaney, M.J. (1993) Early post-natal experience alters hypothalamic cortico-tropin-releasing factor (CRF), mRNA, median eminence CRF content and stress-induced release in adult rats. *Brain Research. Molecular Brain Research, 18,* 195–200.

Plotsky, P.M., Owens, M.J. & Nemeroff, C.B. (1995) Neuropeptide alterations in mood disorders. In: *Psychopharmacology: The Fourth Generation of Progress* (eds F. E. Bloom & D. J. Kupfer). Raven Press, New York.

Poynton, A.M., Kartsounis, L.D. & Bridges, P.K. (1995) A prospective clinical study of stereotactic subcaudate tractotomy. *Psychological Medicine, 25,* 763–770.

Price, L.H., Charney, D.S. & Heninger, G.R. (1985) Effects of tranylcypromine treatment on neuroendocrine, behavioural and autonomic responses to tryptophan in depressed patients. *Life Science, 37,* 809–818.

Price, L.H., Charney, D.S., Delgado, P.L. *et al.* (1989) Effects of desipramine and fluvoxamine treatment on the prolactin response to tryptophan. *Archives of General Psychiatry, 46,* 625–631.

Raadsheer, F.C., Hoogendijk, W.J.C., Stam, F.C. *et al.* (1994) Increased numbers of corticotropin-releasing hormone expressing neurons in the hypothalamic paraventricular nucleus of depressed patients. *Neuroendocrinology, 60,* 436–444.

Rabins, P.V., Pearlson, G.D., Aylward, E. *et al.* (1991) Cortical magnetic resonance imaging changes in elderly inpatients with major depression. *American Journal of Psychiatry, 148,* 617–620.

Ralph, M.R. & Hurd, M.W. (1995) Circadian pacemakers in vertebrates. In: *Circadian Clocks and Their Adjustment* (eds D. J. Chadwick & K. Ackrill) *CIBA Foundation Symposium, 183,* 67–87. CIBA Foundation, London.

Robbins, T. & Everitt, B. (1995) Central norepinephrine neurones and behaviour. In: *Psychopharmacology: The Fourth Generation of Progress* (eds F. E. Bloom & D. J. Kupfer), pp. 363–372. Raven Press, New York.

Robinson, D.S., Richels, K., Feighner, J. *et al.* (1990) Clinical effects of the 5-HT$_{1A}$ partial agonists in depression: a composite analysis of buspirone in the treatment of depression. *Journal of Clinical Psychopharmacology, 10* (Suppl. 3), 67S–76S.

Rubin, R.T., Poland, R.E., Lesser, I.M. *et al.* (1987) Neuroendocrine aspects of primary endogenous depression. IV. Pituitary–thyroid axis activity in patients and matched control subjects. *Psycho-neuroendocrinology, 12,* 333–347.

Rubin, R.T., Phillips, J.J., Sadow, T.F. *et al.* (1995) Adrenal gland volume in major depression. *Archives of General Psychiatry, 52,* 213–218.

Rupprecht, R., Rupprecht, C., Rupprecht, M. *et al.* (1989) Triiodothyronine, thyroxine, and TSH response to dexamethasone in depressed patients and normal controls. *Biological Psychiatry, 25,* 22–32.

Sack, R.L. & Lewy, A.J. (1986) Desmethyl-imipramine treatment increases melatonin production in humans. *Biological Psychiatry, 21,* 406–409.

Sandyk, R. (1986) L-Dopa induced 'serotonin syndrome' in a Parkinsonian patient on bromo-criptine (letter). *Journal of Clinical Psychopharmacology, 6,* 194–194.

Sapolsky, R.M. (1989) Hypercortisolism among socially subordinate wild baboons originates at CNS level. *Archives of General Psychiatry, 46,* 1047–1051.

Sapolsky, R.M. (1990) Adrenocortical function, social rank and personality among wild baboons. *Biological Psychiatry, 28,* 862–872.

Schatzberg, A.F. & Schildkraut, J.J. (1995) Recent studies on norepinephrine systems in mood disorders. In: *Psychopharmacology: The Fourth Generation of Progress* (eds F. E. Bloom & D. J. Kupfer), pp. 911–920. Raven Press, New York.

Seckl, J.R. & Fink, G. (1992) Antidepressants increase glucocorticoid and mineralocorticoid receptors in RNA expression in the rat hippocampus *in vivo. Neuroendocrinology, 55,* 621–626.

Sham, P. (1996) Genetic epidemiology. *British Medical Bulletin, 52,* 408–433.

Shapira, B., Yagmur, M.J. & Gropp, C. *et al.* (1992a) Effect of chlomipramine and lithium on fenfluramine induced hormone release in major depression. *Biological Psychiatry, 15,* 975–983.

Shapira, B., Lerer, B. & Kindler, S. *et al.* (1992b) enhanced serotonergic responsivity following electroconvulsive therapy in patients with major depression. *British Journal of Psychiatry, 160,* 223–229.

Shapira, B., Cohen, J., Newman, M.E. *et al.* (1993) Prolactin response to fenfluramine and placebo challenge following maintenance pharma-cotherapy withdrawal in remitted depressed patients. *Biological Psychiatry, 33,* 531–535.

Sharma, R.P., Janicak, P.G., Javaid, J. I. *et al.* (1990) Platelet MAO inhibition, urinary MHPG, and leukocyte beta-adrenergic receptors in depressed patients treated with phenalzine. *American Journal of Psychiatry*, **147**, 1318–1321.

Sharp, T., Branwell, S.R., Lambert, P. & Grahame-Smith, D.G. (1991) Effects of short- and long-term administration of lithium on the release of endogenous 5HT in the hippocampus of the rat *in vivo* and *in vitro*. *Neuropharmacology*, **30**, 977–984.

Shopsin, B., Gershon, S., Goldstein, M. *et al.* (1975) Use of synthesis inhibitors in defining a role of biogenic amines during imipramine treatment in depressed patients. *Psychopharmacology*, **1**, 239–249.

Shopsin, B., Friedman, E. & Gershon, S. (1976) Parachlorophenylalanine reversal of tranylcypromine effects in depressed patients. *Archives of General Psychiatry*, **33**, 811–819.

Siever, L.J., Murphy, D.L., Slater, S., de la Vega, E. & Lipper, S. (1984) Plasma prolactin changes following fenfluramine in depressed patients compared with controls: an evaluation of central serotonergic responsivity in depression. *Life Science*, **34**, 1029–1039.

Sternbach, H. (1991) The serotonin syndrome. *American Journal of Psychiatry*, **148**, 705–713.

Sulser, F. (1984) Regulation and function of noradrenaline receptor systems in brain. Psychopharmacological aspects. *Neuropharmacology*, **23**, 255–261.

Swayze, V.W., Andreasen, N., Alliger, R.J. *et al.* (1990) Structural brain abnormalities in bipolar affective disorder. *Archives of General Psychiatry*, **47**, 1054–1059.

Tanaka, Y., Hazama, H., Fukuhara, T. & Tsutui, T. (1982) Computerized tomography of the brain in manic-depressive patients: a controlled study. *Folia Psychiatrica Neurologica (Japan)*, **36**, 137–144.

Thompson, C., Mezey, G., Corn, T. *et al.* (1985) The effect of desipramine upon melatonin and cortisol secretion in depressed and normal subjects. *British Journal of Psychiatry*, **147**, 389–393.

Thompson, C., Franey, C., Arendt, J. & Checkley, S.A. (1988) A comparison of melatonin secretion in depressed patients and normal subject. *British Journal of Psychiatry*, **152**, 260–265.

Upadhyaya, A.K., Pennell, I., Cowen, P.J. *et al.* (1991) Blunted growth hormone and prolactin responses to L-tryptophan in depression, a state-dependent abnormality. *Journal of Affective Disorders*, **21**, 213–218.

Watson, S.P. & Girdlestone, D. (1996) TiPS receptor and ion channel nomenclature. *Trends in Pharmacological Sciences*, **17**, 1–44.

Willis, L., Thomas, P., Garry, P.J. & Goodwin, J. (1989) A prospective study of response to stressful life events in initially health elders. *Journal of Gerontology*, **42**, 627–630.

Willner, P. (1995) Dopaminergic mechanisms in depression and mania. In: *Psychopharmacology: The Fourth Generation of Progress* (eds F. E. Bloom & D. J. Kupfer), pp. 921–932. Raven Press, New York.

Wirz-Justice, A. (1995) Biological rhythms in mood disorder. In: *Psychopharmacology: The Fourth Generation of Progress* (eds F. E. Bloom & D. J. Kupfer), pp. 999–1018. Raven Press, New York.

Wu, J.C. & Bunney, W.E. (1990) The biological basis of an antidepressant response to sleep deprivation and relapse: Review and hypothesis. *American Journal of Psychiatry*, **147**, 14–21.

Wu, J.C., Gillin, J.C., Buchsbaum, M.S. *et al.* (1992) Effect of sleep deprivation on brain metabolisms in depressed patients. *American Journal of Psychiatry*, **149**, 538–543.

Young, S.N., Ervin, F.R., Pihl, R.O. *et al.* (1989) Biochemical aspects of tryptophan depletion in primates. *Psychopharmacology*, **98**, 508–511.

Young, E.A., Haskett, R.F., Murphy-Weinberg, V. & Watson, S.J. (1991) Loss of glucorcorticoid fast feedback in depression. *Archives of General Psychiatry*, **48**, 693–699.

4 A psychosocial model of depression: implications for management

TIRRIL O. HARRIS

In the last decade it has become increasingly accepted that the aetiology of depression is multifactorial. Its psychosocial origins are now recognized by those for whom formerly biological factors were the sole consideration. There is, however, a considerable gap between acknowledgement that something contributes to onset or perpetuation of a condition and translating that knowledge into practical management strategies. While this gap may merely indicate a scarcity of the resources necessary to effect this translation, it can also sometimes reflect the fact that, despite repeated reference to the importance of a particular factor, understanding of the process at stake is incomplete, and the implications thus not followed through. Much of social psychiatry deals with gross demographic variables such as age, sex and marital status, the relevance of which, when planning for the individual patient, is often not immediately apparent. The rest consists largely of narrowly focused subtopics such as negative cognitions, social support or negative life events, and these are often defined differently so that integrating them into a meaningful whole is not easy. Furthermore, much work uses rather mechanical definitions of these factors; for example, frequency of contact, rather than anything more qualitative about the relationship, is still often used as an index of good social support, so that the emotional meaning of any findings may not emerge with full strength. This chapter will summarize recent work on the role of psychosocial factors in depression in a way which highlights the emotional meaning of the various experiences identified as predictive across the lifespan. It will also draw out the implications of this psychosocial perspective for the management of depression.

Depression, life events and meaning

Meaning depends on the method of measurement

Studies on life events perhaps exemplify more than those in other areas the way in which research reports can often fail to convey the full meaning of their findings. A life event is a substantial change in life style or prospects, such as job change, engagement to be married or news of examination failure that can be precisely dated. 'Events' are contrasted with 'incidents' ('hassles' if negative or 'uplifts' if positive), which can be dated in a similar way but which are not considered to involve the same degree of change. However, clusters of incidents recurring over a prolonged period may constitute a substantial enough ongoing problem to be classified as a 'difficulty': continuing drops of rain through the roof can amount to a housing difficulty, and repetitive tiffs to a marital one.

Many studies still utilize a checklist questionnaire approach to data collection (see for example the classic Social Readjustment Rating Scale, Holmes & Rahe, 1967) with the respondents ticking a checklist of predefined experiences (such as house-move or birth of a child) if they have occurred in a defined period. The underlying notion was that changes to the usual routines could be stressful, but this approach fails to consider the context and the way in which this can alter the meaning of what is described as the same event. For example, a birth: a planned first pregnancy in a secure marital and financial situation has a totally different meaning from an unplanned pregnancy for a single parent who is already coping with three children, cramped housing and a shortage of money; both, however, would rate the same score on the checklist system. Work based on face-to-face semistructured interviews can address the shortcomings of this approach. For example, the Interview for Recent Life Events (Paykel *et al.*, 1969, 1980); and the Life Events and Difficulties Schedule (LEDS; Brown & Birley, 1968, Brown & Harris, 1978) and the latest edition of the Psychiatric Epidemiology Research Interview (PERI) (Dohrenwend *et al.*, 1993). These, particularly the LEDS, attempt to capture these variations in context without specifically taking account of the emotional appraisal of the individual concerned. Bias may arise if a person who has developed depression is asked about the meaning of events in his/her life, with his/her depression colouring the accounts. The LEDS uses a contextual method of rating based on knowledge of a wide range of circumstances surrounding each event. A judgement is made by the investigator about the likely meaning of each event for the person concerned, on the basis of what most people would feel in such a situation given personal background, prior plans and current circumstances, but ignoring what the person reports as their actual reaction to the event. This judgement has to be ratified by a consensus group of other raters blind to the key outcome variable(s). The rationale for using this type of judgement is that through understandable fear of bias, common sense and empathy have been underutilized on the grounds that they somehow interfere with strict scientific enquiry although they are powerful measuring rods; and that if bias can be minimized, such contextual ratings could enrich research. These ratings thus deal with specific meaning, in the sense of taking into account the specific circumstances surrounding a particular event or difficulty, but they reduce bias by ignoring the person's subjective account. In fact the latter can be deliberately compared with the contextual rating for the same event to gauge whether the person is responding in a manner that exaggerates or minimizes its stressfulness, compared with the reactions expected from others with similar backgrounds. A set of rules laid out in training manuals embodies decades of these consensus decisions and ensures high rates of interrater reliability for the contextual ratings (Tennant *et al.*, 1979; Parry *et al.*, 1981).

Provoking agents for depression: loss, humiliation and entrapment

Events

There are two ways in which this approach has thrown light on the links between life stress and depression. First, it has revealed crucial items that are missing from existing checklists, particularly revelations and disclosures of sensitive information about the self and other close ties. These include finding out that a child has been involved in criminal activities, although as yet unknown to the police, or declaring one's homosexuality to parents. Second, it has shown that, in a sense, these lists contain too many items, as only a small proportion of the life events listed have relevance for depressive onset. Progress here has been through ever-increasing specificity. From the initial definition of an event in terms of the change entailed, the focus moved to the undesirability of that change (Sarason *et al.*, 1978), especially to its long-term threat or unpleasantness above a certain severity threshold. This has distinguished 'severe events' from other, more minor, undesirable ones; the negative implications of which only last a few days, since the latter were no more common among the recently depressed than in the general population (Brown *et al.*, 1973). Thus events such as routine house moves, which were not rated severe, were not associated with depression. Nor were events which were severe in the short term, such as finding a breast lump and learning from biopsy within 2 weeks that it was benign. Whereas 19% of women in a representative British inner city population experienced at least one of these severe events in a nine-month period (Brown & Harris, 1978), figures for those in similar communities with recent onset of depression ranged from 91% (Brown *et al.*, 1986) to 62% (Bebbington *et al.*, 1984). Comparable figures for psychiatric patients with neurotic unipolar depression ranged from 73% (Brown *et al.*, 1994a) to 39% (Bebbington *et al.*, 1988), while those for psychiatric patients with melancholic or psychotic unipolar depression ranged from 58% (Brown & Harris, 1978) to 37% (Bebbington *et al.*, 1988). As will be discussed later the different rates among patients may well be due to different proportions, with first episodes between the different samples reported.

Later research focused even more specifically on what was depressogenic. The severe loss events which precede depression were distinguished from the severe dangers where as yet there has been no loss, for example a child's acute asthma attack. The latter tend to precede anxiety disorders without comorbid depression (Finlay-Jones & Brown, 1981; Brown *et al.*, 1987). An important aspect of this definition of a severe loss was that it included not only severe losses of people and material possessions but also of cherished ideas, for example of the trustworthy nature of close others. Examples of such 'losses of cherished idea' include discovering a partner's extramarital affair or one's close friend's continued failure to repay a substantial loan from another. The insights gained into the importance for depression of the 'revelation events' omitted from standard stress checklists were thus amplified by the parallel findings on the importance of loss of cherished ideas about the fidelity and honesty of the people we rely on. More recently it has become apparent that as a predictor of depression, the concept of loss, needs further refinement. It is really only severe loss events with an element of humiliation or entrapment, or the finality of a death that play the crucial depressogenic role (Brown *et al.*, 1995). Thirty-one per cent of women in the general population with at least one such event became depressed. Other losses, even if substantial, such as job losses involving considerable financial hardship or adult children emigrating to the Antipodes were followed by a much lower rate of depressive onset—only 5%. However, it is important to note here that if such a job loss resulted from dismissal, or if such an emigration involved some estrangement from the parent, then a rating of humiliation would be very likely. Moreover, if there had already been a financial difficulty, the job loss might also prove to be 'entrapping'. It might underline the improbability of climbing out of the debt trap, thus embodying the loss of a cherished idea, namely the hope of paying off all the creditors. In those instances, therefore, the rate of depressive onset might be expected to be closer to 30% than to 5%.

Difficulties

As mentioned earlier, difficulties are ongoing problems such as overcrowded housing or violent interpersonal relationships, lasting at least 4 weeks, which may or may not give rise to severe events. When they do so, this is often experienced as an entrapment. Another set of insights has arisen in connection with difficulties through the concentrated empathic listening required of the investigator by the LEDS process of data collection. It seems that even in the absence of an event, such difficulties, if involving more than physical health problems and if rated on the top three points of severity ('major difficulties'), were more common before depressive onset than in the general community (termed 'major difficulties', see Brown & Harris, 1978). The reason why these major difficulties, which by definition must have been continuing for at least 2 years, could come to provoke depression at that particular point was not clear. Detailed exploration of the data suggested that some reassessment-forcing experience (a minor event or even a positive incident) might have caused the women to reappraise the unpleasantness of situations they had been avoiding facing for some time. Thus one woman with a cold and unsupportive partner became depressed when her younger sister announced her engagement to a successful, warm, young man, as if only then by comparison could she see her own situation clearly. Another became depressed shortly after an uncomplicated routine operation which was common among many non-depressed women. The experience of being well cared for in the relative security of hospital was in stark contrast to her daily experience of living in extremely poor housing conditions. On return home she may perhaps have become more aware at some level of being trapped in her housing, and this may have predicated the onset of depression. The key phrase here, however, is 'at some level', in that it would appear that women quite often register something about their circumstances without necessarily being able to put it into words. One female psychiatric patient was quite able to be specific in interview about the date she had first become depressed but reported no depressogenic events or difficulties in that period. However, at follow-up 2 years later she was able to give us information about the date her husband's extramarital affair had started which she had not possessed at first interview because he was still witholding it from her at that stage. It had happened 5 weeks before the onset of her depression. Certainly women often comment with gratitude at the end of an interview that they can now see certain things about their lives much more clearly as a result of having to focus on answering the detailed questions, that is they have begun to develop a coherent narrative of their life.

The issue of 'endogenous' depression

Although the majority of depressions are preceded by such provoking agents, it is important to register that in secondary and tertiary treatment centres around one-quarter will appear unprovoked, in the sense of having no preceding severe event or difficulty. In some cases the patients report having felt very upset by something most people would find only mildly distressing (such as an adult child moving across town away from home, but without any argument, or a mother's surgical operation for an illness that was in no way life-threatening)—in other words they have subjectively experienced a minor event as if it were severe and this has happened just before onset. However, in other cases there is little evidence of any provocation at all: not even a small incident can be recalled to have preceded onset in the key period.

Previously it was thought that such unprovoked episodes had a distinctive symptom morphology, which was more severe and included melancholic or psychotic features (Carney *et al.*, 1965), but careful studies with clearer, less confounded definitions of events and depressive subtypes did not confirm this perspective (Leff *et al.*, 1970; Paykel *et al.*, 1971, 1984; Brown *et al.*, 1979; Roy *et al.*, 1985; Bebbington *et al.*, 1988). A more recent study suggests that while first episodes of melancholic-psychotic depression resemble the neurotic subtype in following after 'provoking agents' as defined above, subsequent episodes of this depressive subtype are more often than not unprovoked. Moreover, there is also a subgroup of neurotic depressions without provoking agents (Brown *et al.*, 1994a). A mechanism involving kindling (Post *et al.*, 1986) has been proposed to account for this, whereby once sensitized by an environmentally provoked first episode depression can be more easily internally triggered.

Depression and vulnerability to life events and difficulties

Vulnerability prior to the event

About one in five of those who experience a severe event and one in three experiencing a humiliation/entrapment event become depressed. Characteristics that render some women more vulnerable to these events have become known as 'vulnerability factors'. In principle these could involve biological as well as psychological and social factors, since hyper-reactivity to stress may also stem from neuroendocrine factors. In practice, however, the term vulnerability factor in the literature on depression has referred to psychosocial factors which increase the likelihood that severe events and major difficuties will be followed by depression. Early explorations (Brown & Harris, 1978) pinpointed, among other characteristics, lack of employment outside the home and the presence of three or more children within it as vulnerability factors, but went on to try to give meaning to these links with work and motherhood by invoking the concept of the 'role identities' available to each woman. These would vary in importance according to her involvement in the different domains of motherhood, sexual partnership, work, housework, sport and other social and recreational activities. This concept, as it were, forms a bridge between gross demographic groupings such as employment status or parenthood and the individual's sense of him/herself. It was argued that the number of such role identities available could prove crucial in protecting someone against the feelings of total hopelessness entailed by depression. A sense of 'hopelessness-specific-to-the-loss' would arise to a minor extent, at least temporarily, even in a person of robust character when faced with a severe event of this kind, but more vulnerable individuals would have a tendency to generalize the hopelessness, until the point where Beck's well-known cognitive triad of clinical depression (the self seems worthless, the world seems pointless and the future hopeless) produces all the further interferences with vegetative and cognitive functions which accompany depression (Beck, 1967; see also Seligman, 1975). One woman when faced with her teenage son's arrest for burglary may berate herself 'isn't that just typical of a child of mine—all I ever touch turns to dross—I can never succeed at anything', while another may stop short of such generalization with thoughts such as 'I must be a really awful mother, but at least I am a good secretary and the dramatics club can't do without me'. (The first, who generalized her negative role performance to all her role-identities became depressed, while the second, who, though very distressed, maintained her self-esteem by reminding herself of her positive performance in other roles, did not reach criteria for clinical depression.)

Although later research has only rarely been able to look at women between the life event and the onset of depression in order to confirm these anecdotal speculations, it has been able to show the importance of this type of negative evaluation of self in role performance (see below) and in predisposing women to a depressive reaction. Thus these early speculations about the protective function of multiple role identities can still prove informative; although over the last 30 years changes in society have altered the meaning of the two particular factors from which the ideas originally arose, and with this altered their potential to render women vulnerable to depression (T.O. Harris, unpublished information). Thus changes concerning the proportion of women in the workforce, the availability of nursery school places and low-cost, easy-to-use contraception have so altered the meaning of work outside the home, and presence of three or more children within it, that these no longer figure as vulnerability factors in the clear way they did in 1970. The most important vulnerability factors are thus the 'other characteristics' briefly referred to above.

Table 4.1 gives a summary of various vulnerability factors for depression reported at different times. They fall mainly into the two broad categories of negative self-evaluation and poor emotional support. The former category is, of course, the low self-esteem which was hypothesized to promote the generalization of hopelessness, and later found to predict a threefold higher rate of depressive onset after a provoking event or difficulty in a 12-month follow-up period—33% compared with 11% (Brown *et al.*, 1986). Sixty per cent of such onset cases exhibited such negative self-evaluation, compared with 30% of the rest of those with comparable stressful experience. In the same sample the second broad type of vulnerability factor, lack of social support, made a similar-sized contribution: 41% without and 4% with an adequate supportive context became depressed after a provoking agent, with 90% of such onset cases lacking adequate support, compared with 34% of the rest of those with at least one comparable severe event or major difficulty. The

Table 4.1 Vulnerability factors that potentiate the effects of severe events and difficulties among women by promoting the generalization of the hopeless feelings induced in anyone by such provoking agents.

Early identified factors: demographic categories/social roles
1 Lack of employment outside the home[1]
2 Presence of 3 or more children under 15 at home[1]
3 Loss of mother by death or long-term separation before age 11[1]

Recent changes in women's role have revealed these to have been only 'indicators' of the more crucial psychic factors listed below

Core vulnerability factors
1 Variants of psychological vulnerability
   (i) Negative evaluation of self[2]
   (ii) Chronic anxiety and subclinical depression[3]

2 Variants of lack of social support
   (i) Intimate confiding with partner[1]
   (ii) Lack of crisis support from core tie[2]
   (iii) Negative elements in core relationships[3]
   (iv) Lack of adequate parental care in childhood[4]

References from [1]Brown and Harris (1978); [2]Brown *et al.* (1986); [3]Brown *et al.* (1990); [4]Bifulco *et al.* (1987).

four variables listed under this second heading either involve a lack of concern with her emotional well-being on the part of members of the individual's core network, such that she cannot really speak freely to anyone about her worries, or else involve distinctly negative features such as coldness, or frequent criticism or arguments (Brown & Harris, 1978; Brown *et al.*, 1986, 1990). All these amount to a lack of support with stressful experiences, but they are also examples of unsuccessful roles in particular relationships. It is therefore not surprising that such poor support is associated with negative self-evaluation (Brown *et al.*, 1986, 1990). However, despite this association, logistic regression shows that both are required to model depressive onset (Brown *et al.*, 1986, 1990). Mention should also be made of further psychological vulnerability indicated by states of chronic anxiety and subclinical (or minor) depression (Brown *et al.*, 1990).

The evolution of ideas about vulnerability can be seen to have followed a similar course to those concerning life stress and depression, starting from work with straightforward social survey items, such as employment status or life change, and moving to the consideration of the emotional meaning of these items in different historical contexts. With hindsight it is easy to see that these two broad types of vulnerability echo the qualities identified as depressogenic among life events, with poor support mirroring exactly what is 'revealed' by revelation events—the absence of a trustworthy close other—and negative self-evaluation resonating with humiliation events. However, this echoing phenomenon only becomes apparent once the critical thresholds for support and self-evaluation have been located, and in the process their mutual influence appreciated. As already mentioned, support can be of many kinds, from the diffuse variety afforded by neighbours in the pub to the intimate type afforded by free and open confiding of private, possibly shameful, thoughts and feelings. It is the latter not the former which has proved protective against severe events. In a similar way this measure of self-evaluation includes, not only the general view of the self and its acceptance or rejection found in quick questionnaires (e.g. Rosenberg, 1965), but also opinions on performance in key roles. It spans a broad dimension (Brown *et al.*, 1990) from the exuberant recounting of successes among those with marked Positive Evaluation of Self (PES) through the modest self-descriptions of those with neither negative nor positive self-evaluation, to the perjorative comments of those with definite Negative Evaluation of Self (NES). It is the latter, not the absence of PES, which has proved a predictor of depressive onset during a 12-month follow up (Brown *et al.*, 1986, 1990). This insight has been confirmed in work contrasting the predictive power of the negatively and positively worded items of self-esteem questionnaires (Miller *et al.*, 1989). Once these depressogenic thresholds were identified, the links reported between social support and self-evaluation (op. cit.) became intuitively easier to understand: pleasant chatter in a pub might add to a person's already good opinion of him/herself but would be unlikely to affect any change in a negative view of the self built around particular shameful feelings too private to voice in such a setting. Talking one-to-one with a trusted friend, who is accepting, despite knowledge of the shaming items, may mitigate the impact of any new humiliation, and so prevent the generalization of hopelessness, and, in the long run, may decrease, or even eliminate, the NES, particularly if the confiding occurs regularly.

Mediating between life event and disorder: the role of coping style after a severe event or difficulty occurs

The vulnerabilities discussed so far have all involved risk factors pertaining before the life event occurs, although it is their role in the immediate aftermath which is proposed as crucial. In addition the important role of both cognitive and pragmatic coping styles should also be registered, since these may be amenable to influence during this critical, mediating period. Both self-blame and 'denial' (a tendency to miss seeing the negative aspects of a situation until it is too late) have been associated with increased risk of depression, as has helplessness in dealing with the situation (Lazarus & Folkman, 1984; Bifulco & Brown, 1996). By contrast 'downplaying', or what is sometimes termed 'suppression' (Vaillant, 1976), augurs well. This type of cognitive coping consists of fully confronting the meaning of the provoking stressor—again note the protective function of developing a narrative—but also involves focusing on some aspect which serves to mitigate its impact. This can occur either in minimizing the negative implications ('My son with cerebral palsy may not be able to move about but at least he is intelligent and sweet-natured. I am so lucky I do not have Mrs P's Down's daughter') or in discovering some new positive aspect to the situation ('One good thing my cancer has done is to bring the whole family back together again'). Because the coping literature has tended to conflate this response with denial, sometimes calling both 'minimization', it is often more difficult for professionals to appreciate the protective role of the former and distinguish it from the depressogenic role of the latter. A key difference between the two captures the essence of the psychotherapeutic concept of 'working through an issue', again via the development of a coherent narrative: in denial this has been avoided and in downplaying largely achieved.

The model of depression and recovery/improvement

So far, the model of depression has been presented in terms of onset, but very similar considerations apply to recovery or improvement, where the role of hope, and its loss or regain, emerges once again. It appears that the processes involved may broadly mirror those leading to onset; in this case by changing circumstances bringing new hope to a situation. Recovery or improvement from depressive conditions that have lasted for 20 weeks or more is highly related to the occurrence of events which, on common sense grounds, would be expected to bring hope, such as being rehoused, receiving a proposal of marriage from a new boyfriend or finding a job after months without one. Moreover, in addition to such 'fresh starts', reduction in the severity of the ongoing difficulty and receiving support with it also played a part (Brown *et al.*, 1988, 1992; Brown, 1993).

These findings concerning social support, already suggested by other interventions (van der Eyken, 1982; Pound & Mills, 1985; Corney, 1987; Elliott *et al.*, 1988), have now been confirmed experimentally in a trial of a befriending intervention with chronically depressed women (T.O. Harris, G.W. Brown & R. Robinson, unpublished information). In these experiments a trained volunteer was paired with a depressed woman with whom she met weekly for at least an hour and encouraged her to treat her as a confidante in the way described above. In other words, she provided additional social support. Recovery/improvement (measured by the Present-State Examination (Wing *et al.*, 1974) related both to experience of a fresh start (or difficulty reduction) and to membership of the befriending rather than control group. Logistic regression suggested there were two other predictors, one involving very poor coping and another involving attachment style (see page 81). As predicted, depressed befriendees paired with volunteers who offered marked, active emotional support did better than those whose volunteer offered less support. Another two reports focusing on chronicity gave a similar picture, but raise an additional issue concerning the relevance of distant past experience for meaning: both in a psychiatric patient sample (Brown *et al.*, 1994b) and in the general population (Brown & Moran, 1994) women with episodes lasting 1 year or more had more often had severe interpersonal difficulties at onset or had suffered severe neglect and/or abuse in childhood. Previous findings had pointed to the former—for example, poor marriages had often figured as prolonging depressive episodes (Rounsaville *et al.*, 1979; Waring & Patton, 1984; Goering *et al.*, 1992; Hickie & Parker, 1992). Other reports had identified different forms of lack of social support as delaying recovery (Mann *et al.*, 1981; Brugha *et al.*, 1990; George *et al.*, 1989), as well as low income and other 'chronic strains' (Huxley *et al.*, 1979). However, the association with childhood adverse experience had not previously been documented and fitted neatly with the emerging perspective.

Meaning from the past: a lifespan model of depression

So far, the model of depression described has involved psychosocial factors which are all current (see the right of Fig. 4.1). In considering the practical implications of this perspective it is bound to be useful to consider the origins of these factors in the present and whether these too can be influenced in a way that can somehow reduce depression. What has emerged is conveyed diagrammatically by the series of arrows, with the continuous line representing the more sociostructural external pathways (strand 1), and the dotted line the more internal psychic ones (strand 2). However, this is not just some mechanistic system whereby one thing leads to another and thence to depression, the various experiences along the lifespan seem to echo each other in terms of meaning. The losses, shame and lack of emotional support found in the period immediately preceding depression often seem to have begun years before.

A pointer to this emerged in early work where loss of the mother either by death or by separation of at least 12 months before the age of 11 years was found to render women more vulnerable to severe events and difficulties (Brown & Harris, 1978). Another study in Walthamstow (North London), expressly designed to explore experiences intervening between such loss of mother and current mental state, suggested it was not the childhood loss itself but the poor quality of relationships with the substitute care-givers that was the critical depressogenic feature. Once again it was the supportiveness of relationships which was so crucial, and this was highlighted by reports from other research teams (Parker & Hadzli-Pavlovic, 1984; Birtchnell *et al.*, 1988). Premarital pregnancy, which seemed to trap women in unsupportive

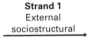

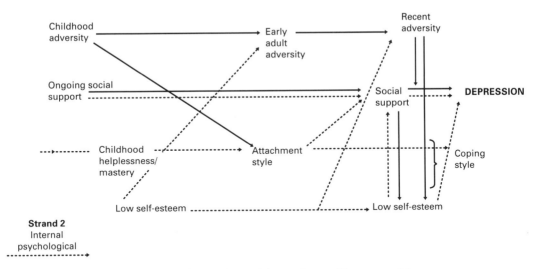

Fig. 4.1 Key psychosocial factors in the aetiology of depression—a lifespan model.

partnerships that they might otherwise not have chosen, turned out to be a more frequent sequel to such lack of adequate replacement care in childhood (Harris *et al.*, 1986, 1987). The Walthamstow study further explored other aspects of the model of depression outlined above by including a measure of the woman's situational helplessness/mastery. This was found to relate both to poor substitute parental care after the maternal loss and to poor support (lack of intimate confiding) in current relationships, as well as to depression (Harris *et al.*, 1990a, 1990b). It seemed that, from early in life, some women had moved from one unsupportive situation to another and seemed unable to be masterful enough to break free of this cycle. This picture was confirmed in an inner city sample (Islington), which looked at sexual abuse and violence from a member of the family as well as at marked parental rejection or neglect; it found such 'childhood adversity' in approximately one-third of the women before the age of 17 years. These women went on to have roughly double the risk of experiencing depression at a clinical level in any one year during adulthood (Bifulco *et al.*, 1987, 1994). Here the adversity and lack of support in childhood was clearly linked, not only with vulnerability such as lack of support and low self-esteem in adulthood (Harris, 1993), but also with severe life events in the current period, particularly those involving humiliation/ entrapment (T.O. Harris & G.W. Brown, unpublished information).

Although the apparent inevitability of moving from early to later adversity emerges powerfully in every sample it is also important to note other pathways

(Rutter, 1987, 1989); some women did seem to have survived potentially damaging childhoods without a psychiatric episode of any kind. Usually they were found to have succeeded in developing a close, confiding relationship without negative elements soon after leaving the childhood home, most often with a sexual partner (Quinton & Rutter, 1984; Brown *et al.*, 1990). Sometimes, however, the fresh start came much later: Mrs A, with three in-patient depressive episodes, two marital separations, two miscarriages, a stillbirth brought on through domestic violence and four children taken into care for adoption, for the first time, had a 10-year period with no depression just before participating in our population survey. At the suggestion of her family doctor in Yorkshire she had, 10 years previously, moved down to London with the only child not removed from her and had met a different sort of boyfriend. She decribed the amazement she felt at how much they had to say to each other: 'Sometimes we talked so much we almost forgot to go to bed.' Sometimes, however, the fresh start can come much earlier, as when Mrs B, as a girl placed for adoption five times previously and sent back to the children's home because she was 'difficult', finally found a more tenacious foster mother when she was 12 years old: 'I think I calmed down when I realized she wasn't going to send me back for not polishing the stairs, or not for anything' she said. Formally adopted after 15 months she made an excellent relationship with her new mother, married, without haste, a most supportive husband and, by the time of the survey, had reached age 48 years with no adult psychiatric episodes despite the multiple repeated abuse up to age 4 years for which she had been removed from her natural parents.

Links between past and present: attachment style and the mutual impact of inner and outer worlds

These two last, brief life-histories exemplify, not only how survival without depression can often be a matter of good fortune, but also how both inner and outer influences may combine to produce a vicious spiral dragging someone down into psychopathology. The parallel continuous and dotted lines across the centre of Fig. 4.1 highlight the complex interplay between internal and external factors in determining the quality of social support available to any individual. On the one hand, externally the range of persons in the close network may include only critical or thick-skinned personalities, unable to empathize with the predicaments in which women typically find themselves. On the other hand, a woman's intrapsychic characteristics may be contributing to her lack of support, either through her fearfulness and hesitation in finding any other friends with a more sympathetic outlook, or through her quarrelsomeness or demanding behaviour driving potential support figures away. In the latter case her style of relating to others (or her attachment style) is as important as her external resources. Until her departure for London Mrs A was trapped in a victim role, not only by the conveyor belt from childhood poverty and a premarital pregnancy (strand 1) but also by her own helpless style (strand 2), which had partly contributed to that pregnancy and kept her in both marriages: the first eroding her self-esteem through the partner's constant infidelity; the second, literally, beating her down still further. The family doctor's successful intervention in advising her to move south somehow fired her with sufficient confidence not only to move but also to build a new relationship. Unfortunately the focus of that particular study was not upon management, so there is no information about the length of time she had been visiting the family doctor and the treatment she received. It is likely that he must have talked to her at some length to give her the confidence to make such a change. Be that as it may, what is documented is that Mrs A, despite her helplessness, did not seem to have exhibited an overall avoidance of, or ambivalence about, relationships with other people. She had had the potential to enjoy friendships with women throughout her life, as also briefly with work colleagues, but circumstances had meant that, more often than not, she was unable to meet up with these people when she most needed their support. In other words, although externally she had received poor social support, her attachment style had been fairly standard for her class and generation. This contrast between 'standard' and 'non-standard' adult attachment styles (Harris & Bifulco, 1991; A.T. Bifulco *et al.*, unpublished information) closely parallels the concept of internal working models of relationships developed by John Bowlby (1988), whose notion of 'secure' and 'insecure' attachment in infancy as the foundation of development and psychopathology has stimulated much recent research. Work in this tradition with adults has mainly rated their attachment security on the basis of how they have cognitively and emotionally processed their childhood relationships (in the Adult Attachment Interview, Main & Goldwyn, 1988), rather than focusing on their current adult ties and whether they show avoidance, ambivalence or enmeshment therein. Studies of the latter type relating non-standard adult attachment style to depression have found it prospectively to predict both onset (A.T. Bifulco *et al.*, unpublished information) and failure to recover (T.O. Harris, G.W. Brown & R. Robinson, unpublished information), even controlling for whether the environment is actually providing good enough support (strand 1). A non-standard attachment style has also been found more commonly among those with childhood adversity (Harris & Bifulco, 1991; Bifulco *et al.*, 1996b). The reason for labouring this point is that, both in the case of Mrs A and in the more general case of any management of depression, it is useful to distinguish the inner and outer origins of poor support in order better to target the way forward. If Mrs A had had a more fearful/avoidant attachment style, she might not have felt able to trust the family doctor enough to take his advice, and might therefore never have had her fresh start. She might have been reached only with a more psychotherapeutic approach. It is perhaps finally worth noting that during her first 6 years Mrs A had a good relationship with her father before his death, only being sent into a home when her mother failed to cope with the bereavement, and was summoned out aged 13 to help this same mother care for the younger siblings born in the interim. Without that early supportive experience with her father, her attachment style might have developed differently to become non-standard. In that case, without intensive psychotherapy, she might never have been able to build a successful relationship with her third partner.

By contrast, Mrs B's adult experience raises none of these issues. On the other hand there is some hint that, until her placement with her adoptive mother, her attachment style in childhood (unfortunately not offically part of that study's measured variables) may not have been standard but rather dismissive, verging on externalizing behaviour or even conduct disorder. At any rate it seems that something about her behaviour caused a succession of foster mothers to return her to the children's home. Certainly in psychiatric patient samples many women recount life-histories where the combination of dependency and acting-out in adulthood has left them with a trail of failed partnerships and unsupportive friendships. In the light of Mrs B's remark about how she 'calmed down', it is difficult not to interpret her adoptive mother's role as changing her early insecure attachment style to standard or secure: in other words, a positive experience along the external strand 1 may have altered the depressogenic potential of a strand-2 factor, her disposition towards disruptive behaviour. This process is, of course, just what emerges as the essential ingredient in many theoretical accounts of psychotherapy. What is important, however, is the insight that the process may not require a professional therapist. In fact, empathic support figures in the continuing social network may be better equipped than experts in the clinic to help counteract the long history of humiliation or neglect suffered by many with depression, and can be enlisted as key allies in the therapeutic process, along the lines of a successful trial of treatment for agoraphobia using husbands and female friends (Oatley & Hodgson, 1987).

These two life-histories provide interesting parallels with another issue, the differing origins of the severe events provoking depression. Some are more clearly contingent upon the subject's own impulsive or argumentative behaviour, whereas others, such as deaths, are clearly independent. The former (contingent) events have been found more frequently among depressed patients with personality disorder of the cluster B variety—that is, dramatic or histrionic (T.O. Harris & G.W. Brown, 1996a,b, unpublished information). In between contingent and independent events are grouped others where the personality of a close relative or friend, usually a partner or child, is crucial in bringing about the event, but some suspicion remains that the subject could have played a more active role in preventing it—in other words, that she was somehow passively involved in its origin. Before managing to escape her conveyor belt, Mrs A seemed to have suffered events of this last type, while as a child Mrs B seemed to have been contributing to her own frequent events in being sent back to the children's home once again—in other words, experiencing contingent events. It is tempting to speculate that without adoption Mrs B might have later left the children's home with something like the histrionic personality found associated with contingent events, and that if she had gone on to have a premarital pregnancy this personality might have become more and more entrenched. This speculation is rendered more plausible when one remembers how borderline personality disorders, despite producing contingent events, have often stemmed from independent environmental abuse and neglect of the kind Mrs B underwent in her first 3 years (Herman *et al.*, 1989). Moreover, borderline personality has been linked with insecure attachment style (of the enmeshed subtype; Patrick *et al.*, 1994).

Implications of this multifactorial aetiological model for management

Before turning to the implications of this psychosocial model for management of depression, it is important to emphasize one of its assumptions that has not so far been spelt out: that physiological changes are assumed to parallel the psychosocial responses, and that pharmacological treatments are in no way seen as unimportant just because the model has not so far incorporated them. It is already pre-eminently a multifactorial model with room to include new factors as they emerge. In fact work is already beginning to illuminate such connections; for example, severe events and difficulties predict a poor response to antidepressant treatment (Lam *et al.*, 1994). Furthermore, experiencing severe events before onset has been linked with higher urinary-free cortisol (Calloway & Dolan, 1989). It is as if a third physiological strand was also inextricably involved in the interplay between strands 1 and 2. A corollary of this is the issue of comorbidity which can be crucial for management decisions. Unfortunately this chapter precludes detailed consideration of comorbidity issues, but it is noteworthy that the model for depression has also been found of relevance in the study of anxiety (Finlay-Jones & Brown, 1981) and alcohol-dependence (Gorman & Brown, 1992), albeit with key variations in meaning. For example, events before anxiety onset tend to involve threat of future loss, rather than humiliations which have already occurred.

In the same way, the central implication of this multifactorial psychosocial model is that even psychosocial treatment should be multimodal. This may not have emerged clearly so far, as the resumé of this model has concentrated on the similarity of meaning emerging from various studies despite their being focused on separate factors within it. Thus the sense of entrapment in a family where there is abuse from a parent figure (childhood adversity) is paralleled by entrapment in a violent marriage (adult adversity); the sense of isolation likely after a humiliation or death event (recent adversity) is paralleled by the isolation likely among those in a crisis without any close confidante (poor social support). The implication is that the sufferer's sense of hopelessness and powerlessness is not purely the result of the depressive episode but has arisen from his or her life context and that confronting all aspects of this— events, difficulties and the tendency to produce them; support available, coping and attachment style—will, in some way, alleviate the intensity of the depressive feelings. Such a thought is hardly new; most treatment programmes in practice now subscribe to such a vision, even if their handbooks seem more focused on a single issue, such as problem-solving or negative cognitions. There are, however, four ways in which this lifespan model can sharpen appreciation of what such a perspective really implies.

A multimodal approach

First, the complexity of the model suggests that confronting the sufferer's hopelessness should occur from whatever direction is possible, that treatment should be multimodal. The fresh start events, engineered by a treatment figure, which change the external world and thereby end the entrapment—for example, rehousing—may, in the short term, be no less effective therapeutically than fresh starts brought about by the patient herself after changing her coping style in response to solution-focused or cognitive therapy. In the long term, however, further severe events may occur in another domain than housing and development of a more masterful coping style may then prove more effective in postponing relapse. Yet in the short term the patient may be incapable of absorbing the cognitive therapy required to increase her mastery until she can see some real shift in her environmental burdens. Taking a similar multimodal perspective, the supportive listening, which may help a patient make sense of her feelings by setting them in context and softening self-derogatory tendencies, should be widely aimed for among all clinical staff, not just the therapist or key worker, whose sickness and holidays can often prove to be setbacks in the recovery process. Relatives can also be enlisted, although this may require special induction (see below). In some settings with scarce resources of professionals befriending may prove a useful alternative, and even where once-a-week therapy is available it may be a helpful adjunct. To set this plea for multimodality more clearly in the context of this chapter, the continuing interplay between strands 1 and 2 means that both should be targeted for change lest by dealing only with one, the door is left open for the other to undo the therapeutic work with the first. Thus, even where the humiliation caused by a poor marital relationship seems more clearly the precipitant of the depressive episode than the family's financial troubles, a treatment package focusing exclusively upon the former might allow the possibility that the next electricity bill would reopen the marital discord, as each member of the couple blamed the other for the new debt.

Assessment of contribution by internal or external factors

In contrast to the generality of the multimodal treatment perspective, the second contribution of this aetiological model is to point up certain specificities; using it at the assessment stage reveals that not everyone responding to a severe event with depression has arrived there by the same route. On the one hand it is possible to ask both of severe events and of poor emotional support how much is due to internal strand-2 factors and how much simply to the environment. In this way the relative distribution of resources between psychotherapy and social intervention can be more clearly planned. Whether the provoking event was independent or contingent upon the patient's agency will be relevant when deciding how best to ensure something similar will not occur again thus preventing symptomatic improvement. Is the poor emotional support the result of the patient's attachment style which endows her with a reluctance to confide in anyone about her difficulties? Or are there external reasons, maybe because her best friend died 2 years previously, and her husband became intolerant after he suffered a stroke and became bedridden 3 years ago, so that she has been unable to get out to meet new friends? Further specificities revealed in using this model in initial assessments would be the different types of non-independent events—whether dependent on the person's active impulsiveness or her passive compliance—and different types of non-standard attachment styles—whether enmeshed in ambivalent relationships with frequent negative interactions, or whether fearful or dismissive of others who could give emotional support, with consequent absence of social ties. The parallels between these contrasting types of event production (or stress generation) and the contrasting types of non-standard attachment styles have already been mentioned when discussing Mrs A and Mrs B, but highlighting these similiarities in talking to the patient about herself can often prove an extra therapeutic tool. Instead of providing treatment for generally dysfunctional attitudes, a more specific focus can be given for impulsive hostile tendencies as opposed to passive self-derogatory ones.

Using the lifespan model to help patients construct their own narrative

The third important feature of this model is its lifespan nature. Again in terms of theory this may seem nothing novel and yet, in practice, many therapies for depression seem to emphasize one end of a person's history more than the other. Some psychoanalytic-based therapies miss opportunities to help the patient deal with the meaning of their life history because they highlight past relationships and largely ignore all current ones bar the transference (that of patient with doctor). By contrast, the focus of interpersonal therapy (Klerman *et al.*, 1984) on current relationships, and of cognitive therapy (Beck *et al.*, 1979) on current dysfunctional attitudes, might often benefit from linking these with childhood adverse experience. As the patient comes to understand that the origins of her current snags and dilemmas in relationships—as formulated in cognitive analytic therapy (Ryle, 1990)—often lie in the past when she was too young to be held to blame and stem from the environment outside herself, she may feel it less demeaning to find herself in her current situation, and her self-esteem may improve. She may also find it less threatening to work on changing herself. This aim of linking past with here and now as a way of understanding hypotheses in psychotherapy has much in common with the 'conversational' therapy model (Goldberg *et al.*, 1984; Hobson, 1985), even though this appears to discourage too great a focus on the past. If these links are made during discussions of concrete memories which revive earlier emotions, it is easier for the patient to understand how she is reliving the past in the present and to feel motivated to change. This applies particularly to parenting style where, despite best intentions, those who experienced childhood adversity often find themselves inflicting similar neglect or abuse upon their own children, who then produce further severe events which, in turn, keep them depressed. One further implication of the model's long time perspective is, however, less encouraging. It would be surprising if a mere 20 therapy sessions, however supportive, could on their own undo the work of 20 or more years. Unfortunately the health services' current cost-reduction-driven plans leave little room to carry out proper tests of the value of longer therapies with longer-term follow-ups. The implications of the model are that the cognitions in strand 2 are highly dependent upon external factors in strand 1; thus if someone is to get off the conveyor belt they need to change more than their automatic negative thoughts; they will need to ensure their current roles will enhance not diminish their identity, and most particularly the role in a core relationship which will reflect back to them a favourable self-image. Again this is often what is done in practice by some therapists, who see the establishment of a supportive marital partnership as a crucial outcome for a patient, but without it being spelt out this may be missed by others.

The potentially unsupportive therapeutic service

The fourth set of implications involves the supportive process itself.

Naturalistic studies in the general population comparing relationships which did and did not prove protective against depression suggest a range of non-supportive responses (Harris, 1992). Their nature may be informative for professionals, both in therapy sessions or encounters on the ward, and in advising relatives. Such failures of support may either involve negative responses to the depressed person's confiding, or anticipated negative responses which have prevented confiding (Table 4.2). The most common are critical responses: 'Well I did warn you; you have only yourself to blame'; or insensitive, thick-skinned reactions: 'It's really not as bad as all that.' Paradoxically, in some cases these responses may embody exactly what the model implies is true. In the first response, that the severe event provoking depression was in some way the result of the individual's own cluster B personality; or in the second response that the individual's low self-esteem has caused her to over-react. The model also implies that to emphasize this part of the truth would be counterproductive at this stage. Building a supportive therapeutic relationship involves developing trust, which takes

Table 4.2 Some key considerations in supportive interactions.

Three questions must be answered positively:
1 Does the patient feel able to confide?
2 Is there a moderately or markedly active emotional response to the confiding by the other person?
3 Is there an absence of definite negative response (such as 'I told you didn't I' or 'Why don't you do the decent thing and agree to their demands')?

Features that might cause one of above answers to be negative
External: Nature of other person who may:
Internal: Patient expects other person to:

Criticize patient for feeling upset about event
Criticize patient's other behaviour/attitudes
Fail to understand implications of event: unempathic
Deny implications of event (because covers up guilt)
Avoid implications of event (because is a co-victim)
Deflect discussion of event to focus on own problems
Side with a third person over event against patient
React falsely: act contradictorily behind patient's back
Fail to maintain confidentiality: gossip
Adopt interfering (even if not critical) stance over event
Be unavailable (for reasons of geography, timetable)
Become too emotional about patient's confidences
Hurry patient into action before emotionally prepared
Try to distract patient — misguided kindness

time and requires the patient to have confidence that disclosure of private shortcomings will not later work against her. Thus opening up to other members of a ward, whether to fellow patients in a group or to key staff members, may feel more difficult than to a therapist or research worker outside the ward. The acceptance of the latter would seem less crucial for the patient since he/she will not be involved in the daily routine of the next few weeks. Furthermore, one of the ways of helping people to open up is to sympathetically ask key questions about what they have experienced, and it may be easier for such an outsider to do this without being experienced as intrusive. Nevertheless, by taking things at the patient's own pace, bearing in mind her attachment style and needs for self validation, ward staff can almost certainly facilitate the assimilation of problematic experiences, which is such a central process in successful psychotherapy (Stiles *et al.*, 1990) and which was referred to above in terms of the capacity to construct a coherent narrative as an essential prerequisite to change. Table 4.2 summarizes possible sources of failures in support. Although these have been identified in the context of everyday relationships, their relevance for management of depression is equally apparent. Concern about other patients' scornful opinions can be as powerful as anxiety about private information reaching rival relatives or neighbours, and worries about professionals passing on shameful secrets to their more critical colleagues, or even siding with visiting relatives, can sometimes impede the therapeutic process unless directly confronted and assuaged.

Before concluding it is important to remember that research has identified subgroups of those with depression where the psychosocial model does not appear to apply (see above), and among whom antidepressant medication has been found effective. Even among those whose history seems to exhibit a classic resemblance to Fig. 4.1, the role of pharmacological interventions may often prove crucial. In managing the depressive outcome of the complex and lengthy psychosocial processes described here, it is important to take no risks and to consider every potential pathway to recovery.

Acknowledgements

The research, on the basis of which this model was developed, was conceived by George W. Brown and supported by the Medical Research Council, the Social Science Research Council (as it then was known) and, in part, by Network I of the John D. and Catherine T. MacArthur Foundation. I am indebted to the many colleagues who participated in the data collection and analysis over the last 28 years, and to the many women who recounted their experiences in detail for us in order to contribute to our understanding.

References

Bebbington, P.E., Stult, E., Tennant, C. & Hurry, J. (1984) Misfortune and resilience: a community study of women. *Psychological Medicine*, **14**, 347–363.

Bebbington, P.E., Brugha, T., MacCarthy, B. *et al.* (1988) The Camberwell Collaborative Depression Study. I: Depressed probands: adversity and the form of depression. *British Journal of Psy-*

chiatry, **152**, 754–765.

Beck, A.T. (1967) *Depression: Clinical, Experimental and Theoretical Aspects.* Staples Press, London.

Beck, A.T., Rush, A., Shaw, B.F. & Emery, G. (1979) *Cognitive Therapy of Depression.* Guilford, New York.

Bifulco, A.T. & Brown, G.W. (1996) Coping and onset of clinical depression. 2: An aetiological model. *Journal of Social Psychiatry and Psychiatric Epidemiology,* **31**, 163–172.

Bifulco, A., Brown, G.W. & Harris, T.O. (1987) Childhood loss of parent, lack of adequate parental care and adult depression: a replication. *Journal of Affective Disorders,* **12**, 115–128.

Bifulco, A., Brown, G.W. & Harris, T.O. (1994) Childhood experience of care and abuse (CECA): a retrospective interview measure. *Child Psychology and Psychiatry,* **35**, 1419–1435.

Bifulco, A.T., Moran, P., Brown, G.W. & Ball, C. (1996a) Cognitive coping and onset of depression in vulnerable London women.

Bifulco, A.T., Brown, G.W., Lillie, A. & Moran, P. (1996b) Adult Attachment Style and Depression: a new measure of ability to make supportive relationships.

Birtchnell, J., Evans, C. & Kennard, J. (1988) Life history factors associated with neurotic symptomatology in a rural community sample of 40–49-year-old women. *Journal of Affective Disorders,* **14**, 271–285.

Bowlby, J. (1988) *A Secure Base: Parent–Child Attachment and Healthy Human Development.* Basic Books, New York.

Brown, G.W. (1993) Life events and affective disorder: replications and limitations. *Psychosomatic Medicine,* **55**, 248–259.

Brown, G.W. & Birley, J.L.T. (1968) Crises and life changes and the onset of schizophrenia. *Journal of Health & Social Behavior,* **9**, 203–214.

Brown, G.W. & Harris, T. (1978) *Social Origins of Depression: A study of Psychiatric Disorder in Women.* Tavistock Press, London and Free Press, New York.

Brown, G.W. & Moran, P. (1994) Clinical and psychosocial origins of chronic depressive episodes. 1: A community survey. *British Journal of Psychiatry,* **165**, 447–456.

Brown, G.W., Sklair, F., Harris, T.O. & Birley, J.L.T. (1973) Life events and psychiatric disorders. 1: Some methodological issues. *Psychological Medicine,* **3**, 74–78.

Brown, G.W., Ni Bhrolchain, M. & Harris, T.O. (1979) Psychotic and neurotic depression. 3: Aetiological and background factors. *Journal of Affective Disorders,* **1**, 195–211.

Brown, G.W., Andrews, B., Harris, T.O., Adler, Z.

& Bridge, L. (1986) Social support, self-esteem and depression. *Psychological Medicine,* **16**, 813–831.

Brown, G.W., Bifulco, A. & Harris, T.O. (1987) Life events, vulnerability and onset of depression: some refinements. *British Journal of Psychiatry,* **150**, 30–42.

Brown, G.W., Adler, Z. & Bifulco, A. (1988) Life events, difficulties and recovery from chronic depression. *British Journal of Psychiatry,* **152**, 487–498.

Brown, G.W., Bifulco, A., Veiel, H. & Andrews, B. (1990) Self-esteem and depression. 2: Social correlates of self-esteem. *Social Psychiatry & Psychiatric Epidemiology,* **25**, 225–234.

Brown, G.W., Lemyre, L. & Bifulco., A. (1992) Social factors and recovery from anxiety and depressive disorders: a test of the specificity hypothesis. *British Journal of Psychiatry,* **161**, 44–54.

Brown, G.W., Harris, T.O. & Hepworth, C. (1994a) Life events and 'endogenous' depression: a puzzle re-examined. *Archives of General Psychiatry,* **51**, 525–534.

Brown, G.W., Harris, T.O., Hepworth, C. & Robinson, R. (1994b) Clinical and psychosocial origins of chronic depression. 2: A patient enquiry. *British Journal of Psychiatry,* **165**, 457–465.

Brown, G.W., Harris, T.O. & Hepworth, C. (1995) Loss, humiliation and entrapment among women developing depression: a patient and non-patient comparison. *Psychological Medicine,* **25**, 7–21.

Brugha, T., Bebbington, P., MacCarthy, B., Sturt, E., Wykes, T. & Potter, J. (1990) Gender, social support and recovery from depressive disorders: a prospective clinical study. *Psychological Medicine,* **20**, 147–156.

Calloway, P. & Dolan, R. (1989) Endocrine changes and clinical profiles in depression. In: *Life Events and Illness* (eds G. W. Brown & T. O. Harris), pp. 139–160. Guilford, New York.

Carney, M.W., Roth, M. & Garside, R.F. (1965) The diagnosis of depressive syndromes and the prediction of ECT response. *British Journal of Psychiatry,* **111**, 659–674.

Corney, R. (1987) Marital problems and treatment outcome in depressed women: a clinical trial of social work intervention. *British Journal of Psychiatry,* **151**, 652–660.

Dohrenwend, B.P., Raphael, K.G., Schwartz, S., Stueve, A. & Skodol, A. (1993) The structured event probe and narrative rating method for measuring stressful life events. In: *Handbook of Stress* (eds L. Goldberger & S. Breznitz), pp. 174–199. Free Press, New York.

Elliott, S.A., Sanjack, M. & Leverton, T.J. (1988)

Parent groups in pregnancy: a preventive intervention for postnatal depression. In: *Marshalling Social Support: Formats, Issues, Processes and Effects* (ed. B. H. Gottlieb), pp. 87–110. Sage, London.

Finlay-Jones, R. & Brown, G.W. (1981) Types of stressful life events and the onset of anxiety and depressive disorders. *Psychological Medicine*, **11**, 803–815.

George, L.K., Blazer, D.G., Hughes, D.C. & Fowler, N. (1989) Social support and the outcome of major depression. *British Journal of Psychiatry*, **154**, 478–485.

Goering, P.N., Lancee, W.J. & Freeman, S.J.J. (1992) Marital support and recovery from depression. *British Journal of Psychiatry*, **160**, 76–82.

Goldberg, D.P., Hobson, R.F., Maguire, G., P. *et al.* (1984) The clarification and assessment of a method of psychotherapy. *British Journal of Psychiatry*, **144**, 567–580.

Gorman, D.M. & Brown, G.W. (1992) Recent developments in life-event research and their relevance for the study of addictions. *British Journal of Addictions*, **87**, 837–849.

Harris, T.O.(1992) Some reflections of the process of social support and nature of unsupportive behaviours. In: *The Meaning and Measurement of Social Support* (eds H. O. F. Veiel & U. Baumann), pp. 171–189. Hemisphere Publishing Corporation, Washington, DC.

Harris, T.O. (1993) Surviving childhood adversity: What can we learn from naturalistic studies? In: *Surviving Childhood Adversity: Issues for Policy and Practice* (eds H. Ferguson, R. Gilligan & R. Torode), pp. 93–107. Social Studies Press, Trinity College, Dublin.

Harris, T.O. (1996) Work, motherhood and mental state in transition: instability of indicator variables and implications for replication studies. (Unpublished information.)

Harris, T.O. & Bifulco, A. (1991) Loss of parent in childhood, and attachment style and depression in adulthood. In: *Attachment Across the Life Cycle* (eds C. M. Parkes & J. S. Hinde), pp. 234–267. Tavistock, London and Routledge, New York.

Harris, T.O. & Brown, G.W. (1996a) The origins of life events preceding onset of depression. 1: Independent events and humiliation/entrapment in the general population. (Unpublished information.)

Harris, T.O. & Brown, G.W. (1996b) The origins of life events preceding onset of depression. 2: Contingent events and dramatic personality disorder in a patient series. (Unpublished information.)

Harris, T.O., Brown, G.W. & Bifulco, A. (1986) Loss of parent in childhood and adult psychiatric disorder: The Walthamstow Study. 1: The role of lack of adequate parental care. *Psychological Medicine*, **16**, 641–659.

Harris, T.O., Brown, G.W. & Bifulco, A. (1987) Loss of parent in childhood and adult psychiatric disorder: The Walthamstow Study. 2: The role of social class position and premarital pregnancy. *Psychological Medicine*, **17**, 163–183.

Harris, T.O., Brown, G.W. & Bifulco, A. (1990a) Depression and situational helplessness/mastery in a sample selected to study childhood parental loss. *Journal of Affective Disorders*, **20**, 27–41.

Harris, T.O., Brown, G.W. & Bifulco, A. (1990b) Loss of parent in childhood and adult psychiatric disorder: a tentative overall model. *Development and Psychopathology*, **2**, 311–328.

Harris, T.O., Brown, G.W. & Robinson, R. (1996) Befriending as an intervention for chronic depression among women in an inner city.

Herman, J., Perry, J. & van der Kolk, B. (1989) Childhood trauma in borderline personality disorder. *American Journal of Psychiatry*, **146**, 490–495.

Hickie, I. & Parker, G. (1992) The impact of an uncaring partner on improvement in non-melancholic depression. *Journal of Affective Disorders*, **25**, 147–160.

Hobson, R.F. (1985) *Forms of Feeling: The Heart of Psychotherapy*. Tavistock, London.

Holmes, T.H. & Rahe, R.H. (1967) The social readjustment rating scale. *Journal of Psychosomatic Research*, **11**, 213–218.

Huxley, P.J., Goldberg, D.P., Maguire, G.P. & Kincey, V.A. (1979) The prediction of the course of minor psychiatric disorders. *British Journal of Psychiatry*, **135**, 535–543.

Klerman, G.L., Weissman, M.M., Rounsaville, B.J., Chevron, R.S. (eds) (1984) *Interpersonal Psychotherapy of Depression*. Basic Books, New York.

Lam, D.H., Green, B., Power, M.J. & Checkley, S. (1994) The impact of social cognitive variables on the initial level of depression and recovery. *Journal of Affective Disorders*, **32**, 75–83.

Lazarus, R.S. & Folkman, S. (1984) *Stress, Appraisal and Coping*. Springer Verlag, New York.

Leff, M.J., Roatch, J.F. & Bunney, W.E. (1970) Environmental factors preceding the onset of severe depressions. *Psychiatry*, **33**, 293–311.

Main, M. & Goldwyn, R. (1988) *Adult Attachment Classification System Version 3.2*. University of California, Berkeley.

Mann, A.H., Jenkins, R. & Belsey, E. (1981) The twelve-month outcome of patients with neurotic illness in general practice. *Psychological Medicine*, **11**, 535–550.

Miller, P.McC., Kreitman, N.B., Ingham, J.O. &

Sashidharan, S.P. (1989) Self-esteem, life stress and psychiatric disorder. *Journal of Affective Disorders*, **17**, 65–76.

Oatley, K. & Hodgson, D. (1987) Influence of husbands on the outcome of their agoraphobic wives' therapy. *British Journal of Psychiatry*, **150**, 380–386.

Parker, G. & Hadzli-Pavlovic, D. (1984) Modification of levels of depression in mother-bereaved women by parental and marital relationships. *Psychological Medicine*, **14**, 125–135.

Parry, G., Shapiro, D.A. & Davies, L. (1981) Reliability of life event ratings: an independent replication. *British Journal of Clinical Psychology*, **20**, 133–134.

Patrick, M., Hobson, P., Castle, D., Howard, R. & Maughan, B. (1994) Personality disorder and the mental representation of early social experience. *Development and Psychopathology*, **6**, 375–388.

Paykel, E.S., Myers, J.K., Diendelt, M.N., Klerman, G.L., Lindenthal, J.J. & Pepper, M.P. (1969) Life events and depression: a controlled study. *Archives of General Psychiatry*, **21**, 753–760.

Paykel, E.S., Prusoff, B.A. & Klerman, G.L. (1971) The endogenous-neurotic continuum in depression, rater independence and factor distributions. *Journal of Psychiatric Research*, **8**, 73–90.

Paykel, E.S., Emms, E.M., Fletcher, J. & Rassaby, E.S. (1980) Life events and social support in puerperal depression. *British Journal of Psychiatry*, **136**, 339–346.

Paykel, E.S., Rao, B.M. & Taylor, C.N. (1984) Life stress and symptom pattern in out-patient depression. *Psychological Medicine*, **14**, 559–568.

Post, R.M., Rubinow, D.R. & Ballenger, J.C. (1986) Conditioning and sensitisation in the longitudinal course of affective illness. *British Journal of Psychiatry*, **149**, 191–201.

Pound, A. & Mills, M. (1985) A pilot evaluation of Newpin—home-visiting and befriending scheme in South London. *A.C.C.P. Newsletter* (4).

Quinton, D. & Rutter, M. (1984) Parents with children in care. 2: Intergenerational continuities. *Journal of Child Psychology and Psychiatry*, **25**, 231–250.

Rosenberg, M. (1965) *The Measurement of Self-esteem: Society and the Adolescent Image.* Princeton University Press, Princeton, NJ.

Rounsaville, B.J., Weissman, M.M., Prusoff, B.A. & Herceg-Baron, R.L. (1979) Marital disputes and treatment outcome in depressed women. *Comprehensive Psychiatry*, **20**, 483–490.

Roy, A., Breier, A., Doran, A.R. & Picar, D. (1985) Life events and depression: relation to subtypes. *Journal of Affective Disorders*, **9**, 143–148.

Rutter, M. (1987) Psychosocial resilience and protective mechanisms. *American Journal of Orthopsychiatry*, **57**, 316–333.

Rutter, M. (1989) Pathways from childhood to adult life. Jack Tizard memorial lecture. *Journal of Child Psychology and Psychiatry*, **30**, 23–51.

Ryle, A. (1990) *Cognitive Analytic Therapy: Active Participation in Change.* John Wiley & Sons, Chichester.

Sarason, I., Johnson, J.H. & Siegel, J.M. (1978) Assessing the impact of life changes: development of the life experiences survey. *Journal of Consulting and Clinical Psychology*, **46**, 932–946.

Seligman, M.E.P. (1975) *Helplessness: On Depression, Development and Death.* W.H. Freeman, San Francisco.

Stiles, W.B., Elliott, R., Firth-Cozens, J.A. *et al.* (1990) Assimilation of problematic experiences by clients in psychotherapy. *Psychotherapy*, **27**, 411–420.

Tennant, C., Smith, A., Bebbington, P. & Hurry, J. (1979) The contextual threat of life events: the concept and its reliability. *Psychological Medicine*, **9**, 525–528.

Vaillant G. (1976) Natural history of male psychological health. The relation of choice of ego mechanisms of defense to adult adjustment. *Archives of General Psychiatry*, **33**, 535–545.

van der Eyken, W. (1982) *Home Star: A Four year Evaluation.* Homestart Consultancy, Leicester.

Waring, E.M. & Patton, D. (1984) Marital intimacy and depression. *British Journal of Psychiatry*, **145**, 641–644.

Wing, J.K., Cooper, J.E. & Sartorius, N. (1974) *The Measurement and Classification of Psychiatric Symptoms.* Cambridge University Press, Cambridge.

5 A cognitive theory of depression

DOMINIC LAM

Cognitive therapy has been seen as one of the most promising innovations in the treatment of depression in the past two decades. Its basic tenet is the cognitive theory in which emotions are seen to be influenced by meanings people ascribe to events in the external world. The depressed individual's cognitive triad (views about the self, the world and the future), negative thoughts and assumptions (rigid or overgeneralized rules) have important contributions to our understanding of how depressed patients construct their internal worlds. Clinically, therapists find that aspects of the theory, such as the cognitive triad and the relationship between thought, mood and behaviour, can help depressed patients describe and make sense of their overwhelming state of mind. The contents of automatic thoughts also enable therapists to have a window into how patients construe their world and work out some general rules or assumptions that have implications for therapy. However, despite the effectiveness of cognitive therapy as a treatment for depression, empirical evidence for the cognitive theory of depression is incomplete.

For the sake of clarity, Beck's cognitive theory for depression can be divided into the descriptive and causal aspects (Beck, 1967; Beck et al., 1979). This chapter consists of three sections: first, an overview of the cognitive theory of depression is presented in order to give an overall picture; then more details of the descriptive and causal aspects of the cognitive theory are elaborated and explained; followed by a review of the empirical evidence. It can be argued that Beck (1983) intended his theories to apply to various levels of depression, both clinical and non-clinical. Hence in this review empirical evidence from both groups has been included. Furthermore, the clinical implications of the cognitive theory for the management of depression is discussed to promote the idea of clinical practice guided by theory.

An overview of the cognitive theory of emotional disorder

Beck's cognitive theory of emotional states spells out how clinical problems such as depression arise (Beck, 1967, 1983; Beck et al., 1979). Figure 5.1 is a

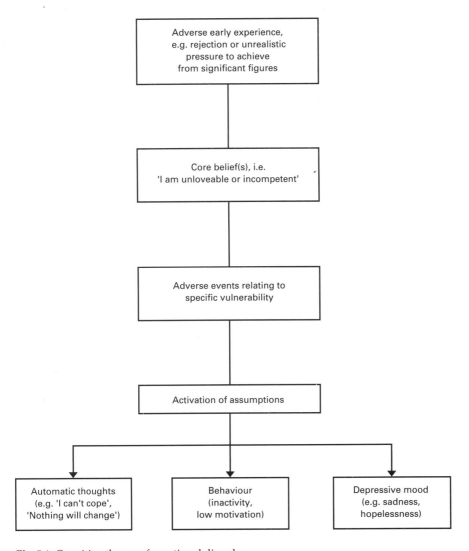

Fig. 5.1 Cognitive theory of emotional disorder.

linear summary of Beck's cognitive theory of emotional states. It is hypo-thesized that certain beliefs about ourselves, other people and events are developed from an early age. These beliefs about ourselves, 'core beliefs', are regarded as truths and are encoded at an early age in linguistically simple forms such as 'I am unloveable or incompetent'. Beck (1983) hypo-thesized that the relevant core beliefs in therapy were related to the themes of loveability or competence (see Table 5.2, p. 114, for more details). It is be-lieved that these core beliefs develop in relation to early experiences, such as traumas and separation, patients' perceived parental attitudes, relationships with peer groups and authority figures and any history of abuse. Beck (1967) hypothesized that early childhood experiences in the form of rejection or authoritarian pressure from significant others can lead to the development of a dependent personality or a value-achiever with little intrinsic sense of self-worth.

Beck *et al.* (1979) proposed the term 'schema' as the stable cognitive patterns that 'maintains a depressed patient's pain-inducing and self-defeating attitudes despite objective evidence of positive factors in his life' (Beck *et al.*, 1979, p. 12). Schema was defined as a functional unit of information processing 'for screening, coding, and evaluating the stimuli that impinge on the organism. It is the mode by which the environment is broken down and organized into its many psychologically relevant facets. On the basis of schemas, the individual is able to … Categorize and interpret his experiences in a meaningful way' (Beck, 1967; p. 283). Both core beliefs and dysfunctional assumptions are hence 'schemata'. Krantz (1985) refined the definition of the schema as the basic rules that are relatively independent of current life circumstances. Furthermore, Beck (1987) hypothesized that 'at the deepest level the conditional phrases starting with "since" are dropped out of the rule, leaving the "core schema" consisting of an absolute concept such as "I am a fraud or incompetent" '.

Dysfunctional assumptions are seen as a permutation of the basic core beliefs in order to cope with the internal world the individual lives in. Hence themes tend to be related to loveableness, acceptance, achievement, or control (Beck, 1983). This, in turn, leads to the vulnerability postulated by cognitive theory. These assumptions are dysfunctional because they are rigid and so prevent the individual's goal attainment in life; for example, a man who experiences unrealistically high parental pressure to achieve may believe that he is incompetent and develop the assumption that, in order to be accepted, he has to be successful all the time. It is thought that the onset of emotional disorders is often preceded by situations relating to individuals' specific vulnerabilities: interpersonal events in dependent individuals and achievement events in achievement-orientated individuals (see Chapter 4). In the case of the man mentioned above, problems may arise if he is trapped in a situation in which he cannot meet his lofty goals. Violation of the rigid rules or assumptions tends to be associated with extreme or excessive emotion. Depression comes about, for example, when adversity occurs that matches the person's vulnerability, threatening the person's sense of self-worth (Beck, 1983). When in a highly emotional state such as depression, individuals tend to have negative automatic thoughts which reflect the content of the idiosyncratic dysfunctional assumptions. Once depression sets in, the individual presents with the classic cognitive, behavioural and affective symptoms. Negative cognitions, depressive behaviour and depressive mood interact with each other to maintain depression; for example, a depressed patient has negative thoughts such as 'I am lazy', 'It's useless trying anything' and 'Everything is just too overwhelmingly difficult'. He lacks motivation and becomes inactive. As a result he has more negative self-denigrating thoughts. He becomes hopeless and more depressed.

Descriptive aspects of the cognitive theory for depression

The descriptive aspects of the cognitive theory for depression consist of: the cognitive triad, thinking errors, and the reciprocal relationship between thought, mood and behaviour. These descriptive aspects of the theory simply propose that a group of phenomena tends to exist in such a way that it constitutes a syndrome. These phenomena disappear when patients are in remission and do not have any causal implications. In this section the details of these three concepts are explained, with an emphasis on the clinical implications of each.

The cognitive triad

The cognitive triad consists of the individual's idiosyncratic view of self, the world and the future. Beck *et al.* (1979) postulated that in depression an individual often views himself as 'defective, inadequate, diseased or deprived. He tends to attribute his unpleasant experience to a psychological, moral or physical defect in himself' (Beck *et al.*, 1979, p. 11). Often he views himself as worthless or inadequate. Beck *et al.* (1979, p. 11) described the depressed person as someone who 'sees the world as making exorbitant demands on him and/or presenting insuperable obstacles to reaching his life goals. He misinterprets his interactions with his animate or inanimate environment as representing defeat or deprivation'. Lastly, Beck *et al.* (1979) described the depressed individual as someone who 'makes long-range projections, he anticipates that his current difficulties or suffering will continue indefinitely. He expects unremitting hardship, frustration and deprivation' (p. 11). The future seems hopeless and gloomy.

Clinical implications

Clinically the cognitive triad provides very useful information for therapists. By paying attention to the cognitive triad, therapists can obtain a sense of how patients see themselves. One rule of thumb in cognitive therapy suggested by Safran *et al.* (1986) is that the important issues or automatic thoughts are those related to the sense of self and self-evaluation. By paying attention to the depressed individuals' world, therapists can obtain much information about interpersonal issues, and in particular therapists can detect the indi-viduals' patterns of interpersonal interactions. These interpersonal interac-tions can be relevant to therapy, which is part of the individual's world, and can interfere with therapy processes. For example, a patient who tends to see other people as critical may perceive the therapist's comments as critical and this may hinder the establishment of a rapport in therapy. Hopelessness is a predictor of suicide (Beck *et al.*, 1975; Kazdin *et al.*, 1983; Dyer & Kreitman, 1984) and the person's view of the future can have enormous implications. Moreover, if the individual is convinced that everything is negative or aversive and will not change, he/she is not going to carry out any homework assign-ment or even come back for future sessions unless his/her hopelessness is labelled and tackled first. In tackling hopelessness, the therapist works with the patient to effect some positive change in one area, which is, in turn, used to challenge the patient's belief that nothing will change.

Empirical evidence

There is much empirical evidence that supports Beck's description of the cognitive triad; for example, depressed individuals are more self-critical than controls (Blatt *et al.*, 1982); they endorse more negative self-referent adject-ives (Bradley & Mathews, 1983; Clifford & Hemsley, 1987; Rude *et al.*, 1988); and they report lower self-esteem (McCauley *et al.*, 1988; Parry & Brewin, 1988). Furthermore, Bradley and Mathews (1988) reported that depressed individuals' negative views of themselves exceed those of remitted depressives and Myers *et al.* (1989) reported that, when depression remitted, individuals have less negative views of themselves. Further evidence of negative sense of self comes from Brewin *et al.* (1992a) who reported that depressed subjects recalled more negative than positive self-referent adjectives. However, when depressed subjects were asked to rate how a series of positive and negative adjectives applied to them the previous week, currently and in general, they rated themselves currently in largely negative terms but in general terms equally in both positive and negative terms. In relation to the depressed 'patient's world view', Blackburn *et al.* (1986) found that depressed patients scored higher than non-depressed controls and remitted depressives on the 'world' subscale of the Cognitive Style Test. Likewise, Greenberg and Beck (1989) found that depressives endorsed less positive depression-relevant world adjectives and more negative depression-relevant adjectives compared with non-depressed controls. With respect to the future, depressed individuals were found to be more hopeless about their future than controls or remitted depressives (Hamilton & Abramson, 1983; Blackburn *et al.*, 1986; Lam *et al.*, 1987).

Cognitive negativity and thinking errors

Beck (1967) hypothesized that systematic thinking errors of depressed patients maintain the patients' validation of their negative concepts. This bias can occur despite objective evidence to the contrary due to individuals making logical errors in their thinking. These errors include: selective abstraction (selecting abstract negative elements of a situation while ignoring other more salient features of the situation); arbitrary inference (drawing a conclusion in the absence of evidence or even when there is evidence to the contrary); overgeneralization; magnification (of negative aspects) and minimization (of the positive aspects); personalization; and dichotomous (black and white) thinking.

Clinical implications

In cognitive therapy, patients are often taught that, for reasons which are not entirely clear, their thinking tends to be idiosyncratic and biased towards negatively evaluating themselves or construing their internal world. Patients are taught to catch and report their negative automatic thoughts. They are taught how to cut through this strong emotional state and step back to evaluate these negative automatic thoughts. They are shown ways to examine evidence objectively for and against their negative thoughts and to look for alternative ways to explain upsetting situations. Cognitive therapists do, however, acknowledge that depressed patients can have real-life difficulties and so problem-solving is often employed when working with overwhelmed depressed patients with real-life difficulties.

Empirical evidence

The evidence that depressed individuals display greater negativity in their thinking is ample; for example, using the Automatic Thoughts Questionnaire (Hollon & Kendall, 1980), depressed subjects scored consistently higher than non-depressed subjects (Blackburn *et al.*, 1986; Dobson & Shaw, 1986; Hollon *et al.*, 1986; Lam *et al.*, 1987). Gotlib (1981) found that depressed patients were significantly more negative about the feedback they had received than psychiatric non-depressed controls. DeMonbreun and Craighead (1977) found that depressed subjects significantly underestimated positive feedback.

However, Beck's theory does not just hypothesize that depressed individuals are negative in their thinking, it also proposes that they make idiosyncratic thinking errors. The evidence for this is relatively scanty because it has been difficult to distinguish reliably between different types of evaluative distortion. For example, Krantz and Hammen (1979) reported that independent judges found it difficult to distinguish reliably between certain depressive cognitive errors postulated by Beck such as arbitrary inference, selective abstraction and overgeneralization. Similarly, Cook and Peterson (1986) reported similar difficulties and they had to collapse together selective abstraction, overgeneralization and magnification and/or minimization into one category. However, there is some evidence of idiosyncratic thinking errors. Depressed subjects are less likely to give depressed-distorted responses according to the Cognitive Bias Questionnaire (Krantz & Hammen, 1979), to justify their causal attribution logically and are more likely to make logical errors in making attribution to personal negative events in the past year (Cook & Peterson, 1986). Lefebvre (1981) measured four types of cognitive errors: catastrophizing, overgeneralization, personalization and selective abstraction. Lefebvre reported that depressed patients scored higher on cognitive errors. Wenzlaff and Grozier (1988) asked depressed and non-depressed students to indicate the extent to which they possessed anxious personality traits and the importance of these traits on a trait scale. Then subjects were given predetermined feedback of success or failure on an ostensible test of social perceptiveness. After feedback, the trait scale was re-administered. Depressed students inflated the importance of social perceptiveness after they had been told that they had done poorly on a test that purportedly measured social perceptiveness. Furthermore, they generalized from the social perceptiveness test results to an overall lowering of their general proficiency. This was taken as evidence of depressed individuals' tendency to self-derogate and to magnify their failings. Golin (1989) asked depressed and non-depressed students to judge the probabilities of positive or negative inferences on 10 hypothetical situations being correct. The situations were other-inferences or self-inferences. Depressed students judged negative self-inferences as more plausible than positive self-inferences. However, one criticism of the above studies is that the experimenter provided dimensions as the basis for inferences. This paradigm can be criticized as artificial and inducing such introspection may disrupt the typical negative, automatic or reflexive processes postulated by Beck *et al.* (1979).

Cognition, mood and behaviour

In his cognitive theory, Beck (Beck *et al.*, 1979) acknowledged that negative cognition may not be the ultimate 'cause' of depression. In fact negative cognitions can be seen as a depressive symptom on a par with affective, behavioural and physiological symptoms. However, an attempt is made to 'make some sense out of the highly diverse phenomena of depression by arranging them in a coherent logical sequence' (Beck *et al.*, 1979; p. 18). Hence the patient's negative constructions of reality can be postulated to be the first link in the chain of depressive symptoms. In the cognitive theory, cognition (thoughts/images), mood and behaviour affect each other. Negative cognitions can maintain, if not lead to, depressive affect. Likewise, behaviour can distract from negative rumination and hence have an impact on cognition and behaviour.

Clinical implications

Theoretically, as mentioned above, Beck (1987) denied making the assumption that cognitions 'cause' depression. However, it is generally accepted that negative cognitions can at least maintain depression and can be an important handle to deal with patients' depression. In therapy, patients are taught this important aspect of the theory in order to understand how emotion can be affected by cognition or behaviour. They are asked to identify their depressive cognitions when depressed in order to make sense of their emotions and, as described below, to examine the idiosyncratic negativity of these cognitions. Similarly, patients are also taught to use certain behavioural skills such as pleasant activity scheduling in order to lift their depressed mood.

Empirical evidence

Evidence to support the view that mood can affect cognition comes from both clinical studies and experimental studies that manipulate non-clinical subjects' mood states. Lloyd and Lishman (1975) reported that in depressed patients the latency for retrieval of unpleasant experiences correlated negatively with their level of depression as measured by Beck Depression Inventory. Clark and Teasdale (1982) took advantage of the diurnal variation of mood in depressed patients to test the effect of mood on recall of personal pleasant or unpleasant memories. Each patient was tested twice, once when in a more depressed phase and once in a less depressed phase of the diurnal variation. Subjects were asked to retrieve a memory when presented with a neutral word. It was found that unpleasant memories were more likely to be retrieved in the more depressed phase. Conversely, negative memories were less likely to be retrieved in the less depressed phase. Experimental studies generally make use of some mood induction procedure to induce a desired mood state and then to test subjects for recall bias. For example, Teasdale and Fogarty (1979) reported that after the subjects' mood was manipulated by a mood induction procedure in a student population, the latency of retrieval of pleasant events was significantly longer than unpleasant events when subjects were depressed. Teasdale and Russell (1983) presented student volunteers with a list containing an equal number of positive, neutral and negative personality trait words. Then the subjects' mood was manipulated by a mood induction procedure.

The authors found that subjects recalled more positive personality trait words when in an elated mood and more negative personality trait words when in a depressed mood.

Similarly there is evidence that cognition can affect mood; for example, mood induction procedures such as reading standardized, negative self-referent statements (Velten, 1968) can lead to a sad mood in 50–70% of subjects, depending on how strict the criteria were for sadness. This can be seen as tentative evidence to support cognition leading to mood. Clark (1983), however, pointed out that in these studies typically subjects were not directly asked how they achieved their sad state. Furthermore, Teasdale and Bancroft (1977) reported that depressed patients became more depressed when they were instructed to think of personally relevant negative thoughts. Conversely, there is evidence that when patients were distracted from negative cognitions, they became less depressed. For example, Teasdale and Rezin (1978) reported single cases of reducing frequency of negative thoughts leading to a significant reduction of depressed mood. A later study (Fennell *et al.*, 1987) replicated Teasdale and Rezin's findings. In both studies, the reduction of depressed mood was associated with the reduction in frequency of negative thoughts, and patients who scored low on the Newcastle Endogenous Scale seemed to have benefited more.

Certain behaviours are reported to be 'antidepressant' in nature. People are generally fairly prompt to offer advice of 'the thing to do when you are depressed'. Rippere (1979) summarized her findings that there seemed to be 'between' and 'within' individual differences in terms of helpfulness of antidepressant behaviours. Certain behaviour such as 'see a friend', 'do something I enjoy', 'talk to someone about how I feel', 'keep busy', seemed to be generally helpful. However, 'take antidepressant', 'crawl away on my own', 'take a rest', and 'read about depression and how to cure it', seemed to be less helpful. Furthermore, Rippere (1981) reported that subjects generally had a good idea of the extent to which people find certain antidepressant behaviour as helpful. Citing evidence that there is a large between-subject difference as to the helpfulness of each antidepressant activity, Rippere (1981) speculated that this common pool of knowledge was likely to be socially transmitted.

Conclusion

The descriptive aspect of the cognitive theory generally has good empirical support. However, it does not make any causal implications. It simply postulates that a group of affective, cognitive and behavioural symptoms coexist in depression. In this sense, negative emotion can be part of the depression syndrome. There has been much debate about the primacy of cognition in depression (see especially Coyne & Gotlib, 1983). However, Beck (1987) has explicitly denied that negative cognition causes depression. Instead, Beck (1987) concedes that 'an accurate view of reality may, in some instances, precipitate or activate a depression … I would argue that the exaggerated negative meanings attached to ongoing experiences are responsible for the buildup and maintenance of the noncognitive symptoms of depression' (p. 11). Unlike the descriptive theory, the causal theory delineates the precipitating as well as the predisposing factors. It is these causal aspects of the cognitive theory that will be discussed below.

The causal aspects of the cognitive theory for depression

In the cognitive theory for depression, early experience is deemed important in the formation of core beliefs and assumptions. In this section, the causal aspects of Beck's cognitive theory are discussed. Then the empirical evidence for these concepts is reviewed. Lastly, clinical implications will be discussed.

Adverse early experience and attachment problems

Bowlby's (1969, 1973, 1980) attachment theory has had an important influence on the way in which the causal aspects of adult emotional problems are regarded by Beck (1983, p. 266), who admitted that 'During 1980 we focused a good deal of attention on the thesis by Bowlby and others that the disruption of social bonding was a critical factor in the production of depression … the principle did seem to hold for cases that we treated over the years'. Even though Beck found a minority of cases (autonomous individuals, see below) that did not fit into this formulation, social bonding seems to be an important aspect in Beck's formulation and warrants a section of this chapter.

Bowlby (1973, 1980, 1988) emphasized the importance of a primary care-giver providing security by being sensitive, reliable and responsive to the infant's needs. By being sensitive and reliable the care-giver shows that the child is accepted, valued and worthwhile. In turn, the child feels safe to explore and to form a positive view of the self. Hence the role of secure attachment is thought to promote independence and foster maturity in social functioning. Insecure attachment is hypothesized to be due to a care-giver's rejection and inconsistent responsiveness. As a result of insecure attachment, a toddler may become anxious or avoidant. Bowlby (1973, 1977, 1980) postulated two types of attachment problems: the 'anxiously attached' and the 'compulsively self-reliant'. The anxiously attached individual seeks close interpersonal contact and displays excessive dependency, while the compulsively self-reliant avoids others and is scornful of intimate interpersonal relationships.

Main *et al.* (1985, pp. 66–67) further refined the attachment concept by elaborating the 'internal working theory'. This was defined as 'a set of conscious and/or unconscious rules for the organization of information relevant to attachment and for obtaining or limiting access to that information, that is, to information regarding attachment-related experiences, feelings and ideations'. The general assumption is that negative childhood experiences would serve as an internal theory or representation of self and others, which provide some sort of a 'blueprint' for later relationships. It is presumed that people with attachment problems will have problematic relationships in later life.

Empirical evidence

The empirical evidence and clinical applications of attachment and early adverse experience leading to vulnerability in childhood have been reviewed extensively elsewhere (Rajecki *et al.*, 1978; Belsky & Nezworski, 1988; Greenberg *et al.*, 1990; Rutter, 1995) and will not be repeated here. In fact Rutter (1995) commented that most of the components of attachment concepts have been found to receive empirical support in studies of children. Furthermore, the general notion of insecure attachment leading to later adult problems is vague and difficult to test empirically. It needs to be better operationalized to yield to empirical testing. Clinically the most important concept of the attachment theory is the 'internal working theory' that serves as a blueprint of further relationships in later life. At one level it makes sense that we have remembered and learned from past experiences which impinge on present relationships, at least in the behavioural repertory of interaction with others in our day-to-day contact and cognitive expectations of people occupying different social roles. However, as Hinde (1988) concluded, problems arise in translating this general notion into more specific hypotheses that are amenable to empirical research.

Adverse early experiences and vulnerable personality types

A more specific and perhaps testable set of theses came from psychotherapeutic observation. Adverse early experiences in the form of perceived parenting style is linked with personality types that are hypothesized to be vulnerable to the development of depression when faced with stressful events in the environment.

Before discussing the link between perceived parenting style and vulnerable personality types, it is important to clarify these personality types. Blatt (1974) described two types of vulnerable individuals: those with anaclitic or dependent traits, and those with introjective or self-critical traits. Similarly, both Arieti and Bemporad (1978) and Beck (1983) postulated two broad subtypes of individuals at risk; those who focus on the interpersonal domain and those who focus on work or a similar achievement-related domain. The former is labelled as the 'dominant other' type and the latter as the 'dominant goal' type by Arieti and Bemporad (1978), and 'sociotropic' and 'autonomous' individuals, respectively, by Beck (1983).

Beck (1983) described the *sociotropic* individual as 'dependent on these social inputs for gratification, motivation, direction and modification of ideas and behaviour. The motif of this cluster is receiving' (p. 272). Arieti and Bemporad (1980) emphasized the failure of the 'dominant other' type to individuate and develop autonomy:

> They do not experience satisfaction directly from effort but only through an intermediary (another person) who gives or withholds reward. They have formed an imagined agreement with the important other that may be called a bargained relationship ..., in which the individual foregoes the independent derivation of gratification in return for the continuance of nurturance and support of the esteemed other. (p. 1360)

Hence the 'sociotropic', 'anaclitic or dependent' and 'dominant other' individuals are greatly reliant on close others as a source of meaning and self-esteem.

Beck (1983) also described the *autonomous* individuals as attaching an irrational amount of importance 'in preserving and increasing his independence, mobility, and personal rights; freedom of choice, action and expression; protection of his domain; and defining his boundary' (p. 272). Arieti and Bemporad (1980) also outline the 'dominant goal' as

> individuals (who) invest their self-esteem in the achievement of some lofty goal and shun any other activities as possibly diverting them from this quest ... The individual believes that the goal will transform his life and possibly himself. Attaining his desired objective will mean that others will treat him in a special way or that he will finally be valued by others. (p. 1361)

A premium is placed on meeting very stringent standards in order to maintain high self-esteem.

Beck (1983) believed patients can change modes from issues of unloveability to incompetence between and even within episodes. Beck *et al.* (1990) labelled these beliefs of basic self-concept as core beliefs. Linguistically these are believed to be encoded in the form of 'I am unlovable or incompetent'. All the above constructs attempt to spell out the characteristics of individuals who are vulnerable to depression and to types of stress which may precipitate a depressive episode in a vulnerable individual. The constructs appeared to be similar even though the terms are different.

More specific hypotheses relating to pathological parenting styles contributing to the vulnerable personality types in later life have been proposed. McClelland *et al.* (1953) pointed out that 'value-achievers' set high but unrealistic standards and are significantly influenced by social approval. They speculated that value-achievers develop these attitudes from 'authoritarian pressure from parents to be ambitious and the resultant motives which originated in external sources show itself as a fear of being unsuccessful' (p. 419). Similarly, Gotlib and Hammen (1992) hypothesized that individuals with insecure attachments may develop dependent personalities and overvaluing interpersonal domains. Adverse parent–child experiences also contribute to the acquisition of negative self-schema, characterized by low self-worth. Moreover, these negative self-schema lead to the development of further negative schemas of expectation of interpersonal negativity and rejection. These hypotheses are more in tune with the cognitive theory relating early experiences to later vulnerability.

Empirical evidence

The empirical evidence linking perceived negative parenting with later adult depression has been reviewed by Blatt and Homman (1992). Instead of repeating the empirical evidence of attachment problems in childhood and non-specific negative perceived parenting in adult depression, this chapter concentrates on the evidence which links specific types of perceived parenting with later vulnerability to self-criticism, autonomy and sociotropy or dependency in adulthood, as suggested by the cognitive theory of depression.

As mentioned above, the vulnerable personality types proposed by Blatt (1974), Arieti and Bemporad (1978) and Beck (1983) are broadly similar. Empirically there is evidence that the various instruments designed to measure these concepts overlap to a large extent. The three better known and more commonly used instruments are the Depressive Experience Questionnaire (DEQ) (Blatt, D'Afflitti & Quinlan, unpublished manuscript); the Sociotropy-Autonomy Scale (Beck *et al.*, 1983); and the Anaclitic and Introjective Dysfunctional Attitudes subscales by Mongrain & Zuroff (1989). As all three scales are used in the studies reviewed in this section and the following section on congruent events, it is worth examining how they relate to each other.

The DEQ (Blatt *et al.*, 1979) yielded three factors: dependency, self-criticism and efficacy. The dependency factor contains themes regarding abandonment, feeling lonely and wanting to be close to and dependent on others; the self-criticism factor contains themes about feeling guilty, failing to meet expectations and standards, and being unable to assume responsibility; the efficacy factor contains themes about high standards and personal goals, inner strength, feelings of independence and pride and satisfaction in one's accomplishments. The Sociotropy-Autonomy Scale (SAS) (Beck *et al.*, 1983) yielded two factors of sociotropy and autonomy: the sociotropy factor relates to themes about disapproval, attachment and pleasing others; and the autonomy factor contains themes about achievement, freedom from control, and preference for solitude. The Anaclitic (dependent) and Introjective (self-critical) Dysfunctional Attitudes subscales were taken from the original Dysfuntional Attitude Scale (DAS) (Weissman & Beck, 1979) by Mongrain and Zuroff (1989).

Robins (1985) found significant correlations between the SAS sociotropy and the DEQ dependency ($r = 0.68$); and SAS autonomy and DEQ self-criticism ($r = 0.39$). Furthermore, Blaney and Kutcher (1991) found high intercorrelations between the DEQ, SAS and Anaclitic DAS factor concerning dependency or sociotropy. However, the intercorrelations between the three scales assessing individuality or self-criticism were less clear. The correlation between Introjective DAS and DEQ self-critical factor was substantial and significant. However, the SAS autonomy factor did not correlate significantly with the DEQ self-criticism. The authors speculated that the SAS autonomy factor appeared to measure counter-dependency rather than individuality.

There is, surprisingly, very little evidence supporting this part of Beck's theory from the traditional cognitive therapy research. Most of the evidence linking perceived problematic parenting and vulnerable personality types in later life comes from research using psychoanalytical perspectives. Given the absence of empirical evidence from the traditional cognitive therapy school and the high intercorrelations between the various instruments, this section concentrates on the more specific hypothesis of perceived parenting and vulnerable personality types in later life using instruments such as the DEQ. Table 5.1 summarizes the studies examining specific perceived parenting relating to self-criticism or sociotropy.

All six studies included assessed perceived parenting retrospectively. Two studies used longitudinal design to control for levels of depression and perceived parenting (Gotlib *et al.*, 1988) and to assess trait self-criticism (Brewin *et al.*, 1992b). Of the six studies, five used non-clinical populations and there was only one study using a clinical population (Gotlib *et al.*, 1988): this did not link perceived parenting with later adult vulnerability type. It is included for two reasons: first, it was longitudinal in design and hence could investigate whether retrospective recall of perceived parenting was a function of the level of depression; and second, the study is the only one using a clinical sample.

The main findings were positive; for example dependent subjects remembered their mothers as dominating and controlling, emphasizing conformity (McCraine & Bass, 1984); maternal overprotectiveness significantly correlated with DEQ dependency in women (Blatt *et al.*, 1992); dependency score in the DEQ was related to perception of a distant relationship with fathers during

Table 5.1 Summary of studies investigating perceived parenting and vulnerable personality types.

Authors	Sample	Instrument	Outcome
McCraine & Bass (1984)	Female nursing students	Depressive Experience Questionnaire (DEQ; Blatt *et al.*, 1979); Strict Control, Conformity and Achievement Control subscale from the Parental Behaviour Form (Kelly & Worrell, 1976); Parental Inconsistency of Love Scale (Schwarz & Zuroff, 1979); Schwarz–Getter Interparental Influence Scale (Schwarz & Zuroff, 1979)	Dependent subjects remembered their mothers as dominating and controlling, emphasizing conformity. Self-critical subjects remembered both of their parents as equally dominant, emphasizing achievement and performance, demonstrating their love inconsistently
Gotlib, *et al.* (1988)	Longitudinal study of 30-month follow-up of 25 postpartum, depressed and 25 matched postpartum, non-depressed women	Beck Depression Inventory (Beck *et al.*, 1961); Parental Bonding Instrument (Parker *et al.*, 1979)	At both T1 and T2 depressed and remitted women reported higher overprotection scores than non-depressed women; at T1 and T2 non-depressed and remitted women reported lower parental caring scores than depressed women
Frost *et al.* (1991)	41 women graduates and their parents	Multidimensional Perfectionism Scale (Frost *et al.*, 1990); Father/mother Trait Scale (Steketee *et al.*, 1985); Brief Symptom Inventory (Derogatis & Melisaratos, 1983)	Mother's perfectionism, correlated with the perfectionism in their daughters; daughters' perception of fathers' harshness correlated with daughters' perfectionism. A combination of mothers' own perfectionism scores and mothers' self-reported harshness accounted for 30% of the daughters' perfectionism. Mothers' perfectionism, was associated with daughters' psychopathology
Blatt *et al.* (1991)	Non-clinical young adults	Beck Depression Inventory (Beck et al., 1961); Parental Bonding Instrument (Parker *et al.*, 1979); Depressive Experience Questionnaire (DEQ; Blatt *et al.*, 1996); Zung Depression Scale (Zung, 1965)	In women, caring by mother and father had a significant negative correlation with DEQ self-criticism; maternal and paternal overprotection correlated with DEQ self-criticism and BDI and Zung depression scores; maternal over-protectiveness significantly correlated with DEQ dependency In men, mother's caring significantly correlated with in only the negative direction; paternal caring correlated significantly only with DEQ self-criticism in negative direction; Maternal overprotection correlated with DEQ self-criticism (not so clear in men)

(Continued.)

Table 5.1 *Continued.*

Authors	Sample	Instrument	Outcome
Brewin *et al.* (1992b)	75 medical students assessed twice with an average interval of 30 months	Depressive Experience Questionnaire (DEQ; Blatt *et al.*, 1976); Family Attitudes Questionnaire (Thomas & Duszynski, 1974); Parental Bonding Inventory (Parker *et al.*, 1979) and Symptom Checklist-90 (Derogatis *et al.*, 1983)	After controlling for mood and social desirability, high levels of trait self-criticism were related to retrospective reports of less satisfactory maternal parenting in terms of level of care and overprotection as well as measures from the Family Attitude Questionnaire
Rosenfarb *et al.* (1994)	132 female subjects	Parent–Child Relations Questionnaire (Siegelman & Roe, 1979); Depressive Experiences Questionnaire (DEQ; Blatt *et al.*, 1976)	Dependency score in the DEQ was related to perception of distant relationship with fathers during development, perceptions of increased parental attention and overindulgence. Self-criticism scores in the DEQ were associated with perceptions of difficulties of affective bond with fathers and peers during childhood, and perceptions of increased paternal power and control

development and perceptions of increased parental attention and overindulgence (Rosenfarb *et al.*, 1994). In relationship to self-criticism, self-critical subjects remembered both of their parents as equally dominant, emphasizing achievement and performance and demonstrating their love inconsistently (McCraine & Bass, 1984); mothers' perfectionism correlated with the perfectionism of their daughters, and daughters' perception of fathers' harshness correlated with daughters' perfectionism (Frost *et al.*, 1991); maternal and paternal overprotection correlated with DEQ self-criticism (Blatt *et al.*, 1992); high levels of self-criticism were related to retrospective reports of less satisfactory parenting and less satisfactory relationships with their parents (Brewin *et al.*, 1992b); and self-criticism scores in the DEQ were associated with perceptions of difficulties of affective bonds with fathers and peers during childhood, and perceptions of increased paternal power and control (Rosenfarb *et al.*, 1994).

In their study, Brewin *et al.* (1992b) investigated self-criticism as a trait and found that subjects who were highly critical at both time 1 and time 2 had significantly worse maternal relationships than other subjects. The authors also reported that the correlation between perceived parenting and self-criticism was much reduced when the level of depression was controlled. However, the authors raised the issue that, if early adverse parenting influences both depression and self-criticism in later adult life, controlling for depression would underestimate the relationship between perceived problematic parenting and self-criticism.

There was some evidence of a gender-specific effect. Three studies used exclusively female subjects (McCraine & Bass, 1984; Frost *et al.*, 1991; Rosenfarb *et al.*, 1994). Blatt *et al.* (1992) investigated the gender effect and commented that the relationship between perceived parenting style and a later adult vulnerable personality type in male subjects was not so clear in their study. In men, mothers' caring significantly correlated with the Beck Depression Inventory (BDI) in the negative direction; paternal caring correlated significantly only with DEQ self-criticism in negative direction, and maternal overprotection correlated with DEQ self-criticism.

The evidence so far has supported the link between perceived problematic parenting style and later vulnerability in adulthood. However, the evidence reviewed has come from retrospective recall of perceived parenting. In retrospective studies, there is a possibility that depressed subjects might report negative parental behaviour as a function of depressive mood. However, it has been argued (Johnson *et al.*, 1982) that depressives do not have a global and indiscriminate tendency to report their childhood experiences in a negative way. This is borne out by the fact that dependent and self-critical individuals did not report indiscriminately on global negative perceived parenting. In the study by Gotlib *et al.* (1988), overprotection and the level of parental care did not change when subjects' depression had remitted.

In a review article on a reappraisal of retrospective reports (Brewin *et al.*, 1993), it was argued that the general unreliability of retrospective reports was exaggerated. Furthermore, one could argue that it was the perception of one's own parents, rather than the actual behaviour of one's parents, that form one's internal working theory, which, in turn, affects one's interaction with the world.

The major problems with the majority of the studies reviewed include the lack of evidence from clinical subjects, the comparative lack of control for mood state and a lack of investigations into whether these vulnerable personality types are truly trait and not state findings. Despite these weaknesses, the findings between perceived parenting and later adult vulnerable personality types seems robust.

Vulnerable personality types and congruent events

Beck (1983) hypothesized that people weave an environment around them in which they can cope. For example, highly sociotropic individuals would invest to the best of their ability in interpersonal domains to ensure that there is someone close in order to feel valued. Similarly, highly autonomous individuals would invest a lot in achieving whatever is important to them in order to be self-sufficient. Furthermore, they develop certain beliefs in response to these core beliefs.

Clinical problems are seen as a result of an event, either social or cognitive, which impinges on a specific vulnerability relating to either issues of loveability or competence: the congruent hypothesis. Both the core belief and conditional beliefs may be activated and further mould subsequent interpretations of an event. This will be followed by intense and emotionally laden automatic thoughts and the person may develop clinical depression.

Empirical evidence

Table 5.2 summarizes the empirical studies that involved identifying vulnerable personality types and investigating whether undesirable events relating to the particular vulnerable personality type (congruent events) lead to emotional problems. Fourteen studies relating to vulnerability types and congruent events are summarized. Eight studies use student samples. Of the eight student sample studies, four are prospective studies (Hammen *et al.*, 1985; Zuroff *et al.*, 1990; Lakey & Thomson-Ross, 1994; Robins *et al.*, 1995). The study by Rude and Burnham (1993) is a cross-sectional study because there was no measurement of depression symptoms at T (at recruitment). In the study by Hammen *et al.* (1985), in addition to the BDI, a formal diagnostic interview was conducted and depression was diagnosed using DSM-III (American Psychiatric Association, 1980) Major Depressive Disorder criteria. However, all the other seven studies used either BDI or the DEQ (Blatt *et al.*, 1976) as an indication of depression. Moreover, the instruments used to measure vulnerable personality types ranged from recall procedures by Teasdale *et al.* (1980); Sociotropy-Autonomy Scale (Beck *et al.*, 1983); to different versions of a Dysfunctional Attitude Scale.

Taken as a whole, the 14 studies summarized in Table 5.2 support the notion that sociotropy or dependency is related to depression. The only exception was the study by Hammen *et al.* (1992) in which bipolar patients were used. Only two studies (Hammen *et al.*, 1989; Segal *et al.*, 1992) found interaction between autonomy, negative achievement events and relapse. The study by Hammen was a small sample and the number of subjects relapsed was even smaller. Of more interest is the study by Segal *et al.* (1992) which needs further replication.

The empirical evidence of congruent events and vulnerable personality types seems more complicated. The timing of the events appears important for the two different types of event. Segal *et al.* (1992) found that relapse was related to the interaction of self-criticism scores and negative achievement events over the whole year but the predicted effect for dependency-orientated patients was only valid when events in the 2 months prior to onset were taken into account. The authors' interpretation was that the impact of interpersonal events was more immediate, whereas achievement-related events might involve worsening of ongoing difficulties over a period of time.

Table 5.2 Summaries of studies investigating congruent events and depression.

Authors	Subjects	Instrument	Results
Hammen *et al.*, 1985	4-month follow-up of a student sample of 46 dependent and 32 self-critical schematic individuals	Recall procedures by Teasdale *et al.* (1980); Beck Depression Inventory (Beck, 1967)	Dependent subgroup showed strong associations between depression and schema-relevant interpersonal events. The predicted pattern for self-critical schematics was observed but was less often statistically significant
Robins and Block (1988)	Cross-sectional study of another student sample of 45 men and 53 women	Sociotropy– Autonomy Scale (Beck *et al.*, 1983); Beck Depression Inventory (Beck, 1967)	Weak support for the specificity of type of event and sociotropy versus autonomy individuals. Autonomy was unrelated to depression and had shown no relationship to any type of event categorized *a priori*, whereas sociotropy was associated with depression level and served as a moderator of the relationship between depression and frequency of negative social events. After partialling out the main effect for sociotropy and for negative social events, the interaction between these two variables accounted for an additional 7% of the variance in the Beck Depression Inventory (BDI), a significant increase in the variance accounted for. However, there was also a significant increase in the BDI variance accounted for by the interaction of sociotropy and negative autonomy events after partialling out their additive effects
Hammen *et al.* (1989)	Currently depressed autonomous and sociotropic unipolar (22 patients) and bipolar (25 patients) depressed patients	Sociotropy– Autonomy Scale (Beck *et al.*, 1983)	Onset of relapse or exacerbation of symptoms in unipolar depression in autonomous subjects who had experienced more achievement events and sociotropic subjects had experienced more interpersonal events. However, congruence hypothesis did not apply for bipolar patients
Segal *et al.* (1989)	6-month follow-up of 40 remitted depressed patients	DAS—need for approval and self-critical factors	Congruent events correlated significantly with depressive symptoms during follow-up for dependent subjects but no significant correlation for congruent events for self-critical subjects
Robins (1990)	41 depressed patients and 44 schizophrenic patients	Sociotropy– Autonomy Scale (Beck *et al.*, 1983)	Highly sociotropic patients reported more recent negative interpersonal events than negative autonomy events. Autonomous subjects did not report more negative autonomy events. No evidence of any congruence among non-depressed schizophrenic patients

(Continued.)

Table 5.2 *Continued.*

Authors	Subjects	Instrument	Results
Zuroff *et al.* (1990)	66 female undergraduates retested 12 months later	Depressive Experience Questionnaire (Blatt *et al.*, 1976); Dysfunctional Attitude Scale (Weissman & Beck, 1979); Beck Depression Inventory (Beck *et al.*, 1961)	After controlling for initial level of depression, majority of dependent and self-critical subjects' worst period involved interpersonal events. Dependency predicted anaclitic state depression and self-criticism predicted introjective state depression
Clark *et al.* (1992)	Cross-sectional study of 600 psychology students	Sociotropy–Autonomy Scale (Beck *et al.*, 1983; Beck Depression Inventory (Beck *et al.*, 1961)	For dysphoric subjects (BDI > 16), sociotrophy significantly interacted with negative social related events but not autonomously related events to predict dysphoria. Autonomy failed to show any significant relation with dysphoria or types of negative life events experienced
Segal *et al.* (1992)	A sample of 59 remitted depressed patients for 1 year	Dysfunctional Attitude Scale (Weissman & Beck, 1979)	Relapse was related to the interaction of self-criticism scores and negative achievement events over the period prior to relapse. The predicted effect for dependency-orientated patients was only valid when events in the 2 months prior to onset were taken into account
Hammen *et al.* (1992)	Followed up a sample of 49 bipolar patients over 18 months	Sociotropy–Autonomy Scale (Beck *el al.*, 1983)	No effect of congruent events in subjects suffering from bipolar depression. However, symptom severity was significantly associated with sociotropy, interpersonal events and the interaction of the two but not for autonomy
Rude and Burnham (1993)	443 students— depression symptoms and life events were measured 4 to 6 weeks later. (A cross-sectional study because no measurement of depression symptoms at T1)	Depressive Experience Questionnaire (Blatt *et al.*, 1976); Sociotropy–Autonomy Scale (Beck *et al.*, 1983); Dysfunctional Attitude Scale (Weissman & Beck, 1979); Beck Depression Inventory (Beck *et al.*, 1961)	With the exception of DAS, all interpersonal/sociotropy scales showed interaction with frequency of interpersonal events but not achievement life events in predicting depressive symptoms. The achievement/autonomous scale yielded no significant interactions with achievement life event frequencies
Lakey and Thomson-Ross (1994)	133 college students in a prospective study of 10 to 12 weeks follow-up	Depressive Experience Questionnaire (Blatt, *et al.*, 1976); Sociotropy–	After controlling for initial level of depression, dependent subjects displayed greater increase of depressive symptoms after interpersonal event but not

(Continued on p. 114.)

Table 5.2 *Continued.*

Authors	Subjects	Instrument	Results
		Autonomy Scale (Beck *et al.*, 1983); College Student Life Events Schedule (Sandler & Lakey, 1982); Beck Depression Inventory (Beck *et al.*, 1961)	achievement events. However self-critical subjects also displayed an increase of depressive symptoms after interpersonal events. There was only a trend for self-critical subjects to display greater increase in depressive symptoms after achievement events. Dysphoric subjects displayed greater increases in depressive symptoms following interpersonal but not achievement events. When the effect of initial dysphoria and interpersonal events was controlled statistically, the power of cognitive variables to predict reactivity was reduced greatly
Bartelstone and Trull (1995)	166 undergraduates including 42 identified as depressed by BDI	Depressive Experience Questionnaire (Blatt *et al.*, 1976); Sociotropy–Autonomy Scale (Beck *et al.*, 1983); Life Experience Scale (Sarason *et al.*, 1978)	Evidence to support congruent event hypothesis by DEQ dependency and SAS sociotropy subscale only
Robins *et al.* (1995)	164 undergraduates in a 1-month longitudinal study	Revised Depressive Experience Questionnaire (Welkowitz, *et al.*, 1985); Sociotropy–Autonomy Scale (Beck *et al.*, 1983); Life Experiences Survey (Sarason *et al.*, 1978); Zung Self-rating Depression Scale (Zung 1965); Beck Depression Inventory (Beck *et al.*, 1961)	Depressive symptom change was predicted by interaction of sociotropy and frequency of negative interpersonal events. However, sociotropy also interacted with achievement to predict depressive symptom change. Similarly autonomy also interacted with both achievement and interpersonal events to predict changes in depressive symptom level. On the whole, findings did not support domain-specific hypotheses. Negative interpersonal events were strongly associated with subjects high in either autonomy or sociotropy
Lam *et al.* (1996)	1-year follow-up of a sample of 37 depressed patients	Dysfunctional Attitude Scale (DAS; Power *et al.*, 1994); Roles and Goals Questionnaire (Lam & Power, 1991)	Adversity in the most invested domain (matching adversity) according to the Roles and Goals Questionnaire and the DAS dependency subscale contributed significantly both to whether or not subjects relapsed and to the number of weeks subjects survived before they relapsed. Most matching adversity were interpersonal events. DAS achievement subscale did not contribute significantly to relapses

Hammen *et al.* (1992) found that sociotropy may relate to symptom severity. The authors argued that with bipolar individuals, the theory of congruent, meaningful, personal events and relapse may not hold. However, once depressed, patients with a sociotropic personality type who have experienced negative interpersonal events and who define their worth in interpersonal relationships may experience more severe depression symptoms, whereas the autonomous individuals may even minimize the severity of their depression.

Another complication relates to the conceptual aspects of vulnerable personality types. Haaga *et al.* (1991) raised the issue of whether sociotropy and autonomy should be construed as dimensional or categorical constructs. Apparently about 37% in the study by Hammen *et al.* (1992) and 65% in that by Goldberg *et al.* (1989) were 'mixed' or unclassifiable. Cognitive theory does not make predictions about them. It could be that individuals who have invested in both interpersonal and achievement domains are less prone to developing depression. Linville (1985) proposed that people vary in the degree of self-complexity. Self-complexity is defined as a function of two factors: the number of self-aspects and the relatedness amongst them. Greater self-complexity is defined as 'cognitively organizing self-knowledge in terms of a greater number of self-aspects and maintaining greater distinction among self-aspects.' The basic assumption is that greater self-complexity moderates the adverse impact of stressful events. For people who have more self-aspects and maintain more distinctions among self-aspects, the impact of negative events is likely to be confined to a smaller aspect of their self-representation. Cognitive theory of vulnerable personality types is based on clinical observation and may not generalize to the non-depressed population. Furthermore, the measure of the stressor (negative events) can also be improved. One could measure the subjective perception of levels of stress, the frequency counts of these negative events or the contextual rating of events by the Life Events and Difficulties Schedule method (Brown & Harris, 1978).

Furthermore, studies have their own problems; for example, the problem with the early study by Hammen *et al.* (1985) is that the initial groupings were based on reported previous significant upsetting events. When subjects were assessed 2 months later, the kappa coefficient was only 0.30, suggesting the classification was temporally unstable. There were also differences in terms of the stringency with which the statistical analysis was carried out. In the Hammen *et al.* (1985) study, the statistical analysis by Hammen's team was of the frequency of events. Presumably the authors could argue that it was not clear in Beck's formulation what level of intensity of events was needed for the onset of depression. Whereas in the other studies (Robins & Block, 1988; Clark *et al.*, 1992; Rude & Burnham, 1993) the authors used more stringent statistical tests such as multiple regression analysis or MANOVA to examine the contribution measures of autonomy and sociotropy and their interaction with congruent events can make to the depression measures.

To sum up, the empirical evidence for congruent events and the onset of a depressive episode for sociotropic or dependent subjects is robust. The majority of the studies reviewed here have produced positive results. However, the evidence is not so clear for the concept of autonomy or self-criticism; only a handful of studies produced positive results. This could partly be due to the fact that the instruments, such as the SAS, are not very good at measuring autonomy. However, all the studies involving patients are of small samples, ranging from 59 to 37 depressed subjects. Again, Hammen *et al.* (1989) used a frequency count as opposed to the interaction of measures of vulnerable personality types and congruent events. Moreover, these studies examined the impact of congruent events on relapses or recurrences of depression as opposed to the onset of the first episode of depression. Hence one can only conclude from these studies that a vulnerable personality and congruent events as a trigger of a depressive episode are only applicable to relapses. There is no evidence relating to the onset of a first episode of depression.

Dysfunctional assumptions

As mentioned above, dysfunctional assumptions are seen as a permutation of the basic core beliefs in order to cope with the internal world in which the individual lives. Hence themes tend to be related to loveability, acceptance, achievement or control. Each patient has a unique set of dysfunctional assumptions which are trait-like and can be latent during a remission. These assumptions are dysfunctional because they are highly rigid and absolutistic, and hence prevent the individual's goal attainment in life. It is through these assumptions that 'the individual attempts to intergrate and assign value to the raw data ... In essence, these basic assumptions form a personal matrix of meaning and value, the backdrop against which everyday events acquire relevance, importance and significance' (Beck *et al.*, 1979, p. 244). Beck *et al.* (1979) hypothesized that people with rigid and extreme dysfunctional assumptions are more prone to depression when faced with relevant adversities.

Empirical evidence

There have been three ways to investigate the trait-like vulnerability of dysfunctional attitudes: (i) cross-sectional studies comparing remitted depressives with normal subjects; (ii) longitudinal studies following a sample of remitted depressives and investigating the relationship of relapse and dysfunctional attitudes; and (iii) treatment studies.

Cross-sectional studies comparing normal controls and recovered depressives have largely yielded negative results. Hamilton and Abramson

(1983), Evans and Rush (1984), Silverman *et al.* (1984), Simons *et al.* (1984) and Blackburn and Smyth (1985) found no difference in the DAS scores between remitted depressives and those who had never been depressed.

However, longitudinal studies have yielded more evidence for Beck's vulnerability theory (Beck *et al.*, 1979). Dysfunctional attitudes were found to predict the subsequent relapse following the successful treatment of depression (Evans *et al.*, 1985; Simons *et al.*, 1986; Rush *et al.*, 1986). Lam *et al.* (1996) reported that in their 1-year follow-up, high levels of dysfunctional dependency attitudes assessed during the index episode when subjects were mildly depressed were associated with shorter survival time. Subjects with higher levels of dependency attitudes on the whole relapsed sooner, even with the effect of adverse events controlled. One explanation for the different findings of cross-sectional and longitudinal studies is that these dysfunctional attitudes remain latent until there is a slight mood disturbance or stress amongst the 'reactives' (Williams, 1984). Hence when subjects are fully remitted, they do not score differently from those who had never been depressed. However, most subjects who have just recovered from an episode of depression have some residual symptoms. It is therefore possible to identify subjects who are more prone to relapses. This explanation is consistent with findings which use mood induction. Miranda and Persons (1988) reported their use of mood induction procedures to distinguish 'reactives' and 'non-reactives'. Mood induction produced a dysphoric mood in both never-depressed and remitted depressives. However, only the remitted depressed endorsed higher scores on dysfunctional attitudes. These studies provide some evidence of dysfunctional assumptions being latent and then activated only by negative emotional states.

Turning to treatment studies, Simons *et al.* (1984) found that when depressed subjects recovered, their change in cognitive measures, including their levels of dysfunctional attitudes, were similar irrespective of whether they received pharmacological treatment or cognitive therapy. The authors postulated that different treatment modalities may work by attacking different facets of a complicated interlocking picture. Williams *et al.* (1990) examined whether dysfunctional attitudes lead to a predisposition to longer-lasting episodes after the onset. They found that more patients in the high dysfunctional attitude scores range remained depressed after 6 weeks.

In summary, there is empirical evidence that dysfunctional assumptions can predict treatment outcome, subsequent relapse and survival time. Furthermore, there is tentative evidence of dysfunctional assumptions being trait-like and activated differentially. This has led Teasdale (1988) to suggest that vulnerability lies in the individual's difference in the patterns of information processing activated in depression: the differential activation hypothesis. Events interpreted as highly aversive and uncontrollable would lead to transient or mild depressed mood. However, the minority who progress to develop depression would access memories or representations of depressing experiences, and the negative interpretative categories and constructs. Hence their depression is often enhanced by negative ruminations even though there is no immediate environmental input.

Clinical implications

Cognitive therapists use a variety of cognitive and behavioural techniques. However, irrespective of the therapeutic techniques used, it is the cognitive theory that distinguishes cognitive therapy from other types of psychotherapy. Within this theory, trainee therapists are taught to conceptualize patients' problems as soon as they begin to work with them. Clinically the causal aspects of the cognitive theory are used for case conceptualization. Case conceptualization is specific, although the actual content is individualized. Person (1994) defined case conceptualization as 'the therapist's hypothesis about the nature of the psychological mechanisms underlying the patient's difficulties' (p. 33). Therapists make use of the case conceptualization in order to have access to the patient's internal world, to provide accurate empathy, to guide intervention strategies and to predict the patient's response to intervention.

Conceptualization consists of making sense of all the longitudinal and cross-sectional data the patient presents in order to understand his/her overt problems. The theory postulates that core beliefs are developed in relation to early experiences, particularly early salient events. Hence therapists take note of any salient childhood events such as traumas and separation, patients' perceived parental attitudes, relationships with peer groups and authority figures and any history of abuse. History of insecure attachment suggests dependency or sociotropic issues, whereas authoritarian pressure from significant figures to be ambitious in early life may lead therapists to hypothesize autonomous vulnerability. The therapist also tries to identify how the patient has always viewed him/herself, what sort of problems the patient has experienced so far as a result of this core belief and how the patient has coped with difficulties.

Furthermore, the cognitive theory of emotional state describes how clinical problems arise. The onset of emotional disorders is often preceded by situations relating to individuals' specific vulnerabilities; for example, interpersonal events in dependent individuals and achievement events in achievement-orientated individuals. Hence, to understand how patients have reached the stage they are at, therapists also need continuously to ask questions about vulnerabilities and undesirable events. In cognitive conceptualization, the undesirable events do not have to be major social adversities. They can be cognitive events that carry special meanings for patients.

Dysfunctional assumptions are important aspects of the cognitive theory as they represent part of the patient's vulnerability to emotional problems. Safran *et al.* (1986) described a useful technique for eliciting core cognitive dysfunctional assumptions: the vertical exploration technique. Vertical exploration is the exploration of the individual's idiosyncratic way of construing events and their perception of the self. Hence therapists may want to explore the meanings of automatic thoughts as well as challenging them. Another important way to elicit dysfunctional assumptions is to look out for patterns of automatic thoughts central for the sense of self and how patients interact with their environment. The process tends to be collaborative. As therapists and patients work collaboratively to agree on the idiosyncratic dysfunctional assumptions, attempts are made to modify these rigid and absolutistic rules intellectually. Furthermore, patients are encouraged also to act against these rules in such a way as to have an experience of a different kind so that there is behavioural, emotional and intellectual learning.

Conclusion

The causal aspects of the cognitive theory for depression have been reviewed. The evidence supporting a pathogenetic parenting style and the formation of vulnerable personality types has mainly come from researchers of the psychoanalytic perspective and from retrospective recall of perceived parenting of non-clinical populations. The findings seem robust and consistent. However, most studies did not control for the effect of the level of depression on such retrospective recall. Hence it is not clear whether such recall is a result of mood.

Turning to studies of vulnerability types and congruent events, there is enough empirical evidence tentatively to support the notion that congruent events are more likely to lead to relapses in depression. Despite the fact that instruments used in the studies reviewed above to measure autonomy and sociotropy were not identical, the effect seems to be robust. The expansion of the cognitive theory of congruent events has advanced the causal theory to an interaction between the intrapsychic and the environment. However, it is still hard to determine the extent to which subjects contribute to the occurrence of an adversity. Perhaps subjects with higher levels of dysfunctional attitudes are more prone to bring about their own adversity. This speculation is supported by the finding of Simons *et al.* (1993) that elevated scores on DAS were associated with the number of objectively defined events occurring prior to the onset of depression. Furthermore, Lam *et al.* (1987) have found that the level of dysfunctional attitudes predicted subjects' length of survival before relapsing due to an adverse event. However, most of the evidence to support sociotropy and autonomy as vulnerable personality types so far are from evidence of relapses in patient populations. It is hard to generalize such findings to the onset of a first episode of depression. It is possible that the experience of depression has lowered the person's level of functioning so much that the person can only invest in one aspect of his/her life.

To sum up, the bulk of the evidence supporting the causal aspects of Beck's cognitive theory for depression either come from cross-sectional or retrospective studies. To test the causal aspects of the cognitive theory, longitudinal studies with long-term follow-up of never-depressed subjects are required.

References

American Psychiatric Association (1980) *Diagnostic and Statistical Manual of Mental Disorders*, 3rd edn. American Psychiatric Association, Washington, DC.

Arieti, S. & Bemporad, J. (1978) *Severe and Mild Depression: The Psychotherapeutic Approach.* Tavistock, London.

Arieti, S. & Bemporad, J. (1980) The psychological organisation of depression. *American Journal of Psychiatry*, **137**, 1360–1365.

Bartlestone, J.H. & Trull, T.J. (1995) Personality, life events and depression. *Journal of Personality Assessment*, **64**, 279–294.

Beck, A.T. (1967) *Depression: Clinical, Experimental, and Theoretical Aspects.* Harper & Row, New York.

Beck, A.T. (1983) Cognitive therapy of depression: New perspectives. In: *Treatment of Depression: Old Controversies and New Approaches* (eds P. J. Clayton & J. E. Barrett), pp. 5–37. Raven Press, New York.

Beck, A.T. (1987) Cognitive models of depression. *Journal of Cognitive Psychotherapy*, **1**, 5–37.

Beck, A.T., Ward, C.H., Mendelson, M., Mock, J. & Erbaugh, J. (1961) An inventory for measuring depression. *Archives of General Psychiatry*, **4**, 53–63.

Beck, A.T., Kovacs, M. & Weissman, A. (1975) Hopelessness and suicidal behaviour: an overview. *Journal of the American Medical Association*, **234**, 1146–1149.

Beck, A.T., Rush, A.J., Shaw, B.F. & Emery, G. (1979) *Cognitive Therapy for Depression.* John Wiley & Sons, New York.

Beck, A.T., Epstein, N., Harrison, R.P. & Emery, G. (1983) *Development of the Sociotropy-Autonomy Scale: A Measure of Personality Factors in Depression.* University of Pennsylvania Press, Philadelphia.

Beck, A.T., Freeman, A. *et al.* (1990) *Cognitive Therapy of Personality Disorder.* Guilford Press, New York.

Belsky, J. & Nezworski, T. (eds). (1988) *Clinical Implication of Attachment.* Erlbaum Associates, Hillsdale, NJ.

Blackburn, I.M. & Smyth, P. (1985) A test of cognitive vulnerability in individuals prone to depression. *British Journal of Clinical Psychology*, **24**, 61–62.

Blackburn, I.M., Jones, S. & Lewin, R.J.P. (1986) Cognitive style in depression. *British Journal of Clinical Psychology*, **25**, 241–251.

Blaney, P.H. & Kutcher, G.S. (1991) Measures of depressive dimensions: are they interchangeable? *Journal of Personality Assessment*, **56**, 502–512.

Blatt, S.J. (1974) Levels of object representation in anaclitic and introjective depression. *Psychoanalytic Studies of the Child*, **29**, 107–157.

Blatt, S.J. & Homman, E. (1992) Parent–child interaction in the etiology of dependent and self-critical depression. *Clinical Psychology Review*, **12**, 47–91.

Blatt, S.J., D'Afflitti, J.P. & Quiulan, D.M. (1979). *Depressive Experience Questionnaire.* Unpublished manual. Yale University, New Haven, CT.

Blatt, S.J., Quinlan, D.M., Chevon, E.S., McDonald, C. & Zuroff, D. (1982) Dependency and self-criticism: psychological dimensions of depression. *Journal of Consulting and Clinical Psychology*, **50**, 113–124.

Blatt, S.J., Quinlan, D.M. & Bers, S. (1992) Depression and the representation of parental behaviour in normal young adults. In: *Parent–child interaction in the etiology of dependent and self-critical depression. Clinical Psychology Review*, **12**, 47–92.

Bowlby, J. (1969) *Attachment and Loss*, Vol. 1. *Attachment* (2nd edn, 1982). Basic Books, New York.

Bowlby, J. (1973) *Attachment and Loss*, Vol. 2. *Separation, Anxiety and Anger.* Hogarth Press, London.

Bowlby, J. (1977) The making and breaking of affectionate bonds: Part 1, Etiology and psychopathology in light of attachment theory. *British Journal of Psychiatry,* **130**, 201–210.

Bowlby, J. (1980) *Attachment and Loss,* Vol. 3. *Loss, Separation and Depression.* Hogarth Press, London.

Bowlby, J. (1988) *A Secure Base: Clinical Implications of Attachment Theory.* Routledge & Kegan Paul, London.

Bradley, B. & Mathews, A. (1983) Negative self-schemata in clinical depression. *British Journal of Psychiatry,* **130**, 201–210.

Bradley, B. & Mathews, A. (1988) Memory bias in recovered clinical depressives. Special Issue: Information processing and emotional disorders. *Cognition and Emotion,* **2**, 235–245.

Brewin, C.R., Smith, A.J., Power, M. & Furnham, A. (1992a) State and trait differences in depressive self-perceptions. *Behaviour Therapy and Research,* **30**, 555–557.

Brewin, C.R., Firth-Cozens, J., Furham, A. & McManus, C. (1992b) Self-criticism in adulthood and recalled childhood experience. *Journal of Abnormal Psychology,* **101**, 561–566.

Brewin, C.R., Andrews, B. & Gotlib, I.H. (1993) Psychopathology and early experience: a reappraisal of retrospective reports. *Psychological Bulletin,* **113**, 82–98.

Brown, G.W. & Harris, T. (1978) *Social Origins of Depression.* Tavistock Publications, London.

Clark, D. (1983) On the induction of depressed mood in the laboratory: evaluation and comparison of the Velten and musical procedures. *Advances in Behaviour Research and Therapy,* **3**, 27–49.

Clark, D.A. & Teasdale, J.D. (1982) Diurnal variation in clincal depression and accessibility of memories of positive and negative experiences. *Journal of Abnormal Psychology,* **91**, 87–95.

Clark, D.A., Beck, A.T. & Brown, K. (1992) Sociotropy, autonomy and life event perceptions in dysphoric and nondysphoric individuals. *Cognitive Therapy and Research,* **16**, 635–652.

Clifford, P.I. & Hemsley, D.R. (1987) The influence of depression on the processing of personal attributes. *British Journal of Psychiatry,* **150**, 98–103.

Cook, L.M. & Peterson, C. (1986) Depressive irrationality. *Cognitive Therapy and Research,* **10**, 293–298.

Coyne, J.C. & Gotlib, I.H. (1983) The role of cognition in depression: A critical appraisal. *Psychological Bulletin,* **94**, 472–505.

DeMonbreun, B.G. & Craighead, W.E. (1977) Distortion of perception and recall of positive and neutral feedback in depression. *Cognitive Therapy and Research,* **1**, 311–329.

Derogatis, L.R. & Melisaratos, N. (1983) The Brief Symptom Inventory: An introductory report. *Psychological Medicine,* **13**, 595–605.

Dobson, K.S. & Shaw, B.F. (1986) Cognitive assessment with major depressive disorders. *Cognitive Therapy and Research,* **10**, 13–29.

Dyer, J.A.T. & Kreitman, N. (1984) Hopelesness, depression and suicidal intent in parasuicide. *British Journal of Psychiatry,* **114**, 127–133.

Evans, G. & Rush, A.J. (1984) Cognitive patterns in symptomatic and remitted unipolar major depression. *Journal of Abnormal Psychology,* **83**, 31–40.

Evans, M., Hollan, S.D., DeRubies, R.J., Piascki, J.M., Tuasson, V.B. & Vye, C. (1985) *Accounting for relapse in a treatment outcome study of depression.* Paper presented at the Annual Meeting of the Association for the Advancement of Behaviour Therapy, November.

Fennell, M.J.V., Teasdale, J.D., Jondes, S. & Damle, A. (1987) Distractions in neurotic and endogenous depression: an investigation of negative thinking in major depressive disorder. *Psychology Medicine,* **17**, 441–452.

Frost, R.O., Marten, P., Lahart, C.M. & Rosenblate, R. (1990) The dimensions of perfectionism. *Cognitive Therapy and Research,* **14**, 449–468.

Frost, R.O., Lahart, C.M. & Rosenblate, R. (1991) The development of perfectionism: a study of daughters and their parents. *Cognitive Therapy and Research,* **15**, 469–489.

Goldberg, J.O., Segal, Z.V., Vella, D.D. & Shaw, B.F. (1989) Depressive personality Milton Clinical Multi Axial Inventory profiles of sociotropic and autonomous subtypes. *Journal of Personality Disorder,* **3**, 193–198.

Golin, S. (1989) Schema congruence and depression: Loss of objectivity in self- and other-inferences. *Journal of Abnormal Psychology,* **98**, 495–498.

Gotlib, I.H. (1981) Self-reinforcement and recall: Differential deficits in depressed and nondepressed psychiatric inpatients. *Journal of Abnormal Psychology,* **90**, 521–530.

Gotlib, I.H. & Hammen, C.L. (1992) *Psychological Aspects of Depression: Towards a Cognitive-Interpersonal Integration.* John Wiley & Sons, Chichester.

Gotlib, I.H., Mount, J.H., Cordy, N.I. & Whiffen, V.E. (1988) Depression and perceptions of early parenting: a longitudinal investigation. *British Journal of Psychiatry,* **152**, 24–27.

Greenberg, M.S. & Beck, A. (1989) Depression vs. anxiety: a test of the content-specificity hypothesis. *Journal of Abnormal Psychology,* **98**, 9–13.

Greenberg, M.T., Cicchetti, D. & Cummings, M.

(eds) (1990) *Attachment in Preschool Year: Theory, Research and Intervention.* University of Chicago Press, Chicago.

Haaga, D.A., Dyck, M.J. & Ernst, D. (1991) Empirical status of cognitive theory of depression. *Psychological Bulletin,* **110**, 215–236.

Hamilton, E.W. & Abramson, L.Y. (1983) Cognitive patterns and major depressive disorder: a longitudinal study in a hospital setting. *Journal of Abnormal Psychology,* **92**, 173–184.

Hammen, C., Marks, T., Mayol, A. & de Mayo, R. (1985) Depressive self-schemas, life stress, and vulnerability to depression. *Journal of Abnormal Psychology,* **94**, 308–319.

Hammen, C., Elliott, A., Gitlin, M. & Jamieson, K.R. (1989) Sociotropy/autonomy and vulnerability to specific life events in patients with unipolar depression and bipolar disorder. *Journal of Abnormal Psychology,* **98**, 154–160.

Hammen, C., Elliott, A. & Gitlin, M. (1992) Stressor, sociotropy and autonomy: a longitudinal study of their relationship to the course of bipolar disorder. *Cognitive Therapy and Research,* **16**, 409–418.

Hinde, R.A. (1988) Continuities and discontinuities. Conceptual issues and methodological considerations. In: *Studies of Psychosocial Risk: The Power of Longitudinal Data* (ed. M. Rutter), pp. 367–383. Cambridge University Press, Cambridge.

Hollon, S.D. & Kendall, P.C. (1980) Cognitive self-statements in depression: development of an Automatic Thoughts Questionnaire. *Cognitive Therapy and Research,* **4**, 383–395.

Hollon, S.D., Kendall, P.C. & Lumry, A. (1986) Specificity of depressiotypic cognitions in clinical depression. *Journal of Abnormal Psychology,* **95**, 52–59.

Johnson, J.E., Petzel, T.P., Dupont, M.P. & Roamno, V.M. (1982) Phenomenological perceptions of parental evaluations in depressed and nondepressed college students. *Journal of Clinical Psychology,* **38**, 56–62.

Kazdin, A.E., French, N.H., Unis, A.S., Esveldt-Dawson, K. & Sherick, R.B. (1983) Hopelessness, depression and suicidal intent among psychiatrically disturbed inpatient children. *Journal of Consulting and Clinical Psychology,* **51**, 504–514.

Kelly, J.A. & Worrell, L. (1976) Parent behaviours related to masculine, feminine and androgenous sex role orientations. *Journal of Consulting and Clinical Psychology,* **44**, 843–851.

Krantz, S.E. (1985) When depressive cognitions reflect negative reality. *Cognitive Therapy and Research,* **9**, 61–77.

Krantz, S. & Hammen, C. (1979) Assessing cognitive bias in depression. *Journal of Abnormal Psy-chology,* **88**, 611–619.

Lakey, B. & Thomson-Ross, L. (1994) Dependency and self-criticism as moderators of interpersonal and achievement stress: the role of initial dysphoria. *Cognitive Therapy and Research,* **18**, 581–599.

Lam, D.H. & Power, M.J. (1991) A questionnaire designed to assess roles and goals: a preliminary study. *British Journal of Medical Psychology,* **64**, 359–374.

Lam, D.H., Brewin, C.R., Woods, R.T. & Beddington, P.E. (1987) Cognition and social adversity in the depressed elderly. *Journal of Abnormal Psychology,* **96**, 23–26.

Lam, D.H., Green, B., Power, M. & Checkley, S. (1996) Dependency, matching adversity and relapse in major depression. *Journal of Affective Disorders,* **37**, 81–90.

Lefebvre, M.F. (1981) Cognitive distortion and cognitive errors in depressed psychiatric and low back pain patients. *Journal of Consulting and Clinical Psychology,* **49**, 517–525.

Linville, P. (1985) Self-complexity and affective extremity: don't put all of your eggs in one cognitive basket. *Social Cognition,* **3**, 94–102.

Lloyd, G.G. & Lishman, W.A. (1975) Effects of depression on the speed of recall of pleasant and unpleasant experiences. *Psychological Medicine,* **5**, 173–180.

Main, M., Kaplan, N. & Cassidy, J. (1985) Security in infancy, childhood and adulthood: a move to the level of representation. In: *Growing Points in Attachment Theory and Research* (eds I. Bretherton & E. Waters), Vol. 50, Society for Research in Child Development Monographs, pp. 60–104. Chicago University Press, Chicago.

McCauley, E., Mitchell, J.R., Burke, P. & Moss, S. (1988) Cognitive attributes of depression in children and adolescents. *Journal of Consulting and Clinical Psychology,* **56**, 903–908.

McClelland, D.C., Atkinson, J.W., Clark, R.H. & Lowell, E.L. (1953) *The Achievement Motives.* Appleton-Century-Croft, New York.

McCraine, C.W. & Bass., J.D. (1984) Childhood family antecedents of dependency and self-criticism: implications for depression. *Journal of Abnormal Psychology,* **93**, 3–8.

Miranda, J. & Persons, J.D. (1988) Dysfunctional attitudes are mood dependent. *Journal of Abnormal Psychology,* **97**, 76–79.

Mongrain, M. & Zuroff, D.C. (1989) Cognitive vulnerability to depressed affect in dependent and self-critical college women. *Journal of Personality Disorders,* **3**, 240–251.

Myers, J.F., Lynch, P.B. & Bakal, D.A. (1989) Dysthymic and hypomanic self-referent effects associated with depressive illness and recovery. *Cognitive Therapy and Research,* **13**, 195–209.

Parker, G., Tupling, H. & Brown, L.B. (1979) A parental bonding instrument. *British Journal of Medical Psychology,* **52**, 1–10.

Parry, G. & Brewin, C.R. (1988) Cognitive style and depression: symptom-related, event-related or independent provoking factor? *British Journal of Clinical Psychology,* **27**, 23–35.

Person, J. (1994) Case conceptualisation in cognitive behavioural therapy. In: *Cognitive Therapy in Action* (eds K. T. Kuehlwein & H. Rosen). Jossey-Bass Publisher, San Francisco.

Power, M.J., Katz, R., McGuffin, P., Duggan, C.F., Lam, D. & Beck, A.T. (1994) The Dysfunctional Attitude Scale (DAS): a comparison of forms a and b and proposal for a new sub-scaled version. *Journal of Research in Personality,* **28**, 263–276.

Rajecki, D.W., Lamb, M.E. & Obmascher, P. (1978) Towards a general theory of infantile attachment: a comparative review of aspects of the social bond. *Brain and Behavioural Sciences,* **1**, 417–436.

Rippere, V. (1979) Scaling the helpfulness of antidepressive activities. *Behaviour Research and Therapy,* **17**, 439–449.

Rippere, V. (1981) Depression, common sense, and psychosocial evolution. *British Journal of Medical Psychology,* **54**, 379–387.

Robins, C.J. (1985) *Construct validation of the Sociotropy–Autonomy Scale: A measure of vulnerability in depression.* Paper presented at the annual meeting of the Eastern Psychological Association, Boston.

Robins, C.J. (1990) Congruence of personality and life events in depression. *Journal of Abnormal Psychology,* **99**, 393–397.

Robins, C.J. & Block, P. (1988) Personal vulnerability, life events and depressive symptoms. *Journal of Personality and Social Psychology,* **54**, 846–862.

Robins, C.J., Hayes, A.M., Block, P., Kramer, R.J. & Villena, M. (1995) Interpersonal and achievement concerns and the depressive vulnerability and symptom specificity hypotheses: a prospective study. *Cognitive Therapy and Research,* **19**, 1–20.

Rosenfarb, I.E., Becker, J., Khan, A. & Mintz, J. (1994) Dependency, self-criticism, and perceptions of socialisation experiences. *Journal of Abnormal Psychology,* **103**, 669–675.

Rude, S.S. & Burnham, B.I. (1993) Do interpersonal and achievement vulnerabilities interact with congruent events to predict depression? Comparison of DEQ, SAS, DAS and Combined Scales. *Cognitive Therapy and Research,* **17**, 531–549.

Rude, S.S., Krantz, S.E. & Rosenhan, D.L. (1988) Distinguishing the dimensions of valence and belief consistency in depressive and non-depressive information processing. *Cognitive Therapy and Research,* **12**, 391–407.

Rush, A.J., Weissenburger, J. & Evans, G. (1986) Do thinking patterns predict depressive symptoms? *Cognitive Therapy and Research,* **10**, 225–236.

Rutter, M. (1995) Clinical implications of attachment concepts: retrospective and prospective. *Journal of Child Psychology and Psychiatry,* **36**, 549–571.

Sandler, I.N. & Lakey, B. (1982) Locus of control as a stress moderator: the role of control perceptions and social support. *American Journal of Community Psychology,* **10**, 65–80.

Sarason, I.G., Johnson, J.H. & Siegel, J.M. (1978) Assessing the impact of life changes: development of the Life Experiences Survey. *Journal of Consulting and Clinical Psychology,* **46**, 932–946.

Schwarz, J.C. & Zuroff, D. (1979) Family structure and depression in female college students: effects of parental conflict, decision making power, and inconsistency of love. *Journal of Abnormal Psychology,* **88**, 398–406.

Sefran, J.D., Vallis, T.M., Segal, Z.V. & Shaw, B.F. (1986) Assessment of core cognitive processes in cognitive therapy. *Cognitive Therapy and Research,* **10**, 509–526.

Segal, Z.V., Shaw, B.F. & Vella, D.D. (1989) Life stress and depression: a test of the congruency hypothesis for life event content and depressive subtype. *Canadian Journal of Behavioural Science,* **21**, 389–400.

Segal, Z.V., Shaw, B.F., Vella, D.D. & Katz, R. (1992) Cognitive and life stress predictors of relapse in remitted unipolar depressed patients: a test of the congruency hypothesis. *Journal of Abnormal Psychology,* **101**, 26–36.

Siegelman, M. & Roe, A. (1979) *Manual: The Parent–Child Relations Questionnaire: II.* City College of New York, New York.

Silverman, J.S., Silverman, J.A. & Eardley, D.A. (1984) Do maladaptive attitudes cause depression: misconception of cognitive theory. *Archives of General Psychiatry,* **41**, 1112.

Simons, A.D., Garfield, S.L. & Murphy, G.E. (1984) The process of change in cognitive therapy and pharmacotherapy for depression. *Archives of General Psychiatry,* **41**, 45–51.

Simons, A.D., Murphy, G.E., Levine, J. & Wetzel, R.D. (1986) Cognitive therapy and pharmacotherapy for depression. *Archives of General Psychiatry,* **43**, 43–50.

Simons, A.D., Angell, K.L., Monroe, S.M. & Thase, M.E. (1993) Cognition and life stress in depression: cognitive factors and the definitions, rating and generation of negative life events. *Journal of Abnormal Psychology,* **102**, 584–591.

Steketee, G., Grayson, J. & Foa, E. (1985) Obsessive-compulsive disorder: differences between washers and checkers. *Behaviour Research and Therapy,* **23**, 197–201.

Teasdale, J. (1988) Cognitive vulnerability to persistent depression. *Cognition and Emotion,* **2**, 247–274.

Teasdale, J. & Bancroft, J. (1977) Manipulation of thought content as a determinant of mood and corrugator EMG in depressed patients. *Journal of Abnormal Psychology,* **86**, 235–241.

Teasdale, J. & Fogarty, S. (1979) Differential effects of induced mood on retrieval of pleasant and unpleasant events from episodic memory. *Journal of Abnormal Psychology,* **88**, 248–257.

Teasdale, J. & Rezin, V. (1978) The effects of reducing frequency of negative thoughts on the mood of depressed patients: tests of a cognitive theory of depression. *British Journal of Social and Clinical Psychology,* **17**, 65–74.

Teasdale, J.D. & Russel, M.L. (1983) Differential effects of induced mood on the recall of positive, negative and neutral words. *British Journal of Clinical Psychology,* **22**, 163–172.

Teasdale, J., Taylor, R. & Fogarty, S. (1980) Effects of induced elation–depression on the accessibility of memories of happy and unhappy experiences. *Behaviour Research and Therapy,* **18**, 339–346.

Thomas, C.B. & Duszynski, K.R. (1974) Closeness to parents and the family constellation in a prospective study of five disease states. *Johns Hopkins Medical Journal,* **134**, 251–270.

Velten, E. (1968) A laboratory task for induction of mood states. *Behaviour Research and Therapy,* **6**, 473–482.

Weissman, A. & Beck, A.T. (1979) *Development and Validation of the Dysfunctional Attitude Scale: A Preliminary Investigation.* Paper presented at the annual meeting of the American Education Research Association.

Welkowitz, J., Lish, J.D. & Bond, R.N. (1985) The Depressive Experiences Questionnaire: revision and validation. *Journal of Personality Assessment,* **49**, 89–94.

Wenzlaff, R.M. & Grozier, S.A. (1988) Depression and the magnification of failure. *Journal of Abnormal Psychology,* **97**, 90–93.

Williams, J.M.G. (1984) *The Psychological Treatment of Depression.* Routledge, London and New York.

Williams, J.M.G., Healy, J.D., Teasdale, J.D., White, W. & Paykel, E.S. (1990) Dysfunctional attitudes and vulnerability to persistent depression. *Psychological Medicine,* **20**, 375–381.

Zung, W.W.K. (1965) A self-rating depression scale, *Archives of General Psychiatry,* **12**, 63–70.

Zuroff, D.C., Igreja, I. & Mongrain, M. (1990) Dysfunctional attitudes, dependency, and self-criticism as predictors of depressive mood states: a 12-month longitudinal study. *Cognitive Therapy and Research,* **14**, 315–326.

6 A psychodynamic-interpersonal model of depression based on attachment theory

GILLIAN E. HARDY

Psychoanalytic (Abraham, 1911; Freud, 1917; Cohen *et al.*, 1954; Mendelson, 1960) and interpersonal theorists (Coyne, 1976a; Brown & Harris, 1978; Klerman & Weissman, 1982; Lewinsohn, 1985) have pointed to the importance of interpersonal processes in promoting and maintaining depression. While the psychoanalytic theorists have described how early childhood experiences of interpersonal processes are important precursors of depression, particularly the quality of the child–parent (usually mother) relationship, interpersonal theorists have tended to focus on the functional role of depression. Interpersonal theories emphasize how problematic interpersonal interactions develop when a person becomes depressed. Psychoanalytic theories have described how parental rejection and lack of warmth and availability can lead to ambivalent feelings towards important figures which, if reactivated in adulthood, result in regression to earlier beliefs of helplessness and hopelessness. Self-esteem and mood are then lowered, feelings of inadequacy and anger are turned inwards, and a depressive episode may be experienced. Interpersonal theorists, in contrast, focus on the current relationship difficulties of the depressed individual. Such difficulties lead to a reduction in social reinforcement (Libet & Lewinsohn, 1973; Weissman & Paykel, 1974) and the pattern of interacting between the depressed person and others becomes confused and unsupportive (Coyne, 1976a).

Despite the abundance of theoretical accounts of depression, research studies of the social and interpersonal context of depression have not been guided by a cohesive theory (Gotlib, 1992), and attempts at synthesis of the research in this area (for example, Segrin & Dillard, 1992) have led to complex and often contradictory conclusions (Burchill & Stiles, 1995). In addition, many writers have not considered depression as a separate illness, but as one element of the array of disturbances a person may display when faced with interpersonal and social difficulties. Strupp *et al.* (1982), for example, wrote, 'the objective of developing relatively specific treatments for relatively specific clinical conditions has been basically alien to psychoanalytic psychotherapy' (p. 217) Although a psychoanalytic clinician observes and describes the same symptoms, mood and behaviours as clinicians from a cognitive or biological background, they understand them in a different way. Part of the problem of producing an inclusive intra- and interpersonal theory of depression is that it requires multiple meanings to be attached to the same phenomena; as Coyne (1985) noted, there is no neutral language to describe depression, viewpoints are not distinct from their data.

In this chapter attachment theory (Bowlby, 1969, 1973, 1980) will be used to move beyond these conflicts in the literature. Attachment theory incorporates both intra-individual or personality mechanisms involved in the aetiology of depression and interpersonal factors that lead to the maintenance and relapse of depression. Although attachment is conceived of as a fundamental human motivation (Baumeister & Leary, 1995), specific early attachment experiences are thought to predispose the individual to depression. These attachment experiences lead to dysfunctional working models about the self, others and relationships, which leave the individual vulnerable to depression when faced with life events that activate the attachment system. Early dysfunctional attachment experiences, it is proposed, can lead to two basic attachment styles that, in turn, can lead to two types of depression based on threats to interpersonal relations and threats to self-esteem (Blatt & Zuroff, 1992). Thus, attachment theory provides a conceptual model within which much of the psychodynamic and interpersonal work in this area can be organized.

Attachment theory

The attachment system

Attachment theory originated from Bowlby's seminal work with infants on the impact of separation from their care-giver (Bowlby, 1969, 1973, 1980). In three volumes entitled *Attachment, Separation and Loss*, Bowlby documented the emotional bond that infants develop with their primary care-giver and the serious consequences that follow if this bond is disrupted. Predictable stages of emotional responses were recorded following separation. These were, first, *protest*, when infants cry, search for their care-givers and resist others' attempts to soothe; second, *despair*, when infants are visibly sad and passive; and third, *detachment*, characterized by a seeming defensive disregard for the care-givers. From this work Bowlby argued that there was a primary motivational system to seek contact with and security from a care-giver. This is known as the attachment system and is evidenced most clearly when situations are seen as dangerous or threatening. Considerable evidence of these elements of attachment behaviour in children has been obtained from naturalistic and laboratory studies (Rutter, 1979; Maccoby, 1980; Bretherton, 1985; Erickson *et al.*, 1985).

Bowlby listed the primary features of the attachment system as a bond with specific individuals who are seen as stronger and wiser, which is enduring and serves the function of protection and survival. The attachment bond has a strong emotional component that can be positive (such as when being renewed) or negative (when threatened or lost). In addition, because attachment behaviour is driven by a primary motivation, attachments develop irrespective of the ability of care-givers to respond appropriately or consistently.

Attachment, security and exploration

In evolutionary terms, the attachment system is seen as providing infants with a means of obtaining protection from danger by keeping them close to their care-giver. If the primary care-givers are responsive and sensitive to a child's attachment signals, then that child will form a 'secure base' from which to manage emotional experience and handle distress (Bowlby, 1988). Such children will then be able to use their care-giver as a base from which to explore their environment. Providing a secure base involves care-givers being both emotionally responsive and providing physical security.

The attachment system, or care-seeking behaviour, is complemented by what Bowlby called 'exploratory behaviour'. If children experience their care-givers as available and responsive, then they will increasingly move further and further away from their care-givers in order to explore and master their environment and establish friendships with a widening net of social contacts (Main, 1983).

Attachment behaviour in adulthood

Bowlby hypothesized that infants and children internalize their attachment experiences and form internal working models of themselves and their relationships with significant others. According to Bowlby these working models are central components of personality:

> … confidence that an attachment figure is likely to be responsive depends on (a) whether the attachment figure is judged to be the sort of person who in general responds to calls for support and protection; and (b) whether or not the self is judged to be the sort of person towards whom anyone in general, and the attachment figure in particular, is likely to respond in a helpful way … as a result, the model of the attachment figure and the model of the self are likely to develop so as to be complementary and mutually confirming.
> (Bowlby, 1973, p. 238)

These internal working models are thought to be enduring structures and so they provide people throughout their lives with the experience of 'felt security' (or insecurity) (Blunstein *et al.*, 1991). Social, interpersonal and exploratory behaviour will be influenced by the experience of security (provided in infancy almost totally by the responsiveness of care-givers) and, as cognitive structures become more sophisticated, increasingly by felt security (which is a product of a person's internal working models).

The attachment pattern established in infancy was also seen by Bowlby as continuing throughout adulthood (Bowlby, 1979). This fundamental need to form and maintain interpersonal bonds, pervading adult life but beginning in infancy with one's primary care-givers, also forms the basis of psychoanalytic thinking (Freud, 1930; Horney, 1945; Guisinger & Blatt, 1994). In a review of the literature, Baumeister and Leary (1995, p. 497) concluded that sufficient evidence exists to support the hypothesis that the 'need to belong is a powerful, fundamental, and extremely pervasive motivation'. Hazan and Shaver (1987) argued that there was a strong case for conceptualizing adult romantic relationships as attachment processes. These separate strands of theoretical and empirical support began what is now a major interest in applying attachment theory to describe, explain and predict adult social behaviour within both normal and psychiatric populations (Bowlby, 1977; Bartholomew & Perlman, 1994).

Attachment theory and depression

According to attachment theory, psychopathology therefore results from deviant patterns of attachment behaviour established early in life, which persist through the influence of internal working models and affect interpersonal relationships in adult life. Bowlby's original work on loss experiences has been used to clarify the processes that underlie the development of depression. Threat of separation from or loss of an attachment figure results, initially, in anger and protest. It is thought that the function of anger is to achieve reunion with the lost figure (Parkes, 1972). If protests go unheeded, then anger gives way to despair and then finally to detachment. These processes are part of normal grieving, but if experienced early in life, or repeatedly without resolution, then despair and detachment become the customary response when a person (child or adult) is faced with a threatening situation. Such responses make the person vulnerable to a sense of helplessness and to depression (Bowlby, 1973). Seligman (1975) showed how this phenomenon of 'learned helplessness' is active in producing depressed states. Attachment theory therefore links depression to: (i) early experiences of care-giving; (ii) expectations and interpretations of others' behaviour; and (iii) current relationship functioning (Carnelley *et al.*, 1994).

Early experiences of caregiving

Early attachment experiences can provide children with models of themselves as loveable and competent, and with models of others as supportive, warm and reliable. Such models are likely to lead children to develop a style of what Ainsworth *et al.* (1978) described as 'secure attachment'. Children who experience their important care-givers as cold, unavailable or inconsistent, in contrast, are likely to develop patterns of 'insecure attachments' through their poor and inflexible working models of themselves in relationships with others.

Psychodynamic understandings of depression also point to the central importance of early experiences. Freud (1917) originally saw depression as the result of the loss of either a loved one or a 'narcissistic need' or an unrelinquished wish to be loved, superior or good (Rapaport, 1959). A basic ambivalence towards the lost person (i.e. the individual feels both love and hate towards the lost person), means grief is not worked through, but the individual maintains anger towards the lost 'object' (person or need), which then is turned inward towards the self. Sustained self anger is then a cause of guilt and depression.

Working models of others

Cognitive theories (see Chapter 5) focus on the depressed person's view of him/herself. Studies based on these theories have shown that depressed people, in comparison to non-depressed people, have a negative view of themselves, the world and the future (Beck, 1967). Some research into depressed people's views of others, however, has produced conflicting findings. Some studies have found that depressed individuals have a negative view of others (Pietromonaco *et al.*, 1992), while others have found that depressed people are more positive about others than about themselves (Bargh & Tota, 1988). These findings are perhaps tapping two underlying dimensions of depression that will be discussed later, and are based on the early experiences of attachment figures being either: (i) rejecting, resulting in people feeling negative about themselves, *but* positive about their attachment figure; or (ii) inconsistent, resulting in people feeling negative about themselves *and* their attachment figures.

Current relationship functioning

The role of intimate relationships in depression is seen as central by many writers from Cohen *et al.* (1954), through the experientialists (Rogers, 1959; Perls *et al.*, 1951) to Coyne (1976b). There is indeed convincing evidence to show that relationships involving depressed people are often distressed; for example, Gotlib and Hooley (1988) concluded that the marital relationships of depressed people tend to be conflictual and unhappy and are characterized by poor communication. Weissman and Paykel (1974) found that depressed women were impaired in their social functioning, expressed hostility and dissatisfaction with their spouses or partners, and that the couples had poor levels of communication. Attachment theory would, of course, predict that the relationships of depressed individuals reflect their past attachment experiences, and are likely to be insecure and problematic.

Coyne's (1976b) model of depression is also based on the communication patterns between a depressed person and her/his close relationships. Coyne conceptualized depression as a response to a disruption in a person's social structure, which eventually comes to be supported and validated by others (Burchill & Stiles, 1995). When first depressed, a person obtains the sympathy and support of their close ones. If the depression continues, then the depressive symptomatology no longer produces concern in others but frustration and a burdensome sense of undischarged responsibility for the depressed person. The spouse or close friend then feels guilty as their concern comes to be tempered by anger, helplessness and a wish to avoid too much or too close a contact with the depressed person. This, in turn, reinforces the depressed person's view of themselves as unloveable and so a vicious circle is set up.

This research has clear implications for choice of treatments in the management of depression; for example, the Interpersonal Treatment (Klerman & Weissman, 1982) used in the National Institute of Mental Health study of depression (Elkin *et al.*, 1989) and the Psychodynamic-Interpersonal treatment (Hobson, 1985; Shapiro & Firth, 1985) used in the Second Sheffield Psychotherapy study (Shapiro *et al.*, 1994) are based on the premise that depression occurs in a social and interpersonal context that needs to be understood for improvement to occur.

Attachment styles and types of depressive experience

There is now substantial evidence to suggest that poor childhood attachment experiences lead to a vulnerability to depression in adulthood (Basic Behavioural Task Force, 1996). This vulnerability can be triggered by a number of life experiences (see Klerman & Weissman, 1982). These have been grouped into two main types: disruptions of interpersonal relations and experiences of failure, guilt or loss of control (see Table 6.1). These, in turn, lead to two forms of depressive reactions, dependent and self-critical (Blatt & Homann, 1992). The dependent depressed individual is someone who relies heavily on others, is fearful of being alone and whose depression is characterized by feelings of loss, abandonment and inability to face the future using their own

Table 6.1 Schematic summary of literature on dependent and self-critical depression styles. (From Blatt, S.J. (1991) Depression and self destructive behaviour in adolescence. In: *Self-Regulatory Behaviour and Risk-Taking: Causes and Consequences* (eds L. P. Lipsett & L. L. Mitnick)). Ablex, Norwood, NJ. Copyright 1991 by Ablex Publishing Corp. Reprinted by permission.

Distal precipitating events (parental styles)	Personality organization (dysphoria)	Proximal precipitating events (life stress)	Clinical disorders
1 Inconsistent, neglectful, rejecting, abandoning and/or overindulgent parents. Anxious/ ambivalent attachment	*Interpersonal vulnerability* Dependent, affectively labile, preoccupied with attachment and interpersonal relations. Use of avoidant defences (denial and repression)	Disruptions of interpersonal relations, experiences of loss, abandonment, and rejection	*Dependent depression* Feeling sad and lonely, rejected, unloved, abandoned. Helpless searching for an object who will care, soothe, feed and provide love. Somatic preoccupation, eating disorders, sexual acting out. Suicide-passive
2 Caring and dependable parents who are able to establish appropriate and constructive limits, set appropriate standards and goals, and provide approval and criticism in constructive ways. Secure attachment	*Relative Invulnerability* Able to form mature, mutual reciprocal relationships. Able to enjoy one's talent and capacities and to accept comfortably one's shortcomings and limitations		Normal grief and sadness (mourning) without protracted, prolonged severe depression
3 Intrusive, controlling, judgemental, punitive parents. Avoidant attachment	*Self-evaluative vulnerability* Striving self-critical, overcompensating; preoccupied with issues of failure/ success, blame and responsibility. Hostile, critical, angry. Use of counteractive defences (projection, reaction formation, overcompensation)	Experiences of failure, guilt diminished self-esteem, loss of control and an impaired sense of mastery. Feeling criticized, unappreciated, and ridiculed	*Self-critical depression* Feelings of worthlessness self-criticism and guilt. Constant striving to compensate for perceived feelings of guilt and inferiority. Serious attempts to hurt self and others. Anti-social delinquency, violence (aggression). Suicide-violent

resources. The self-critical depressed person, in contrast, is fearful of disapproval by others, strives for perfection and suffers from feelings of unworthiness, failure and guilt. The attachment styles that result in these two types of depression have been called, respectively, anxious/ambivalent and avoidant

(Ainsworth *et al.*, 1978; although see Main *et al.*, 1985 for an alternative termi-nology). These attachment styles or interpersonal strategies develop from and reflect the responsiveness of the person's care-giver. If the care-giver responds negatively to an infant's demands, then the infant will learn to avoid expres-sion of internal states, but will have a sense that the relationship with the care-giver is predictable, at least in a cognitive or causal sense. However, such an individual will not learn to use and understand her/his emotions; an avoidant pattern of engagement with others is developed. If, on the other hand, a care-giver is inconsistent, the infant will not be able to organize her/his behaviour nor develop a sense of mastery within interpersonal relation-ships, and will have intense feelings of insecurity for long periods. Such experiences lead to ambivalent interpersonal attachments, in which there is intense emotional expression, but little ability to observe and make use of causal relationships between events. The links between these two attachment styles and dependent and self-critical depression are shown in Table 6.1 (taken from Blatt, 1991) and are discussed below.

This summary of two types of depression represents the views of many interpersonal, psychodynamic and cognitive writers; for example, Arieti and Bemporad (1978) state that when depressed the person is trying either: (i) to (re)gain the love and attention of a 'dominant other' on whom the individual feels dependent for support, self-esteem and well-being (anxious/ambiva-lent); or (ii) to be reassured of her/his worth and be free of guilt following failure to reach a self-imposed goal of impossibly high standards (avoidant). Arieti and Bemporad called these two forms of depression 'dominant other' and 'dominant goal', respectively. Blatt and Zuroff (1992) describe two forms of depression that result when there are disruptions to interpersonal relation-ships (anaclitic depression) or threats to self-integrity and self-esteem (introjective depression). Finally, Beck (1983) distinguished between 'sociotropic depression', where there is a vulnerability to loss or disruptions in interpersonal relationships (anxious/ambivalent), and 'autonomous de-pression', which is characterized by fear of failure and criticism and loss of control (avoidant). Although these writers have many different components to their theories, the basic distinction between the two forms of depression remains similar.

Anxious/ambivalent attachments and dependent depression

Early experiences of individuals with anxious/ambivalent attachments are characterized primarily by inconsistent parenting. Sometimes the child's needs are attended to and sometimes not; sometimes quickly, sometimes slowly; sometimes overindulgently, but often not. The care-giver is frequently intru-sive, but again can be unpredictably absent or abandoning. Children of such care-givers give frequent affective signals of distress, which are maintained because they are partially reinforced (Crittendon, 1992). However, these children are not able to learn any consistently effective way of signalling to others. As a result, they remain dependent on their care-giver and fail to develop a sense of their own capacities or self-esteem. This later translates into a preoccupation with relationships, beliefs that they are relatively ineffective, difficulty in judging the seriousness of situations and displays of extreme feelings; for example, Arieti and Bemporad (1980) emphasize how anxious/ambivalent individuals fail to individuate and develop autonomy.

These experiences and strategies become built into the person's internal working models of the self, others and interpersonal relationships. Such working models Blatt (1991) calls Personality Organization (see Table 6.1) and predispose the individual to respond to certain stressful life events with a depressive reaction, particularly events with an interpersonal component, such as the experience of loss, abandonment or rejection. Such events assume greater salience if the individual sees him/herself as being responsible for them, or if the individual sees her/himself as being dependent on the other person. Indeed, there is some evidence that individuals may be differentially vulnerable to different types of life events (Hammen *et al.*, 1985).

The content of anxious/ambivalent depressed people's experience is therefore one of sadness, loneliness, helplessness and dependency. This has been called dependent or anaclitic depression by Blatt and Zuroff (1992). Such people have no satisfactory sense of themselves or their future, without reliance on protection and support from another. However, although they desire close interpersonal contact, there is also evidence that when they are in close relationships, they see their partners as less positive, supportive and intimate than do non-depressed individuals. Even so, because of their dependency and felt need for others, they have great difficulty in expressing anger or dissatisfaction. Similarly, the partner of the depressed individual experiences hostility, disappointment and dependency, but feels unable to resolve such issues openly (Coyne, 1976b). So, a cycle of need, expectancy and disappointment in interpersonal relationships develops.

Avoidant attachments and self-critical depression

Care-givers who respond predictably to their children's need, but in a way that increases discomfort, are likely to produce avoidant attachments in their children. Such care-givers may be unavailable, or they may be intrusive and controlling, but they consistently either fail to respond or their responses are poor. The children then learn to ignore their own feelings because this will result in uncomfortable reactions from their care-giver. They take responsibility for managing situations, avoid meaningful interactions with others and are preoccupied with controlling events. These individuals are often very self-critical, preoccupied with success and feel guilty and responsible for any failures they encounter. They tend to avoid close interactions with other people and invest in achievements rather than relationships. Emotional expression is limited, but underneath the desire for success is the belief that this will bring approval and a sense of being valued by others.

If such avoidant people experience failure or loss of control, then their fragile self-esteem is significantly impaired and dysphoric mood results. The content of their depressive thoughts is of self-deprecation and guilt. They feel that they have not lived up to their own self-imposed standards, and they will inevitably lose the respect and love of those around them. Blatt and Zuroff (1992) have called this form of depression self-critical or introjective.

Links with self-esteem and emotional functioning

The concepts of self-esteem and affect regulation have often been referred to in the preceding descriptions of attachment theory and types of depression. Indeed, in both psychodynamic and interpersonal theories, loss of self-esteem is one of the central symptoms of a depressive episode and one of the vulnerability factors for depression. Affect, such as anger, disappointment, guilt and sadness, is also described in psychodynamic interpretations of depression. Experientialists, although they would reject many of the psychodynamic understandings of such phenomena, see psychological distress, including depression, as a result of the meanings people attach to their mood or affect (Greenberg *et al.*, 1993).

Self-esteem refers to our views of whether other people value, respect and like us. To have low self-esteem is to say that we feel that others have little regard for us, that they do not like us or think we have little to offer to them or to society in general. The concept is interpersonal in that it reflects individuals' views of themselves in relation to others. This concept is, of course, part of what Bowlby called the 'internal working model'. It develops based on our experiences of how others, especially care-givers, have responded to us. In securely attached children, care-givers have generally responded positively, consistently and responsively to demands and needs, giving children the sense that they are valued and loved and confident that their requests for support or help will be met. Such children develop positive and robust self-esteem. In contrast, children who are unsure whether care-givers will respond helpfully and with affection, or who know that any displays of upset or need will be rejected, are fundamentally less sure about their place or survival in the world. As they grow, their self-esteem remains fragile. Although they may develop strategies for avoiding the pain of not feeling valued, if these are challenged too strenuously then the early feelings of rejection and disappointment are likely to resurface resulting in low self-esteem. Anxious/ambivalent people and avoidant people, respectively, depend on closeness with others and success for self-esteem.

There are significant differences in the emotional functioning of anxious/ambivalent and avoidant individuals. Anxious/ambivalent people tend to show a great deal of emotional lability. They are anxious about being ignored or abandoned, need reassurance and demand emotional investment from other people. It is this that often leads others to feel annoyed and trapped, resulting in the depressed pattern of interacting described by Coyne (1976b). The emotions expressed by the anxious/ambivalently depressed person are what the experientialists call the automatic 'activation of dysfunctional emotion schemas' (Greenberg *et al.*, 1993). By this they mean that certain situations or actions automatically activate particular emotional responses without the individual consciously appraising the situation, for example, perceived loss or rejection will inevitably result in feelings of anger and protest, whatever the context.

Avoidant individuals avoid emotional expression both in themselves and from others. They do not utilize the emotional information available to them, and exhibit what the experientialists call 'dysfunction in symbolizing'. When faced with a potentially upsetting or difficult situation, avoidant people will ignore their physiological experiences of emotion (such as increased heart rate associated with anger). They have failed to develop an effective language for expressing how they are feeling and consequently, when depressed, experience emptiness and flatness, rather than grief or anger.

Implications for clinical practice

There now exists compelling evidence for many aspects of attachment theory's hypotheses concerning the development of depression. Depression not only comprises specific symptomatology, but also affects quality of life pervasively, especially in the area of interpersonal relationships. It is a recurrent disorder, and the emotional and relationship deficits that occur within a depressive episode are likely to contribute to future relapse (Brown *et al.*, 1977; Barnett & Gotlib, 1988; Hooley & Teasdale, 1989; Marcus & Nardone, 1992). Moreover, depression runs in families; children of depressed mothers are twice as likely to suffer from depression than children of non-depressed mothers (Hammen, 1991). It can be concluded safely that vulnerability to depression begins in childhood and is dependent upon the context or environment within which the at-risk person finds themselves. Whilst biological and cognitive factors may contribute to the aetiology and maintenance of the condition, interpersonal factors constitute a common theme across all models, whether this be at the stage of early life experiences resulting in a vulnerability for depression, or the later family dynamics of a depressed person maintaining a depressive cycle.

For the clinician interpersonal issues are therefore important to assess at three stages: vulnerability factors, mechanisms of change in treatment, and maintaining treatment gains. These will be considered in turn.

Vulnerability factors

Using attachment representations and style as a focus, the depressed person's vulnerability can be assessed in two ways: their self concept and their interpersonal history. Poor relationships with care-givers in childhood may lead to insecure attachments. This, in turn, may leave the individual excessively dependent on others and fearful of rejection or abandonment (anxious/ambivalent), or rejecting of close relationships and fearful of being controlled or hurt. Both of these experiences lead to a fragile self-concept.

The anxious/ambivalent person when depressed is likely to have a lowered sense of self-worth and feel that they have little to contribute to the world; for example, they may feel that they 'have nothing of value to contribute to a relationship, group or even society at large' (Gilbert, 1992). Following the loss of a confiding relationship (associated with onset of a depressive episode, Brown & Harris, 1978), anxious/ambivalent people often feel that they are not sufficiently interesting to be worthy of the attention or concern of anyone, including that of the person they have just lost. The anxious/ambivalent person needs closeness to others to maintain any sense of self-esteem.

The avoidant person has feelings of personal inadequacy. To avoid these feelings, such a person invests in some demanding (and often unrealizable) goal. Depression follows failure to reach this goal, with the linked fear that other people will no longer show respect or liking. The avoidant person, when faced with failure, may also feel loss of belief in self-control or ability to change things and begin to feel hopeless about the future.

The interpersonal history of both anxious/ambivalent and avoidant individuals is likely to include a pattern of dysfunctional relationships. The mother–child interactions of depressed mothers, when compared to interactions with non-depressed mothers, are less positive, more critical and show less involvement (Rutter, 1990). A depressed woman often chooses a depressed partner and the marriages of depressed people, on the whole, are more stressful, more conflictual and are more likely to break down (Gotlib & Hooley, 1988). Assessment of current attachment style and attachment representations of care-givers can give the clinician a good picture of interpersonal functioning and of more general life functioning (i.e. exploratory behaviour).

Mechanisms of change

The aims of an interpersonal-psychodynamic treatment are to understand and modify the problems that have arisen as a result of disturbances of significant personal relationships. The primary mechanisms through which change is assumed to occur are: (i) through the relationship and dialogue between the therapist and patient; and (ii) through the expression of feelings associated with difficult experiences from past, current and therapeutic relationships. These mechanisms are described in a generic model of psychotherapy (Garfield & Bergin, 1986) in which the therapeutic contract, the therapeutic intervention (which in interpersonal therapies involves the expression of feelings and relationship difficulties) and the therapeutic bond (patient–therapist relationship) contribute to therapeutic self-realizations (such as insight, resolution of conflicts) and the patient's self-relatedness (their personality, or their attachment internal working model). These, in turn, influence the outcome of psychotherapy.

In treatment the interpersonal issues facing the patient will be reflected in the relationship that develops between the patient and the therapist. This provides the therapist with material for exploring, understanding and modifying relationship difficulties. The methods for achieving this will not be described in this chapter, but involve the therapist developing conversational strategies that enable the patient to disclose and re-experience problematic feelings in relationships, develop a language for expressing these feelings, understand the nature, origins and consequences of the feelings and seek new solutions to the interpersonal problems (Rounsaville & Chevron, 1982; Hobson, 1985; Greenberg *et al.*, 1993).

Maintenance of treatment gains

It has been argued throughout this chapter that depression is a developmental disorder in the sense that vulnerability is established early in childhood, patterns of relationship functioning and beliefs about the self are developed from these early experiences through working models, and these show stability over time (McCrae & Costa, 1988; van Ijzendoorn, 1995). The close relationships of depressed individuals are more stressful and less secure than those of non-depressed individuals, leading to greater vulnerability to subsequent depressive episodes (Merikangas *et al.*, 1985). However, if depressed people have supportive marriages, they are more likely to maintain treatment gains than depressed people with conflictual marriages, and single people (i.e. those without attachment figures) are the depressed group least likely to maintain treatment gains (Hardy *et al.*, 1996).

This points to the importance of considering marital and family relationships and support networks of the depressed person even when in remission (see Chapter 4 on social theories of depression). Equally, the interactive style of the depressed person will suggest what sort of life stressors will increase their likelihood for another depressive episode. Understanding the attachment process and increasing the flexibility of the attachment response in the patient will reduce the likelihood of relapse. In addition, the clinician should be a responsive attachment figure for the patient both during treatment and through the follow-up period.

Summary

It is clear that interpersonal contexts, both historical and current, influence the nature and course of depression. Attachment theory provides a powerful framework for organizing current knowledge of these influences. Early caregiving experiences help determine the way people see themselves and their styles of interacting with others. These 'internal working models' of the self and others make individuals vulnerable to stressful events that threaten their interpersonal relationships or their self-esteem. It has been suggested that two types of depression result from these different life events: dependent and self-critical depression. In addition, the depressed person's interactions with others help to maintain depressive symptomatology, and increase the likelihood of future depressive episodes.

This conceptual framework, initially developed by Bowlby, but expanded and further articulated by many researchers since, links together both traditional psychodynamic and social psychological models of depression. It represents an overarching and powerfully practical approach to understanding some of the causes and consequences of depression. The value of this approach for preventing and treating depression is great, although it is only recently that researchers and clinicians have begun to recognize how valuable it is.

References

Abraham, K. (1911) Notes on the psycho-analytic investigation and treatment of manic-depressive insanity and allied conditions. Reprinted in: *Essential Papers on Depression* (ed. J.C. Coyne) (1985). New York University Press, New York.

Ainsworth, M.D.S., Blehar, M.C., Waters, E. & Wall, S. (1978) *Patterns of Attachment: A Psychological Study of the Strange Situation.* Erlbaum, Hillsdale, NJ.

Arieti, S. & Bemporad, J.R. (1978) *Severe and Mild Depression: The Therapeutic Approach.* Basic Books, New York.

Arieti, S. & Bemporad, J.R. (1980) The psychological organization of depression. *American Journal of Psychiatry,* **137**, 1356–1365.

Bargh, J. & Tota, M.E. (1988) Context-dependent automatic processing in depression: accessibility of negative constructs with regard to self but not others. *Journal of Personality and Social Psychology,* **54**, 925–939.

Barnett, P.A. & Gotlib, I.H. (1988) Psychosocial functioning and depression: distinguishing among antecedents, concomitants, and consequences. *Psychological Bulletin,* **104**, 97–126.

Bartholomew, K. & Perlman, D. (1994) *Attachment Processes in Adulthood: Advances in Personal Relationships*, Vol. 5. Jessica Kingsley, London.

Basic Behavioral Task Force (1996) Basic behavioral science research for mental health: vulnerability and resilience. *American Psychologist*, **51**, 22–28.

Baumeister, R.F. & Leary, M.R. (1995) The need to belong: desires for interpersonal attachments as a fundamental human motivation. *Psychological Bulletin*, **117**, 497–529.

Beck, A.T. (1967) *Depression: Causes and Treatment.* University of Philadelphia Press, Philadelphia, PA.

Beck, A.T. (1983) *Cognitive Therapy and the Emotional Disorders*. International Universities Press, New York.

Blatt, S.J. (1991) Depression and destructive risk-taking behavior in adolescence. In: *Self-regulatory Behavior and Risk-taking: Causes and Consequences* (eds L. P. Lipsett & L. L. Mitnick), pp. 285–309. Ablex, Norwood, NJ.

Blatt, S.J. & Homann, E. (1992) Parent–child interaction in the etiology of dependent and self-critical depression. *Clinical Psychology Review,* **12**, 47–91.

Blatt, S.J. & Zuroff, D.C. (1992) Interpersonal relatedness and self definition: two prototypes for depression. *Clinical Psychology Review,* **12**, 527–562.

Blunstein, D.L., Walbridge, M.M., Friedlander, M.L. & Palladino, D.E. (1991) Contributions of psychological separation and parental attachment to the career development process. *Journal of Counseling Psychology*, **38**, 39–50.

Bowlby, J. (1969) *Attachment and Loss*, Vol. 1. *Attachment*. Basic Books, New York.

Bowlby, J. (1973) *Attachment and Loss*, Vol. 2. *Separation, Anxiety and Anger*. Basic Books, New York.

Bowlby, J. (1977) The making and breaking of affectional bonds. Part 1: Etiology and psychopathology in the light of attachment theory. *British Journal of Psychiatry*, **130**, 201–210.

Bowlby, J. (1979) *The Making and Breaking of Affectional Bonds*. Tavistock Press, London.

Bowlby, J. (1980) *Attachment and Loss*, Vol. 3. *Loss, Separation and Depression*. Basic Books, New York.

Bowlby, J. (1988) *A Secure Base: Parent–child Attachment and Healthy Human Development*. Basic Books, New York.

Bretherton, I. (1985) Attachment theory: retrospect and prospect. *Monographs of the Society for Research in Child Development*, **50**, 3–35.

Brown, G.W. & Harris, T. (1978) *Social Origins of Depression*. Free Press, New York.

Brown, G.W., Harris, T. & Copeland, J.R. (1977) Depression and loss. *British Journal of Psychiatry*, **130**, 1–18.

Burchill, S.A.L. & Stiles, W.B. (1995) *Interpersonal processes in depression: What do we know now?* Manuscript. Department of Psychology, Miami University, Oxford, Ohio.

Carnelley, K.B., Pietromonaco, P.R. & Jaffe, K. (1994) Depression, working models of others, and relationship functioning. *Journal of Personality and Social Psychology*, **66**, 127–140.

Cohen, M.B., Baker, G., Cohen, R., Fromm-Reichmann, F. & Weigert, E.V. (1954) An intensive study of twelve cases of manic-depressive psychosis. Reprinted in: *Essential Papers on Depression* (ed. J.C. Coyne) (1985). New York University Press, New York.

Coyne, J.C. (1976a) Depression and the response of others. *Journal of Abnormal Psychology*, **85**, 186–193.

Coyne, J.C. (1976b) Towards an interactional description of depression. *Psychiatry*, **39**, 28–40.

Coyne, J.C. (1985) Ambiguity and controversy: an introduction. In: *Essential Papers on Depression* (ed. J.C. Coyne), pp. 311–330. New York University Press, New York.

Crittendon, P.M. (1992) Treatment of anxious attachment in infancy and early childhood. *Developmental Psychopathology*, **4**, 575–602.

Elkin, I., Shea, M.T., Watkins, J.T. *et al.* (1989) National Institute of Mental Health Treatment of Depression Collaborative Research Program: general effectiveness of treatments. *Archives of General Psychiatry*, **46**, 971–982.

Erickson, M.F., Sroufe, L.A. & Engeland, B. (1985) The relationship between quality of attachment and behavior problems in pre-school in a high risk sample. *Monographs of the Society for Research in Child Development*, **50**, 147–166.

Freud, S. (1917) Mourning and melancholia. Reprinted in: *Essential Papers on Depression* (ed. J.C. Coyne) (1985). New York University Press, New York.

Freud, S. (1930) *Civilization and its Discontents* (trans. J. Riviere). Hogarth Press, London.

Garfield, S.L. & Bergin, A.E. (eds) (1986) *Handbook of Psychotherapy and Behavior Change*, 3rd edn. John Wiley & Sons, New York.

Gilbert, P. (1992) *Counselling for Depression*. Sage Publications, London.

Gotlib, I.H. (1992) Interpersonal and cognitive aspects of depression. *Current Directions in Psychological Science*, **1**, 149–154.

Gotlib, I.H. & Hooley, J.M. (1988) Depression and marital distress: current status and future directions. In: *Handbook of Personal Relationships* (ed. S. Duck), pp. 543–570. John Wiley & Sons, New York.

Greenberg, L.S., Rice, L.N. & Elliott, R. (1993)

Facilitating Emotional Change. Guilford Press, New York.

Guisinger, S. & Blatt, S.J. (1994) Individuality and relatedness: Evolution of a fundamental dialectic. *American Psychologist,* **49,** 104–111.

Hammen, C. (1991) Generation of stress in the course of unipolar depression. *Journal of Abnormal Psychology,* **100,** 555–561.

Hammen, C., Marks, T., Mayol, A. & deMayo, R. (1985) Depressive self-schemas, life stress, and vulnerability to depression. *Journal of Abnormal Psychology,* **94,** 308–319.

Hardy, G.E., Barkham, M. & Stiles, W.B. (1996) *The impact of marital status on the outcome of treatment for depression.* Manuscript. Psychological Therapies Research Centre, University of Leeds.

Hazan, C. & Shaver, P. (1987) Romantic love conceptualised as an attachment process. *Journal of Personality and Social Psychology,* **52,** 511–534.

Hobson, R.F. (1985) *Forms of Feeling.* Tavistock Press, London.

Hooley, J.M. & Teasdale, J.T. (1989) Predictors of relapse in unipolar depressives: expressed emotion, marital distress, and perceived criticism. *Journal of Abnormal Psychology,* **98,** 229–235.

Horney, K. (1945) *Our Inner Conflicts: A Constructive Theory of Neurosis.* Norton, New York.

Klerman, G.L. & Weissman, M.M. (1982) Interpersonal psychotherapy: Theory and research. In: *Short-term Psychotherapies for Depression* (ed. J. Rush), pp. 89–106. John Wiley & Sons, New York.

Lewinsohn, J. (1985) A behavioral approach to depression. Reprinted in: *Essential Papers on Depression* (ed. J.C. Coyne), pp. 150–180. New York University Press, New York.

Libet, J. & Lewinsohn, P.M. (1973) The concept of social skill with reference to the behavior of depressed persons. *Journal of Consulting and Clinical Psychology,* **40,** 304–312.

Maccoby, E.E. (1980) *Social Development: Psychological Growth and the Parent–child Relationship.* Doubleday, New York.

Main, M. (1983) Exploration, play, and cognitive functioning related to infant–mother attachment. *Infant Behavior and Development,* **6,** 167–174.

Main, M., Kaplan, N. & Cassidy, J. (1985) Security in infancy, childhood and adulthood: A move to the level of representation. *Monograph of the Society for Research in Child Development,* **50,** 66–104.

Marcus, D.K. & Nardone, M.E. (1992) Depression and interpersonal rejection. *Clinical Psychology Review,* **12,** 433–449.

McCrae, R. & Costa, P. (1988) Recalled parent–child relations and adult personality. *Journal of Personality,* **56,** 427–434.

Mendelson, M. (1960) *Psychoanalytic Concepts of Depression.* Thomas, Springfield, IL.

Merikangas, K.R., Pruscoff, B.A., Kupfer, D.J. & Frank, E. (1985) Marital adjustment in major depression. *Journal of Affective Disorders,* **9,** 5–11.

Parkes, C.M. (1972) *Studies of Grief in Adult Life.* International Universities Press, New York.

Perls, F.S., Hefferline, R.F. & Goodman, P. (1951) *Gestalt Therapy: Excitement and Growth in the Human Personality.* Julian Press, New York.

Pietromonaco, P.R., Rook, K.S. & Lewis, M.A. (1992) Accuracy of perceptions of interpersonal interactions: effects of dysphoria, friendship, and similarity. *Journal of Personality and Social Psychology,* **63,** 247–259.

Rapaport, D. (1959) Edward Bibring's theory of depression. Reprinted in: *Essential Papers on Depression* (ed. J. C. Coyne) (1985). New York University Press, New York.

Rogers, C.R. (1959) A theory of therapy, personality, and interpersonal relationships, as developed in the client-centered framework. In: *Psychology: A Study of Science,* Vol. 3, 184–256 (ed. S. Koch). Basic Books, New York.

Rounsaville, B.J. & Chevron, E. (1982) Interpersonal psychotherapy: clinical applications. In: *Short-term Psychotherapies for Depression* (ed. J. Rush), pp. 107–142. John Wiley & Sons, New York.

Rutter, M. (1979) Maternal deprivation, 1972–1978: New findings, new concepts, new approaches. *Child Development,* **50,** 283–305.

Rutter, M. (1990) Commentary: some focus and process considerations regarding effects of parental depression on children. *Developmental Psychology,* **26,** 60–67.

Segrin, C. & Dillard, J.P. (1992) The interactional theory of depression: a meta-analysis of the research literature. *Journal of Social and Clinical Psychology,* **11,** 43–70.

Seligman, M.E.P. (1975) *Helplessness: On Depression, Development and Death.* W.H. Freeman, San Francisco, CA.

Shapiro, D.A. & Firth, J.A. (1985) *Exploratory therapy manual for the Sheffield Psychotherapy Project (SAPU Memo 733).* University of Sheffield.

Shapiro, D.A., Barkham, M., Rees, A., Hardy, G.E., Reynolds, S. & Startup, M. (1994) Effects of duration and severity of depression on the effectiveness of cognitive-behavioral and psychodynamic-interpersonal psychotherapy. *Journal of Consulting and Clinical Psychology,* **62,** 522–534.

Strupp, H.H., Sandell, J.A., Waterhouse, G.J.,

O'Malley, S.S. & Anderson, J.L. (1982) Psychodynamic therapy: Theory and research. In: *Short-term Psychotherapies for Depression* (ed. J. Rush). John Wiley & Sons, New York.

van Ijzendoorn, M.H. (1995) Adult attachment representations, parental responsiveness, and infant attachment: a meta-analysis on the predictive validity of the Adult Attachment Interview. *Psychological Bulletin*, **117**, 387–403.

Weissman, M.M. & Paykel, E.S. (1974) *The Depressed Woman: A Study of Social Relationships*. University of Chicago Press, Chicago.

7 Efficacy of psychodynamic, interpersonal and experiential treatments of depression

DAVID A. SHAPIRO

Before the rise of cognitive-behavioural therapy in the 1970s, psychological treatments of depression were confined to the broad range of psychodynamic, interpersonal and experiential approaches reviewed in this chapter. Although diverse, these typically share an emphasis upon empathic attention to, and consideration of, the patient's emotions and subjective experiences as being necessary to the alleviation of depression. Research has focused on brief (a maximum of about 6 months of weekly sessions) forms of these treatments, with some attention also paid to extensions of treatment at a reduced frequency in an effort to prevent relapse or recurrence of depression.

Psychodynamic therapy (Luborsky, 1984; Strupp & Binder, 1984) derives from psychoanalysis, as developed by Freud and his associates. Key elements include *uncovering unconscious processes* via *interpretation* and the emphasis upon the re-enactment of significant processes in the *transference*, or here-and-now relationship between patient and therapist. The origin of *interpersonal* therapy (Klerman *et al.*, 1984) can be traced to the work of Harry Stack Sullivan (Perry, 1982). Its central idea is that depression arises in an *interpersonal context*, the *clarification and renegotiation* of which will reduce the intensity of depressive symptoms. Brief and structured forms of psychodynamic therapy increasingly share this emphasis, leading to the adoption for research purposes of the designation, *psychodynamic-interpersonal* therapy. As described by Hardy (see Chapter 6), this synthesis accords well with recent theoretical developments using attachment theory to account for psychopathology, including depression. The defining characteristics of *experiential* therapy are its emphasis on the facilitation of the patient's *experiencing* as its key task, and on the *therapeutic relationship* as curative. Rogers' (1951) Client-Centred Therapy, Perls *et al.*'s (1951) Gestalt Therapy, Gendlin's (1981) Focusing, and Greenberg *et al.*'s (1993) Process Experiential Therapy are leading examples.

A shared feature of all these methods is that their primary conceptual origins are with clinical practice rather than, as in the case of cognitive-behavioural methods (Chapter 8), an external, non-clinical body of scientific theory and knowledge. Until recently, high-quality controlled trials of these methods were rare. This lack is now being remedied. Trials with defined diagnostic groups using manuals to specify the treatment procedures, together with ratings of therapists' adherence and competence to establish that these have been delivered with integrity, are now feasible.

Much of the evidential base for these procedures comes from process research analysing the components of treatment and their relationship to its effects (Elliott, 1995; Shapiro, 1996). Accordingly, clinical trials will be reviewed alongside studies of the mechanisms of change. A drawback of the latter must be acknowledged at the outset, however. The scientific focus of much process research has been on understanding the treatment rather than the disorder; consequently, diagnostic issues are frequently de-emphasized, although many studies include a substantial proportion of patients with at least mild or moderate depression. Strictly speaking, the specific applicability of many of these findings to formally diagnosed depression remains to be demonstrated, although there is seldom prima-facie evidence to doubt this.

Major systematic reviews

An overview of evidence from trials of psychodynamic, interpersonal and experiential therapies of depression can be gained from systematic reviews (meta-analyses). This approach to reviewing literature was introduced to the health care domain via reviews of psychological treatments in mental health (Smith & Glass, 1977; Smith *et al.*, 1980; Shapiro & Shapiro, 1982). Robinson *et al.* (1990) produced a landmark review of depression treatments. Psychodynamic and interpersonal treatments are discussed in the practice guidelines of the American Psychiatric Association (1993) and the US Agency for Health Care Policy and Research (Depression Guideline Panel, 1993), the latter guideline incorporating findings of a new systematic review. Roth and Fonagy (1996) were commissioned by the UK Department of Health to inform a review of psychotherapy services with an analysis of outcome research, including a detailed analysis of depression treatments.

Early meta-analytic reviews of depression treatments encompassing psychodynamic methods alongside other approaches produced mixed results. Neitzel *et al.* (1987) found no relationship between treatment type and outcome. In contrast, Dobson (1989) found 'other psychotherapies', many of which were dynamic therapies, to be inferior to cognitive therapy.

Robinson *et al.* (1990) highlighted studies comparing four types of psychotherapy of depression. Their bibliography suggests that the 'general verbal' category mainly comprised psychodynamic and experiential methods. This category yielded outcomes that were inferior to those for cognitive, behavioural and cognitive-behavioural methods. However, investigators' allegiance to one or other of the therapeutic methods under test, assessed from comments in the introductory section of each report, was strongly related to the outcome of a given study: investigators tended to find in favour of their preferred method. Statistical correction for allegiance abolished the differences between treatment categories. This reflects the fact that most researchers who have compared psychotherapies of depression are more expert in, and committed to, cognitive, behavioural and cognitive-behavioural methods than to psychodynamic, interpersonal and experiential approaches.

The legitimacy of this statistical correction is open to debate, however. Proponents of cognitive and behavioural approaches (Giles, 1993) argue that investigator allegiance merely reflects the weight of objective evidence for their methods. Jacobson and Hollon (1996) attribute allegiance effects to differences in expertise or perspective rather than any attempt to bias the nature of the findings. This shows the need for more research by investigators with allegiance to dynamic and interpersonal methods, or by teams comprising advocates of each of the treatments being compared, in order to level the playing field.

The United States Public Health Service's Agency for Health Care Policy and Research commissioned a review using Bayesian statistical methods to derive from published data the probability that each of several treatment methods will be successful in the treatment of a depressed patient (Depression Guideline Panel, 1993). Overall efficacy percentages of 55.3, 34.8, 56.6 and 52.3 were obtained for behavioural, dynamic, cognitive, and interpersonal therapies, respectively. However, these percentages were based on just six trials of dynamic therapy and a single trial, the National Institute of Mental Health (NIMH) study reviewed below, of interpersonal therapy. Behavioural and cognitive therapies were represented by 10 and 12 trials, respectively. A comparison, based on eight trials, of dynamic therapy with other forms of psychotherapy found it slightly less effective (−7.8%). These figures suggest that dynamic therapy may be marginally inferior to other methods, but the extent of evidence available for inclusion was restricted by the data-analytic strategy followed (Roth & Fonagy, 1996).

Psychodynamic therapy

Psychodynamic therapy applies the central principles of psychoanalysis in a focused, relatively brief treatment, typically lasting for fewer than 30 weekly sessions (Alexander, 1954; Sifneos, 1972; Malan, 1976; Luborsky, 1984; Strupp & Binder, 1984). Psychoanalysis itself developed into a long-term, intensive treatment aimed not at removing single symptoms or problematic behaviours, but attempting to restructure the entire personality (Roth & Fonagy, 1996). Psychodynamic therapy, in contrast, assumes that increasing the patient's insight into, or understanding of, emotional difficulties and personal problems will resolve unconscious conflict, thereby alleviating symptoms. Insight is achieved through interpretation of the patient's behaviour and talk during treatment sessions. Problematic internal states, including feelings, desires and beliefs that are in conflict with one another, are believed to be encoded in patterns of interpersonal relationships which are brought to the patient's attention within the treatment situation and in relation to the therapist. Unlike the stereotype of the passive, often silent psychoanalyst, the modern psychodynamic therapist works actively to identify recurrent patterns of behaviour related to hypothesized unconscious conflicts. Conscious insight is viewed by contemporary psychodynamic therapists as less important than the emotional experience of the therapist's acceptance of thoughts and feelings previously considered intolerable by the patient (Roth & Fonagy, 1996).

Clinical trials

Three reviews focusing on short-term, dynamically orientated psychotherapy have appeared since 1991 (Svartberg & Stiles, 1991; Crits-Christoph, 1992; Anderson & Lambert, 1995). Of these reviewers, Crits-Christoph (1992), whose inclusion criteria were the strictest, gave the most favourable verdict, and Svartberg and Stiles (1991) the least favourable. However, since each includes only a minority of studies of depression alongside trials of other disorders, these studies are best considered individually.

Hersen *et al.* (1984) found that time-limited psychodynamic therapy was equally as effective as social skills training and amitriptyline. Therapists were all highly experienced and 'true believers' in the method they used within the trial. None the less, fewer than half the patients in each treatment were deemed clinically improved after an initial 12-week period or following a further period of 6 months' maintenance treatment.

McLean and Hakstian (1979) found dynamic psychotherapy to be less effective than behaviour therapy on six out of 10 outcome measures, and less effective than amitriptyline on three measures, despite the use for both psychotherapies of experienced therapists working with their preferred treatment; for example, on the Beck Depression Inventory (BDI), patients treated with dynamic and behaviour therapy recorded means of 17 and 10 after treatment, both groups having started treatment with means of 27. Limiting the treatment to between eight and 12 sessions may have disadvantaged the dynamic treatment (Crits-Christoph, 1992). This is consistent with trends in the data reported by Hersen *et al.* (1984), whose dynamic therapy patients improved less markedly over the first 6 weeks of treatment but had caught up over 6 months of maintenance therapy.

Kornblith *et al.* (1983) found group dynamic therapy as effective as behavioural self-control methods. Covi and Lipman (1987) found dynamic group therapy less effective than both group cognitive-behavioural therapy alone and cognitive-behavioural therapy combined with medication. Three comparisons of psychodynamic and cognitive-behavioural therapies delivered in group formats to elderly, depressed patients have been reported. Gallagher and Thompson (1982) found similar improvement over the course of behavioural, cognitive, or 'relational/insight' therapy, but superior maintenance of gains over the year following treatment was detected amongst those receiving the former two treatments, despite small samples of just 10 patients in each group. Steuer *et al.* (1984) found psychodynamic therapy less effective than cognitive-behavioural therapy on one of three outcome measures, the BDI, whilst Thompson *et al.* (1987) found no difference between psychodynamic, behavioural and cognitive therapy groups.

In summary, trials comparing brief psychodynamic therapy with other psychological treatments of depression have generally found its efficacy to be similar to that of the comparison treatments, although a minority of results appear slightly to favour the contrasted treatments. More trials are urgently needed to guide the choice between psychodynamic treatments and other methods, especially medication.

Mechanisms of change in psychodynamic therapy

Henry *et al.* (1994) reviewed evidence on an issue that is central to the claims of psychodynamic theory and practice in the treatment of depression as of other disorders: the effects of interpretations, specifically *transference interpretations* linking the patient's responses to the therapy or therapist to core conflicts, which are the chief technical focus of psychodynamic therapy. Several findings challenge the core assumptions of psychodynamic theory. The more recent, methodologically sound work, suggests that as far as transference interpretations are concerned, more is not better and may even be damaging (Piper *et al.*, 1991; Henry *et al.*, 1993), at least in brief therapy. Frequent transference interpretations may cause patients to feel criticized and so to withdraw. Four studies of patients' responses to transference interpretations were consistent in showing that transference interpretations do not elicit the expected greater affective response or deeper experiencing on the part of the patient. However, this may reflect the fact that most interpretations offered by therapists are not judged by experts to be accurate. Recent evidence suggests that transference interpretations may only be effective when judged to be accurate, and delivered relatively infrequently to more highly functioning patients (Henry *et al.*, 1994). Henry *et al.* (1993) noted the perils of inflexible, mechanistic adherence to treatment procedures such as transference interpretations on the part of newly trained therapists. In contrast, experienced therapists have gained the opportunity to learn how to deliver treatment elements in a responsive manner (Stiles & Shapiro, 1989), attuned to the patient's subtle communication of readiness, or otherwise, to absorb constructively the challenging information often contained within interpretations.

The benefits of accurate rather than inaccurate interpretations can only be properly assessed if the patient's problems can be formulated in a reliable and reproducible way. Progress is now being made in this direction; for example, a series of papers demonstrated substantial convergence among seven operational measures of transference-related constructs applied to a single sample interview (Luborsky *et al.*, 1994); for example, the plan formulation method (Curtis *et al.*, 1995) describes the manner in which a patient will work in the therapeutic relationship to disconfirm individual pathogenic beliefs, overcome problems and achieve goals. Therapist interventions compatible with a plan formulated in object relations terms predicted in-session patient progress (Tishby & Messer, 1995).

Interpersonal therapy

A useful account of interpersonal therapy (IPT) is given by Weissman and Markowitz (1994). In addition to the adult major depression of interest to us here, these authors also review the developing use of IPT with related populations (including depressed adolescents, depressed patients with HIV, dysthymic patients), as well as with other psychiatric disorders such as drug abuse and bulimia.

IPT is based on the assumption (Sullivan, 1953) that depression occurs in an environmental, more specifically interpersonal, context and that clarifying and renegotiating the context associated with the onset of symptoms is important to recovery (Weissman *et al.*, 1981). This approach builds on extensive evidence linking stress and life events with the onset of depression. It focuses on the patient's present relationships rather than seeking origins of problems in the past, although overall patterns in the patient's interpersonal relationships are identified by reviewing previous depressive episodes, early family relationships, and previous significant relationships and friendship patterns.

The therapist is active, supportive and quite didactic in style. Treatment begins with a diagnostic or explanatory phase, highlighting the ways in which the patient's current functioning, social relationships and expectations may have influenced his/her depression. The patient is given the sick role, which excuses from overwhelming social obligations but requires the patient to work in treatment to return to full functioning. The approach is educational, linking depressive symptoms to one of four interpersonal domains: grief, interpersonal role disputes, role transitions or interpersonal deficits. In the second phase of treatment the therapist follows strategies specific to one of the four domains. If grief is the focus, for example, the therapist aids mourning and the uptake of new relationships and activities to make good the loss. In the final phase of treatment, attention is focused on the gains achieved and on a preventive approach to identifying and overcoming depressive symptoms arising in the future.

Acute trials of IPT

Two major trials of IPT as acute treatment have been reported. DiMascio *et al.* (1979; see also Weissman *et al.*, 1979) found that IPT and imipramine were equally effective in reducing the symptoms of unipolar depressives overall. At the level of symptom clusters, it was apparent that the drug was very rapidly effective in reducing sleep disturbance, whilst IPT was more rapid than pharmacotherapy in reducing mood disturbance and apathy. This suggests that patients with predominantly vegetative complaints may do better with pharmacotherapy, whilst IPT may be especially useful for patients with predominantly emotional complaints and mood disturbance. The effects of the two treatments in combination were essentially additive. One year later, most patients were asymptomatic, with no differences between the groups, although many had received further drug and/or psychotherapeutic treatment (Weissman *et al.*, 1981). There was evidence, however, that IPT resulted in better social functioning at 1-year follow-up, suggesting a long-term benefit not apparent after 4 months of treatment.

The National Institute of Mental Health's Treatment of Depression Collaborative Research Program (TDCRP) has attracted widespread media and professional attention because of its unprecedented scale and, in some respects, disappointing results. Across three treatment sites, IPT was compared with Beck *et al.*'s (1979) Cognitive Therapy (CT), the then standard tricyclic antidepressant imipramine, and a control condition in which placebo tablets were accompanied by a clinical management protocol identical to that used with the active drug. Patients met criteria for major depressive disorder. Elkin (1994) presents an overview of the study and its findings.

Therapists adhered to the requirements of the different treatment protocols (Hill *et al.*, 1992). However, there were essentially no efficacy differences in respect of depressive symptoms, overall functioning (Elkin *et al.*, 1989) or specific areas of functioning targeted by each of the psychotherapies (Imber *et al.*, 1990), as measured at the end of treatment between IPT, cognitive-behavioural therapy and imipramine. For example, IPT was no more effective than the other treatments in enhancing patients' social adjustment. Interestingly, amongst patients whose social adjustment was relatively good at the outset of treatment, IPT was more effective than the other treatments, suggesting that good social functioning is required for patients to take advantage of interpersonal strategies to recover from depression (Sotsky *et al.*, 1991).

The response of depressive symptoms to imipramine was somewhat more rapid than to the psychological treatments (Watkins *et al.*, 1993). Twelve weeks into treatment, those receiving medication were doing significantly better than those receiving the psychotherapies, although this difference was slight (and no longer statistically reliable) 4 weeks later.

Patients were subdivided into groups presenting with relatively severe vs. relatively mild depressive symptoms, and again into groups with relatively severe vs. relatively mild impairment of functioning (Elkin *et al.*, 1989). These analyses revealed that amongst relatively severely depressed patients, active medication was substantially more effective than placebo, with the two psychotherapies achieving intermediate results which remained indistinguishable from one another. The placebo condition yielded surprisingly good outcomes amongst mildly depressed patients.

The main findings were broadly confirmed by subsequent re-analysis using state-of-the-art statistical techniques to include all data points for all patients within a single analysis (Gibbons *et al.*, 1993). However, the greater power of this analysis yielded somewhat stronger conclusions regarding the comparative efficacy of the treatment conditions among more severe patients; among those who were more severely depressed before treatment, imipramine and IPT were superior to CT and placebo; among those who were both more severely depressed and more functionally impaired before treatment, imipramine was superior to both psychological treatments and the placebo condition (Elkin *et al.*, 1996).

In contrast to the modest effect of treatment conditions on outcomes in this study there were findings that perfectionistic, self-critical patients did less well in all treatments. In addition, the quality of the therapeutic relationship, measured early in therapy, predicted improvement, especially amongst those patients who were moderately perfectionistic; the therapeutic relationship did not strongly predict outcome amongst patients who were either highly self-critical or not at all self-critical (Blatt *et al.*, 1996). Moderately self-critical patients may be thought of as those most ready to engage most fully in a therapeutic relationship whose goal is personal change, and it is these patients who are most affected by the quality of that relationship.

Patients were followed for 18 months after the end of treatment (Shea *et al.*, 1992a). In common with other studies of short-term depression treatments, relatively small percentages (19% of those receiving imipramine, 20% of those receiving placebo, 26% of those receiving IPT, and 30% of those receiving CT) of those with follow-up data both met a stringent recovery criterion post-treatment and did not relapse at any time over the follow-up period. Although there were no statistically significant differences, CT appeared to do somewhat better overall than the other treatments during the follow-up. However, the results of such a 'naturalistic' follow-up, in which patients are free to take up further treatments, are notoriously difficult to interpret. For example, focusing on the relapse rate of those initially making a good response to treatment may result in a biased comparison because different types of patients respond to each treatment. In addition, sample sizes were too small to detect modest effects with any confidence.

Controversy concerning the TDCRP has arisen mainly from adherents of cognitive-behavioural and pharmacological treatments, for each of whom the findings could be considered somewhat disappointing. From a carefully reasoned cognitive-behavioural viewpoint, Jacobson and Hollon (1996) pointed to evidence suggestive of differential effectiveness of the psychological treatments at the participating sites, especially among the more severe patients. Although the anonymity of each site is protected for confidentiality reasons, therapists at the site with best CT outcomes were also rated (non-significantly) more competent in CT than those at the other two sites (Elkin *et al.*, 1996). Were this site to be the one generally considered to have greatest expertise in, and commitment to, CT the results could be interpreted to suggest that the efficacy of CT was underestimated by the inclusion of the other two sites.

From a pharmacotherapeutic perspective, Klein (1996) suggested that the TDCRP's pharmacotherapy condition was not optimally conducted, noting that patients who dropped out of the pharmacotherapy condition were rated by their therapists as having shown inferior compliance with medication. Klein and Ross's (1993) reanalysis of TDCRP data found a clear advantage to IPT over CT in patients with more severe depression. Klein (1996) interprets this finding, alongside those of Sotsky *et al.* (1991), as suggesting that psychotherapies may be counterproductive if they focus on areas of difficulty for the patient, and are at their most helpful when providing emotional support, usable coping skills and success experiences (Frank & Frank, 1991).

A further piece of evidence concerning indications for IPT was obtained by Prusoff *et al.* (1980). It was found that patients with endogenous depression responded better to either pharmacotherapy alone or to IPT with pharmacotherapy than to IPT alone; whereas patients whose depression was not endogenous responded better to either IPT alone or the combined treatment than to pharmacotherapy alone.

More generally, comparisons between psychotherapies and drug treatments become outmoded as new drug therapies are adopted. For example, if serotonin re-uptake inhibitors are more widely tolerated because of lower side-effect profiles than tricyclics, the range of patients who can be effectively treated by medication may be broader than it was when the drug-psychotherapy comparisons of the 1970s and 1980s were undertaken. Equally, of course, that literature will be outdated by advances in psychotherapeutic treatment.

Trials of maintenance IPT

Studies of continuation or maintenance treatment (offered after remission of the acute episode in order to prevent relapse or recurrence of depression) must be distinguished from studies (such as that by Shea *et al.*, 1992a, discussed above) examining the extent to which gains made during the treatment of a depressive episode are sustained over the months following treatment termination.

Interpersonal therapy was first tested in an 8-month continuation trial with depressed women who had responded to 4–6 weeks of amitriptyline (Klerman *et al.*, 1974). On entering the continuation phase, patients were randomized to weekly IPT or a low-contact control condition. Two months later, patients were further randomized to continuing medication, placebo or no tablets. Thus there were six arms to the trial. Findings indicated that continuing pharmacotherapy prevented relapse and worsening of symptoms (Paykel *et al.*, 1975), whilst IPT benefited social adjustment (Weissman *et al.*, 1974).

In a study by Frank *et al.* (1990), patients in at least their third depressive episode were given a combination of imipramine and IPT. This combined treatment was continued for 17 weeks after symptomatic remission. In the maintenance phase, patients were randomized to one of five treatment conditions: a maintenance form of IPT—monthly sessions—was offered alone, or in combination with continued imipramine at the full dosage used in acute treatment (mean 200 mg per day), or in combination with placebo; and medication clinic visits were offered with full imipramine medication or with placebo.

Monthly IPT sessions substantially lengthened the time between episodes amongst patients not receiving active medication, represented by mean survival times of 82 and 74 weeks for the two groups receiving IPT vs. 45 weeks for those receiving placebo alone. However, monthly IPT sessions had little impact on those receiving active medication, whose mean survival times were 131 and 124 weeks, respectively, with and without IPT. This result suggests that continuing medication at the acute dosage level is the best way to prevent a recurrence. However, the alternative of monthly IPT sessions is worth considering as a less toxic alternative, although one carrying greater risk of recurrence. Monthly IPT sessions did not appear to reduce the risk of recurrence amongst those receiving active medication.

Overview of IPT efficacy

Research from two major American groups has identified IPT as a promising treatment of the acute, continuation and maintenance phases of depression. The number of trials is less impressive than their quality and the consistency of their results. In addition, the NIMH's TDCRP suggested that IPT at least equals the more extensively researched cognitive-behavioural methods, although debate continues concerning this study's delivery of CT.

Effective components of IPT

There is promising evidence linking the technical integrity of IPT to its effects. O'Malley *et al.* (1988) found that supervisors' ratings of an early IPT treatment session, encompassing the quality of problem-orientated strategies, quality of techniques, general IPT skills, and overall session quality, predicted depressed patients' self-rated change and clinician ratings of the patient's apathy at the end of treatment, over and above the effects of patients' pretreatment characteristics.

Frank *et al.*'s (1991) further analysis of the 1990 study (Frank *et al.*, 1990) of maintenance IPT examined the contribution of the quality of IPT sessions to the length of time that formerly depressed patients, not receiving active medication, remained well during the 3-year maintenance period. Sessions were rated for the specificity and purity of IPT interventions. Patients whose sessions were rated more specifically interpersonal did much better than those whose sessions were rated less so, with median times to recurrence of 102 vs. 18 weeks, respectively. This finding could not be explained in terms of other patient characteristics, such as severity of depression or comorbid personality disorder, that might be suspected of influencing both recurrence and therapists' behaviour. Nor was it due to consistent differences between therapists in their use of IPT techniques with all their patients. Rather, it appeared to reflect the dyadic process between patient and therapist. It is of interest that the survival times of those with high-quality IPT sessions were quite similar to those of patients receiving medication.

Psychodynamic-interpersonal therapy

As psychodynamic therapy has grown more focused and its emphasis upon interpersonal processes and problems has become more explicit, the term *Psychodynamic-interpersonal* has come into use to differentiate this approach more clearly from earlier psychodynamic methods with their greater emphasis on intrapsychic conflicts; for example, this designation fits the methods of Luborsky (1984) and Strupp and Binder (1984). In the treatment of depression, the second Sheffield Psychotherapy Project (SPP2; Shapiro *et al.*, 1994, 1995) compared a psychodynamic-interpersonal (PI) method, based on Hobson's (1985) 'Conversational Model' with cognitive-behavioural (CB) therapy.

The Sheffield PI treatment uses a psychodynamic theory of relationship disturbances in which the therapeutic relationship is used as a vehicle for understanding and modifying interpersonal difficulties which are viewed as primary in the origins of depression. The therapist's contributions include adopting a negotiating style, developing a language of mutuality, using metaphor to enhance the immediacy of experienced affect, focusing on here-and-now experiences, and offering hypotheses to express understanding of the patient's experiences. These hypotheses are based on psychodynamic and interpersonal concepts, but are offered tentatively as aids to the patient's self-understanding rather than being delivered authoritatively as revealed truth.

A positive bond between patient and therapist is maintained, and challenging or unwelcome ideas are not pursued at the expense of this. The patient–therapist relationship is seen as a microcosm of the patient's relationships outside treatment, and a readily available source of data concerning the patient's problems in relating to others and of hypotheses with which to build a new understanding of these. For example, Kohut's analysis of the role of narcissism in human development (Mollon & Parry, 1984) may enable the therapist to help a patient to understand his or her apparent need for appreciative 'mirroring' by others, including—during treatment sessions—the therapist. Similarly, attachment theory (see Chapter 6) serves the therapist as a source of hypotheses concerning the patient's responses to experienced or feared loss. Manifestations of the patient's attachment patterns within the therapeutic relationship can now be assessed reliably (Mallinckrodt *et al.*, 1995).

Outcomes of the second Sheffield Psychotherapy Project

Within SPP2, 117 patients completed either eight or 16 weekly sessions of either PI or CB therapy in a randomized design. Each patient scored 16 or more on the BDI, attained an Index of Definition on the Present-State Examination of at least five (indicative of current psychiatric disorder), and had met DSM-III (American Psychiatric Association, 1980) criteria for a major depressive episode during the 3 months preceding treatment. Prior to randomization, patients were stratified into three levels of depression severity. To separate for scientific purposes the effects of the specific treatment methods from the influence of personal characteristics of therapists choosing to practise each method, five research clinical psychologists sympathetic to both approaches were trained to carry out both PI and CB therapies. Their adherence to the contrasting treatment protocols was established via ratings of randomly selected sessions (Startup & Shapiro, 1993).

On most measures, CB and PI therapies were equally effective, regardless of severity of depression or the duration of treatment, however, the BDI showed a modest advantage to CB over PI therapy. Irrespective of the treatment method used, more severely depressed patients responded better to 16 than to eight sessions (Shapiro *et al.*, 1994). A 1-year follow-up suggested that eight sessions of PI therapy may be insufficient to secure subsequent maintenance of gains, with patients in that condition reporting more depressive symptoms than those in the other three groups (Shapiro *et al.*, 1995).

Findings also indicated that not all patients may benefit equally from PI therapy: consistent with a review by Shea *et al.* (1992b), those with comorbid cluster C personality disorders (avoidant, dependent or obsessive-compulsive personalities) did less well in PI therapy, whereas this comorbidity had no effect on response to CB therapy (Hardy *et al.*, 1995a). Similarly, response to PI therapy was reduced amongst patients approaching treatment with a less psychological approach to the treatment of psychological problems, whereas these prior attitudes had no effect on response to CB therapy (Hardy *et al.*, 1995b).

Mechanisms of psychodynamic-interpersonal therapy

In a strategic approach to delineating the mechanisms of psychotherapeutic change (Shapiro, 1995), both quantitative and qualitative methods are used to identify factors contributing to the effects of PI therapy in depression, systematically contrasted with CB therapy. Before linking these process parameters to outcome, it is necessary to assess fully the similarities and differences between the two treatments across time: illustrative examples follow. Quantitative findings have included that by Agnew *et al.* (1997) in which the quality of the relationship between patient and therapist strongly predicted the extent of clinical improvement achieved by the patient. Stiles *et al.* (1997) plotted therapists' intentions on a session-by-session basis in both PI and CB therapies. Distinctive features of PI therapy included an extended 'working phase' in the middle sessions of treatment involving a gradually increasing focus on encouraging change and a gradually decreasing focus on affect, consistent with a gradual shift from exploration to implementation.

Ongoing work on the Sheffield data is assessing the role of therapists' responsiveness to the requirements and characteristics of individual patients in shaping the outcomes of treatment. For example, Hardy *et al.* (in press) found that therapists used more affective and relationship-orientated interventions with patients whose attachment style (see Chapter 6) had been assessed as anxious-ambivalent, particularly (but not solely) in PI therapy. Therapists used more cognitive treatment methods with avoidant patients in PI therapy, although not as markedly as in CB therapy. These differing patterns of therapist response were made without knowledge of the questionnaire data on which the attachment classification was based. Outcomes of the three attachment groups were approximately equivalent, consistent with a view that the differences in treatment implementation reflected appropriate responsiveness to clients' attachment styles.

Reynolds *et al.* (1996) analysed session-by-session changes over the course of PI and CB therapies in the patient's post-session mood and evaluation of the treatment session itself. Early in treatment, PI sessions were less smooth (i.e. more tense and uncomfortable) and less focused on problem-solving, but PI sessions changed more rapidly than CB sessions on these dimensions, so that later in the treatment sessions of both, treatments were equivalently positive. Similarly, patients rated their relationship with their therapists slightly worse in early PI sessions and slightly better in later PI sessions, in comparison with the corresponding CB sessions. These findings are consistent with the hypothesis, derived from the assimilation model (Stiles et al., 1990), that early sessions of PI treatment involve the uncovering and exploration of potentially distressing, warded off or avoided material, whilst later in treatment both methods converge on applications of new understandings—albeit different understandings—to solving the presenting problems.

Stiles et al. (1995) also conceptualized the goal of the Sheffield PI therapy of depression as being to *promote the patient's assimilation of problematic experiences* (Stiles *et al.*, 1990). This goal is achieved through the following five tasks.

1   Build a therapeutic relationship characterized by trust and mutuality on the basis of which the patient is encouraged and enabled to experience rather than to ward off problematic feelings.

2   Promote more intense experiencing and more open expression and exploration of feelings.

3   Draw attention to patient patterns of feeling and activity which result from difficulties in experiencing, expression, or interpersonal relationships.

4   Promote the patient's self-understanding of difficulties by linking patterns of feeling and activity within the therapeutic relationship with patterns in significant relationships outside therapy.

5   Explore and experiment with alternative activities using the therapeutic relationship as the vehicle.

Stiles *et al.* (1995) illustrated this analysis with case material concerning an individual patient's assimilation of a single theme—her difficulty in expressing feelings—that appeared to be an aspect of her successfully treated depression. The therapist's pursuit of tasks 2, 3 and 4 above, and the patient's associated progress toward assimilation of the problematic theme, were revealed in the session transcripts.

Experiential therapy

Experiential approaches covered in a review by Greenberg *et al.* (1994) include client-centred therapy (Rogers, 1951), Gestalt therapy (Perls *et al.*,

1951), the experiential approaches of Gendlin (1981) and Mahrer (1983), and a cluster of emotionally focused expressive approaches (Janov, 1970; Pierce *et al.*, 1983). Existential approaches (e.g. Bugental, 1978; Yalom, 1980) fall within their scope but coverage is limited by a lack of research. All define the facilitation of the patient's *experiencing* as the key therapeutic task, and view the therapeutic relationship as potentially curative. The relationship with the therapist provides the patient with a new, emotionally validating experience and an opportunity to discriminate between past and present and to discover and own experience.

In the past 15 years, new, more structured and active experiential therapies have emerged (e.g. Greenberg *et al.*, 1993). These incorporate specific procedures, such as the Gestalt therapy technique of the 'empty chair' in which the patient alternately takes the role of the self and of the other party to a problematic relationship. Such procedures are designed to promote the patient's processing of problematic emotions, and their well-specified components lend themselves to productive empirical research.

Trials of experiential therapy

Greenberg *et al.* (1994; enlarged by Elliott, 1996) present a meta-analysis of research on the effectiveness of experiential therapies. This literature is not extensive, but its findings are broadly supportive. Unfortunately for present purposes, experiential therapies have traditionally neglected diagnostic issues and so in many studies an indeterminate proportion of patients are likely to have met criteria for major depression. Sixty-three studies were analysed, including 27 with waiting-list or no-treatment conditions, and 31 studies comparing experiential therapies with other treatments. These ranged from psychoeducational interventions or treatment-as-usual conditions to cognitive, behavioural or psychodynamic therapies.

A mean pre-post effect size of 1.13 standard deviation units, and a mean control-referenced effect size of 1.04 standard deviation units, indicated substantial overall efficacy. Such effects place the average treated patient beyond the 80th percentile of control patients. Four studies of depression yielded pre-post effect sizes of 1.22, 1.35, 1.52 and 1.18 standard deviation units, thoroughly representative of the overall, mixed-diagnosis population embraced by the meta-analysis. The average difference between experiential and other treatments was essentially zero. A more specific comparison was made between experiential and cognitive and behavioural methods. Seventeen studies yielded an overall effect size advantage of 0.23 standard deviation units in favour of cognitive and behavioural treatments over experiential treatments. Although suggestive, this difference was significantly smaller than the 0.40 criterion for a clinically meaningful advantage of one treatment over another (Elliott *et al.*, 1993).

Illustrative studies available in English include a trial of the empty chair method, which demonstrated its superiority to a psychoeducational control group in yielding clinically meaningful improvements in symptoms of depression and anxiety, as well as interpersonal difficulties (Paivio & Greenberg, 1995). In a study of group therapies for major depressive disorder, Beutler *et al.* (1991) found that cognitive therapy and Focused Expressive Psychotherapy (Daldrup *et al.*, 1988) using directed fantasy and the empty chair technique, achieved overall benefits similar to those of a non-directive condition in which patients were supported and encouraged to use their own initiative to overcome problems via weekly telephone contacts and self-help readings.

Importantly, however, different patients prospered under each treatment, in accordance with the authors' predictions based on theories of personality: behavioural and symptom-orientated procedures of cognitive therapy were most helpful to 'externalizing' patients, those who control stress poorly, are irritable and impulsive, and tend to blame others. In contrast, these patients were not helped by the non-directive approach. Furthermore, 'internalizing' patients (who blame themselves, as is typical of many with depression), did worst with cognitive therapy and best with non-directive therapy. In addition, patients showing high 'resistance potential' fared best with non-directive therapy and worst with focused expressive therapy.

Change mechanisms of experiential therapy

Task analysis is a process research strategy that involves the detailed study of the processes that individuals actually use to perform tasks. It focuses on understanding the process of task solution and building explanatory models of the mechanisms involved therein. For example, Greenberg and Foerster (1996) focused on the resolution of 'unfinished business' (dissatisfaction about the nature of relationships in the past and associated feelings of disappointment, resentment, and grief) by the empty chair technique (Paivio & Greenberg, 1995).

Greenberg and Foerster (1996) used a 'rational-empirical' methodology of repeatedly cycling between rational conjecture and empirical observations to develop an intervention manual and to identify the components of the patient's resolution performance. A refined model of the change process developed in this fashion was validated by comparing 11 successful and 11 unsuccessful attempts at resolution. Four components, including intense expression of feeling, expression of need, shift in the representation of the other person, and self-validation or understanding of the other, were found to discriminate between successful and unsuccessful attempts.

This approach to experiential therapy in particular has demonstrated the benefits of analysing this treatment as a non-uniform, differentiated process in which patient and therapist engage in varied activities with specific impacts at different points (Greenberg *et al.*, 1994).

Overview of experiential therapy

Greenberg *et al.* (1994) conclude that experiential therapies have promise in the treatment of depression. They also warn of hindering factors identified in the literature, including therapist intrusion or pressure, therapist misatunement, insufficient therapist direction, and patient concerns such as lack of perceived safety, confusion or distraction. They note that highly autonomous or reactant patients may react negatively to the more directive experiential therapies, whereas more dependent or externally orientated patients may react negatively to unstructured, non-directive therapies.

Postscript: the wider context of psychotherapy research

Our understanding of what makes for effective psychological treatment of depression is usefully informed by considering the broader literature relating the processes of psychological treatments to their effects. A comprehensive overview of studies linking features or elements of treatment to clinical outcomes was conducted by Orlinsky *et al.* (1994). This review incorporated over 2000 findings, and yielded consistent evidence identifying factors that contribute to treatment efficacy. These factors are highly congruent with the findings already reviewed in this chapter, and include the following points.

1 *Implementation of the therapeutic 'contract'*: the patient's understanding and acceptance of the rationale and procedures of therapy; the patient's verbal activity; the therapist's skill and adherence to the treatment model. These findings argue for clear, explicitly structured treatment approaches that are well explained to the patient and competently followed by the therapist. This recommendation is supported, for example, by Frank and colleagues (1991) findings on therapists' contributions to the success of IPT.

2 *Procedures followed within therapy*: patients' focus on life problems and core personal relationships, and therapists' focus on patient problems, and, with sufficient tact and caution, on patients' emotional reactions during sessions; therapists' experiential confrontation and interpretation may also be beneficial, but this appears to depend on the patient's readiness to accept these interventions; patients' co-operation (as opposed to resistance) and positive affective arousal. These findings point to productive elements within psychodynamic, interpersonal and experiential therapies of depression and offer guidelines concerning their delivery.

3 *The quality of relationship between patient and therapist*, or 'therapeutic alliance', including role investment, coordination between the participants,

communicative contact and affective attitude. These findings are especially powerful from the patient's perspective, with a clear implication for management that if the patient does not feel positive about the relationship with the therapist, treatment will not succeed.

4 *The patient's openness (as opposed to defensiveness)*: this implies that therapists must foster this by making therapy as 'safe' as possible, confirmed by findings that critical or hostile responses by therapists interfere markedly with the treatment process and result in poor outcomes. These findings may explain why comorbid personality disorders impair the response of depressed patients to these treatments.

5 *The patient's experiencing of positive impacts within sessions*, which therapists (significantly) may fail to perceive although they are apparent to patients themselves and to outside observers.

In summary, the circumstances in which psychological treatment of depression is likely to succeed include the following: a well-structured treatment, skilfully delivered in the context of a safe, positive relationship between patient and therapist, in a manner responsive to the patient's requirements and productive of positive feelings during sessions, that focuses on the patient's key problem areas, will be effective with a patient who is open and ready to change.

Conclusions

There is reasonably good evidence for the efficacy of brief, structured forms of psychodynamic, interpersonal and experiential therapy in reducing the severity of depression or ending depressive episodes. This evidence comes from a variety of sources, including controlled trials, comparisons with other treatments of known efficacy, and single-group pre-post studies showing changes of comparable magnitude to those shown by other treatments independently supported by controlled trials. The evidence is patchy rather than comprehensive, however. It is likely to remain so, unless resources comparable to those made available by the pharmaceutical industry for drug trials become available for psychological treatment research. In addition, there is a pressing need for exponents of these treatment methods to become more skilled in, and committed to, the research enterprise. The use of these treatments in less-intensive formats over the months following successful treatment to prevent relapse or recurrence of depression warrants further study, based on promising results obtained with IPT.

As noted by Persons *et al.* (1996), the American Psychiatric Association's (1993) practise guideline offers an incomplete evaluation of psychodynamic therapy, overlooking the evidence of similarity in its effects to those of behavioural and drug treatments. When directly compared in 'head-to-head' trials with cognitive-behavioural therapies or drug treatments, these treatments do not fare badly. For example, cognitive-behavioural treatments may enjoy a slight advantage over the methods reviewed here, but any difference is small and may well reflect the preferences and skills of the majority of researchers rather than substantially inferior effectiveness. Persons *et al.* (1996) also note that the guideline overstates the argument that more severely or endogenously depressed out-patients require drug treatment (since the evidence on this point is in fact mixed) as well as the case for combining antidepressant medication with psychotherapy (unsupported by the majority of comparative studies).

Useful implications for the treatment of depression can be derived from the wider field of research on the processes of change in these treatments as applied to patient populations, including those not diagnosed with depression. For example, the evidence underscores the skill and sensitivity required for psychodynamic interpretations to be experienced as helpful rather than hindering or undermining. There is also evidence that the formation and maintenance of a positive relationship between patient and therapist is of paramount importance in determining the outcome of treatment, and may outweigh the specific techniques used. Comparison, in the Sheffield depression research, with cognitive-behavioural treatment, highlights many features in common between these two approaches whilst also identifying specific points of difference. For example, it may be that the methods considered here are less universally accepted by patients bringing differing attitudes and personality difficulties to the treatment of their depression than are cognitive-behavioural methods.

From an empirical researcher's perspective, the future of psychodynamic, interpersonal and experiential therapies of depression looks rosier than ever before. This is just as well, given the current demand for evidence-based treatment services (Aveline *et al.*, 1995). Evidence already to hand indicates that these methods have a place in the treatment of depression; extension and refinement of that evidence over the coming decade will assuredly define more clearly the indications for these treatments and their modes of action.

References

Agnew, R.M., Stiles, W.B., Hardy, G.E. *et al.* (1997) Alliance structure and relations with psychotherapy outcome assessed by the Agnew Relationship Measure (ARM).

Alexander, F. (1954) Psychoanalysis and psychotherapy. *Journal of the American Psychoanalytic Association*, **11**, 722–733.

American Psychiatric Association (1980) *Diagnostic and Statistical Manual of Mental Disorders*, 3rd edn. American Psychiatric Association, Washington, DC.

American Psychiatric Association (1993) Practice guideline for major depressive disorder in adults. *American Journal of Psychiatry*, **150** (Suppl. 4), 1–126.

Anderson, E.M. & Lambert, M.J. (1995) Short-term dynamically oriented psychotherapy: a review and meta-analysis. *Clinical Psychology Review*, 15, 503–514.

Aveline, M., Shapiro, D.A., Parry, G. & Freeman, F. (1995) Building research foundations for psychotherapy practice. In: *Research Foundations for Psychotherapy Practice* (eds M Aveline & D. A. Shapiro), pp. 301–322. John Wiley & Sons, Chichester.

Beck, A.T., Rush, A.J., Shaw, B.F. *et al.* (1979) *Cognitive Therapy of Depression*. Guilford, New York.

Beutler, L.E., Engle, D., Mohr, D. *et al.* (1991) Predictors of differential response to cognitive, experiential, and self-directed psychotherapeutic procedures. *Journal of Consulting and Clinical Psychology*, **59**, 333–340.

Blatt, S.J., Zuroff, D.C., Quinlan, D.M. & Pilkonis, P.A. (1996) Interpersonal factors in brief treatment of depression: further analyses of the National Institute of Mental Health Treatment of Depression Collaborative Research Program. *Journal of Consulting and Clinical Psychology*, **64**, 162–171.

Bugental, J.F.T. (1978) *Psychotherapy and Process: The Fundamentals of an Existential-humanistic Approach*. Random House, New York.

Covi, L. & Lipman, R.S. (1987) Cognitive-behavioral group psychotherapy combined with imipramine in major depression. *Psychopharmacology Bulletin*, **23**, 173–176.

Crits-Christoph, P. (1992) The efficacy of brief dynamic psychotherapy: a meta-analysis. *American Journal of Psychiatry*, **149**, 151–158.

Curtis, J.T., Silberschatz, G., Sampson, H. & Weiss, J. (1994) The plan formulation method. *Psychotherapy Research*, **4**, 197–207.

Daldrup, R.J., Beutler, L.E., Engle, D. & Greenberg, L.S. (1988) *Focused Expressive Psychotherapy: Freeing the Overcontrolled Patient*. Guilford Press, New York.

Depression Guideline Panel (1993) *Clinical Practice Guideline: Depression in Primary Care*, Vol. 2. *Treatment of Major Depression*. Agency for Health Care Policy and Research Publication no. 93–0551. US Department of Health and Human Services, Rockville, MD.

DiMascio, A., Weissman, M., Prusoff, B., Neu, C., Zwilling, M. & Klerman, G. (1979) Differential symptom reduction by drugs and psychotherapy in acute depression. *Archives of General Psychiatry*, **36**, 1450–1456.

Dobson, K.S. (1989) A meta-analysis of the efficacy of cognitive therapy for depression. *Journal of Consulting and Clinical Psychology*, **57**, 414–419.

Elkin, I. (1994) The NIMH Treatment of Depression Collaborative Research Program: where we began and where we are. In: *Handbook of Psychotherapy and Behavior Change*, 4th edn, 114–139 (eds A. E. Bergin & S. L. Garfield). John Wiley & Sons, New York.

Elkin, I., Shea, M.T., Collins, J.F. *et al.* (1989) National Institute of Mental Health Treatment of Depression Collaborative Research Program: general effectiveness of treatments. *Archives of General Psychiatry*, **46**, 971–982.

Elkin, I., Gibbons, R.D., Shea, M.T. *et al.* (1996) Science is not a trial (but it can sometimes be a tribulation). *Journal of Consulting and Clinical Psychology*, **64**, 92–103.

Elliott, R. (1995) Therapy process research and clinical practice: practical strategies. In: *Research Foundations for Psychotherapy Practice*, pp. 49–72 (eds M. Aveline & D. A. Shapiro). John Wiley & Sons, Chichester.

Elliott, R. (1996) Are Client-centered/experiential therapies effective? A meta-analysis of outcome research. Paper presented at the Annual Meeting of the Society for Psychotherapy Research, Amelia Island, Florida, June 1996.

Elliott, R., Stiles, W.B. & Shapiro, D.A. (1993) Are some psychotherapies more equivalent than others? In: *Handbook of Effective Psychotherapy* (ed. T.R. Giles), pp. 455–479. Plenum Press, New York.

Frank, E., Kupfer, D.J., Perel, J.M. *et al.* (1990) Three year outcomes for maintenance therapies in recurrent depression. *Archives of General Psychiatry*, **47**, 1093–1099.

Frank, E., Kupfer, D.J., Wagner, E.F., McEachran, A.B. & Cornes, C. (1991) Efficacy of interpersonal psychotherapy as a maintenance treatment of recurrent depression: contributing factors. *Archives of General Psychiatry*, **48**, 1053–1059.

Frank, J.D. & Frank, J.B. (1991) *Persuasion and Healing: A Comparison to Psychotherapy*. Johns Hopkins University Press, Baltimore.

Gallagher, D.E. & Thompson, L.W. (1982) Treatment of major depressive disorder in older adult patients with brief psychotherapies. *Psychotherapy: Theory, Research and Practice*, **19**, 482–490.

Gendlin, E.T. (1981) *Focusing*, 2nd edn. Bantam Books, New York.

Gibbons, R.D., Hedeker, D., Elkin, I. *et al.* (1993) Some conceptual and statistical issues in analysis of longitudinal psychiatric data. *Archives of General Psychiatry*, **50**, 739–750.

Giles, T.R. (ed.) (1993) *Handbook of Effective Psychotherapy*. Plenum Press, New York.

Greenberg, L.S. & Foerster, F.S. (1996) Task analysis exemplified: the process of resolving unfinished business. *Journal of Consulting and Clinical Psychology*, **64**, 439–446.

Greenberg, L., Rice, L.N. & Elliott, R. (1993) *Facilitating Emotional Change: The Moment-by-Moment Process*. Guilford, New York.

Greenberg, L., Elliott, R. & Lietaer, G. (1994) Research on experiential psychotherapies. In:

Handbook of Psychotherapy and Behavior Change (eds S. L. Garfield & A. E. Bergin), pp. 509–539. John Wiley & Sons, New York.

Hardy, G.E., Barkham, M., Shapiro, D.A., Stiles, W.B., Rees, A. & Reynolds, S. (1995a) Impact of Cluster C personality disorders on outcomes of contrasting brief psychotherapies for depression. *Journal of Consulting and Clinical Psychology*, **63**, 997–1004.

Hardy, G.E., Barkham, M., Shapiro, D.A., Reynolds, S., Rees, A. & Stiles, W.B. (1995b) Client beliefs, expectancy and outcome in cognitive-behavioural and psychodynamic-interpersonal psychotherapy. *British Journal of Clinical Psychology*, **34**, 555–569.

Hardy, G.E., Stiles, W.B., Barkham, M. & Startup, M. (in press) Therapist responsiveness to client interpersonal styles during time-limited treatments for depression. *Journal of Consulting and Clinical Psychology*.

Henry, W.P., Strupp, H.H., Butler, S.F., Schacht, T.E. & Binder, J.L. (1993) The effects of trzaining in time-limited dynamic psychotherapy: changes in therapist behavior. *Journal of Consulting and Clinical Psychology*, **61**, 434–440.

Henry, W.P., Strupp, H.H., Schacht, T.E. & Gaston, L. (1994) Psychodynamic approaches. In: *Handbook of Psychotherapy and Behavior Change*, 4th edn (eds A. E. Bargin & S. L. Garfield), pp. 467–508. John Wiley & Sons, New York.

Hersen, M., Bellak, A.S., Himmelhoch, J.M. & Thase, M.E. (1984) Effects of social skill training, amitriptyline, and psychotherapy in unipolar depressed women. *Behavior Therapy*, **15**, 21–40.

Hill, C.E., O'Grady, K.E. & Elkin, I. (1992) Applying the Collaborative Study Psychotherapy Rating Scale to rate therapist adherence in cognitive-behavior therapy, interpersonal therapy, and clinical management. *Journal of Consulting and Clinical Psychology*, **60**, 73–79.

Hobson, R.F. (1985) *Forms of Feeling: The Heart of Psychotherapy*. Basic Books, New York.

Imber, S.D., Pilkonis, P.A., Sotsky, S.M. *et al.* (1990) Mode-specific effects among three treatments for depression. *Journal of Consulting and Clinical Psychology*, **58**, 352–359.

Jacobson, N.S. & Hollon, S.D. (1996) Prospects for future comparisons between drugs and psychotherapy: lessons from the CBT-vs.-pharmacotherapy exchange. *Journal of Consulting and Clinical Psychology*, **64**, 104–108.

Janov, A. (1970) *The Primal Scream: Primal Therapy, the Cure for Neurosis*. Dell, New York.

Klein, D.F. (1996) Preventing hung juries about therapy studies. *Journal of Consulting and Clinical Psychology*, **64**, 81–87.

Klein, D.F. & Ross, D.C. (1993) Reanalysis of the National Institute of Mental Health Treatment of Depression Collaborative Research Program general effectiveness report. *Neuropsychopharmacology*, **8**, 241–251.

Klerman, G.L., DiMascio, A., Weissman, M.M., Prusoff, B.A. & Paykel, E.S. (1974) Treatment of depression by drugs and psychotherapy. *American Journal of Psychiatry*, **131**, 186–191.

Klerman, G.L., Weissman, N.M., Rounsaville, B.J. & Chevron, E.S. (1984) *Interpersonal Psychotherapy of Depression*. Basic Books, New York.

Kornblith, S.J., Rehm, L.P., O'Hara, M.W. & Lamparski, D.M. (1983) The contribution of self-reinforcement training and behavioral assignments to the efficacy of self-control therapy for depression. *Cognitive Therapy and Research*, **7**, 499–527.

Luborsky, L. (1984) *Principles of Psychoanalytic Psychotherapy: A Manual for Supportive-Expressive Treatment*. Basic Books, New York.

Luborsky, L., Popp, C., Barber, J.P. & Shapiro, D.A. (eds) (1994) Special issue: seven transference-related measures. *Psychotherapy Research*, **4**, 151–286.

Mahrer, A.R. (1983) *Experiential Psychotherapy: Basic Practises*. Brunner/Mazel, New York.

Malan, D.H. (1976) *The Frontier of Brief Psychotherapy*. Plenum Press, New York.

Mallinckrodt, B., Gantt, D.L. & Coble, H.M. (1995) Attachment patterns in the psychotherapy relationship: development of the client attachment to therapist scale. *Journal of Counseling Psychology*, **42**, 307–317.

McLean, P.D. & Hakstian, A.R. (1979) Clinical depression: comparative efficacy of outpatient treatments. *Journal of Consulting and Clinical Psychology*, **47**, 818–836.

Mollon, P. & Parry, G. (1984) The fragile self: narcissistic disturbance and the protective function of depression. *British Journal of Medical Psychology*, **57**, 137–145.

Neitzel, M.T., Russell, R.L., Hemmings, K.A. & Gretter, M.L. (1987) Clinical significance of psychotherapy for unipolar depression: a meta-analytic approach to social comparison. *Journal of Consulting and Clinical Psychology*, **55**, 156–161.

O'Malley, S.S., Foley, S.H., Rounsaville, B.J. *et al.* (1988) Therapist competence and patient outcome in interpersonal psychotherapy of depression. *Journal of Consulting and Clinical Psychology*, **56**, 496–501.

Orlinsky, D.E., Grawe, K. & Parks, B.K. (1994) Process and outcome in psychotherapy: noch einmal. In: *Handbook of Psychotherapy and*

Behavior Change, 4th edn (eds A. E. Bergin & S. L. Garfield), pp. 270–376. John Wiley & Sons, New York.

Paivio, S. & Greenberg, L.S. (1995) Resolving 'unfinished business': efficacy of experiential therapy using empty chair dialogue. *Journal of Consulting and Clinical Psychology*, **63**, 419–425.

Paykel, E.S., DiMascio, A., Haskell, D. & Prusoff, B.A. (1975) Effects of maintenance amitriptyline and psychotherapy on symptoms of depression. *Psychological Medicine*, **5**, 67–77.

Perls, F.S., Hefferline, R.F. & Goodman, P. (1951) *Gestalt Therapy*. Julian Press, New York.

Perry, H.S. (1982) *Psychiatrist of America: The life of Harry Stack Sullivan*. Belknap Press of Harvard University Press, Cambridge, MA.

Persons, J.B., Thase, M.E. & Crits-Christoph, P. (1996) The role of psychotherapy in the treatment of depression: review of two practice guidelines. *Archives of General Psychiatry*, **53**, 283–290.

Pierce, R.A., Nichols, M.P. & DuBrin, J.R. (1983) *Emotional Expression in Psychotherapy*. Gardner Press, New York.

Piper, W.E., Azim, F.A., Joyce, S.A. & McCullum, M. (1991) Transference interpretations, therapeutic alliance and outcome in short-term individual psychotherapy. *Archives of General Psychiatry*, **48**, 946–953.

Prusoff, B.A., Weissman, M.M., Klerman, G.L. & Rounsaville, B.J. (1980) Research diagnostic criteria subtypes of depression: their role as predictors of differential response to psychotherapy and drug treatment. *Archives of General Psychiatry*, **37**, 796–801.

Reynolds, S., Stiles, W.B., Barkham, M., Shapiro, D.A., Hardy, G.E. & Rees, A. (1996) Acceleration of changes in session impact during contrasting time-limited psychotherapies. *Journal of Consulting and Clinical Psychology*, **64**, 577–586.

Robinson, L.A., Berman, J.S. & Neimeyer, R.A. (1990) Psychotherapy for the treatment of depression: a comprehensive review of controlled outcome research. *Psychological Bulletin*, **100**, 30–49.

Rogers, C.R. (1951) *Client-Centered Therapy*. Houghton Mifflin, Boston.

Roth, A. & Fonagy, P. (1996) *What Works for Whom: A Critical Review of Psychotherapy Research*. Guilford Publications, New York.

Shapiro, D.A. (1995) Finding out how psychotherapies help people change. *Psychotherapy Research*, **5**, 1–13.

Shapiro, D.A. (1996) Models of change in psychotherapy. *Current Opinion in Psychiatry*, **9**, 177–181.

Shapiro, D.A. & Shapiro, D. (1982) Meta-analysis of comparative therapy outcome research: a replication and refinement. *Psychological Bulletin*, **92**, 581–604.

Shapiro, D.A., Barkham, M., Rees, A. *et al.* (1994) Effects of treatment duration and severity of depression on the effectiveness of cognitive-behavioral and psychodynamic-interpersonal psychotherapy. *Journal of Consulting and Clinical Psychology*, **62**, 522–534.

Shapiro, D.A., Rees, A., Barkham, M. *et al.* (1995) Effects of treatment duration and severity of depression on the maintenance of gains following cognitive-behavioral and psychodynamic-interpersonal psychotherapy. *Journal of Consulting and Clinical Psychology*, **63**, 378–387.

Shea, M.T., Elkin, I., Imber, S.D. *et al.* (1992a) Course of depressive symptoms over follow-up: findings from the National Institute of Mental Health Treatment of Depression Collaborative Research Program. *Archives of General Psychiatry*, **49**, 782–787.

Shea, M.T., Widiger, T.A. & Klein, M.H. (1992b) Comorbidity of personality disorders and depression: implications for treatment. *Journal of Consulting and Clinical Psychology*, **60**, 857–868.

Sifneos, P.E. (1972) *Short-term Psychotherapy and Emotional Crisis*. Harvard University Press, Cambridge, MA.

Smith, M.L. & Glass, G.V. (1977) Meta-analysis of psychotherapy outcome studies. *American Psychologist*, **32**, 752–760.

Smith, M.L., Glass, G.V. & Miller, T.I. (1980) *The Benefits of Psychotherapy*. Johns Hopkins University Press, Baltimore.

Sotsky, S.M., Glass, D.R., Shea, M.T. *et al.* (1991) Patient predictors of response to psychotherapy and pharmacotherapy: findings in the NIMH Treatment of Depression Collaborative Research Program. *American Journal of Psychiatry*, **148**, 997–1008.

Startup, M.J. & Shapiro, D.A. (1993) Therapist treatment fidelity in Prescriptive vs. Exploratory psychotherapy. *British Journal of Clinical Psychology*, **32**, 443–456.

Steuer, J.L., Mintz, J., Hammen, C.L. *et al.* (1984) Cognitive-behavioral and psychodynamic group psychotherapy in treatment of geriatric depression. *Journal of Consulting and Clinical Psychology*, **52**, 180–189.

Stiles, W.B. & Shapiro, D.A. (1989) Abuse of the drug metaphor in psychotherapy process-outcome research. *Clinical Psychology Review*, **9**, 521–543.

Stiles, W.B., Elliott, R., Lewellyn, S.P. *et al.* (1990) Assimilation of problematic experiences by clients in psychotherapy. *Psychotherapy*, **27**, 411–420.

Stiles, W.B., Shapiro, D.A., Harper, H. & Morrison, L.A. (1995) Therapist contributions to psychotherapeutic assimilation: an alternative to the drug metaphor. *British Journal of Medical Psychology,* **68,** 1–13.

Stiles, W.B., Startup, M., Hardy, G.E. *et al.* (1996) Therapist session intentions in cognitive-behavioral and psychodynamic-interpersonal psychotherapy. *Journal of Counseling Psychology,* Vol. 43, **4,** 402–414.

Strupp, H.H. & Binder, J.L. (1984) *Psychotherapy in a New Key: A Guide to Time-limited Dynamic Psychotherapy.* Basic Books, New York.

Sullivan, H.S. (ed.) (1953) *The Interpersonal Theory of Psychiatry.* W.W. Norton, New York.

Svartberg, M. & Stiles, T.C. (1991) Comparative effects of short-term psychodynamic psychotherapy: a meta-analysis. *Journal of Consulting and Clinical Psychology,* **59,** 704–714.

Thompson, L.W., Gallagher, D. & Breckenridge, L.S. (1987) Comparative effectiveness of psychotherapies for depressed elders. *Journal of Consulting and Clinical Psychology,* **55,** 385–390.

Tishby, O. & Messer, S.B. (1995) The relationship between plan compatibility of therapist interventions and patient progress: a comparison of two plan formulations. *Psychotherapy Research,* **5,** 76–88.

Watkins, J.T., Leber, W.R., Imber, S.D. *et al.* (1993) NIMH Treatment of Depression Collaborative Research Program: temporal course of symptomatic change. *Journal of Consulting and Clinical Psychology,* **61,** 858–864.

Weissman, M.M. & Markowitz, J.C. (1994) Interpersonal therapy: current status. *Archives of General Psychiatry,* **51,** 599–606.

Weissman, M.M., Klerman, G.L., Paykel, E.S., Prusoff, B.A. & Hanson, B. (1974) Treatment effects on the social adjustment of depressed patients. *Archives of General Psychiatry,* **30,** 771–778.

Weissman, M.M., Prusoff, B.A., DiMascio, A. *et al.* (1979) The efficacy of drugs and psychotherapy in the treatment of acute depressive episodes. *American Journal of Psychiatry,* **136,** 555–558.

Weissman, M.M., Klerman, G.L., Prusoff, B.A. *et al.* (1981) Depressed outpatients: results one year after treatment with drugs and/or interpersonal psychotherapy. *Archives of General Psychiatry,* **38,** 51–55.

Yalom, I.D. (1980) *Existential Psychotherapy.* Basic Books, New York.

8 The efficacy of cognitive-behavioural therapy

EDWARD WATKINS AND RUTH WILLIAMS

Cognitive-behavioural therapy (CBT) is the generic term for a variety of short-term psychological therapies which are based upon the importance of thinking and behaviour in generating and maintaining emotional disorders. Specifically, cognitive therapy, first described by Beck *et al.* (1979), was probably the first psychological therapy to be demonstrated as effective with modern research methods in the treatment of depression and it has since received considerable interest from the scientific community, having been taken up and studied in numerous cultures and populations, spawning a variety of new methods and techniques to deal with other problems. Much of this chapter will focus upon studies of Beck's Cognitive Therapy, although in practice and in different clinical contexts a variety of cognitive and behavioural methods are in use.

CBT uses a combination of behavioural and cognitive techniques to help an individual cope with symptoms and deal with life problems. For example, therapy may start by combating inactivity and withdrawal by monitoring and planning activities and proceed into examining the specific interpretations he/she is making in the context of such activity. As therapy proceeds, the focus moves on to examine the themes underlying these specific interpretations to examine and challenge the individual's underlying attitudes and beliefs which relate to their problems. CBT differs from some other therapies in being educative and non-mysterious in character. Beck uses the term 'collaborative empiricism' to describe the particular nature of the therapeutic relationship which is neither directive nor authoritative, as in traditional behaviour therapy nor aloof and dogmatically interpretative as in psychodynamic therapy. The central idea is that the patient and therapist work together to examine and test out the usefulness of the way the patient is thinking and behaving in order to achieve therapeutic goals. An important role is given to the carrying out of intersession tasks designed to help change both thought and behaviour. Therapeutic success is often directly correlated with the degree to which the patient complies in carrying out these assignments. Beck has suggested that the patient needs practice in dealing with some 70 episodes of negative thinking to learn the necessary skills. In the process the patient learns some general principles about the way they may become and remain depressed which may help them to deal differently with problems in the future. CBT is a short-term therapy, initially designed to be carried out over 12–20 sessions in 3–6 months. Recently, both briefer and longer, more intensive packages have been devised, in response to the varieties of need with which depressed patients present.

CBT has been demonstrated to be a generally effective treatment for depression in the large number of studies that have accumulated since the original study of Rush *et al.* (1977). It has performed well in trials comparing minimal treatment controls and other treatments (Dobson, 1989). It has generally produced greater improvement in depressive symptomatology than no treatment or waiting-list controls (Comas-Diaz, 1981; Gallagher & Thompson, 1982; Wilson, *et al.*, 1983).

Comparisons with pharmacotherapy have yielded less clearcut results, principally because of methodological difficulties. Individual studies have involved relatively few patients and studies have been carried out in prestigous university centres where patients and therapists employed may not have been representative of those in more usual settings. Many studies comparing CBT and pharmacotherapy have lacked drug-placebo controls, so it was not possible to determine whether the patients were pharmacologically responsive. Furthermore, the administration of pharmacotherapy has not been adequately operationalized; in many studies patient compliance or plasma medication levels were not monitored, such that the adequacy of the pharmacotherapy was not checked (Hollon *et al.*, 1991). As a result of these difficulties, although many clinical trials have demonstrated CBT and pharmacotherapy to be of comparable efficacy for depression (e.g. Rush *et al.*, 1977; Blackburn *et al.*, 1981; Murphy *et al.*, 1984; Hollon *et al.*, 1992a), to some critics this hypothesis has still not been adequately tested. In addition, little is known as yet about the effectiveness of CBT relative to other forms of psychological intervention. Robinson *et al.* (1990) carried out a comprehensive review of controlled outcome research comprising all types of psychotherapy for depression using meta-analysis. Results indicated an advantage for CBT methods over strictly behavioural and 'general verbal' psychotherapies. The authors raise the point, however, that there is a relationship between 'allegiance' to school of therapy and outcome. When this is corrected for, the comparative benefit for CBT disappears. Whilst we would agree that there might be a therapeutic impetus to be gained through therapist allegiance, we would not agree that this should necessarily be counted as error.

The one recent and larger study which sought to control for some of these difficulties was the National Institute of Mental Health (NIMH) Treatment of Depression Collaborative Research Program (Elkin *et al.*, 1989). This study compared imipramine, CBT, interpersonal psychotherapy and a psychological placebo control therapy in treating depression in three different sites away from university clinics. This study found overall few significant differences between treatments, but for the relatively more severe patients those receiving medication did best, and patients with placebo only did worst, with the two psychotherapies intermediate. On several measures CBT did only as well as the placebo control and much less well than pharmacotherapy. However, the adequacy of the execution of the CBT at different sites has been questioned in this study. Many of the therapists were relatively inexperienced and supervision was deliberately less intense. Large differences were seen between sites: at one site, pharmacotherapy outperformed CBT, but at another site the different treatments were equally effective. This suggests that there were differences in the skill in application of CBT between sites. Thus there are possible methodological problems with the administration of CBT in this study.

In all, therefore, the relative performance of CBT and pharmacotherapy in treating depression is still an open question. Where therapists have adequate training and supervision, it is most likely that the two treatments will prove to be of overall comparable efficacy. The more controlled studies, utilizing experienced pharmacologists and monitoring compliance and plasma medication levels, demonstrated little superiority for either CBT or pharmacotherapy in the treatment of depression (Murphy *et al.*, 1984; Hollon *et al.*, 1992a). What is clear is that no controlled study of outcome of CBT in depression has had a negative result. Whatever the relative merits of CBT to pharmacotherapy, it is clearly an effective treatment. Perhaps the more important issues to address are the differences in responsiveness within a 'depressed' sample in different settings, the identification of the 'responder' and the development of methods to cope with non-responders.

When examining the efficacy of CBT, two issues are of importance. First, a distinction needs to be made between CBT applied alone and CBT applied in combination with other treatments, principally pharmacotherapy. When considering the efficacy of a treatment in a research study, comparison with another validated treatment may be most helpful, but in clinical practice knowing whether the addition of another treatment will produce further symptomatic improvement may be of more benefit. Therefore this chapter will draw attention to studies of CBT alone and CBT in combination with other treatments. Second, CBT is constantly evolving and new modifications are made for specific difficulties. When considering the efficacy of CBT in depression, a distinction is necessary between the original approach of individual sessions in the Beck format (Beck *et al.*, 1979) and more specialist approaches. Some recent developments will be briefly mentioned at the end of this chapter.

Treatment settings

Primary care

In primary care settings, CBT has been demonstrated to be at least as effective as other interventions (Blackburn *et al.*, 1981; Scott & Freeman, 1992), and a useful adjunct to normal general practice care (Teasdale *et al.*, 1984), and in at least one setting, superior to normal general practice care (Ross & Scott, 1985). Since depressive illness makes up around 10% of consecutive consultations in primary care (Blacker & Clare, 1987) and the longer depression is untreated, the more chance there is of a chronic treatment-refractory depressive disorder developing (Scott *et al.*, 1992), the increased availability of CBT in primary care settings may be a development to be actively considered.

In one of the earliest investigations of CBT in the UK in Edinburgh, Blackburn *et al.* (1981) compared CBT and antidepressant medication in patients with major depressive disorder in psychiatric out-patient and general practice settings. They found that patients receiving CBT in general practice did better than patients receiving antidepressants. There were difficulties with this study however. It has been suggested that the administration of medication in primary care was inadequate. Furthermore, patients were not randomly allocated to therapists.

Teasdale *et al.* (1984) compared treatment-as-usual in a general practice setting in Oxford, with treatment-as-usual plus CBT, for patients with major depressive disorder. At completion of treatment, patients receiving cognitive therapy were significantly less depressed than the comparison group, both on blind ratings of symptom severity made by psychiatric assessors and on a self-report measure of depression. Three out of 17 patients given the combined treatment failed to improve at all; the remaining 14 improving substantially to a non-depressed status. The treatment-as-usual group, which included medication and advice from the general practitioner (GP), contained only four patients who improved to a non-depressed status, with five out of 17 patients failing to improve at all, and the remaining eight patients ending in a mildly to moderately depressed state. Fennell and Teasdale (1987) identified a group of quick responders to CBT who produced a 50% improvement in symptomatology within one or two sessions only. These findings indicate both the importance of individual differences in response to treatment and the high proportion of patients benefiting from the combined approach. They also pointed the way to the development of abbreviated treatments for some patients in primary care.

Ross and Scott (1985) randomly allocated depressed patients in a general practice health centre in inner city Liverpool, to individual CBT, group CBT (each having 12 sessions) or a treatment-as-usual group. Both CBT groups did significantly better than the treatment-as-usual group. There were no significant differences between the group or individual CBT. Treatment improvements were maintained at 12-month follow-up.

In a more recent study which suggests an improved outcome (at least in Edinburgh) in the treatment of depression by GPs in the community, Scott and Freeman (1992) compared randomized allocation to an abbreviated individual CBT, amitriptyline, social work counselling and routine GP care for 121 major depressive disorder patients in 14 primary care practices in Edinburgh. They found that all treatment groups produced marked improvement in depressive symptoms over 16 weeks, with only small advantages for specialist treatments over GP care. However, as Jan Scott points out (Scott J. *et al.*, 1994), there are some important questions about this study, including failure to control for chronicity of depression (the CBT group had significantly longer duration of depression), failure to monitor the adequacy of the CBT intervention and absence of follow-up. Such shortcomings limit the conclusions to be drawn from this study.

There have been some other successful developments to produce abbreviated courses of CBT for depression in primary care (Miranda & Munoz, 1994; Scott C.S. *et al.*, 1994). With the need for cost-effectiveness, short but effective treatments in primary care are likely to become increasingly important.

Miranda and Munoz (1994) randomly assigned 150 public care medical patients in San Francisco to either an 8-week CBT course or a control condition. The patients fulfilled criteria for minor depression (depressed mood or anhedonia plus one or more depressive symptoms, insufficient to meet major depressive disorder). The CBT group showed reductions in symptoms which persisted over 1 year. They also reported less somatic symptomatology and missed fewer appointments with their primary care provider in the following year.

Scott C.S. *et al.* (1994) have piloted a short CBT consisting of six weekly sessions each lasting 20 min (a total of 2 h of therapy) carried out by GPs themselves. With a sample of seven major depressive disorder patients (more severely depressed than in comparable studies) a mean fall of 15 points (47%) was seen on the Beck Depression Inventory (BDI) and a mean fall of 14.7 points (54%) seen on the Hamilton Rating Scale for Depression (HRSD). Four of the subjects showed at least 50% change in depression ratings during treatment. Only one of the seven patients was on antidepressant medication. Although small and lacking a control group, this study does demonstrate the potential for CBT to make a large impact on the population of depressed primary care patients, within the financial and time constraints of such a service, although caution is warranted in the interpretation of these results, especially due to the absence of follow-up. Results of primary care studies are summarized in Table 8.1.

Table 8.1 Studies of CBT in primary care.

Study group	n	HRSD at start	Treatment	Controls
Blackburn *et al.* (1981)	24	17	12–20 sessions	Tricyclic
Teasdale *et al.* (1984)	34	19	12–20 sessions	TAU
Ross & Scott (1985)	51	–	12 sessions individual or group	TAU
Scott & Freeman (1992)	121	18	Eight sessions	Tricyclic SW counselling GP care
Miranda & Munoz (1994)	150	–	Eight sessions ×2 h	WL
Scott *et al.* (1994)	7	27	Six ×20 min sessions	Uncontrolled

HRSD, Hamilton Rating Scale for Depession;
TAU, treatment as usual;
SW, social worker;
WL, waiting List.

Another development of interest is the evaluation of minimal contact bibliotherapy in the treatment of depressed individuals in the community. A great deal of self-help written material is currently available, much of it espousing a cognitive-behavioural approach. One book about depression, *Feeling Good* by David D. Burns (1980) is commonly used as an adjunct to individual therapy and patients often find it useful. (A revised version is now available called *The Feeling Good Handbook*, Burns, 1995). Jamison and Scogin (1995) were the first to conduct a controlled trial of the effectiveness of the original book, as a stand-alone treatment with a group of 80 community volunteers diagnosed from the HRSD as suffering from major depression. The experimental group showed a statistically and clinically highly significant improvement in symptoms relative to a waiting list control group, and these changes were maintained at 3 months' follow-up. At the end of the 'treatment' period, 70% of the experimental group (in comparison with 3% of the control group) no longer reached criteria for major depression. These findings, if replicated, could suggest a straightforward solution to the problem of scale in reaching the large numbers of depressed individuals presently untreated in the community.

Out-patient settings

The majority of controlled outcome studies already quoted in this chapter, testify to the effectiveness of CBT for depression in out-patient settings. CBT

Table 8.2 Studies of CBT in secondary care (out-patients).

Study group	n	HRSD at start	Controls
Rush *et al.* (1977)	41	22	Tricyclic
Backburn *et al.* (1981)	40	19	Tricyclic Combination
Murphy *et al.* (1984)	70	20	Tricyclic Combination Placebo
Beck *et al.* (1985)	33	21	Combination
Elkin *et al.* (1989)	250	19	Tricyclic IPT Placebo + CM
Hollon *et al.* (1992a, b)	64	24	Tricyclic Combination
Jacobson *et al.* (1996)	150	18	BA AT

HRSD, Hamilton Rating Scale for Depression;
Combination, tricyclic + CT;
IPT, interpersonal psychotherapy;
CM, clinical management;
BA, behavioural activation;
AT, BA + work on automatic thoughts.

for out-patients has been shown to be effective in a range of countries: the US (e.g. Rush *et al.*, 1977); UK (e.g. Blackburn *et al.*, 1981); Australia (e.g. Wilson *et al.*, 1983); and Canada (Jacobson *et al.*, 1996). Studies of outcome for depressed patients in secondary care out-patient settings are summarized in Table 8.2. Later in this chapter further data will be discussed bearing upon extent of improvement and other questions of interest about this group of patients.

In-patient settings

Controlled studies of CBT in in-patient settings are few as yet but again there are suggestions for the effectiveness of CBT. Patients on psychiatric wards are more likely to have greater severity and chronicity of depression and more associated psychopathology. Examination of CBT with in-patients therefore also provides information about the use of CBT with more severely depressed patients. The studies of CBT with this population do not compare CBT alone with other treatments but are interested in whether CBT added to medication can significantly improve treatment outcome. The results are generally positive; the addition of CBT to standard in-patient treatment, including pharmacotherapy, often improves outcome at either discharge or follow-up (Miller *et al.*, 1989; Bowers, 1990; Scott, 1992). Treatment developments have also been made in this setting; Scott (1992) has developed a version of CBT for use with drug-refractory chronic depression patients which, by taking account of the special needs of these patients, has greatly increased their symptom improvement. Thus, a specially designed CBT managed to produce improvements in patients who had been depressed for at least 2 years and had failed to respond to all other standard anti-depressant treatments.

Miller *et al.* (1989) compared standard in-patient treatment (pharma-cotherapy, hospital milieu, management sessions) with standard therapy plus CBT and standard therapy plus social skills training. The treatments began in hospital and continued for 4 months on an out-patient basis after discharge. All groups showed significant improvements at discharge. There were no significant differences at discharge between groups but after 4 months, the CBT and social skills treatment groups had less symptoms than the stand-ard treatment group. Similarly, Bowers (1990) demonstrated that a CBT plus medication group produced lower clinical ratings of depression at discharge than a medication alone or a medication plus relaxation group. Scott (1992) showed that the addition of 15 sessions of standard CBT to a combined pharmacotherapy treatment for chronically depressed patients, produced a statistically significant improvement in symptoms (mean change HRSD of 12, mean change in BDI of 16), although the clients were not clinically recov-ered and half the sample reported minimal change.

A specifically modified version of CBT (Scott, 1992) produced much bet-ter results; a mean change in HRSD of 14 and mean change in BDI of 24 (52–57%) and significant subjective and objective change in 69% of patients. This treatment adopted a 'CBT milieu' approach. Increased attention was focused on action-orientated techniques and on patients' responses to, and engagement with, therapy. CBT sessions were shorter and more frequent (20 min, three times a week) and nursing staff adopted CBT techniques into their everyday interactions with the patients. Thus some staff would have the role of encouraging patients to perform tasks, others would collaborate with patients in making plans or give reinforcement for their efforts. All staff would try and test negative cognitions whenever they became apparent. There were also sessions with the patient's families. As yet untested in controlled evaluation, the chronicity of the group studied by Scott and her colleagues indicates that such an intensive combined approach can yield powerful effects, although the *specificity of these effects for this modified CBT needs to be studied.* Replications and extensions of this approach would be of great value.

Depressed patients suitable for CBT

Although the greatest scientific attention has been given to major depression, CBT has been shown to be effective for a range of depressive conditions: symptomatic community volunteers (Wierzbicki & Bartlett, 1987); adolescents (Reynolds & Coats, 1986); elderly populations (Gallagher & Thompson, 1982); minor depression (Miranda & Munoz, 1994); primary major depressive disorder (Blackburn *et al.*, 1981; Kovacs *et al.*, 1981; Elkin *et al.*, 1989); residual symptoms of depression (Fava *et al.*, 1994) and chronic drug-refractory depressed patients (Scott, 1992). The usefulness of CBT with bipolar depression and psychotic depression is, as yet, little explored. Recent studies of CBT as an adjunctive treatment with medication in schizophrenic populations (e.g. Garety *et al.*, 1994) would suggest that these areas could be fruitfully investigated. Although CBT may not act on primary causes and symptoms of these disorders, it may be useful to deal with secondary problems.

Attempts to determine whether CBT is more or less effective for any particular types of depressed patient have not been particularly successful. Approaches to the question of who will respond to CBT can be broadly split into two factors: *prognostic* factors—what factors predict who will do best with CBT?—and *prescriptive* factors—which treatment will best help this individual?

The evidence gathered has tended to generate some prognostic factors but few prescriptive factors. The factors which have been considered in response to treatment range from sociodemographic variables (age, sex, marital status), to diagnostic and course of depression variables (endogenous, situational, severity, chronicity), to function and personality variables (IQ, personality disorder, attitudes to treatment and self).

Prescriptive factors

No sociodemographic factors have been demonstrated to favour the choice of one therapy over another in a range of studies (McLean & Hakstian, 1979; Jarrett *et al.*, 1991; Sotsky *et al.*, 1991).

Attempts to demonstrate that different types of depression would respond better to CBT or pharmacotherapy have also been inconclusive. Beck's cognitive model for depression would seem to be most applicable to depressions that are reactive to life events. Gallagher and Thompson's (1982) results which suggested that more non-endogenously depressed elderly patients (80%) responded to CBT than endogenous depressed patients (33%) are consistent with this view. However, both Blackburn *et al.* (1981) and Kovacs *et al.* (1981) found that an endogenous/non-endogenous distinction did not separate responders from non-responders to CBT alone. Sotsky *et al.* (1991) found that endogenous depression predicted more improvement with all interventions

(CBT, interpersonal therapy, imipramine and placebo control). Again, endogeneity did not distinguish CBT from the other treatments. Similarly, depressed patients with higher pretreatment stress levels do not respond better to CBT than to imipramine (Garvey *et al.*, 1994). Therefore, overall, factors which would suggest a depression of a situational/reactive nature, do not favour a differential responsiveness to CBT. It may be that CBT can produce change irrespective of original causation *through its impact upon the vicious cycles which maintain depression.*

Severity of depression has been considered as a possible prescriptive factor for different therapies, with pharmacotherapy recommended for more severe patients and CBT recommended for milder depression (Paykel, 1994). This suggestion carries some face value in that it may well be argued that for CBT to be effective, patients require some flexibility of thinking and mood and some willingness to attempt new behavioural tasks. In the most severe depressions, the rigidity of negative thinking and intractability of depressed mood, coupled with fatigue and inertia, are likely to act against ability to collaborate in CBT. In such cases, pharmacotherapy may act to potentiate a condition where CBT can be more effective. The differential response to CBT and pharmacotherapy for severe depression is supported by Elkin *et al.*'s (1989) finding that CBT was inferior to imipramine for more severely depressed patients. This, however, is not conclusive evidence when the methodological problems mentioned earlier are considered. Thase *et al.* (1991a) have specifically examined the effects of CBT in an open uncontrolled study with more severely (Hamilton Rating Scale of > 20) and less severely depressed patients. Poorer response to CBT was seen in the more severe patients but both groups experienced similar, robust and clinically significant reductions in depressive symptoms leading the authors to the conclusion that treatment needs to be maintained over a longer duration for those patients who start treatment at a more severe level of depression, rather than to the alternative view that CBT is ineffective. Thase *et al.* (1991b) report successful results with a modified intensive CBT for 16 endogenously and severely depressed in-patients treated without medication. Treatment consisted of a maximum of 20 sessions given on a daily frequency over 4 weeks. Thirteen patients were characterized as responders making highly significant changes on measures of depression. The authors comment that relapse rate was high in individuals who did not receive continuation CBT therapy after discharge fron hospital. More research is clearly needed to shed further light upon this question. It would seem that where therapists are well trained and supervised to maintain morale and persistence with a severe group, highly clinically significant changes can be achieved.

Thase and colleagues' (1991b) study is one of the very few that have utilized CBT without medication in a severely depressed group. More frequently a combined treatment is used, particularly in in-patient settings. This combination has been shown to be effective, although questions are still unanswered as to whether a combined treatment is more effective than a single treatment. Miller *et al.* (1989) found that a combined treatment for depressed in-patients showed an advantage 4 months after discharge and out-patient treatment. Scott (1992) showed that combined CBT and pharmacotherapy with a chronic depressed group produced better improvement (42% change) in comparison to a study utilizing CBT alone with a similar group in primary care (Fennell & Teasdale, 1982; 24% change). Miller *et al.* (1990) demonstrated that depressed in-patients with high pretreatment Dysfunctional Attitude Scores responded poorly to pharmacotherapy alone, but responded much better to pharmacotherapy plus CBT.

However, Beck *et al.* (1985) in out-patient samples found no difference between the effectiveness of CBT alone and CBT in combination with pharmacotherapy. Murphy *et al.* (1984) and Hollon *et al.* (1992a) found no significant differences between CBT alone, pharmacotherapy alone and the combined treatment but non-significant differences did favour the combined treatment. This non-statistically significant difference is, however, of clinical significance. Perhaps with larger samples, there would be sufficient statistical power to demonstrate a statistical difference. Again, the setting and the severity or type of depression may explain the differences between these studies. In clinical practice, though, combined treatment probably has its benefits, particularly amongst the more severe patients, and there are no antagonistic effects.

Prognostic factors

Attempts to determine prognostic factors for CBT have been more successful, although many of these factors are probably not specific to CBT. Most demographic factors do not predict response to CBT. Thase *et al.* (1994) demonstrated that depressed men and women tended to have comparable responses to CBT. One factor that has been demonstrated as predictive in several studies is marital status. It appears that having a partner improves a patient's response to CBT (Jarrett *et al.*, 1991; Sotsky *et al.*, 1991).

The most prognostic factor that has been found is the severity of pretreatment depression (Blackburn *et al.*, 1981; Elkin *et al.*, 1989; Jarrett *et al.*, 1991; Sotsky *et al.*, 1991). The more depressed the patient, the less likely they are to respond to CBT, although, as has been suggested above, this may be an artefact of the chosen length or intensity of treatment. The effect of initial severity does not appear to be specific to CBT: the more severe the depression, the less effective pharmacotherapy will also be. Hollon (as quoted in Fennell & Teasdale, 1982) developed a seven-item scale of Global Chronicity and Severity which predicted 39% of outcome variance for depressed subjects treated either with medication or CBT in the Rush *et al.* (1977) study. Scores of 4 or more predicted poor treatment outcome.

The Global Chronicity/Severity Index comprises these seven items:

1 Beck Depression Inventory (BDI) $\geqslant$ 30;
2 duration of current episode is greater than 6 months;
3 inadequate response to previous treatment;
4 previous episodes, at least two;
5 associated psychopathology;
6 overall impairment is Moderate or Severe (rated by clinician);
7 poor estimated tolerance for life stress.

This scale is clearly multifactorial and there is potential for further investigation of the weight of these different factors in predicting outcome in different samples.

Some functional and personality factors are also important indicators for prognosis for CBT. While many suppose that intelligence is required for CBT, studies that have examined this variable have not found it to be predictive, although level of education has been associated with drop-out (Blackburn *et al.*, 1981). Much may depend upon the flexiblity of the therapist in devising techniques for those with less education. Considerable interest has emerged for the use of CBT in mildly learning-disabled patients (Williams & Moorey, 1989). Whilst personality (as measured by scores on the Eysenck Personality Questionnaire) did not predict outcome with CBT (McLean & Hakstian, 1979; Kovacs *et al.*, 1981), personality disorders have been reported as being a negative indicator for straightforward CBT for depression (Tyrer *et al.*, 1993) and this view is commonly promoted. This finding is probably related to the difficulties in engaging such patients in therapy, the more extreme attitudes and behaviours they tend to display, the limited flexibility they show and their greater difficulty in reporting thoughts and feelings. However, Shea *et al.* (1990), reporting the interaction of personality disorders with treatment for depression in the NIMH study, found that personality-disordered patients did as well or slightly better than those without personality disorders in the CBT group only. The specificity of this negative finding in the Shea study is interesting because it could be that CBT's emphasis upon collaboration might be more acceptable for some patients with personality problems. However, the concept of personality disorder clearly encompasses a dimension of severity; it may be that the most extreme cases are difficult to engage in any therapy. However, one might also argue that in such instances the definition of satisfactory outcome might need to take into account the degree of dysphoria normally experienced by an individual with a highly dysfunctional personality outside of a depressed episode.

Various studies indicate the importance of patient's attitudes prior to treatment in predicting outcome. The Dysfunctional Attitude Scale (DAS), a 40-item questionnaire which measures unhelpful attitudes concerning perfectionism and a need for approval (Weissman, 1979), has been particularly implicated in predicting response to CBT. The stronger the unhelpful attitudes endorsed by patients, the less responsive they are to CBT (Keller, 1983; Simons *et al.*, 1986; Jarrett *et al.*, 1991; Sotsky *et al.*, 1991). This cognitive measure does not, however, simply predict response to CBT; Sotsky *et al.* (1991) also found that low DAS scores predicted better responses to imipramine and placebo-control. It did appear, however, that in addition to this general predictive effect, this measure was a more powerful predictor for CBT. DeRubeis *et al.* (1990) demonstrated that whilst the DAS score changed both with CBT and pharmacotherapy, only in CBT did mid-treatment change on the DAS predict subsequent change in depressive symptoms. This finding is one of the very few to date that demonstrate a specifically cognitive mediation for change in CBT.

Another predictor for response to CBT is initial endorsement of the cognitive model and any subsequent expectation of improvement this may produce. Sotsky *et al.* (1991) found that high expectations of improvement predicted better outcome, whatever the treatment. More specifically, Fennell and Teasdale (1987) found that patients who showed a positive response to a booklet outlining the CBT approach, *Coping with Depression*, showed a much greater improvement over the next 12 sessions of therapy. Thus the extent to which the CBT model is congruent with the individual's own beliefs or the extent to which the individual is open to look at things in another way may be significant. These hypotheses suggest fruitful avenues for further research.

In conclusion, there is little evidence for prescriptive discriminations between CBT and other treatments for most depressed patients. Endogeneity/ severity/situational factors do not predict which treatment will be more effective for patients. Psychotic depression and bipolar illness currently strongly indicate pharmacotherapy rather than CBT. Less severe depression, less dysfunctional attitudes, greater expectations of improvement and being married/having a partner are all factors which are related to a good outcome in CBT. These factors may partially explain why some personality-disordered patients who tend to lack these factors, respond poorly to straightforward CBT approaches. More research into the identification of characteristics of patients who are likely to respond to CBT is clearly needed. Current best practice relies upon a frank discussion of different approaches with the patient to arrive at a choice acceptable to the individual.

In addition, therapists commonly take a 'let's try it and see' approach, offering a trial of five or six sessions before a review to decide on whether or not to take it further.

Magnitude of treatment effects

The majority of controlled outcome studies have examined treatment effects using two measures. The first is the Beck Depression Inventory (BDI), a self-report, 21-item questionnaire listing depressive symptomatology (Beck *et al.*, 1961). The second is the Hamilton Rating Scale for Depression (HRSD; Hamilton, 1960), a clinician-rated measure. The outcome is then reported in terms of percentage change from pretreatment to post-treatment on average scores on these measures for each treatment group. Studies have demonstrated a range in percentage change following CBT; between 48 and 80% change in BDI scores and between 64 and 77% change on Hamilton Ratings (Rush *et al.*, 1977; Blackburn *et al.*, 1981; Murphy *et al.*, 1984; Beck *et al.*, 1985; Elkin *et al.*, 1989; Hollon *et al.*, 1992a). The average scores change from around 30 pretreatment to around 10 post-treatment on the BDI and from between 20 and 25 pretreatment to around 7 post-treatment on the HRDS. Such a change in scores is equivalent to a change from severe-moderate depression to mild depression-euthymic. This size of therapeutic impact is similar to that found for antidepressant medication (Lader, 1996; and see Chapter 11).

Most studies have also reported a percentage treated to full remission, as assessed by BDI and HRSD scales, and these range from 63 to 82% in the earlier studies where perhaps CBT has been best executed, falling to 51% in the Elkin *et al.* (1989) study, where, as has been observed, competency may have been lower and variable between sites. Whilst we have expressed enthusiasm about this approach, there is clearly no room for complacency. The treatment effect sizes (0.85–0.96 reported in a meta-analysis carried out by Robinson *et al.*, 1990) are, on average, less than for cognitive-behavioural treatment of anxiety and to obtain the best results it would seem that considerable investment in training and supervision is required. Many have also reported that a small minority of patients do not respond at all or become worse with CBT. Shea *et al.* (1992a) rather sadly reflect upon the outcome of their hugely expensive, multicentre NIMH study that 16 weeks of the therapies studied was insufficient for most patients to reach full recovery and lasting remission. That being said, it is clear that CBT has a treatment effect that can produce remission in at least one half of depressed out-patients and significant clinical improvements in the majority of such patients.

Time-course of treatment effect

Short term

Cognitive therapy has been found to be an effective short-term treatment for both depressed in-patients and out-patients, producing effective results in the acute episode of depression (Rush *et al.*, 1977; Blackburn *et al.*, 1981; Murphy *et al.*, 1984; Elkin *et al.*, 1989; Hollon *et al.*, 1992a). The time-course of short-term change, where it has been studied, seems to be, on average, similar to the time-course for pharmacotherapy with tricyclic drugs, although, as has been observed, there is also a great range of variability, with some patients making marked changes with one or two sessions.

Long term

As more studies have shown a significant short-term treatment effect for depression, interest has shifted to maintenance of treatment effects. It has been recognized that depression frequently returns in affected individuals so the challenge now may be not so much short-term improvement but long-term maintenance. The model for CBT would suggest that underlying attitudes are shifted or that patients learn skills that may help them to deal with future problems. There is some limited evidence that this hope may be justified.

A series of studies have followed up the controlled treatment studies of CBT for up to 2 years, using scores on the BDI as the criterion for a return of depression (Kovacs *et al.*, 1981: 56% of CBT group had BDI >16 over 1 year; Blackburn *et al.*, 1986: 23% of CBT group had BDI >10 over 2 years; Simons *et al.*, 1986: 20% of CBT group had BDI >16 over 1 year; Evans *et al.*, 1992: 18% of CBT group had BDI >16 over 2 years). Several of these studies have methodological problems, most particularly the lack of a maintenance medication group in the pharmacotherapy group and small samples. Furthermore, the studies differ in assessment methods, timing of assessments and even inclusion criteria for follow-up groups. None the less, all these studies show that the CBT groups do better than other treatments after 1 or 2 years following termination of therapy and suggest that CBT does indeed have a sustained effect beyond the end of therapy which helps to protect individuals from relapse. The Evans *et al.* (1992) study, the most recent and best designed in this series, included a group who continued on medication for 1 year of the study beyond termination of active therapy in the CBT groups. Using a definition of relapse as a BDI score of 16 or greater and/or return to treatment, within the 2-year follow-up period, 21% of the CBT group relapsed, compared to 50% of a pharmacotherapy group without maintenance medication (i.e. active treatment halted at the point when CBT ended) and 32% of a pharmacotherapy group with maintenance medication for the first year. This mirrors many of the reported results, with short-term CBT producing about half the probability of relapse with short-term pharmacotherapy and approximately equal effects with long-term maintenance of medication. These results indicate that a short-term therapy can produce some lasting change, comparable to continued pharmacotherapy, which persists in the absence of the therapy. This is consistent with the suggestion in the cognitive model of depression that CBT may alter underlying assumptions that produce vulnerability to depression. It is also consistent with the idea that CBT teaches patients coping skills to handle future difficulties. Again, however, a cautionary note must be added, in that in the above Evans study the percentages quoted refer only to those patients who were successfully treated and therefore entered the follow-up stage. If one takes the non-responders into account, the long-term outcome would show that many more patients from the sample originally entering the treatment study relapse or remain depressed.

The question remains whether the reduced return of symptoms in CBT is reduced relapse or reduced recurrence of depression. *Relapse* is the return of symptoms associated with the current treated episode and *recurrence* is the onset of a new episode of depression (Klerman, 1978). An untreated moderate depression usually has a natural course of 6–9 months and therefore such a length of time makes a suitable cut-off between relapse and recurrence. Ending antidepressant medication within this initial 6–9 months, even following rapid remission, carries a higher risk of a return of symptoms than terminating medication beyond this period. This is consistent with the concept of an ongoing process of depression, which medication suppresses rather than removes. Because most of the return of symptoms in the studies quoted occurs in the first 6 months after discharge, it has been argued that these studies have been assessing relapse rather than recurrence (Hollon *et al.*, 1991, 1993). The results are indicative of a *relapse prevention* function for CBT for depression. However, Hollon *et al.* (1991, 1993) do raise one methodological problem with these results; because the follow-up studies have assessed patients who completed therapy successfully, a filtering effect may occur, with the pharmacotherapy group successfully treating more difficult patients and then subsequently showing less effectiveness in preventing relapse. This is one possible explanation of the results and until it is tested, it cannot be argued for sure that CBT has a differential relapse-prevention effect. None the less, it is clear that CBT does have a good record in reducing symptom return up to 2 years after discharge.

Ludgate (1991), in an uncontrolled retrospective study quoted in Ludgate (1994), followed up 80 unipolar depressed patients, 3 and 5 years after CBT. Using the criteria for affective disorder as a measure for recurrence, 52% of the sample had a recurrence of depression within the 5 years. With a criterion of a 'return of symptoms of equal or greater severity to the index episode', 32% of the sample had a recurrence of depression over 5 years. This suggests that the improved effects for CBT shown for preventing relapse are maintained over longer periods of time, indicating that CBT may also protect against recurrence. Thus during a long time period following discharge, patients undergoing CBT showed a return of symptoms comparable to those continuing medication for the 5-year period. However, Ludgate's patients attended the Centre for Cognitive Therapy in Philadelphia and are a highly selected group, so generalizations from this sample must be guarded. Furthermore, there is still much room for improvement because between one-third and a half of patients successfully treated with CBT, again suffered from depression within 5 years.

Table 8.3 shows results of follow-up studies of controlled clinical trials of CBT for depression.

Table 8.3 Follow-up studies of CBT for depression.

Study group	Months	Outcome % relapsed
Kovacs *et al.* (1981)	12	Tricyclic 82% vs. CT 56% (NS)
Blackburn *et al.* (1986)	12	Tricyclic 78% vs. CT 23% vs. Combination 12% (S)
Simons *et al.* (1986)	12	Tricyclic 67% vs. Combination 43% (S) vs. CT + placebo 18% (S)
Evans *et al.* (1992)	24	Tricyclic discountinued 50% vs. CT 21% (S) vs. combination 15% (S) Tricyclic continued 32%
Shea *et al.* (1992)	18	Tricyclic 50% vs. CT 36% vs. IPT 33% (NS)

IPT, interpersonal psychotherapy.
S, significance levels.

Special issues

Availability of treatment

Whilst many of the key ideas of CBT (e.g. collaborative approaches, empirical testing, formulation of hypotheses, activity structuring and challenging of thoughts) are relatively simple and likely to improve the general approach of any mental health care professional to their patients, the effective practice of CBT is much more complex. Effective use of CBT requires considerable training, practice and supervision. The selection and monitoring of therapists to guarantee high levels of skill and experience is a core part of many of the treatment studies quoted. With less experienced therapists, less effective results would be expected (cf. Elkin *et al.*, 1989). Beck himself developed a training course for postqualification psychologists that runs full-time over a year. No course in the UK offers such intensive training, most courses being day-release, professional development courses. Little is known about the effectiveness of this relatively dilute dose of training for the different professional groups that are trained. Economic pressures preclude the development of more time-intensive courses at present, although basic training courses are beginning to incorporate more of the principles of the CBT approach as the research evidence grows. Such courses that exist are scarce, with demand far exceeding supply. In consequence, qualified therapists are few and far be-tween, although the provision of a register in the UK will at least allow moni-toring and access to those who are trained. At present, access is relatively more available in some geographical areas of the NHS than others. This has implications for waiting-list time and ease of referral. With a longer waiting list, some depressed patients will have significantly improved before reaching treatment, others will have significantly worsened. In a time- and therapist-intensive therapy, such problems are clearly greater than in pharmacotherapy-based approaches. Mechanisms for prioritizing patients may be required under these circumstances as well as funding being made available for training. However, even in an ideal economy, the prevalence of depression would suggest that CBT is never going to be a treatment for all. It would seem that many patients can benefit from bibliotherapy, abbreviated courses in primary care, group approaches, etc., allowing the more expert staff to devote time to those who are unable to use these less supported methods.

Whilst the availability of training is scarce, therapists and counsellors abound who espouse the practice of CBT. The practice of *caveat emptor* should be borne in mind by purchasers and referrers, who are becoming more conscious of quality indices. Exposure to an inept therapist will do nothing for the optimism of a depressed patient and will add to the problems of future therapists for this patient. The managing clinician may also be faced with the problem of deciding whether the patient has received a proper trial. Detailed enquiry into the nature of the work undertaken in previous episodes of therapy may shed some light upon this question.

Cost-effectiveness

The cost-effectiveness of CBT relative to other treatments is a highly relevant question, with an increase in market forces becoming apparent in the NHS. If CBT is of comparable effectiveness to pharmacotherapy, but requires the extra costs of training and paying for a number of sessions between therapist and patient, should it be used?

A number of issues are pertinent to this question. First, the exact cost of CBT relative to other treatments is unclear. Ross and Scott (1985) concluded that CBT could be applied cost-effectively in general practice, whilst Scott and Freeman (1992) concluded that the additional costs of any specialist treat-ments (at least twice as much as routine GP care) were not commensurate with their clinical superiority over routine GP care. However, in this latter study, the time difference between administering a course of CBT and administering a course of medication was only 3.6h. Second, as patient choice in therapy has increased, a preference towards psychological therapies and away from pharmacotherapy has become evident. Indeed, patients' dislike of medication may be a major factor in attrition rates in drug studies. However, drop-out rates for CBT in the major outcome studies vary between 5 and 38% (Hollon *et al.*, 1992a), suggesting that CBT also has a considerable attrition factor to address. Third, it is clear that CBT can help some patients who are not responsive or who are unable to take medication for some reason. Fourth, CBT appears to have additional effects beyond treating the acute episode of depression, all of which have cost-benefit implications. Reducing somatization and failures to attend in a primary care setting are likely greatly to improve the general efficiency of a GP surgery. Most importantly, the relapse prevention effects suggested for CBT would reduce return of depression compared to pharmacotherapy. This would reduce the costs involved in repeating treatments and reduce the financial effects of depression, for example, loss of man-hours and efficiency at work. Furthermore, successful CBT appears to remove the need for the expenses of maintaining antidepressant medication for many years.

A major factor in treatment cost is treatment duration. A major advantage of CBT is that it has a brief but flexible length. Substantial treatment effects can be seen within four sessions and often therapists do not exceed 20 sessions of treatment. However, with more difficult and intractable problems, longer courses of therapy can be utilized if required. Returning to the question of who responds well to CBT, perhaps the most useful practical predictor, is a patient's response to the initial sessions. Patients who respond to initial sessions are highly likely to respond much more. Using a time-limited contract can greatly enhance the efficiency of treatment and improve cost-effectiveness.

Future developments

When considering CBT and its place in treating depression, the standard CBT approach as outlined by Beck (Beck *et al.*, 1979) has been the main focus of this chapter because it is the method that has received the most scientific attention. However, a number of developments in CBT, relevant to the treatment of depression, are evolving. One set of developments involve shifting CBT beyond just a 'here and now' approach, to investigate more fully the patterns of thoughts and behaviours that characterize patients. By examining the models that people construct of themselves and the world from childhood onwards, better understanding of chronic problems can be achieved. Such approaches incorporate all the standard CBT repertoire but add more consideration of imagery, experiential techniques and interpersonal factors, drawing upon techniques from Gestalt and psychodynamic therapies. Others are developing the cognitive-behavioural model itself and increasing our understanding of the conceptual basis of CBT (Teasdale, 1993; Teasdale & Barnard, 1993). Such approaches may be particularly useful for treating both chronically depressed and dysthymic patients and for managing personality disorders associated with depression and chronic dysphoria (Beck *et al.*, 1990; Young, 1990; Linehan, 1993).

Another set of developments concern the relapse prevention function of CBT. Fava *et al.* (1994) have demonstrated the value of CBT in reducing residual symptoms, following successful treatment with medication. Reducing these residual symptoms by CBT produced a lower rate of relapse at 2-year follow-up (15% vs. 35%, although not statistically significant). Hollon *et al.* (1992b) are investigating the use of CBT for euthymic populations to reduce the risk of future depression. Teasdale *et al.* (1995) have proposed an attentional retraining programme to prevent relapse in remitted depressed patients. These developments will improve our ability to focus intervention on the problems most intractable in the treatment of depression. As these new approaches are refined and tested in controlled treatment studies, the efficacy of CBT for dealing with a wider range of aspects of depression will become clearer.

Conclusions

This chapter has focused upon research in relation to the efficacy of CBT in the treatment of depression. We have argued for the general efficacy of the approach with a wide and expanding range of depressed patients and have pointed to some problems in its training and supervision implications with some suggested answers in the way expertise may become more focused upon resistant problems as knowledge grows about the treatment of depression. Much of the research to date has compared CBT with pharmacotherapy, the standard treatment approach. Rather little is known about the relative efficacy of CBT and other psychological approaches, although procedural similarities between differing therapies are becoming more evident and some have suggested that CBT may become an integrative therapeutic model which will come to embrace more and more techniques developed from differing theoretical perspectives. It will have become clear that CBT is more than a static series of operations but a whole scientific approach closely tied in to the developing psychology of human emotion; this relationship is leading to fruitful developments in method and process. Perhaps this is the main secret of its continuing success beyond the first decade of its youthful enthusiasm and of the extent to which it continues to dominate the field of applied clinical psychology and to attract the interest of the mental health professions.

Cognitive therapy based upon Beck's theory of depression is now a standard treatment of depressive illness of mild to moderate severity presenting in primary and secondary care. In these patients and settings, CBT and antidepressant medication may be of equivalent therapeutic efficacy. CBT may (unlike antidepressant medication) continue to have beneficial effects, even after treatment is withdrawn. Despite their apparent therapeutic equivalence, patient preference for the two treatment modalities varies and more research is needed into the indications for each form of treatment and the possible interactions between them. Much more research is needed upon the role of CBT in the treatment of severe depression and manic depressive illness for which CBT cannot yet be recommended.

All doctors treating mildly and moderately depressed patients should have access to a CBT service because for some patients this will be the most effective and acceptable treatment.

References

Beck, A.T., Ward, C.H., Mendelson, M., Mock, J. & Erbaugh, J. (1961) An inventory for measuring depression. *Archives of General Psychiatry,* **4,** 561–571.

Beck, A.T., Rush, A.J., Shaw, B.F. & Emery, G. (1979) *Cognitive Therapy of Depression.* Guilford Press, New York.

Beck, A.T., Hollon, S.D., Young, J.E., Bedrosian, R.C. & Budenz, D. (1985) Treatment of depression with cognitive therapy and amitriptyline. *Archives of General Psychiatry,* **42,** 142–148.

Beck, A.T., Freeman, A., Pretzer, J. *et al.* (1990) *Cognitive Therapy of Personality Disorders.* Guilford Press, New York.

Blackburn, I.M., Bishop, S., Glen, A.I.M., Whalley, L.J. & Christie, J.E. (1981) The efficacy of cognitive therapy in depression: a treatment trial using cognitive therapy and pharmacotherapy, each alone and in combination. *British Journal of Psychiatry,* **1399,** 181–189.

Blackburn, I.M., Eunson, K.M. & Bishop, S. (1986) A two-year naturalistic follow-up of depressed patients treated with cognitive therapy, pharmacotherapy and a combination of both. *Journal of Affective Disorders,* **10,** 67–75.

Blacker, C.V.R. & Clare, A.W. (1987) Depressive disorder in primary care. *British Journal of Psychiatry,* **150,** 737–751.

Bowers, W.A. (1990) Treatment of depressed inpatients: Cognitive therapy plus medication, relaxation plus medication and medication alone. *British Journal of Psychiatry,* **156,** 73–78.

Burns, D.D. (1980) *Feeling Good: The New Mood Therapy.* Signet, New York.

Burns, D.D. (1995) *The Feeling Good Handbook.* Penguin, New York.

Comas-Diaz, L. (1981) Effects of cognitive and behavioural group treatment on the depressive symptomatology of Puerto Rican women. *Journal of Consulting and Clinical Psychology,* **49,** 627–632.

DeRubeis, R.J., Hollon, S.D., Grove, W.M., Evans, M.D., Garvey, M.J. & Tuason, V.B. (1990) How does cognitive therapy work? Cognitive change and symptom change in cognitive therapy and pharmacotherapy for depression. *Journal of Consulting and Clinical Psychology,* **58,** 862–869.

Dobson, K. (1989) A meta-analysis of the efficacy of cognitive therapy for depression. *Journal of Consulting and Clinical Psychology,* **57,** 414–419.

Elkin, I., Shea, M.T., Watkins, J.T. *et al.* (1989) NIMH Treatment of Depression Collaborative Research Program. 1: General effectiveness of treatments. *Archives of General Psychiatry,* **46,** 971–982.

Evans, M.D., Hollon, S.D., DeRubeis, R.J. *et al.* (1992) Differential relapse following cognitive therapy and pharmacotherapy for depression. *Archives of General Psychiatry,* **49,** 802–808.

Fava, G.A., Grandi, S., Zielezny, M., Canestrari, R. & Morphy, M.A. (1994) Cognitive behavioural treatment of residual symptoms in primary major depressive disorder. *American Journal of Psychiatry,* **151,** 1295–1299.

Fennell, M.J.V. & Teasdale, J.D. (1982) Cognitive therapy with chronic, drug-refractory depressed out-patients: a note of caution. *Cognitive Therapy and Research,* **6,** 455–460.

Fennell, M.J.V. & Teasdale, J.D. (1987) Cognitive therapy for depression: individual differences and the process of change. *Cognitive Therapy and Research,* **11,** 253–271.

Gallagher, D.E. & Thompson, L.W. (1982) Treatment of major depressive disorder in older adult outpatients with brief psychotherapies. *Psycho-*

therapy: Theory, Research and Practice, **19**, 482–490.

Garety, P.A., Kuipers, E.A., Fowler, D. *et al.* (1994) Cognitive behavioural therapy for drug-resistant psychosis. *British Journal of Medical Psychology*, **67** (3), 259–271.

Garvey, M.J., Hollon, S.D. & DeRubeis, R.J. (1994) Do depressed patients with higher pretreatment stress levels respond better to cognitive therapy than imipramine? *Journal of Affective Disorders*, **32**, 45–50.

Hamilton, M. (1960) A rating scale for depression. *Journal of Neurology, Neurosurgery and Psychiatry*, **12**, 52–62.

Hollon, S.D., Shelton, R.C. & Loosen, P.T. (1991) Cognitive therapy and pharmacotherapy for depression. *Journal of Consulting and Clinical Psychology*, **59**, 88–99.

Hollon, S.D., DeRubeis, R.J., Evans, M.D. *et al.* (1992a) Cognitive therapy and pharmacotherapy for depression: singly and in combination. *Archives of General Psychiatry*, **49**, 774–781.

Hollon, S.D., DeRubeis, R.J. & Seligman, M.E.P. (1992b) Cognitive therapy and the prevention of depression. *Applied and Preventive Psychology*, **1**, 89–95.

Hollon, S.D., Shelton, R.C. & Davis, D.D. (1993) Cognitive therapy for depression: conceptual issues and clinical efficacy. *Journal of Consulting and Clinical Psychology*, **61**, 270–275.

Jacobson, N.S., Dobson, K.S., Truax, P.A. *et al.* (1996) A component analysis of cognitive-behavioral treatment for depression. *Journal of Consulting and Clinical Psychology*, **64**, 295–304.

Jamison, C. & Scogin, F. (1995) The outcome of cognitive bibliotherapy with depressed adults. *Journal of Consulting and Clinical Psychology*, **63**, 644–650.

Jarrett, R.B., Eaves, G.G., Grannemann, B.D. & Rush, A.J. (1991) Clinical, cognitive and demographic predictors of response to cognitive therapy for depression: a preliminary report. *Psychiatry Research*, **37**, 245–260.

Keller, K.E. (1983) Dysfunctional attitudes and cognitive therapy for depression. *Cognitive Therapy and Research*, **7**, 437–444.

Klerman, G.L. (1978) Long term treatment of affective disorders. In: *Psychopharmacology: A Generation of Progress* (eds M. Lipton, A. Dimascio & K. Killam), pp. 1303–1313, Raven Press, New York.

Kovacs, M., Rush, A.J., Beck, A.T. & Hollon, S.D. (1981) Depressed outpatients treated with cognitive therapy or pharmacotherapy. *Archives of General Psychiatry*, **38**, 33–39.

Lader, M.H. (1996) Tolerability and safety: essentials in antidepressant pharmacotherapy. *Journal of Clinical Psychiatry*, **J7** (Suppl. 2), 39–44.

Linehan, M.M. (1993) *Cognitive-Behavioural Treatment of Borderline Personality Disorder*. Guilford Press, New York.

Ludgate, J.W. (1994) Cognitive behavioural therapy and depressive relapse: justified optimism or unwarranted complacency? *Behavioural and Cognitive Psychotherapy*, **22**, 1–11.

McLean, P.D. & Hakstian, A.R. (1979) Clinical depression: comparative efficacy of outpatient treatments. *Journal of Consulting and Clinical Psychology*, **47**, 818–836.

Miller, I.W., Norman, W.H., Keitner, G.I., Bishop, S.B. & Dow, M.G. (1989) Cognitive-behavioural treatment of depressed inpatients. *Behavior Therapy*, **20**, 25–47.

Miller, I.W., Norman, W.H. & Keitner, G.I. (1990) Treatment response of high cognitive dysfunction: depressed inpatients. *Contemporary Psychiatry*, **30**, 62–71.

Miranda, J. & Munoz, R. (1994) Intervention for minor depression in primary care patients. *Psychosomatic Medicine*, **56**, 136–142.

Murphy, G.E., Simons, A.D., Wetzel, R.D. & Lustman, P.J. (1984) Cognitive therapy and pharmacotherapy, singly and together in the treatment of depression. *Archives of General Psychiatry*, **41**, 33–41.

Paykel, E.S. (1994) Psychological therapies. *Acta Psychiatrica Scandinavica*, **89**, 35–41.

Reynolds, W.M. & Coats, K.I. (1986) A comparison of cognitive-behavioural therapy and relaxation training for the treatment of depression in adolescents. *Journal of Consulting and Clinical Psychology*, **54**, 653–660.

Robinson, L.A., Berman, J.S. & Neimeyer, R.A. (1990) Psychotherapy for the treatment of depression: a comprehensive review of controlled outcome research. *Psychological Bulletin*, **108**, 30–49.

Ross, M. & Scott, M. (1985) An evaluation of the effectiveness of individual and group cognitive therapy in the treatment of depressed patients in an inner city health centre. *Journal of the Royal College of General Practitioners*, **35**, 239–242.

Rush, A.J., Beck, A.T., Kovacs, M. & Hollon, S.D. (1977) Comparative efficacy of cognitive therapy and pharmacotherapy in the treatment of depressed outpatients. *Cognitive Therapy and Research*, **1**, 17–37.

Scott, A.I.F. & Freeman, C.P.L. (1992) Edinburgh primary care depression study: treatment outcome, patient satisfaction, and cost after 16 weeks. *British Medical Journal*, **304**, 883–887.

Scott, C.S., Scott, J.L., Tacchi, M.J. & Jones, R.H.

(1994) Abbreviated cognitive therapy for depression: a pilot study in primary care. *Behavioural and Cognitive Psychotherapy*, **22**, 57–64.

Scott, J. (1992) Chronic depression: can cognitive therapy succeed when other treatments fail? *Behavioural Psychotherapy*, **20**, 25–36.

Scott, J., Eccleston, D. & Boys, R. (1992) Can we predict the persistence of depression? *British Journal of Psychiatry*, **161**, 633–637.

Scott, J., Moon, C.A.L., Blacker, C.V.R. & Thomas, J.M. (1994) A.I.F. Scott and C.P.L. Freeman's 'Edinburgh Primary Care Depression Study'. *British Journal of Psychiatry*, **164**, 410–415.

Shea, M.T., Pilkonis, P.A., Beckham, E. *et al.* (1990) Personality disorders and treatment outcome in the NIMH Treatment of Depression Collaborative Research Program. *American Journal of Psychiatry*, **147**, 711–718.

Shea, M.T., Elkin, I., Imber, S.D. *et al.* (1992) Course of depressive symptoms over follow-up: findings from the NIMH Treatment of Depression Collaborative Research Program. *Archives of General Psychiatry*, **49** (10), 782–787.

Simons, A.D., Murphy, G.E., Levine, J.L. & Wetzel, R.D. (1986) Cognitive therapy and pharmacotherapy for depression: sustained improvement over one year. *Archives of General Psychiatry*, **43**, 43–48.

Sotsky, S.M., Glass, D.R., Shea, M.T. *et al.* (1991) Patient predictors of response to psychotherapy and pharmacotherapy: findings in the NIMH Treatment of Depression Collaborative Research Program. *American Journal of Psychiatry*, **48**, 997–1008.

Teasdale, J.D. (1993) Emotion and two kinds of meaning: cognitive therapy and applied cognitive science. *Behaviour Research and Therapy*, **31**, 339–354.

Teasdale, J.D. & Barnard, P.J. (1993) *Affect, Cognition and Change*. Lawrence Erlbaum Associates, Hove and London.

Teasdale, J.D., Fennell, M.J.V., Hibbert, G.A. & Amies, P.L. (1984) Cognitive therapy for major depressive disorder in primary care. *British Journal of Psychiatry*, **44**, 400–406.

Teasdale, J.D., Segal, Z. & Williams, J.M.G. (1995) How does cognitive therapy prevent depressive relapse and why should attentional control (mindfulness) training help? An information processing analysis. *Behaviour Research and Therapy*, **33**, 25–39.

Thase, M.E., Simons, A.D., Cahalane, J., McGeary, J. & Harden, T. (1991a) Severity of depression and response to cognitive behavior therapy. *American Journal of Psychiatry*, **148**, 784–789.

Thase, M.E., Bowler, K. & Harder, T. (1991b) Cognitive behavior therapy of endogenous depression. Part 2: Preliminary findings in 16 unmedicated inpatients. *Behavior Therapy*, **22**, 469–477.

Thase, M.E., Reynolds, C.F., Frank, E. *et al.* (1994) Do depressed men and women respond similarly to cognitive behavioural therapy? *American Journal of Psychiatry*, **151**, 500–505.

Tyrer, P., Seivewright, N., Ferguson, B., Murphy, S. & Johnson, A.L. (1993) The Nottingham study of neurotic disorder: effect of personality status on response to drug treatment, cognitive therapy and self-help over two years. *British Journal of Psychiatry*, **162**, 219–226.

Weissman, A. (1979) The Dysfunctional Attitude Scale: a validation study. *Dissertation Abstracts International*, **40**, 1389–1390.

Wierzbicki, M. & Bartlett, T.S. (1987) The efficacy of group and individual cognitive therapy for mild depression. *Cognitive Therapy and Research*, **11**, 337–342.

Williams, J.M.G. & Moorey, S. (1989) The wider application of cognitive therapy: the end of the beginning. In: *Cognitive Therapy in Clinical Practice: An Illustrative Casebook* (eds J. Scott, J. M. G. Williams & A. T. Beck), pp. 227–250. Routledge, London.

Wilson, P.H., Goldin, J.C. & Charbonneau-Powis, M. (1983) Comparative efficacy of behavioural and cognitive treatments of depression. *Cognitive Therapy and Research*, **7**, 111–124.

Young, J.E. (1990) *Cognitive Therapy for Personality Disorders: A Schema-focused Approach*. Professional Resource Exchange, Sarasota, FL.

9 The efficacy of antidepressant medication

MALCOLM H. LADER

The term depression can apply to a transient mood, a sustained change in affect, a symptom, a syndrome or a psychiatric disorder. It is a common and chronic condition; most patients experiencing an initial episode of depression will succumb to a recurrence. It is symptomatically distressing, patients reporting an ineffable and all-pervading depth of despair and hopelessness far beyond normal experience. Physical, social and personal role functioning is greatly impaired, comparable to or even worse than the handicaps associated with physical illnesses such as hypertension, diabetes and arthritis (Wells *et al.*, 1989). Suicide is often a risk. Major depression is often associated with other disorders such as anxiety disorders, dysthymia and physical illnesses, and such comorbidity worsens the prognosis (Wells *et al.*, 1992). Even in the milder cases, partial remission not full recovery is the usual outcome (Ormel *et al.*, 1993).

Depressive disorders can be divided into five main conditions, although overlap may occur: major depression, dysthymia, bipolar-disorder depressed, cyclothymia and unspecified depressive disorder. This chapter will concentrate on major depression, although the drug treatment is quite similar for bipolar depressives. Resistant depression is dealt with in Chapter 11 (see also Sokolov & Joffe, 1995).

The toll exacted by depression necessitates the condition being taken seriously, especially at the primary care level where it is often missed or its significance overlooked. Vigorous treatment must be instituted early, adequate dosages attained, compliance encouraged, and the course of treatment prolonged rather than curtailed. An increasingly wide range of antidepressant medication is becoming available although, as will be seen later, improvements relate to side-effect profile, tolerability and safety; efficacy remains only limited, and effectiveness in practice unchanged. The use of medication has always to be set into the context of wider management, with sympathetic counselling, improvement of psychosocial circumstances, and more formal psychological treatments where appropriate and available.

Historical background

In the late 1940s, imidodibenzyl derivatives were investigated as antihistamines and antiparkinsonian compounds and re-evaluated a few years later as possible antipsychotics. One, imipramine, was found to be disappointing as an antipsychotic but to have genuine antidepressant (as opposed to stimulant) properties. The parameters of efficacy were explored and the side-effect profile established. Numerous other similar tricyclic compounds were synthesized (TCAs) and introduced over the years including amitriptyline, dothiepin, clomipramine and lofepramine. Variants, the so-called 'atypical' antidepressants, appeared, with a range of different pharmacological properties. The search for more selective compounds led first to compounds acting primarily on noradrenergic mechanisms, for example maprotilene, and to those more selective for serotonin such as zimeldine (later withdrawn). A series of selective serotonin re-uptake inhibitors (SSRIs) have appeared, although they vary in their selectivity. They have a different and somewhat better-tolerated side-effect profile and are currently the focus of a vigorous debate concerning their comparative risk/benefit ratios *vis-à-vis* the TCAs and an even more heated controversy concerning relative cost-effectiveness (Edwards, 1995).

The other major group of antidepressants is the monoamine oxidase inhibitors (MAOIs). The first, iproniazid, was developed as an antituberculosis medication and was found to make patients euphoric. Antidepressant properties were discerned but the side-effects and hazardous drug and dietary interactions greatly trammelled the use of these drugs. More recently, selective and reversible inhibitors of MAO have been developed and one, moclobemide, has been introduced into clinical use.

In the 35 or so years since the introduction of imipramine and iproniazid, much has been learned about the clinical use of antidepressant medication. Some practical questions remain, relating to topics such as compliance and the utility of plasma concentration monitoring. But the paramount puzzle has not been answered, namely, the mode of action of these drugs. A plethora of both short- and long-term biochemical effects have been catalogued but it remains a complete mystery how these effects are translated into a clinical response.

These drugs lead to a worthwhile improvement in about 70% of unselected patients with a depressive disorder. However, many of these patients would improve spontaneously or with help, support and counselling (Brown & Khan, 1994). Despite this, as has become apparent over the years, careful choice of patient can maximize drug-placebo-non-drug treatment differences. The use of powerful drugs like the antidepressants to treat minor fluctuations in mood or psychological problems in general is to be deprecated.

Pharmacokinetic considerations

In practice, these mainly revolve around the usefulness of monitoring plasma concentrations of the various antidepressants. This is still a controversial issue. By and large, the relationship between daily dose and levels of drug and its major metabolites is a tenuous one because of wide variations in the metabolizing capabilities of individual patients (e.g. for clomipramine, Balant-Gorgia *et al.*, 1991). Low plasma concentrations are associated with poor response and high ones with adverse effects. What remains unclear is whether high concentrations are associated with a poor clinical response, in other words, whether a therapeutic 'window' can be discerned. Even where such a relationship across patients has been found, it is usually too weak statistically to influence a clinical decision. Estimation of the plasma concentration of an antidepressant in an individual patient remains a help in evaluating a side-effect or excluding total non-compliance, rather than in facilitating clinical response.

Pharmacokinetic data may also help obviate dangerous drug interactions. Many antidepressants and other drugs are metabolized via common cytochrome P450 pathways so that potential interactions can be predicted (Taylor & Lader, 1996). This is particularly important with some of the SSRIs, such as fluoxetine and paroxetine.

The pharmacokinetics of the SSRIs has been studied in some detail but more with respect to potential drug interactions rather than the correlation between clinical efficacy and plasma concentrations (van Harten, 1993). Data so far suggest that plasma concentrations bear little relationship to clinical response for any of the SSRIs.

Clinical uses and efficacy

Brown and Khan (1994) recently averred, 'Although antidepressants are clearly effective, when used in common practice their effectiveness is not astounding' (p. 342). Even in patients who meet criteria for a moderately severe depressive syndrome, the type of depression considered most responsive to antidepressants, the improvement rate with antidepressants is only around 70%. Furthermore, in these same patients the response rate to placebo is between 30 and 40%. 'Improvement' and 'response' rate are not defined, and this uncovers a fundamental problem in assessing efficacy and effectiveness. Efficacy usually reflects the mean drug-placebo difference on a standard rating scale, usually the Hamilton Depression Scale (Hamilton, 1960). A meta-analysis carried out in the early 1980s by the Australian and New Zealand College of Psychiatrists found that both the tricyclic and the newer antidepressants were associated with an effect size of 1.5, placebo with 0.8, in patients with 'endogenous' depression (Quality Assurance Project, 1983). The figures for 'neurotic' depression were 1.5 and 1.1, respectively. Thus, antidepressants on average effect an improvement of much less than one effect size. (One effect size is one standard deviation of the initial severity level ratings (say, 4–6 points on the Hamilton).) However, clinicians are not primarily concerned with average responses in groups of patients. They choose a treatment on the probability that it will result in a clinically useful improvement—for example, recovery with discharge of the patient from in-patient, out-patient or primary care. The figures given earlier would suggest that, even with carefully chosen patients, this probability with a TCA is around 2 in 3, compared with 1 in 3 for placebo. For less typically 'core' patients, the response probability rises from about 1 in 2 to 2 in 3, hardly an earth-shattering therapeutic manoeuvre!

The phenomenon of the placebo response needs further qualification. In most trials, this epithet is applied to the improvement seen in the placebo-treated group. However, it is comprised of several elements of which the most important are natural remission, spontaneous fluctuations and true placebo response. Thus, 80–90% of depressive episodes naturally remit and the coincidence of this with treatment will overestimate the real efficacy. Secondly, patients tend to seek help when their condition is worsening, so spontaneous fluctuations in severity without genuine remission will tend to be towards improvement; again, efficacy is overestimated. Finally, the true placebo response is improvement consequent on the administration of a dummy medication and its psychological implications. It can only be assessed by including a 'no-treatment' group (Quality Assurance Project, 1983).

The newer antidepressants do not have increased efficacy. Indeed, the clinical impression is that they may have marginally less efficacy. This is probably a complex indirect reflection of their better-tolerated side-effect profile. The argument runs as follows: SSRIs are being perceived as having fewer and less severe side-effects than the TCAs. Therefore, many prescribers will try them in patients to whom they would not normally give TCAs, because of these side-effects. However, these patients, being less typical depressives, tend to be less responsive than typical moderate to severely depressed patients and respond less. Certainly, inspection of the data bases for some of the newly marketed antidepressants suggests that drug-placebo differences are narrowing. This is so for the newer drugs but also true to a lesser extent for the long-established comparators such as imipramine.

Clinical trials are generally carried out on patients who meet criteria for major depression. This comprises a syndrome including both psychological and somatic symptoms. Most important are a sustained depressed mood and loss of interest or pleasure. The syndrome persists for at least 2 weeks, although in practice most depressives in clinical trials have been ill for much longer than this. The third criterion is that the condition produces impairment in social, occupational or other important areas of functioning (American Psychiatric Association, 1994).

Spurious estimates of mean efficacy can be obtained by relying too heavily on a single rating scale. For example, the Hamilton Depression Scale has several items such as anxiety, psychic and somatic (numbers 10 and 11) and insomnia (4, 5 and 6) which will respond to sedatives. Therefore, it is necessary to assess a medication on the core depressive items such as mood, guilt and suicide. An alternative is to use the Montgomery–Asberg Depression Rating Scale which is a 'purer' depression scale (Montgomery & Asberg, 1979).

The depressive episode phase of a bipolar manic-depressive disorder also responds to antidepressants at about the same efficacy rate as major depressive disorder. However, bipolar depressives tend to remit spontaneously so the antidepressant seems to act to expedite that remission. Indeed, the role of antidepressant medication in precipitating mania remains controversial (Wehr & Goodwin, 1987; Sulzer & Cummings, 1989).

At the extreme of the severity continuum, psychotic depressives tend to do relatively poorly with antidepressants. Although the placebo response rate is very low, only about a third of such patients with hallucinations and delusions will respond to a TCA, but twice that proportion to electroconvulsive therapy (ECT) or to the combination of a TCA and an antipsychotic drug (Khan *et al.*, 1991). These patients are in severe anguish, function poorly if at all, and may develop physical complications because of self-neglect, so rigorous treatment is essential.

At the other end of the severity continuum, milder cases of depression often show little response to antidepressants (Stewart *et al.*, 1983; Paykel *et al.*, 1988). Part of this reflects the mildness of the condition, so rating scores are relatively low initially, leaving little scope for much improvement, and also a high placebo response and spontaneous remission rate. However, some apparently mild cases do have biological features, such as poor sleep, indifferent appetite, muted libido, and vague aches and pains. These patients often show a gratifying response to an antidepressant. Similarly, antidepressants may be effective even where the depression appears to be an understandable reaction to life-stresses (Paykel & Priest, 1992).

One study compared problem-solving (essentially directive counselling), amitriptyline (150mg at night) and placebo (including general support, encouragement and detailed progress-monitoring) in patients with major depression in primary care (Mynors-Wallis *et al.*, 1995). By week 12, 60% of patients given problem-solving had recovered compared with 52% on amitriptyline and 27% in the placebo group.

The category of 'atypical depression' has been bandied about in antidepressant literature for many years, with particular reference to the MAOIs.

Unfortunately, it has not been clearly defined until fairly recently. An early mention related to 'anxiety hysteria with secondary atypical depression' (West & Dally, 1959). The usual features are irritability, somatic anxiety, hypochondriasis and phobic symptoms, often with 'reverse' vegetative symptoms such as increase in sleeping, appetite and weight, and mood worse in the evenings. These patients do best with an MAOI (Quitkin *et al.*, 1993).

Long-term therapy

Increasing emphasis is being placed on long-term treatment. This is generally divided into two types, although the distinction is not always easy to make in practice (Thase & Sullivan, 1995) (Fig. 9.1). Relapse is common in patients who have apparently responded to treatment. This is typically about 50% of

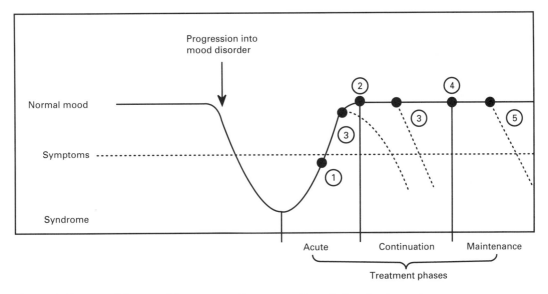

Fig. 9.1 A diagram of five possible outcomes (1, response; 2, remission; 3, relapse; 4, recovery; and 5, recurrence) during the three phases of treatment of depression (acute, continuation and maintenance).

responders and suggests that the clinical mode of action of antidepressants, in these patients at least, is to control or suppress symptoms until natural remission takes place. If natural remission does not ensue (10–20% of patients), then maintenance drug treatment may be needed indefinitely.

The second type of long-term therapy is to prevent recurrence of depression, prophylaxis. This assumes that full recovery has taken place, i.e. that the patient is euthymic without treatment but is constantly at risk of a further episode. The long-term antidepressant is then used to 'prevent' that recurrence. However, this prevention of clinical symptoms might not be true prophylaxis at all but rather the control of symptoms in the episode, which therefore remains subclinical.

Prien and Kupfer (1986) reviewed the studies to that date which evaluated the effectiveness of antidepressants in preventing relapse. The overall conclusion was that the relapse rate on placebo during a 2- to 8-month period of observation was 50% as compared with around 25% on active drug, mostly a TCA. Belsher and Costello (1988) point out the need to control for number of previous episodes, duration of normal mood before entering the comparative clinical trial and clear definitions of recovery and relapse, with regular follow-up interviews, rather than relying on medical records.

Similar methodological considerations occur in prophylactic trials. The need for a carefully defined period of recovery from the previous period of depression is paramount. Relapse is commonest in the first 4 weeks after discontinuing an antidepressant but there is still some risk up to 4 months. Accordingly, a symptom-free period of 4–6 months is the minimum and removes almost all risk of labelling a relapse as a failure of prophylaxis.

Discontinuation of the antidepressant in a placebo-controlled study should not be abrupt as a short-lived withdrawal with autonomic symptoms may confuse the clinical picture as well as jeopardize the double-blind procedures.

Other considerations are adequate criteria for illness recurrence and sufficient previous morbidity for a prophylactic effect to be manifest within 2–3 years (Montgomery & Montgomery, 1992).

Imipramine is the best-studied drug with respect to prophylaxis. The larger studies have shown a significant superiority. One study involved 75 patients treated with imipramine, placebo or interpersonal therapy and followed up for 3 years after a 20-week symptom-free period (Frank *et al.*, 1990). Only 22% of imipramine-treated patients had a further episode compared with 78% on placebo and 62% given interpersonal therapy.

Out-patients with major depressive disorder in the National Institute of Mental Health Treatment of Depression Collaborative Study received either cognitive behaviour therapy, interpersonal therapy, imipramine plus clinical management or placebo plus clinical management (Shea *et al.*, 1992). After 16 weeks of treatment, follow-ups were conducted at 6, 12 and 18 months. Response rates were equal in the four groups varying between 19% and 30%, i.e. surprisingly low. Between a third and a half relapsed subsequently, emphasizing the need for sustained treatment.

Evaluation of the SSRIs long-term has involved large numbers of patients. A rigorous study using fluoxetine in unipolar depression recruited 456 patients treated openly (Montgomery *et al.*, 1988). Of these, 220 responded and remained well for 18 weeks. They were then allocated randomly and double-blind either to continue on fluoxetine or to switch to placebo for 1 year. Those on fluoxetine had a 26% risk of developing a new episode, those on placebo over twice this risk. Similar are available for paroxetine, sertraline and citalopram. The data from a combined relapse/recurrence prevention trial over a year comparing paroxetine and placebo are shown in Fig. 9.2 . Signifi-

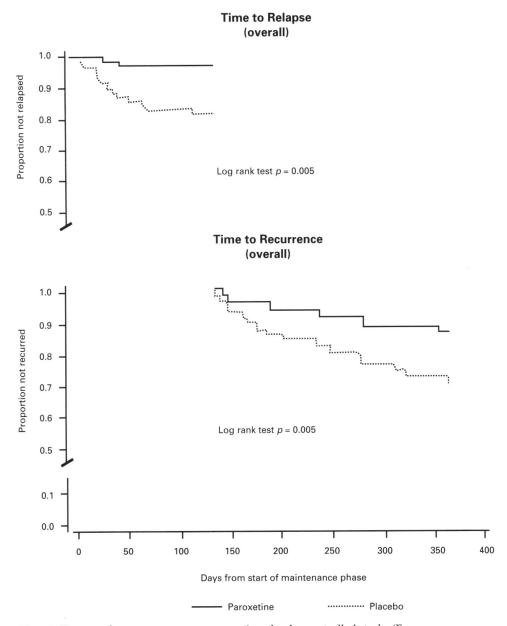

Fig. 9.2 Time to relapse or recurrence, paroxetine placebo-controlled study. (From Montgomery, S.A. & Montgomery, D.B. (1992) Prophylactic treatment in recurrent unipolar depression. In: *Long-term Treatment of Depression* (eds S. Montgomery & F. Rouillon), pp. 53–79. Copyright John Wiley & Sons Limited. Reproduced with permission.)

cant effects were found for both therapeutic effects (Montgomery & Montgomery, 1992).

Dosage considerations

The dosage of antidepressant is often inadequate for full efficacy. This is particularly so in primary care where dosages of TCAs may be as low as a third of the recommended level, particularly in women (Munizza *et al.*, 1995). By contrast, dosages of SSRIs in primary care usually attain recommended levels (Donoghue, 1995). The reason for this is mainly to avoid side-effects (Beaumont *et al.*, 1996). However, there are few good dose-effect studies with the antidepressants (Quitkin, 1985). A further complication is that the dosages prescribed by psychiatrists tend to be higher in the USA than in Europe. Doses of 150 mg of a typical TCA are deemed adequate in the UK and Continental Europe, with 225 mg and, rarely, 300 mg reserved for in-patients who have failed to respond to the lower dose. In the USA, the accepted therapeutic range starts at 225 mg and goes up to 300 mg and beyond.

The recommended dosage does not depend on efficacy alone. The risk/benefit ratio is the relevant attribute at each dose level. Also, dosages are attained in a sequence, usually of increase, occasionally a decrease in the unduly sensitive. Thus, complex algorithms are needed but few if any of these dosage schemata are supported by clear data. Accordingly, the time-honoured schedules persist, usually obtained using the older TCAs, where dosage titration reflected tolerability rather than efficacy. A further obfuscatory influence is the ostensible delay in onset of action which makes dosage titration even more of a hit-and-miss affair.

One dose-ranging study has explored the dosage requirements of fluoxetine. Fluoxetine showed marginal efficacy at doses as low as 5 mg daily, but full efficacy was not reached until 20 mg daily (Wernicke *et al.*, 1988).

It was generally accepted that when a patient has recovered from a depressive episode, a lower dose can be used in maintenance and prophylaxis. There are few data to support this and most recent long-term studies have opted to use full doses throughout. Moreover, one study does suggest more efficacy for maprotiline at 75 mg (half dose) than 37.5 mg (quarter dose) (Rouillon *et al.*, 1989).

Evidence is slightly clearer for a dose relationship with the MAOIs. High doses of phenelzine are more effective than low doses (Robinson *et al.*, 1978; Pare, 1985), and this tends to correlate with degree of inhibition of MAO in platelets.

Although dose-effect relationships are difficult to establish with respect to efficacy, clear relationships are usually discernible between dose levels and side-effects such as dry mouth and constipation with the TCAs, nausea and dizziness with the SSRIs, and postural hypotension with the MAOIs. Indeed, the astute clinician often titrates dosage against incipient side-effect rather than efficacy.

Compliance issues

Psychiatric patients are notoriously poor compliers. Most comply poorly in not taking their medication at all, taking lower than prescribed dosages, taking medication as required rather than on a continuous basis, and stopping treatment prematurely. In one study, two-thirds of patients prescribed a TCA were no longer taking their medication after 4 weeks (Johnson, 1981). A variety of factors may lead to poor compliance. The most important is severe side-effects which, coupled with delay in apparent response, can lead to disillusionment and then demoralization in an already depressed patient. At the least, the patient reduces the dosage to tolerable, and sometimes inefficacious, levels; at the most, the medication is stopped often without admitting this to the prescribing doctor. The cessation of medication can be after just one dose, the sedation, dizziness or other side-effect leading the patient to conclude that the treatment did not 'agree' with him or her.

Another reason is the patient refusing to acknowledge that they are suffering from a mental illness, regarding this as a weakness or a stigma. Taking medication comes to symbolize this, so it is refused.

Education is the key to improving compliance (Fernando & Kazarian, 1995). This should be aimed at relatives, friends and carers as well as the patient. Written material is preferable to verbal instruction as the information given can be carefully prepared to minimize jargon and psychobabble, and because patients find it difficult to attend to and concentrate on the spoken word.

Patterns of response

Depression is a complex conglomeration of symptoms and signs affecting many psychological and bodily functions. Response to antidepressants is also complex, with some features leading and some lagging. Overall, response tends to be fairly smooth when drug-related but more variable when spontaneous or placebo-related (Quitkin *et al.*, 1984).

One detailed study looked specifically at patterns of improvement in depressed in-patients using frequent observations (Lader *et al.*, 1987). A longitudinal study of 70 depressed patients established differential rates of recovery of the various components of depression over the first few weeks of hospitalization. Clinical progress was monitored by self- and observer-ratings of mood, a symptom Q-sort, and tests of psychomotor and cognitive functioning.

Deficits in mood and cognition were substantially reduced after patients had spent 5 weeks in hospital. Marked differences emerged in the *severity* and *rate* of response of various components of the depressive illness. Sad affect, lack of interest, hopelessness, helplessness, suicidal thinking and somatic dysfunction rapidly recovered. An intermediate rate was observed for low self-esteem, sleep disturbances, cognitive slowing, impulsivity, emotional blunting, self-criticism, anhedonia, and subjective memory complaints. Specific features like guilt, intropunitive anger, acquiescence, low expectancies, indecision, suspicion, hostility, diminished libido and anxiety remitted slowly. After 5 weeks, performance on psychomotor, immediate memory and paired-associate learning tasks reached a plateau.

It was apparent that the response of some items was fairly prompt, raising questions about the belief that response to antidepressants is delayed, the subject of the next topic.

A study from the USA considered patterns of response in severely de-pressed in-patients categorized as full responders or non-responders (Katz *et al.*, 1987). In responders, improvement overall and in depressed mood, cognitive impairment, anxiety and physical signs was apparent as early as 1 week, whereas retardation and somatization were only significantly improved by 2 weeks. The differences between this and the previous study probably relate to differences in criteria for improvement, the former using clinical as well as statistical criteria.

Delay in response

From the earliest clinical experience with the TCAs and the MAOIs, it was apparent that the depressed mood was slow to lift in the course of the therapeutic response. This has led to oft-repeated statements concerning the delay in the onset of action of antidepressants and the search, usually disappointing, for fast-acting agents (Norman & Leonard, 1994).

A thorough search of the literature by Danjou *et al.* (1994) identified 127 clinical trials which were appropriate for analysis with respect to onset of action defined as 'the first assessment with a statistical difference vs. placebo'. If no placebo difference ensued, then the onset of action was taken as the duration of the study. The mean onset of action for the TCAs was 3 weeks; for SSRIs, 3.1 weeks; and for MAOIs, 6 weeks. By far the largest number of studies (41) involved imipramine, and a weak positive relationship ($r = 0.48$) was found between onset of action and dose, being longer at higher dose. This presumably reflects the time taken to titrate the dose upwards. Conversely, data with venlafaxine showed a correlation (-0.52) in the opposite direction, believed due to the ability to attain high and effective doses rapidly. A re-working of such analyses using only fixed dosage data would be very informative, as it would obviate titration delays.

Manifestly, one reason for delay in onset of response reflects the time taken to attain therapeutic dosages. This is only a minor factor as the delays with the SSRIs fluoxetine (17 studies) and paroxetine (17 studies) were the same as with the TCAs, and yet most patients start treatment on a standard dose which is not increased.

A second factor concerns the detection of response. Various scales may be differentially sensitive to different symptomatic components. For example, the Hamilton Depression Scale has three items relating to sleep which would be sensitive to early actions of sedative antidepressants.

A more important factor concerns the pooling of data from eventual responders and non-responders (Potter & Manji, 1994). Thus, patients who show no response will introduce a delay into the composite curve of the total group. Again, analysis of data from responders only would be useful and would probably show an onset of action around 1–2 weeks for both TCAs and SSRIs.

After having taken all the above factors into account, it cannot be gainsaid that depressed patients take time to improve when treated with an antidepressant. This delay has been attributed to biochemical adaptive changes which take time to develop after the immediate changes in amine neurotransmitter disposition.

Prediction of response

In his original account, Kuhn (1958) observed that the closer the patient approximated to the classic 'endogenous depressive', the more likely was an adequate response. That remains the firm clinical impression. Nevertheless, up to 30% of such patients fail to show an adequate response and are termed 'refractory' (Guscott & Grof, 1991; Sokolov & Joffe, 1995).

Antidepressants are effective across a wide range of severity, all but the mildest forms responding to at least some extent (Paykel *et al.*, 1988). However, recurrent brief depressions appear to be fairly unresponsive to antidepressant medication (Kasper *et al.*, 1995). At the other end of the continuum, patients with psychotic (delusional) depression tend to need either the addition of an antipsychotic drug to the antidepressant or the use of ECT.

A coruscating review by Joyce and Paykel (1989) concludes that the TCAs are broad-spectrum drugs 'that convey therapeutic benefit over a wide range of depressions and some anxiety disorders' (p. 95). The patient with a good premorbid personality, an insidious onset of illness, psychomotor retardation, and intermediate in severity and endogeneity but without psychotic features is most likely to respond. The MAOIs were regarded as an important option in previous responders, and as a second-line treatment in refractory depression, and in patients with marked anxiety/panic features. Biological predictors were relatively uninformative.

The advent of the SSRIs has not changed this overall assessment. Efficacy is similar to that of the TCAs, as is the type of patient who responds. Sometimes newer drugs have modified or additional indications in the data sheet, but this usually reflects proven efficacy in that subgroup of patients rather than differential efficacy.

Non-endogenous depression remains more difficult to treat than patients with classical 'endogenous' depression. Even then, more severe symptoms including weight loss were predictive of better response (Parker *et al.*, 1985). Another important predictor of good response was the break-up of an intimate relationship in the 12 months preceding treatment.

Early signs of response predict later full response. Thus, improvement in overall depressed state as well as on depressed mood, cognitive impairment, anxiety and physical symptoms was apparent after a week in ultimate responders. Retardation and somatization improvements were also predictive but only after 2 weeks (Katz *et al.*, 1987).

Duration of treatment

The length of time needed for antidepressant treatment has become a topic of debate recently. The tendency has been to recommend longer and longer courses of treatment as the recurrent/chronic nature of depression has become increasingly appreciated and the risk of relapse on premature withdrawal better quantified. The criteria for relapse and recurrence have been discussed by Paykel (1994) and by Kupfer and Frank (1992), and can be set against the background of the natural history of depressive illnesses (Angst, 1992). Thus, about 15–20% of depressives become chronic and about 15% commit suicide. After the onset of the illness, about 20% of the subsequent lifetime is spent in episodes (Angst, 1992). Between episodes, many patients remain symptomatic, but 20% suffer only one episode. A UK study of 70 patients showed that remission was quite rapid with 70% doing so within 6 months (Ramana *et al.*, 1995). However, 40% relapsed over the subsequent 10 months. Greater initial severity predicted longer time to remission and greater risk of relapse.

The NIMH Collaborative Program on the Psychobiology of Depression concentrated on in-patients in special research centres (Keller *et al.*, 1982a). Two-thirds recovered within the first 4 months but 26% were still not recovered at 1 year; 21%, at 2 years; and 12%, at 5 years (Keller *et al.*, 1992). After remission, 12% relapsed within a month; a quarter, within 3 months; but only 30%, by a year (Keller *et al.*, 1982b). After relapse, recovery was less likely than initially.

Residual symptoms after the initial response are predictive of relapse if medication is discontinued: about a third of patients fall into this category of partial responders (Kupfer & Spiker, 1981). Even mild symptoms are predictive of relapse. Withdrawal of therapy is safe only after the patient has been free of symptoms for 16–20 weeks (Prien & Kupfer, 1986).

The definition of relapse is, itself, non-standard. Sometimes it refers to a recurrence of symptoms, sometimes to an operational change, such as admission to hospital. The borderline between relapse of the current episode and development of a new episode also involves an arbitrary decision. A symptom-free interval of 16–20 weeks is generally taken as indicating that the initial attack has resolved and that the risk is of a recurrence.

Discontinuing treatment

Although there is a plethora of studies investigating the initiation and maintenance of antidepressant treatment, very few address the issue of discontinuing medication. Greden (1993) recommends that the schedule should be gradual, over several weeks or even a few months. After long-term maintenance, the tapering period should be even longer. He opines 'that the brain requires months rather than days or weeks to adjust to the changes associated with stopping a medication'.

TCAs with anticholinergic potency, particularly amitriptyline, require special care because of the problem of cholinergic rebound (Dilsaver & Greden, 1984). Symptoms include gastrointestinal distress, restless sleep with vivid nightmares, frequent awakenings, and anxiety and agitation.

The withdrawal of an MAOI should also be gradual. However, this is because the usual episode length in patients who respond to an MAOI may be much longer than in more typical patients responding to a TCA or an SSRI (Robinson *et al.*, 1991). Furthermore, relapse may be particularly slow to resolve after the MAOI withdrawal.

The above refers to planned discontinuation of treatment after successful response. Dropout refers to unplanned discontinuation, often early in treatment and most commonly related to treatment failure and/or intolerable side-effects. Indeed, the dropout rate due to side-effects has been used as a crude indicator of tolerability (Lader, 1988). Dropout rates due to side-effects in patients on TCAs tend to be higher than those on SSRIs (Song *et al.*, 1993). In one meta-analysis of 42 randomized comparative controlled studies, the dropout rate due to side-effects was 19% in those on TCAs, 15% in those on SSRIs ($P<0.01$) (Montgomery *et al.*, 1994). Another meta-analysis of 62 studies yielded dropout rates of 18.8% in patients on TCAs as compared with 14.4% in those given SSRIs ($P<0.001$) (Anderson & Tomenson, 1995).

Comorbidity

Depression is often encountered in conjunction with other psychiatric conditions, particularly anxiety in its various forms (Keller & Hanks, 1995). The unitary view considers the two disorders to be a single entity expressing both groups of symptoms concurrently or over time separately. Or the presence of one condition may make the onset of the second, ostensibly independent, condition more likely. Third, comorbidity may just reflect the chance concatenation of two common conditions (Cassano & Michelini, 1995). Angst and colleagues (1990) in their detailed longitudinal study in Zurich showed that primarily anxious individuals were more likely to develop comorbid depression as follow-up than vice versa. Comorbidity occurs between depression and panic disorder, and generalized anxiety disorder (Cassano *et al.*, 1992), as well as with social and simple phobia, obsessive-compulsive disorder, and probably post-traumatic stress disorder.

Concern about the use of benzodiazepines in the treatment of anxiety disorders, particularly in the long term, has led to a convergence of treatment stratagems in these comorbid conditions. Antidepressants of various types are widely used in these disorders, not only to treat the depressive component but increasingly as effective therapy for the panic, anxiety or obsessive-compulsive elements. In particular, drugs acting on serotonin seem effective (Burrows *et al.*, 1994). However, more systematic evaluations are needed to establish the degree of efficacy in these comorbid conditions. The use of antidepressants to treat 'pure' anxiety disorders lies outside the scope of this chapter.

Special groups

The young

Reservations have been expressed about the efficacy of TCAs in the treatment of childhood depression. A meta-analysis of 12 studies revealed no significant effect vs. placebo, either on mean response or number of responders (Hazell *et al.*, 1995). Data on SSRIs and MAOIs are insufficient to allow any conclusions to be drawn. Nevertheless, clinical experience still supports the use of antidepressants in selected cases (Kaplan & Hussein, 1995).

The elderly

The antidepressants in general are of proven efficacy in the treatment of the elderly depressive. Indeed, several regulatory authorities ask for a substantial minority of patients in the clinical trials of a new drug to be elderly in order to establish efficacy and tolerability in this age group. Dosages are generally low, at least initially, and dosage escalation should be gradual. This is because of complex pharmacokinetic changes in the elderly, particularly in those aged over 85 years.

A complicating factor is the effect of cognition of both depression and antidepressants. However, cognitive function in general is not disproportionately impaired in the elderly as compared with younger depressives, although the speed of performance may fall (Tarbuck & Paykel, 1995). The use of TCAs with anticholinergic effects may further impair performance although SSRIs seem better tolerated in general (e.g. Fairweather *et al.*, 1993). For this reason, the SSRIs or other newer drugs (e.g. lofepramine, nefazodone) are increasingly preferred to standard TCAs (Dufour *et al.*, 1994).

The physically ill

The TCAs have many effects on many bodily systems and some of these may compromise organ function. The best-known are the cardiovascular effects, and special precautions are needed when treating depressed patients with cardiovascular disease (Glassman & Stage, 1994). The SSRIs are usually to be preferred. Renal and hepatic impairment are other conditions where care should be taken in choosing an antidepressant and its dosage (Hale, 1993).

Almost all antidepressants lower the convulsive threshold so epileptics may have their condition exacerbated. Many other physical conditions may affect the side-effect profile of individual drugs—for example, diabetes and parkinsonism. Finally, drug interactions may occur, and again patterns vary from drug to drug (Taylor & Lader, 1996).

Personality factors

These have been largely neglected until recently. Akiskal (1995) has reviewed the relationships between temperaments and depression and concluded that recognition of the importance of various personality factors reduced the heterogeneity of major depressive disorders as presently defined. One efficacy study suggested that patients who failed to respond to both a TCA and an MAOI given at various times were more likely to have an abnormal personality than those who did respond (Shawcross & Tyrer, 1985).

Antidepressants and suicide

Drug addicts

Some concern has been expressed about the abuse potential of antidepressants, particularly the more stimulant ones. In France, the antidepressant amineptine appeared to be associated with some risk (Castot, 1990). However, the risk with other antidepressants seems vanishingly small, and antidepressants should never be withheld from depressed drug addicts because

Table 9.1 Fatal poisonings and deaths per million defined daily doses for deaths from single antidepressants, by groups of drug. Values in parentheses are 95% confidence intervals.

Antidepressant	Observed deaths, 1987–92	Expected deaths, 1987–92	Mean defined daily dose (mg) 1987–92	χ^2 value	Deaths per million defined daily doses, 1987–92
Tricyclic drugs	1563	1346	94	34.98	16.63 (1.36 to 1.50)*
Monoamine oxidase inhibitors	12	41	28	20.51	0.43 (0.19 to 0.60)*
Atypical drugs	26	62	165	20.90	0.16 (0.34 to 0.74)*
Selective serotonin re-uptake inhibitors	5	56	66	46.45	0.08 (0.03 to 0.23)
All antidepressants	1606	1606	89		1.26

$P < 0.001$ (difference from all by χ^2 test).

of this fear (Pagliaro & Pagliaro, 1995). The relationship between antidepressants and suicide has excited much controversy which continues unabated. One issue concerns the relative safety of antidepressants (Jick et al., 1995). It is unfortunate that the drugs given to potentially suicidal patients can themselves prove fatal in overdose. League tables have been published of the fatal overdoses associated with various antidepressants (deaths per million prescriptions or per defined daily dose) (e.g. Henry et al., 1995) (Table 9.1). However, these data may reflect *perceived* as well as *actual* safety, as practitioners may favour one drug over another for any patient with a risk of attempting suicide. This, added to the limitations of official suicide statistics (O'Donnell & Farmer, 1995), renders interpretation difficult. Despite this, it is clear that the newer drugs, in particular the SSRIs and lofepramine, are much less toxic than the standard TCAs. Among the TCAs, dothiepin may be particularly hazardous (Buckley et al., 1994).

The strategy of prescribing an SSRI instead of a TCA in the prevention of suicide was examined by Freemantle and colleagues (1994). They concluded that a high price would be paid for a total switch to an SSRI to prevent suicide but that the newer tricyclics (e.g. lofepramine) are more cost-effective in this regard. A storm of protest followed, touching on many issues (Correspondence, 1994). The debate continues, characterized more by heat than by light!

A second issue concerns whether antidepressant treatment can itself worsen depressive symptoms and release suicidal thoughts and impulses (Damluji & Ferguson, 1988). Attention focused on fluoxetine with several studies supporting or refuting the hypothesis that this drug may induce *de novo* suicidal ideation (see Teicher et al., 1993). These authors suggest 'that antidepressants may redistribute suicide risk, attenuating risk in some patients who respond well, while possibly enhancing risk in others who respond more poorly' (p. 187).

Comparison of antidepressants

The advent of the SSRIs has opened up a massive, on-going debate concerning their merits *vis-à-vis* the TCAs. Similarly, but on a much more muted note, the introduction of the selective and reversible inhibitor of MAO, moclobemide, has led to comparisons with the old MAOIs. This has coincided with an insistence in many countries that cost-effectiveness must be a major factor in the choice of medication. The SSRIs are more expensive than the older TCAs, most of which are available as generics. Many elements enter the comparative arguments, including side-effect profile, tolerability and compliance, safety in overdose (Henry & Martin, 1987), and usefulness in special groups such as the elderly.

The one aspect which hardly enters into the equation is efficacy, the focus of this chapter. Some atypical antidepressants such as nomifensine (withdrawn some years ago), trazodone and perhaps mianserin have been found less effective than imipramine in meta-analyses (Müller *et al.*, 1994). Another meta-analysis concluded that the SSRIs were slower in action than TCAs but were equal in efficacy by 6 weeks, except on sleep items (Bech, 1990). A review some years ago concluded that TCAs are still preferable in patients who have responded to them previously, and in patients where plasma concentration monitoring might be helpful (Rudorfer & Potter, 1989).

More recently, Song *et al.* (1993) analysed 63 randomized controlled trials comparing an SSRI with an older antidepressant. No difference in efficacy was found. A similar exercise identified 55 double-blind studies and found no differences in efficacy between five SSRIs and comparator TCAs (Anderson & Tomenson, 1994). There was some suggestion in the data that the TCAs had the edge over the SSRIs in the more severely depressed patients and with in-patients. This was due to a clinically significant lower efficacy for paroxetine in those patients. Another meta-analysis indicated that trazodone, buproprion, fluoxetine and imipramine were all equally effective compared with placebo (Workman & Short, 1993).

It is not surprising that efficacy differences among the antidepressants are marginal, if they exist at all. With about a third of patients non-responders and a third placebo responders, the efficacy 'window' is quite narrow. Reduced efficacy would have to be substantial to be detected, as would enhanced efficacy.

The debate continues with respect to the relative merits of various antidepressants. For example, Edwards (1995), after a detailed review of the topic, concludes, 'In the light of existing knowledge, the decision as to whether to use SSRIs as first-line treatment for depression and the opinion as to whether the benefits are worth the cost must remain as value judgements' (pp. 156–7). By contrast, Harrison (1994) avers: 'But for the first line treatment of patients seen every day in surgeries and psychiatric clinics, new is better' (p. 1281). In my experience, if one actually asks patients for their opinion, they generally prefer to take an SSRI rather than a TCA.

Individual antidepressants

It is not the purpose of this chapter to review the individual drugs in detail. Recourse can be made to standard textbooks (e.g. Lader & Herrington, 1996; Schatzberg & Nemeroff, 1995). The reader will also find useful the recent reviews and papers on individual drugs in Table 9.2.

Table 9.2 Antidepressant drugs: reviews and key references.

Drug	Reference
Tricyclic antidepressants	
Clomipramine	McTavish and Benfield (1990)
Dothiepin	Lancaster and Gonzalez (1989a)
Lofepramine	Lancaster and Gonzalez (1989b)
Selective serotonin re-uptake inhibitors	
Citalopram	Milne & Goa (1991)
Fluoxetine	Wernicke *et al.* (1988)
Fluvoxamine	Wilde *et al.* (1993)
Paroxetine	Dechant and Clissold (1991)
	Holliday and Plosker (1993)
Sertraline	Murdoch and McTavish (1992)
Selective serotonin/noradrenaline re-uptake inhibitors	
Venlafaxine	Artigas (1995)
	Cowen (1995)
	Holliday and Benfield (1995)
Serotonin re-uptake inhibitor and antagonist	
Nefazodone	Rickels *et al.* (1994)
Reversible inhibitors of MAO	
Moclobemide	Fitton *et al.* (1992)
	Priest and Schmid-Burgk (1994)
	Moll *et al.* (1994)
Brofaromine	Volz *et al.* (1995)
Amine precursors	
Tryptophan	Kaufman and Philen (1993)

Conclusions

Depression is a common and distressing condition. It is associated with impairment of psychosocial functioning—education, occupational, marital and social—which tends to persist (Coryell *et al.*, 1993). It imposes medical, social and economic burdens on the community: one estimate was that the annual costs of depression in the USA total $43.7 billion, comprising 28% direct costs (medical care, etc.), 17% mortality costs including suicide, and 55% indirect costs such as loss of work capacity (Greenberg *et al.*, 1993).

Despite this, treatment is often barely adequate. One survey showed that less than one-third of depressed out-patients used antidepressant medication (Wells *et al.*, 1994). The need for more education among the public and also primary care practitioners, who see the bulk of depressed patients, is manifest (Paykel & Priest, 1992). However, in the harsh economic climate that now prevails, justification for the use of all but the cheapest drugs is demanded by our political masters. Increasingly, pharmacoeconomic considerations are entering not only into the use of newer antidepressants but also in their licensing (Wilde & Whittington, 1995). Let us strive to ensure that our choice of antidepressant medication remains a wide one so that patients can receive the drug that suits them best. And in the long run, let us hope that inducements remain to encourage the development and introduction of novel agents of enhanced efficacy.

References

Akiskal, H.S. (1995) Toward a temperament-based approach to depression: implications for neurobiologic research. In: *Depression and Mania: From Neurobiology to Treatment* (eds G. L. Gessa, W. Fratta, L. Pani & G. Serra), pp. 99–112. Raven Press, New York.

American Psychiatric Association (1994) *Diagnostic criteria for DSM-IV.* American Psychiatric Association, Washington, DC.

Anderson, I.M. & Tomenson, B.M. (1994) The efficacy of selective serotonin re-uptake inhibitors in depression: a meta-analysis of studies against tricyclic antidepressants. *Journal of Psychopharmacology*, 8, 238–249.

Anderson, I.M. & Tomenson, B.M. (1995) Treatment discontinuation with selective serotonin reuptake inhibitors compared with tricyclic antidepressants: a meta-analysis. *British Medical Journal*, 310, 1433–1438.

Angst, J. (1992) How recurrent and predictable is depressive illness? In: *Long-term Treatment of Depression* (eds S. Montgomery & F. Rouillon), pp. 1–13. Wiley, Chichester.

Angst, J., Vollrath, M., Merikangas, M.R. & Ernst, C. (1990) Comorbidity of anxiety and depression in the Zurich cohort study of young adults. In: *Comorbidity of Mood and Anxiety Disorders* (eds J. Maser & R. Cloninger). American Psychia-

tric Press, Washington, DC., pp. 123–137.

Artigas, F. (1995) Selective serotonin/noradrenaline reuptake inhibitors (SNRIs). Pharmacology and therapeutic potential in the treatment of depressive disorders. *CNS Drugs*, 4, 79–89.

Balant-Gorgia, A.E., Gex-Fabry, M. & Balant, L.P. (1991) Clinical pharmacokinetics of clomipramine. *Clinical Pharmacokinetics*, 20, 447–462.

Beaumont, G., Baldwin, D. & Lader, M. (1996) A criticism of the practice of prescribing subtherapeutic doses of antidepressants for the treatment of depression. *Human Psychopharmacology*, 11, 283–291.

Bech, P. (1990) A meta-analysis of the antidepressant properties of serotonin reuptake inhibitors. *International Review of Psychiatry*, 2, 207–211.

Belsher, G. & Costello, C.G. (1988) Relapse after recovery from unipolar depression: a critical review. *Psychology Bulletin*, 104, 84–96.

Brown, W.A. & Khan, A. (1994) Which depressed patients should receive antidepressants? *CNS Drugs*, 1, 341–347.

Buckley, N.A., Dawson, A.H., Whyte, I.M. & Henry, D.A. (1994) Greater toxicity in overdose of dothiepin than of other tricyclic antidepressants. *Lancet*, 343, 159–162.

Burrows, G.D., Judd, F.K. & Norman, T.R. (1994) Differential diagnosis and drug treatment of panic disorder, anxiety and depression. *CNS Drugs*, **1**, 119–131.

Cassano, G.B. & Michelini, S. (1995) Pharmacological treatment of depression and comorbid anxiety disorders. In: *Depression and Mania: From Neurobiology to Treatment* (eds G. L. Gessa, W. Fratta, L. Pani & G. Serra), pp. 113–125. Raven Press, New York.

Cassano, G.B., Savino, M. & Perugi, G. (1992) Comorbidity of mood disorders and anxiety states: implications for long-term treatment. In: *Long-term Treatment of Depression* (eds S. Montgomery & F. Rouillon), pp. 229–243. John Wiley, Chichester.

Castot, A. (1990) Sur consommation d'amineptine. Analyse de 155 cas. Bilan de l'enquête officielle cooperative des centres regionaux de pharmacovigilance. *Therapie*, **45**, 399–405.

Correspondence (1994) Selective serotonin reuptake inhibitors. *British Medical Journal*, **309**, 1082–1085.

Coryell, W., Scheftner, W., Keller, M., Endicott, J., Maser, J. & Klerman, J.L. (1993) The enduring psychosocial consequences of mania and depression. *American Journal of Psychiatry*, **150**, 720–727.

Cowen, P. (1995) Venlafaxine: a new class of antidepressant drug. *Prescriber*, **June**, 19–26.

Damluji, N.F. & Ferguson, J.M. (1988) Paradoxical worsening of depressive symptomatology caused by antidepressants. *Journal of Clinical Psychopharmacology*, **8**, 347–349.

Danjou, P., Weiller, E. & Richardot, P. (1994) Onset of action of antidepressants: a literature survey. In: *Critical Issues in the Treatment of Affective Disorders* (eds S.Z. Langer, N. Brunello, G. Racagni & J. Mendlewicz), pp. 136–153. Karger, Basel.

Dechant, K.L. & Clissold, S.P. (1991) Paroxetine: a review of its pharmacodynamic and pharmacokinetic properties, and therapeutic potential in depressive illness. *Drugs*, **41**, 225–253.

Dilsaver, S.C. & Greden, J.F. (1984) Antidepressant withdrawal phenomena. *Biological Psychiatry*, **19**, 237–256.

Donoghue, J.M. (1995) A comparison of prescribing patterns of selective serotonin reuptake inhibitors in the treatment of depression in primary care in the United Kingdom. *Journal of Serotonin Research*, **1**, 47–51.

Dufour, H., Wertheimer, J., Baumann, P. & Bertschy, G. (1994) Efficacy and safety of antidepressants in the elderly. In: *Critical Issues in the Treatment of Affective Disorders* (eds S. Z. Langer, N. Brunello, G. Racagni & J. Mendlewicz), pp. 44–51. Karger, Basel.

Edwards, J.G. (1995) Drug choice in depression: selective serotonin reuptake inhibitors or tricyclic antidepressants? *CNS Drugs*, **4**, 141–159.

Fairweather, D.B., Kerr, J.S., Harrison, D.A., Moon, C.A. & Hindmarch, I. (1993) A double blind comparison of the effects of fluoxetine and amitriptyline on cognitive function in elderly depressed patients. *Human Psychopharmacology*, **8**, 41–47.

Fernando, M.L.D. & Kazarian, S.S. (1995) Patient education in the drug treatment of psychiatric disorders. *CNS Drugs*, **3**, 291–304.

Fitton, A., Faulds, D. & Goa, K.L. (1992) Moclobemide: a review of its pharmacological properties and therapeutic use in depressive illness. *Drugs*, **43**, 561–596.

Frank, E., Kupfer, D.J. & Perel, J.M. *et al.* (1990) Three-year outcomes for maintenance therapies in recurrent depression. *Archives of General Psychiatry*, **47**, 1093–1099.

Freemantle, N., House, A., Song, F., Mason, J.M. & Sheldon, T.A. (1994) Prescribing selective serotonin reuptake inhibitors as strategy for prevention of suicide. *British Medical Journal*, **309**, 249–253.

Glassman, A.H. & Stage, K.B. (1994) Depressed patients with cardiovascular disease: treatment considerations. *CNS Drugs*, **1**, 435–440.

Greden, J. (1993) Antidepressant maintenance medications: when to discontinue and how to stop. *Journal of Clinical Psychiatry*, **54** (Suppl. 8), 39–45.

Greenberg, P.E., Stiglin, L.E., Finkelstein, S.N. & Berndt, E.R. (1993) The economic burden of depression in 1990. *Journal of Clinical Psychiatry*, **54**, 405–418.

Guscott, R. & Grof, P. (1991) The clinical meaning of refractory depression: a review for the clinician. *American Journal of Psychiatry*, **148**, 695–704.

Hale, A.S. (1993) New antidepressants: use in high-risk patients. *Journal of Clinical Psychiatry*, **54** (Suppl. 8), 61–70.

Hamilton, M. (1960) A rating scale for depression. *Journal of Neurology, Neurosurgery and Psychiatry*, **23**, 56–62.

Harrison, G. (1994) New or old antidepressants? New is better. *British Medical Journal*, **309**, 1280–1282.

Hazell, P., O'Connell, D., Heathcote, D., Robertson, J. & Henry, D. (1995) Efficacy of tricyclic drugs in treating child and adolescent depression: a meta-analysis. *British Medical Journal*, **310**, 897–901.

Henry, J.A. & Martin, A.J. (1987) The risk-benefit assessment of antidepressant drugs. *Medical Toxicology*, **2**, 445–462.

Henry, J.A., Alexander, C.A. & Sener, E.K. (1995) Relative mortality from overdose of antidepressants. *British Medical Journal,* **310**, 221–224.

Holliday, S.M. & Benfield, P. (1995) Venlafaxine: a review of its pharmacology and therapeutic potential in depression. *Drugs,* **49**, 280–294.

Holliday, S.M. & Plosker, G.L. (1993) Paroxetine: a review of its pharmacology, therapeutic use in depression and therapeutic potential in diabetic neuropathy. *Drugs and Aging,* **3**, 278–299.

Jick, S.S., Dean, A.D. & Jick, H. (1995) Antidepressants and suicide. *British Medical Journal,* **310**, 215–218.

Johnson, D.A.W. (1981) Depression: treatment compliance in general practice. *Acta Psychiatrica Scandinavica,* **63** (Suppl. 290), 447–453.

Joyce, P.R. & Paykel, E.S. (1989) Predictors of drug response in depression. *Archives of General Psychiatry,* **46**, 89–99.

Kaplan, C.A. & Hussein, S. (1995) Use of drugs in child and adolescent psychiatry. *British Jounal of Psychiatry,* **166**, 291–298.

Kasper, S., Stamenkovic, M. & Fischer, G. (1995) Recurrent brief depression: diagnosis, epidemiology and potential pharmacological options. *CNS Drugs,* **4**, 222–229.

Katz, M.M., Koslow, S.H. & Maas, J.W. *et al.* (1987) The timing, specificity and clinical prediction of tricyclic drug effects in depression. *Psychological Medicine,* **17**, 297–309.

Kaufman, L.D. & Philen, R.M. (1993) Tryptophan: current status and future trends for oral administration. *Drug Safety,* **8**, 89–98.

Keller, M.B. & Hanks, D.L. (1995) Anxiety symptom relief in depression treatment outcomes. *Journal of Clinical Psychiatry,* **56** (Suppl. 6), 22 29.

Keller, M.B., Shapiro, R.W., Lavori, P.W. & Wolfe, N. (1982a) Recovery in major depressive disorder: analysis with the life table and regression models. *Archives of General Psychiatry,* **39**, 905–910.

Keller, M.B., Shapiro, R.W., Lavori, P.W. & Wolfe, N. (1982b) Recovery in major depressive disorder: analysis with the life table. *Archives of General Psychiatry,* **39**, 911–915.

Keller, M.B., Lavori, P.W. & Mueller, T.I. *et al.* (1992) Time to recovery, chronicity, and levels of psychopathology in major depression: a 5-year prospective follow-up of 431 subjects. *Archives of General Psychiatry,* **49**, 809–816.

Khan, A., Noonan, C. & Healey, W. (1991) Is a single tricyclic antidepressant trial an active treatment for psychotic depression? *Progress in Neuropsychopharmacology and Biological Psychiatry,* **15**, 765–770.

Kuhn, R. (1958) The treatment of depressive states with G22355 (imipramine hydrochloride). *American Journal of Psychiatry,* **115**, 459–463.

Kupfer, D.J. & Frank, E. (1992) The minimum length of treatment for recovery. In: *Long-term Treatment of Depression* (eds S. Montgomery & F. Rouillon), pp. 33–52. Wiley, Chichester.

Kupfer, D.J. & Spiker, D.G. (1981) Refractory depression: prediction of non-response by clinical indicators. *Journal of Clinical Psychiatry,* **42**, 307–312.

Lader, M. (1988) Fluoxetine efficacy vs. comparative drugs: an overview. *British Journal of Psychiatry,* **153** (Suppl. 3), 51–58.

Lader, M. & Herrington, R. (1996) *Biological Treatments in Psychiatry,* 2nd edn. Oxford University Press, Oxford.

Lader, M., Lang, R.A. & Wilson, G.D. (1987) *Patterns of Improvement in Depressed In-patients.* Oxford University Press, Oxford.

Lancaster, S.G. & Gonzalez, J.P. (1989a) Dothiepin: a review of its pharmacodynamic and pharmacokinetic properties, and therapeutic efficacy in depressive illness. *Drugs,* **38**, 123–147.

Lancaster, S.G. & Gonzalez, J.P. (1989b) Lofepramine: a review of its pharmacodynamic and pharmacokinetic properties, and therapeutic efficacy in depressive illness. *Drugs,* **37**, 123–140.

McTavish, D. & Benfield, P. (1990) Clomipramine: an overview of its pharmacological properties and a review of its therapeutic use in obsessive compulsive disorder and panic disorder. *Drugs,* **39**, 136–153.

Milne, R.J. & Goa, K.L. (1991) Citalopram: a review of its pharmacodynamic and pharmacokinetic properties, and therapeutic potential in depressive illness. *Drugs,* **41**, 450–477.

Moll, E., Neumann, N., Schmid-Burgk, M., Stabl, M. & Amrein, R. (1994) Safety and efficacy during long-term treatment with moclobemide. *Clinical Neuropharmacology,* **17** (Suppl. 1), S74–S87.

Müller, H.-J., Fuger, J. & Kasper, S. (1994) Efficacy of new generation antidepressants: meta-analysis of imipramine-controlled studies. *Pharmacopsychiatry,* **27**, 215–223.

Montgomery, S.A. & Asberg, M. (1979) A new depression scale designed to be sensitive to change. *British Journal of Psychiatry,* **134**, 382–389.

Montgomery, S.A. & Montgomery, D.B. (1992) Prophylactic treatment in recurrent unipolar depression. In: *Long-term Treatment of Depression* (eds S. Montgomery & F. Rouillon), pp. 53–79. John Wiley, Chichester.

Montgomery, S.A., Dufour, H. & Brion, S. *et al.* (1988) The prophylactic efficacy of fluoxetine in unipolar depression. *British Journal of Psychiatry,* **3**, 69–76.

Montgomery, S.A., Henry, J. & McDonald, G. *et al.* (1994) Selective serotonin reuptake inhibitors: meta-analysis of discontinuation rates. *International Clinical Psychopharmacology*, **9**, 47–53.

Munizza, C., Tibaldi, G., Bollini, E., Pirfo, E., Punzo, F. & Gramaglia, F. (1995) Prescription pattern of antidepressants in out-patient psychiatric practice. *Psychological Medicine*, **25**, 771–778.

Murdoch, D. & McTavish, D. (1992) Sertraline: a review of its pharmacodynamic and pharmacokinetic properties, and therapeutic potential in depression and obsessive-compulsive disorder. *Drugs*, **44**, 604–624.

Mynors-Wallis, L.M., Gath, D.H., Lloyd-Thomas, A.R. & Tomlinson, D. (1995) Randomised controlled trial comparing problem solving treatment with amitriptyline and placebo for major depression in primary care. *British Medical Journal*, **310**, 441–445.

Norman, T.R. & Leonard, B.E. (1994) Fast-acting antidepressants: can the need be met? *CNS Drugs*, **2**, 120–131.

O'Donnell, I. & Farmer, R. (1995) The limitations of official suicide statistics. *British Journal of Psychiatry*, **166**, 458–461.

Ormel, J., Oldehinkel, T., van Brilman, E. & den Brink, W. (1993) Outcome of depression and anxiety in primary care. *Archives of General Psychiatry*, **50**, 759–766.

Pagliaro, L.A. & Pagliaro, A.M. (1995) Abuse potential of antidepressants: does it exist? *CNS Drugs*, **4**, 247–252.

Pare, C.M.B. (1985) The present status of monoamine oxidase inhibitors. *British Journal of Psychiatry*, **146**, 576–584.

Parker, G., Tennant, C. & Blignault, I. (1985) Predicting improvement in patients with non-endogenous depression. *British Journal of Psychiatry*, **146**, 132–139.

Paykel, E.S. (1994) Relapse, recurrence and chronicity in depression. In: *Critical Issues in the Treatment of Affective Disorders* (eds S. Z. Langer, N. Brunello, G. Racagni & J. Mendlewicz), pp. 9–20. Karger, Basel.

Paykel, E.S. & Priest, R.G. (1992) Recognition and management of depression in general practice: consensus statement. *British Medical Journal*, **305**, 1198–1202.

Paykel, E.S., Hollyman, J.A., Freeling, P. & Sedgwick, P. (1988) Predictors of therapeutic benefit from amitriptyline in mild depression: a general practice placebo-controlled trial. *Journal of Affective Disorders*, **14**, 83–95.

Potter, W.Z. & Manji, H.K. (1994) Clinical onset of antidepressant action: implications for new drug development. In: *Critical Issues in the Treatment of Affective Disorders* (eds S.Z. Langer, N. Brunello, G. Racagni, J. Mendlewicz), pp. 118–126. Karger, Basel.

Prien, R.F. & Kupfer, D.J. (1986) Continuation drug therapy for major depressive episodes: how long should it be maintained? *American Journal of Psychiatry*, **143**, 18–23.

Priest, R.G. & Schmid-Burgk, W. (1994) Moclobemide in the treatment of depression. *Reviews in Contemporary Pharmacotherapy*, **5**, 35–43.

Quality Assurance Project (1983) A treatment outline for depressive disorders. *Australian and New Zealand Journal of Psychiatry*, **17**, 129–146.

Quitkin, F.M. (1985) The importance of dosage in prescribing antidepressants. *British Journal of Psychiatry*, **147**, 593–597.

Quitkin, F.M., Rabkin, J.G., Ross, D. & Stewart, J.W. (1984) Identification of true drug response to antidepressants. *Archives of General Psychiatry*, **41**, 782–786.

Quitkin, F.M., Stewart, J.W. & McGrath, P.J. *et al.* (1993) Columbia atypical depression. *British Journal of Psychiatry*, **163** (Suppl), 30–34.

Ramana, R., Paykel, E.S., Cooper, Z., Hayhurst, H., Saxty, M. & Surtees, P.G. (1995) Remission and relapse in major depression: a two-year prospective follow-up study. *Psychological Medicine*, **25**, 1161–1170.

Rickels, K., Schweizer, E., Clary, C., Fox, I. & Weise, C. (1994) Nefazodone and imipramine in major depression: a placebo-controlled trial. *British Journal of Psychiatry*, **164**, 802–805.

Robinson, D.S., Nies, A., Ravaris, L., Ives, J.O. & Bartlett, D. (1978) Clinical pharmacology of phenelzine. *Archives of General Psychiatry*, **35**, 629–635.

Robinson, D.S., Lerfald, S.C. & Bennett, B. *et al.* (1991) Continuation and maintenance treatment of major depression with the monoamine oxidase inhibitor phenelzine: a double-blind placebo-controlled discontinuation study. *Psychopharmacology Bulletin*, **27**, 31–39.

Rouillon, F., Phillips, R. & Serrurier, D. *et al.* (1989) Rechutes de depression unipolaire et efficacite de la maprotiline. *L'Encephale*, **XV**, 527–534.

Rudorfer, M.V. & Potter, W.Z. (1989) Antidepressants: a comparative review of the clinical pharmacology and therapeutic use of the 'newer' vs. the 'older' drugs. *Drugs*, **37**, 713–738.

Schatzberg, A.F. & Nemeroff, C.B. (eds) (1995) *The American Psychiatric Press Textbook of Psychopharmacology*. American Psychiatric Press, Washington, DC.

Shawcross, C.R. & Tyrer, P. (1985) Influence of personality on response to monoamine oxidase inhibitors and tricyclic antidepressants. *Journal of Psychiatric Research,* **19**, 557–562.

Shea, M.T., Elkin, I. & Imber, S.D. *et al.* (1992) Course of depressive symptoms over follow-up: findings from the National Institute of Mental Health Treatment of Depression Collaborative Research Program. *Archives of General Psychiatry,* **49**, 782–787.

Sokolov, S.T.H. & Joffe, R.T. (1995) Practical guidelines for combination drug therapy of treatment-resistant depression. *CNS Drugs,* **4**, 341–350.

Song, F., Freemantle, N. & Sheldon, A. *et al.* (1993) Selective serotonin reuptake inhibitors: meta-analysis of efficacy and acceptability. *British Medical Journal,* **306**, 683–687.

Stewart, J.W., Quitkin, F.M., Liebowitz, M.R. McGrath, P.J., Harrison, W.M. & Klein, D.F. (1983) Efficacy of desipramine in depressed outpatients: response according to reserch diagnostic criteria diagnoses and severity of illness. *Archives of General Psychiatry,* **40**, 202–207.

Sulzer, D.L. & Cummings, J.L. (1989) Drug-induced mania-causative agents, clinical charactristics and management: a retrospective analysis of the literature. *Medical Toxicology and Adverse Drug Experience,* **4**, 127–143.

Taylor, D. & Lader, M. (1996) Cytochromes and psychotropic drug interactions. *British Journal of Psychiatry,* **168**, 529–532.

Tarbuck, A.F. & Paykel, E.S. (1995) Effects of major depression on the cognitive function of younger and older subjects. *Psychological Medicine,* **25**, 285–296.

Teicher, M.H., Glod, C.A. & Cole, J.O. (1993) Antidepressant drugs and the emergence of suicidal tendencies. *Drug Safety,* **8**, 186–212.

Thase, M.E. & Sullivan, L.R. (1995) Relapse and recurrence of depression. A practical approach for prevention. *CNS Drugs,* **4**, 261–277.

van Harten, J. (1993) Clinical pharmacokinetics of selective serotonin reuptake inhibitors. *Clinical Pharmacokinetics,* **24**, 203–220.

Volz, H.-P., Gleiter, C.H., Struck, M. & Müller, H.-J. (1995) Brofaromine: insight into the nature of drug development. *CNS Drugs,* **3**, 1–8.

Wehr, T.A. & Goodwin, F.K. (1987) Can antidepressants cause mania and worsen the course of affective illness? *American Journal of Psychiatry,* **144**, 1403–1411.

Wells, K.B., Stewart, A. & Hays, R.D. *et al.* (1989) The functioning and well-being of depressed patients: results from the Medical Outcomes Study. *Journal of the American Medical Association,* **262**, 914–919.

Wells, K.B., Burnam, M.A., Rogers, W., Hays, R. & Camp, P. (1992) The course of depression in adult outpatients: results from the Medical Outcomes Study. *Archives of General Psychiatry,* **49**, 788–794.

Wells, K.B., Katon, W., Rogers, B. & Camp, P. (1994) Use of minor tranquilizers and antidepressant medications by depressed outpatients: results from the Medical Outcomes Study. *American Journal of Psychiatry,* **151**, 694–700.

Wernicke, J.F., Dunlop, S.R. & Dornseif, B.E. *et al.* (1988) Low-dose fluoxetine therapy for depression. *Psychopharmacology Bulletin,* **24**, 183–188.

West, E.D. & Dally, P.J. (1959) Effects of iproniazid in depressive syndromes. *British Medical Journal,* **i**, 1491–1492.

Wilde, M.I. & Whittington, R. (1995) Paroxetine: a pharmacoeconomic evaluation of its use in depression. *Pharmacoeconomics,* **8**, 62–81.

Wilde, M.I., Plosker, G.L. & Benfield, P. (1993) Fluvoxamine: an updated review of its pharmacology, and therapeutic use in depressive illness. *Drugs,* **46**, 895–924.

Workman, E.A. & Short, D.D. (1993) Atypical antidepressants vs. imipramine in the treatment of major depression: a meta-analysis. *Journal of Clinical Psychiatry,* **54**, 5–12.

10 The adverse effects of antidepressant medication

DAVID TAYLOR

Antidepressants are a chemically diverse group of drugs with a wide range of pharmacological actions. As a consequence, antidepressants are associated with a great many adverse effects, both predictable and idiosyncratic.

The severity and frequency with which these adverse effects occur with individual drugs are important considerations for three pressing reasons. First, antidepressants have broadly equivalent efficacy, thus drug choice is based largely on differences in their adverse effects. Second, the adverse effects of these drugs have a major impact on patient tolerability and therefore adherence to prescribed regimens. Third, some adverse effects are life-threatening in overdose, making some agents potential aids to suicide in those patients already relatively more likely to make a suicide attempt.

This chapter reviews the adverse effects associated with the four major groups of antidepressants: monoamine oxidase inhibitors (MAOIs), tricyclic antidepressants (TCAs), selective serotonin re-uptake inhibitors (SSRIs) and the so-called 'atypical' antidepressants.

In each case, adverse effects common to all members of a group will be stressed, but important differences between individual drugs within a group will also be emphasized. Summary tables are included for ease of reference and to allow comparisons between groups to be made. Tables are also used to recommend drugs to be used in conditions such as epilepsy and pregnancy, where some antidepressants may be strictly contra-indicated. Clinically relevant adverse drug interactions are outlined and summarized in a table.

Monoamine oxidase inhibitors

In many Western countries, four MAOIs are available: isocarboxazid, phenelzine and tranylcypromine, the 'traditional' or non-reversible MAOIs; and moclobemide, a reversible inhibitor of monoamine oxidase (RIMA). Another RIMA, brofaromine, which has broadly similar properties to moclobemide, reached a late stage of development before being discarded. Despite a shared mode of action, traditional MAOIs and RIMAs differ widely in the adverse effects they produce and so will be considered separately.

Table 10.1 Comparison of adverse effects of MAOIs.

Drug	Sedation	Weight changes	Anticholinergic	Hypotension
Isocarboxazid	+	↓	++	+
Phenelzine	+	↑	++	+
Tranylcypromine	−	−	+	+
Moclobemide	−	−	−	−

Traditional MAOIs

The most common adverse effects of traditional MAOIs are hypotension (often causing dizziness), and anticholinergic effects such as dry mouth, constipation, blurred vision and difficulty in micturition (Table 10.1). Both of these effects are dose dependent and tend to lessen in severity with time. The anticholinergic effects are usually less severe than those seen with TCAs (Bass & Kerwin, 1989). Mild sedation occurs with some MAOIs such as phenelzine but rarely with tranylcypromine, which is more likely to exhibit a stimulant action and may cause insomnia. This may be because tranylcypromine is structurally similar to amphetamine and is partly metabolized to amphetamine, at least after an overdose (Dollery, 1991).

Other common adverse effects include headache (Zisook, 1984) and changes in weight. Isocarboxazid may cause weight loss (Davidson & Turnbull, 1982); and substantial weight gain occurs with phenelzine (Evans *et al.*, 1982). Other adverse effects of MAOIs occur much less frequently. Neurological adverse effects such as weakness, numbness and parasthesia may be seen (McEvoy, 1995), leading some authors to suggest that pyridoxine should be given to all patients taking MAOIs (Krishnan, 1995). Peripheral oedema has been associated with all MAOIs although it is thought to be less common with tranylcypromine (Krishnan, 1995); and it appears not to respond to diuretics.

Iproniazid is well known to be hepatotoxic and has now been withdrawn from the market in many countries. Other hydrazine compounds such as phenelzine and isocarboxazid may occasionally be associated with altered liver function tests but these changes are usually benign (Zisook, 1984). Progressive necrotizing hepatocellular damage may occur, though this is rare (McEvoy, 1995); regular checks of liver function are therefore essential.

Sexual dysfunction is sometimes observed with MAOI therapy. However, symptoms such as low libido, impotence and delayed or absent orgasm occur as a result of depression itself, thus making any direct association between a drug and sexual dysfunction difficult to establish. Nevertheless, the number of reports of sexual dysfunction (e.g. Evans *et al.*, 1982; Zisook, 1984; Jacobson,

1987) make the association very likely. The true incidence of MAOI-induced sexual dysfunction is virtually impossible to estimate because reports of such adverse effects are rarely volunteered by patients. An increase in central serotonergic function may be responsible for these adverse effects and the serotonergic antagonist cyproheptadine has been suggested (Krishnan, 1995) as a suitable remedial treatment.

MAOIs may, in rare instances, be implicated as a cause of speech defects. Phenelzine was reported to have caused 'speech blockage' in a 45-year-old woman who had not experienced this problem while taking tranylcypromine (Goldstein & Goldberg, 1986), and tranylcypromine has been associated with severe stuttering in a 14-year-old girl (Duffy, 1994).

Withdrawal

In general, any psychotropic drug given regularly for more than 4–6 weeks should be withdrawn slowly—usually over 2 weeks or more. This is particularly important with MAOIs, especially tranylcypromine, with which withdrawal reactions can occur following abrupt discontinuation (Tyrer, 1984). Symptoms include headache, nightmares and paraesthesia; occasionally more severe symptoms such as psychosis and delirium result from abrupt withdrawal of an MAOI (Lejoyeux *et al.*, 1996). Cautious, slow dose tapering is therefore advised.

Toxicity in overdose

Overdose with MAOIs may have serious consequences and is sometimes fatal. Symptoms vary but usually include agitation, tachycardia, muscular rigidity and coma (Williams *et al.*, 1995). Hypotension occurs with hydrazine compounds, whereas tranylcypromine causes hypertension (Dollery, 1991). Tranylcypromine overdose may also present with unusual signs such as delirium and thrombocytopenia (Chatterjee & Tosyali, 1995). Signs of overdose may take several hours to develop and may persist for up to 2 weeks (McEvoy, 1995). Death may be due to pulmonary and cerebral oedema (Lichtenwalner *et al.*, 1995).

Food interactions

The interactions between MAOIs and foodstuffs containing tyramine has been comprehensively reviewed (e.g. Blackwell *et al.*, 1967). Tyramine is produced by degradation of protein and is present in many foods and drinks. Ingested tyramine is normally metabolized by monoamine oxidase and causes few problems. In those taking MAOIs, ingested tyramine is not deactivated and may cause hypertension, headache, subarachnoid haemorrhage and death (the severity of the reaction is related to the amount consumed) (Anon., 1976).

Debate now centres on the exact frequency and severity or clinical importance of this interaction. Pare (1985), reviewing the conflicting evidence relating to this issue, noted that there had only been 17 reports of food interactions involving phenelzine and none of these were fatal. With tranylcypromine, seven deaths had been reported but in only two of these could a definite relationship with dietary indiscretion be established. The author went on to calculate the risk of death due to dietary interaction as one per 14 000 patient-years; a small incidence compared to the risk of suicide in untreated depressives. Bass and Kerwin (1989) concurred, stating that 'fears about the interaction have been grossly exaggerated'.

The range of foodstuffs forbidden to patients taking MAOIs may also have been exaggerated. Sullivan and Shulman (1984) averred that only four foods should be absolutely prohibited: mature cheese, pickled fish, concentrated yeast extracts, and (the rarely eaten) broad bean pods; other 'forbidden' foods could be taken in true moderation. This conclusion was based on a survey and literature review. Using measurements of tyramine content of over 100 foodstuffs, Shulman *et al.* (1989) came to very similar conclusions, adding only sauerkraut and (possibly) aged meats to the realistic prohibited list.

Drug interactions

MAOIs are involved in a large number of clinically important drug interactions. Serious interactions (usually hypertensive crises) may occur with pethidine, laevodopa, many antidepressants and a variety of sympathomimetic agents such as amphetamine and ephedrine. A comprehensive list of known drug interactions can be found in the relevant manufacturer's data sheet or package insert, and in Bazire (1996).

More recently reported interactions include that between isocarboxazid and venlafaxine (Klysner *et al.*, 1995) and between phenelzine and venlafaxine (Heisler *et al.*, 1996). Serotonin syndrome (diaphoresis, restlessness, rigidity and changes in mental state) appeared to have occurred in both instances.

Use in special patient groups

There are few published data on the use of MAOIs in special patient groups. This is undoubtedly because of their relatively early introduction.

Epilepsy. MAOIs are thought not to reduce seizure threshold (Skowron & Stimmel, 1992; Stimmel & Dopheide, 1996). One study found that no seizures occurred in 132 patients treated with MAOIs (Rabkin *et al.*, 1984). Seizures may occur as a result of hypertensive crisis and myoclonic movements are sometimes seen in patients on MAOIs. Neither of these effects represents a lowering of the seizure threshold. Overall, MAOIs appear to be safe to use in epilepsy although there are few conclusive data to confirm this.

Pregnancy. The danger of hypertensive crisis makes the use of MAOIs in pregnancy inadvisable. In addition, MAOIs have been suggested as human teratogens (Miller, 1991) and phenelzine is teratogenic in animals (Poulson & Robson, 1964).

Breastfeeding. Published data on the use of MAOIs in lactation are very limited. It is thought that small amounts of MAOI may be excreted into breast milk (Rowan, 1976) but little more is known. MAOIs should not, therefore, be given to breastfeeding mothers.

RIMAs—Moclobemide

Adverse effects

Moclobemide's pharmacological action is limited to the reversible inhibition of monoamine oxidase-A. Because of this, adverse effects are few and infrequent: in clinical trials dropouts due to side-effects were uncommon and only nausea occurred with a higher frequency (10%) than placebo (Fitton *et al.*, 1992). Other adverse effects observed in clinical practice include insomnia, dizziness and headache; activation (e.g. agitation and restlessness) also seems to occur in some patients taking moclobemide, although the incidence of all of these events is around 10% or less (Baldwin & Rudge, 1994). Confusion and asymptomatic rises in liver enzymes may be associated with moclobemide but these are rare (Freeman, 1993).

Unlike many other antidepressants, moclobemide appears not to impair psychomotor performance (Tiller, 1990) or to cause sexual dysfunction (Philipp *et al.*, 1993). Moclobemide, perhaps because of its short duration of action, does not suppress REM sleep, while it lengthens overall sleep time in depressed patients (Monti, 1989). This is in contrast to standard MAOIs, which are known to abolish REM sleep and cause profound rebound on withdrawal. Brofaromine is also short-acting but it does suppress REM sleep (Steiger *et al.*, 1987).

Clinical experience with moclobemide indicates that tyramine reactions (including hypertensive crisis) may occur. Coutler and Pillans (1995) have reported six cases of hypertension related to moclobemide use and a controlled rise in blood pressure was induced by the combination of Bovril (containing tyramine) and moclobemide (Taylor *et al.*, 1995).

Withdrawal

Withdrawal reactions have not been reported following abrupt withdrawal of moclobemide. Slow withdrawal is, however, advised.

Overdose

If taken alone, moclobemide appears to be safe in overdose (Freeman, 1993). Symptoms include drowsiness and disorientation (Fitton *et al.*, 1992). Deaths have occurred from serotonin syndrome after overdose of moclobemide and an inhibitor of serotonin re-uptake (Neuvonen *et al.*, 1993).

Drug interactions

Moclobemide is involved in few clinically important drug interactions. Cimetidine decreases moclobemide metabolism (Zimmer *et al.*, 1990) and so the dose of moclobemide should be halved. Moclobemide should not be given with SSRIs because of the danger of serotonin syndrome and because SSRIs and moclobemide are poorly tolerated when co-administered. Theoretical interactions with opiates such as pethidine (meperidine), dextromethorphan and dextropropoxyphene should be noted. This caution is based on experience with other, standard MAOIs but may have relevance since there has been one case report of serotonin syndrome occurring with pethidine and moclobemide (Gillman, 1995).

Moclobemide may safely be given with many sympathomimetics and TCAs (Fitton *et al.*, 1992).

Special patient groups

Epilepsy. Moclobemide appears to be safe in epilepsy: no seizures have been reported, even following overdoses of up to 7–8G (Myrenfors *et al.*, 1993).

Pregnancy. Data on the use of moclobemide in pregnancy are limited. Because of this and the small risk of hypertension, moclobemide should not be used in pregnancy.

Breastfeeding. Moclobemide is excreted only in small amounts into breast milk (Pons *et al.*, 1990) but is not considered to be the drug of first choice in postpartum depression (Duncan & Taylor, 1995b).

Table 10.2 Comparison of adverse effects of tricyclic drugs.

Drug	Sedation	Cardiotoxicity	Anticholinergic effects
Amitriptyline	+++	+++	+++
Amoxapine	++	+	++
Clomipramine	++	+++	++
Desipramine	+	++	++
Dothiepin	+++	+++	++
Doxepin	+++	++	++
Imipramine	++	+++	+++
Lofepramine	+	+	+
Nortriptyline	+	++	++
Protriptyline	–	+++	++
Trimipramine	++++	+++	++

Tricyclic antidepressants

The adverse effects of TCAs are well known and have been widely described over the past 30 years or so (Table 10.2). The majority of these adverse effects can be predicted from the diverse pharmacology demonstrated by this group of drugs: they are antagonists at cholinergic, histaminic and alpha-adrenergic receptors and have a quinidine-like effect on cardiac tissue. Thus, constipation, sedation, hypotension and cardiac conduction changes, respectively, are commonly found with tricyclic drugs. Differences between drugs are largely due to minor differences in chemical structure.

Sedation is caused by all tricyclic drugs, with the notable and sole exception of protriptyline, which has stimulant properties. In general, tertiary amine drugs such as amitriptyline, dothiepin, doxepin and trimipramine are the most sedative. Secondary amines such as desipramine and nortriptyline are the least sedative. Lofepramine is metabolized to desipramine and is also only mildly sedative.

Sedation is most profound when starting therapy and tends to wear off over a period of several weeks. This property may be considered advantageous in patients with prominent anxiety and insomnia. However, because all tricyclics have both long plasma half-lives and active metabolites, the sedation caused by a single night-time dose is often prolonged. Many patients experience difficulty in awakening and may be drowsy throughout the morning and even in the afternoon. This obviously has important implications for those who need to drive, operate machinery or work on skilled tasks. In the longer term, subjective feelings of sedation resolve but reaction times may continue to be extended.

Anticholinergic effects are common and include constipation, dry mouth, blurred vision, tachycardia and urinary hesitancy. No tricyclic drug is free from these adverse effects although secondary amines are relatively less likely to give rise to profound symptoms. Because of these effects, tricyclics are contraindicated in narrow-angle glaucoma and in patients with a history of urinary retention. Anticholinergic side-effects are said to wear off in time, but many patients report problems with constipation and dry mouth after months or years of treatment.

Cardiovascular effects are also common with tricyclics. Blockade of α_1-adrenoreceptors induces postural hypotension which is often severe enough to engender dizziness and even falls (Ray, 1992). Secondary amines are again less likely to cause severe problems and there is some evidence to suggest that nortriptyline rarely causes hypotension even in the elderly (Kragh-Sorensen, 1982).

Tricyclic drugs have complex effects on cardiac tissue: their quinidine-like membrane-stabilizing activity provokes a slowing in impulse conduction which may lead to a benign lengthening of PR, QRS and QTC intervals, amongst others. Tricyclics may suppress premature contractions and have a beneficial effect in those predisposed to certain cardiac dysrhythmias. How-ever, their quinidine-like effect represents the most serious aspect of their overall toxicity: tricyclics may precipitate, especially in overdose, bundle branch block, complete heart block and a bewildering array of other serious dysrhythmias. The cardiac effect of tricyclics has been comprehensively reviewed by Warrington *et al.* (1989). There are few, cogent data compar-ing the pro-arrhythmic potential of tricyclic antidepressants and the relative danger of sudden death with their use. Perhaps the best indication of relative cardiac toxicity is provided by overdose data. This is discussed later.

A reduction in cardiac contractility has been reported to occur with tricyclic drugs. However, evidence suggesting a deleterious effect (e.g. precipitating or worsening cardiac failure) is equivocal. It is now generally held that TCAs may safely be used in cardiac failure. However, since the introduction of newer antidepressants such as the SSRIs, the use of tricyclics in heart failure has become unnecessary. Tricyclics are also associated with a wide range of other adverse effects. In common with other antidepressants, they can precipitate mania in susceptible individuals. They can also cause hyponatraemia (Com-mittee on Safety of Medicines, 1994) and sexual dysfunction, which is prob-ably most likely to occur when a potent inhibitor of serotonin re-uptake such as clomipramine is used (Hawley & Smith, 1994).

Tricyclics are well known to cause weight gain and increased appetite, possibly by increasing insulin activity (Winston & McCann, 1972). Tremor is sometimes reported, although frank dyskinesias are much less common. Rare, idiosyncratic adverse effects include hepatitis, rashes and various blood dyscrasias.

Withdrawal. Anxiety, headache and tremor are seen after the discontinuation of a short course of TCAs and accompanied by increased production of MHPG (Charney *et al.*, 1984). Much more serious withdrawal symptoms are seen after several years of TCA treatment: symptoms include confusion, incontinence, nausea and convulsions may be due to supersensitive muscarinic receptors (Dilsaver & Greden, 1984). In addition, there are a few case reports (e.g. van Sweden, 1988) describing the emergence of cardiac arrhythmias after TCA discontinuation.

Interaction. Most interactions with which tricyclic drugs are involved are readily predicted from their pharmacology. Thus, tricyclics show additive pharmacodynamic interactions with sedatives (including alcohol), anticholinergics, hypotensives and antiarrhythmics. With MAOIs, hypertension and central nervous system (CNS) excitation may occur. The metabolism of tricyclics is inhibited by disulfiram, calcium channel blockers, cimetidine, phenothiazines, and most SSRIs. An increased frequency and severity of adverse effects may result. Carbamazepine and phenytoin may increase the rate of tricyclic metabolism and reduce efficacy.

Toxicity in overdose. Tricyclic antidepressants, with the exception of lofepramine, may cause death if taken in large doses such as those taken in suicide bids. Their toxicity is probably a consequence of their arrhythmogenic potential, but anticholinergic effects and profound CNS depression may also play a part along with rarer complications such as respiratory difficulties and acid–base disturbances (Pinder, 1990). Convulsions sometimes occur, especially with amoxapine and maprotiline.

Relating the number of deaths by overdose to the number of prescriptions issued for a drug gives some idea of relative toxicities, although other factors (variability in use of particular drugs in patient types; inherent ability of drugs to promote or prevent suicide attempts) are also important and difficult to evaluate. It is now accepted that some tricyclics, such as desipramine, dothiepin and amitriptyline, have greater inherent toxicity and are relatively more dangerous in overdose (Cassidy & Henry, 1987; Power *et al.*, 1995). Lofepramine, in stark contrast, seems to be safe in overdose despite desipramine being the drug's major metabolite. The reasons for this are not clear.

The profound and unarguable toxicity of tricyclic compounds is seen by some as sufficient reason to prevent their use now that safer alternatives are available. After all, why should a patient at risk of suicide be prescribed the means with which to accomplish the task? Others argue that any patient intent on suicide will find the means to do so whether or not they are prescribed a tricyclic, and that tricyclics are well known to be cheap and effective. Individual prescribers need to come to their own conclusions at this dilemma. Lofepramine, a safe tricyclic drug, stands out as a suitable compromise.

Use in special patient groups

Epilepsy. Tricyclics have been associated with seizures both in clinical use and following overdose, thus indicating a threshold-lowering effect. Firm, conclusive data on the relative incidence of seizures are lacking (Duncan & Taylor, 1995a) but amoxapine and maprotiline (essentially a tricyclic) probably have the greatest effect on seizure threshold (Wedin *et al.*, 1986). Where possible, tricyclic drugs should not be used in patients with seizure disorders.

Pregnancy. Tricyclics have been widely used in pregnancy and, despite a number of case reports suggesting human teratogenicity, are considered the safest antidepressant drugs to use in pregnancy: extensive epidemiological studies have failed to show an association with birth defects (Robinson G.E. *et al.*, 1986; Lee & Donaldson, 1995). Nevertheless, they should not be used in the first trimester of pregnancy unless absolutely necessary. Moreover, tricyclics should be gradually withdrawn before delivery so as to avoid withdrawal symptoms in the newborn.

Breastfeeding. Because of the high incidence of postpartum depression and the long history of TCA use, these drugs have been relatively well studied in breastfeeding mothers. As expected, tricyclics are excreted in breast milk and infants are commonly exposed to the drug taken by the mother. However, often no drug can be detected in the infant's serum and where detectable, serum concentrations are extremely low (Duncan & Taylor, 1995b). Adverse events are infrequent and development does not seem to be impaired (Buist & Janson, 1995). Tricyclics are therefore recommended in breastfeeding mothers. Doxepin, however, should be avoided because of its association with infant respiratory depression (Matheson *et al.*, 1985).

Specific serotonin re-uptake inhibitors

Since the introduction of fluvoxamine in the mid-1980s, the group of drugs known as the SSRIs has gradually grown in size. The SSRIs available in most western countries in 1996 are: citalopram, fluoxetine, fluvoxamine, paroxetine and sertraline. Their growing popularity can be seen to be a result of their perceived low toxicity, relatively good tolerability and generally slight adverse effects. Comparative efficacy and tolerability data on SSRIs and TCAs are reviewed in Chapter 9.

The most common and clinically important adverse effects of SSRIs are nausea, insomnia and a collection of 'activation' symptoms usually described as 'nervousness', 'agitation' or 'anxiety' (Table 10.3). The precise incidence of these effects is difficult to establish. Variation in reported incidence can be

Table 10.3 Comparison of adverse effects of SSRIs.

Drug	Nausea	Anticholinergic effects	Sedation	EPSE
Citalopram	++	−	−	+/−
Fluoxetine	++	−	−	+/−
Fluvoxamine	+++	−	+	+/−
Paroxetine	++	+	+	+
Sertraline	++	−	−	+/−

accounted for by the way in which information was gathered (for example, by self-reporting or from direct questioning) and by different dosing schedules used in different studies and reviews. In addition, adverse effects are generally more common at the beginning of treatment, so making the time of reporting most important. This imprecision makes difficult any meaningful comparison of the incidence of common adverse effects with individual drugs.

Data on the use of citalopram in short-term trials (Lundbeck, 1995) indicate that nausea occurs in 21.4% of patients and insomnia in 18.8%, although in the latter case this figure did not differ significantly from placebo. An earlier meta-analysis (Dencker & Hopfner Petersen, 1989) indicated that nausea and/or vomiting occurred in 20% of patients taking citalopram. Fluoxetine has been reported to cause nausea in 22.9% of patients, insomnia in 15.5% and nervousness in 14.5% (Pande & Sayler, 1993). In contrast, an early estimate of the frequency of adverse effects occurring with fluvoxamine (Benfield & Ward, 1986) listed nausea as occurring in 37% of patients, agitation in 16% and insomnia in 15%. A later review (Wagner *et al.*, 1992), which included data on more than 24000 patients, found the incidence of nausea with fluvoxamine to be 15.7%, and insomnia and agitation to occur in less than 5%. Many clinicians have noted that fluvoxamine frequently causes an unacceptable degree of nausea and its use has declined substantially in the UK.

With paroxetine, the incidence of nausea has been quoted to be 23% (Caley & Weber, 1993), although insomnia and nervousness appear to be uncommon (less than 15%). With sertraline, nausea occurs in 27% of patients, insomnia in 14% and anxiety in 8% (Grimsley & Jann, 1992)

The incidence figures quoted here, given the caveats outlined, give the clinician little guidance in drug choice. Nevertheless, it is important to note that individual experience and tolerability vary widely and that nausea, insomnia and nervousness all tend to decline in severity as treatment progresses. The short-term (1–3 weeks) use of benzodiazepines is recommended for those who suffer severe activation. A drug holiday or the use of cisapride (Bergeron & Blier, 1994), but not with P4503A4 inhibitor fluoxetine, may help reduce the severity of nausea. Whilst SSRIs are accepted generally to be activating and to cause insomnia in some, others may experience symptoms of sedation such as somnolence or drowsiness. This adverse effect is most commonly seen with paroxetine which has been reported to cause sedation, particularly with regard to driving ability. SSRIs are dispensed in many countries with a label cautioning against driving if affected. However, studies appear to indicate that SSRIs, including paroxetine, do not adversely affect driving performance (North West Regional Drug Information Service, 1995).

All SSRIs can cause sexual dysfunction. Men may suffer a lowering of libido, and may have difficulty maintaining an erection. Orgasm may be delayed or be absent. Women may also suffer lack of libido and anorgasmia. Again, an accurate assessment of comparative incidence cannot be made, but all SSRIs have been reported to cause sexual dysfunction. This effect may be a result of enhanced serotonergic activity: SSRI-induced anorgasmia appears to be ameliorated by the serotonin antagonist cyproheptadine (Arnott & Nutt, 1994; Lauerma, 1996)

SSRIs are sometimes, albeit infrequently, associated with dry mouth and constipation, perhaps reflecting their relative selectivity for the serotonergic system compared with tricyclic antidepressants. Paroxetine is most commonly associated with these adverse effects (Grimsley & Jann, 1992) and, indeed, has the greatest anticholinergic activity (Hyttel, 1994). It should be noted that dry mouth and constipation appear to occur with all SSRIs, despite very poor anticholinergic activity with some drugs. This may indicate that alterations in serotonin function are at least in part responsible.

Extrapyramidal adverse effects such as dystonia and parkinsonism are rarely associated with the use of SSRIs (Arya, 1994). The reasons for the occurrence of these effects are unclear (although the serotonin and dopamine system are known to be linked) and the true incidence difficult to establish. Paroxetine is possibly the most likely of the SSRIs to cause extrapyramidal effects (Consumers' Association, 1993) but there are few comparative data to confirm this.

Hyponatraemia, with concomitant inappropriate secretion of antidiuretic hormone, is a rare but well recognized adverse effect of many antidepressant drugs including the SSRIs (Thomas & Verbalis, 1995). This adverse effect seems only to occur in elderly patients and is usually benign (e.g. dizziness and weakness). Occasionally, disorientation and delirium have been reported (Thornton & Resch, 1995). Sodium levels return to normal after withdrawal of the offending drug.

In recent years, debate has raged over the association between the use of SSRIs and the occurrence of suicide ideation and suicide attempts. A meta-analysis (Beasley *et al.*, 1991) has shown that fluoxetine was not associated with an increase in suicide and it is now widely accepted that SSRIs do not provoke suicidal ideation or suicide (Montgomery, 1992).

Unlike other groups of antidepressants, SSRIs do not cause weight gain.

Fluoxetine sometimes causes weight loss, especially in those who are overweight.

Other adverse effects linked to the use of SSRIs include transient head-ache, diarrhoea and sweating, and rare events such as rash (especially with fluoxetine) and vasculitis. In addition, hair loss has been associated with the use of fluoxetine (Seifritz *et al.*, 1995) and sertraline (Bourgeois, 1996).

Withdrawal. Abrupt withdrawal of an SSRI may bring about a withdrawal syndrome. Symptoms include delirium, malaise, incoordination, nausea, fatigue and dizziness (Lazowick & Levin, 1995). Skin disorders may occur on abrupt withdrawal of sertraline (Leiter *et al.*, 1995) and extrapyramidal symp-toms have been reported following withdrawal of fluoxetine (Stoukides, 1991). A flu-like withdrawal syndrome has been described in patients withdrawing from paroxetine (Lejoyeux *et al.*, 1996), in some cases despite slow withdrawal over 7–10 days.

Some debate surrounds the issue of which SSRI is most likely to cause a withdrawal syndrome. Fluoxetine, because of its long plasma half-life, was originally thought not to induce withdrawal symptoms but several (some-times delayed) withdrawal reactions have been described (e.g. Einbinder, 1995). Paroxetine is widely believed to be particularly liable to cause a with-drawal reaction. All SSRIs should therefore be withdrawn cautiously and slowly; usually over a period of 2 weeks or more.

Overdose. It is well known that SSRIs are safe in overdose. This is probably because of their specific mode of action and their lack of effect on cardiac tissue. Remarkably few deaths have been reported following overdose of an SSRI alone. Symptoms of overdose include vomiting, agitation, seizures and, less often, loss of consciousness (Anon., 1993; Grimsley & Jann, 1992; Baldwin & Johnson, 1995). SSRIs may be dangerous if taken in overdose with other drugs which potentiate the serotonergic system since life-threatening serotonin syndrome may result (Neuvonen *et al.*, 1993).

More recently, the safety of citalopram in overdose has been brought into question. Östrom *et al.* (1996) have reported six deaths following citalopram overdose where, in each case, high plasma levels of citalopram appeared to be the cause of death. A possible effect on cardiac QT interval was suggested as the primary toxic mechanism.

Interactions. Knowledge of the range of drug interactions in which SSRIs are involved has grown substantially since their introduction and it is now well recognized that they have the potential to cause serious adverse interactions. SSRIs are inhibitors of a variety of hepatic cytochrome P450 (CYP) enzymes: most SSRIs inhibit CYP2D6, fluvoxamine inhibits CYP1A2 and fluoxetine inhibits CYP3A4. As a consequence of this activity, all SSRIs (with the possible exception of citalopram) may increase plasma levels of co-administered tricyclic antidepressants and engender serious adverse effects (Taylor, 1995). Fluvoxamine may raise levels of caffeine and theophylline, and fluoxetine has been reported to increase levels of clozapine (and possibly other anti-psychotics), cyclosporin and terfenadine (Taylor & Lader, 1996). Fluvoxamine, sertraline and paroxetine also increase clozapine plasma concentrations (Centurrino *et al.*, 1996), but the author's experience with citalopram suggests no important altering of clozapine plasma levels. SSRIs may also increase levels of some anticonvulsants, propranolol and warfarin. Pharmacodynamic interactions may occur with tryptophan.

Interactions may also occur following discontinuation of an SSRI, especially fluoxetine, which has a long plasma half-life and an active metabolite with an even longer half-life. If stopping treatment with an SSRI, manufacturer's information should be consulted before starting any drug known to interact with SSRIs.

SSRIs are also involved in serious pharmacodynamic interactions with MAOIs (Ciraulo *et al.*, 1995). Fatal serotonin syndrome has been reported when fluoxetine and an MAOI were given together, and so MAOIs and SSRIs should never be coprescribed. Interactions may occur after discontinuation of either type of drug: fluoxetine has a long half-life; MAOIs have a long duration of action. Prescribers are advised to consult manufacturers' literature before changing from an SSRI to an MAOI, or vice versa.

Use in special patient groups

Epilepsy. SSRIs probably do not alter seizure threshold to a clinically important extent, although this is the subject of some debate. They are thought to be safe to use in epilepsy (Duncan & Taylor, 1995a). Interactions with some anticonvulsants (notably carbamazepine and phenytoin) have been reported and so caution is advised.

Pregnancy. Available data on the use of SSRIs in pregnancy are limited, but the drugs seem not to be teratogenic. However, on account of the lack of data and the absence of large prospective studies, and because fluoxetine has been linked with an increased rate of miscarriage (Pastuszak, 1993), SSRIs should usually be avoided in pregnancy.

Breastfeeding. SSRIs are lipid-soluble drugs which would be expected to be excreted in breast milk, an expectation confirmed for fluoxetine (Isenberg, 1990). Neither the acute effects on the neonate nor the long-term effects on development are known. SSRIs should therefore be avoided in breastfeeding mothers (Duncan & Taylor, 1995b).

Atypical antidepressants

Antidepressant drugs which do not fall readily into the classes so far described are usually referred to as 'atypical'. They may have different chemical structures (e.g. non-tricyclic) or different modes of action (e.g. dopamine re-uptake inhibition) or both, and have little in common with each other. Since this group of drugs is so heterogeneous, each compound will be considered separately.

Bupropion

Bupropion is an inhibitor of dopamine re-uptake which is widely used in the USA. It has few, if any, sedative, anticholinergic, hypotensive or cardiotoxic properties (Rudorfer & Potter, 1989). Most of bupropion's adverse effects are related to overstimulation of dopaminergic function: insomnia, agitation, nausea, weight loss and psychosis can occur (Reynolds, 1996). Bupropion should be withdrawn slowly to avoid precipitating a withdrawal reaction.

Acute toxicity in overdose is less profound than that seen with tricyclics (Hayes & Kristoff, 1986). Bupropion should not be given with MAOIs, dopamine precursors or agonists (e.g. those used in Parkinson's disease) or to those at risk of seizures since it decreases seizure threshold in a dose-dependent fashion (Reynolds, 1996). There are few safety data relating to the use of bupropion in pregnancy and so its use should be avoided. Bupropion accumulates in breast milk but infant exposure is minimal (Briggs *et al.*, 1993). Further studies are needed before bupropion can be recommended for breastfeeding mothers.

Viloxazine

Viloxazine is an antidepressant with an unknown mode of action which is marketed in the UK and Europe. It is not widely used, probably because of doubts over its efficacy (Bazire, 1996). Nausea, vomiting and headache (sometimes severe or migraine-like) are commonly reported adverse effects (Reynolds, 1996).

Mianserin

Mianserin is a tetracyclic compound which is an antagonist at $alpha_2$, $5\text{-}HT_{1A}$, $5\text{-}HT_2$ and $5\text{-}HT_3$ receptors. It is not currently available in the USA. Adverse effects of mianserin are usually mild—only sedation is frequently reported, albeit with impairment of psychomotor function (Peet & Behagel, 1978). Blood dyscrasias have also been described (some of them fatal, particularly in the elderly) and so monthly blood monitoring is recommended when mianserin is started (Committee on Safety of Medicines, 1985). Mianserin is safe in over-dose (Chand *et al.*, 1981) and appears to lack cardiotoxicity. Convulsions have been reported to occur in patients taking mianserin, but a true association has not been shown and its effect on seizure threshold is uncertain (Edwards & Glen-Bott, 1983).

Venlafaxine

Venlafaxine is a relatively new antidepressant which inhibits the re-uptake of serotonin and noradrenaline but, unlike tricyclics, has little or no affinity for alpha adrenoceptors, cholinergic or histaminic receptors. Nevertheless, its adverse effect profile includes nausea, dry mouth, headache, sedation and constipation. Nausea has been reported to occur in 44% of patients (Lecable *et al.*, 1995), although combining data from several studies indicates that the true incidence is nearer 30% and that it occurs mainly in the first 2 weeks of treatment (Danjou & Hackett, 1995). Cisapride appears to ameliorate nausea caused by venlafaxine (Russel, 1996). Dry mouth, constipation, sedation, insomnia, headache and nervousness all occur in more than 15% of patients given venlafaxine (Ellingrod & Perry, 1994) and are very probably treatment-related. Perhaps as a result, the rate of withdrawal from treatment because of adverse effects is similar to that seen with imipramine (Shrivastava *et al.*, 1994).

Elevation of blood pressure may occur at higher doses of venlafaxine (>200 mg daily) (Danjou & Hackett, 1995). Close monitoring of blood pressure is essential for those on higher doses and venlafaxine should not be given to those with hypertension. As with other antidepressants, abrupt cessation of venlafaxine may precipitate a withdrawal reaction. A syndrome of headache, nausea, abdominal distension and fatigue has been described (Farah & Lauer, 1996). Venlafaxine does not appear to inhibit strongly any of the cytochrome enzymes and is not highly protein-bound (Ellingrod & Perry, 1994). Few adverse drug interactions are therefore predicted. However, venlafaxine is metabolized by cytochrome P450IID6, an enzyme which is strongly inhibited by a number of drugs including fluoxetine.

Venlafaxine appears to have little, if any, cardiotoxicity. Limited data indicate that venlafaxine is safe in overdose, although seizures have been reported (Woo *et al.*, 1995). Venlafaxine should not be used in epilepsy, pregnancy or breastfeeding because of the absence of convincing safety data.

Milnacipran has a similar action to venlafaxine but little is reported of its adverse effect profile in English language literature. It is marketed in Portugal and France.

Mirtazapine

Mirtazapine is a novel antidepressant with unusual pharmacological activity: it is an antagonist at presynaptic alpha$_2$ receptors and at 5-HT$_2$, 5-HT$_3$ and H$_1$ receptors. These actions result in enhanced serotonergic transmission (via 5-HT$_{1A}$ receptors) and this is thought to be responsible for its antidepressant activity. The adverse effects of mirtazapine have been comprehensively reviewed (Davies & Wilde, 1996). Sedation, dry mouth, increased appetite and weight gain occur quite frequently (10–20% of patients) but the drug seems to be better tolerated than amitriptyline. Preliminary data suggest mirtazapine is safe in overdose (Hoes & Zeijpveld, 1996) and seems to have little or no effect on seizure threshold. This latter observation needs more conclusive examination since H$_1$ receptor antagonists are known to reduce seizure threshold.

Trazodone

Trazodone is a weak inhibitor of serotonin re-uptake and an antagonist at 5-HT and alpha$_1$ adrenoreceptors. It has no anticholinergic activity. This pharmacology predicts adverse effects such as sedation and a lowering of blood pressure. Indeed, sedation and dizziness (due to hypotension) are the most frequently reported adverse effects (Brogden *et al.*, 1981). Sedation is particularly common, especially at higher doses.

Trazodone appears to lack the profound cardiotoxicity of tricyclic drugs but dysrhythmias have occasionally been reported (Schatzberg & Nemeroff, 1995). Overdose with trazodone alone is not usually fatal.

Some sexual problems are associated with the use of trazodone. Priapism is a rare but frequently reported problem (Thompson *et al.*, 1990) and increased libido and spontaneous orgasm (Purcell & Ghurye, 1995) have been described.

Abrupt or rapidly tapered withdrawal of trazodone may give rise to withdrawal symptoms which include malaise, myalgia, nausea and restless legs syndrome (Otani *et al.*, 1994). Very slow withdrawal is therefore recommended: over 1 month or more, where possible. Trazodone exhibits additive pharmacodynamic interactions with other sedatives (including alcohol) and hypotensive agents. Combination with SSRIs or MAOIs should be avoided because of the risk of serotonin syndrome.

Trazodone probably does not lower seizure threshold (Wedin *et al.*, 1986). Convulsions have been reported in overdose in one patient, but were perhaps related to hyponatraemia (Balestrieri *et al.*, 1992). Data on the use of trazodone in pregnancy and lactation are limited.

Table 10.4 Comparison of adverse effects of atypical antidepressants.

Drug	Toxicity in overdose	Sedation	Hypotension	Anticholinergic effects
Bupropion	+	−	−	−
Mianserin	−	++	−	+
Mirtazapine	−	++	−	+
Nefazodone	−	+	+	−
Trazodone	+	+++	++	−
Venlafaxine	−	++	−	+
Viloxazine	−	+	−	−

Nefazodone

Nefazodone is chemically related to trazodone but is a less potent antagonist at alpha$_1$ receptors. Its activity in depression is thought to be due to inhibition of serotonin re-uptake and antagonism of 5-HT$_2$ receptors.

Adverse effects are mild and infrequent. Somnolence, nausea, dry mouth and dizziness are reported in around 5–10% of patents leading to dropout rates similar to those seen with fluoxetine and placebo (Preskorn, 1995). Other workers have estimated that these adverse effects are seen in 10–20% of subjects (Robinson *et al.*, 1996). Nefazodone appears to cause less hypotension than trazodone, although this suggestion needs confirmation by direct comparison. Sexual dysfunction and seizures are very rarely reported with nefazodone (Canadian ADR Newsletter, 1996; Preskom, 1995). Indeed, nefazodone is thought not to induce seizures (Laird & Benfield, 1995) and may be considered to be safe in epilepsy.

Like trazodone, nefazodone should be withdrawn slowly to avoid the development of withdrawal phenomena. Nefazodone appears to be safe in overdose (Lader, 1996).

Nefazodone is a very weak inhibitor of cytochrome P450IID6 and P450IA2. It is a potent inhibitor of P4503A4 (Robinson *et al.*, 1996) and so should not be given with alprazolam, astemizole, terfenadine, cisapride or cyclosporin.

There are few data on the use of nefazodone in pregnancy and lactation. It should therefore be avoided.

References

Anon. (1976) MAOI's and food — fact and fiction. *Adverse Drug Reaction Bulletin*, **58**, 200–203.

Anon. (1993) Selective serotonin re-uptake inhibitors for depression? *Drug and Therapeutics Bulletin*, **31**, 57–59.

Anon. (1995) Can SSRI's affect driving ability? *Materia Medica*, Nov. 1995. North West Regional Drug Information Service, Manchester, UK.

Anon. (1996) Nefazodone: adverse drug reaction profile. *Canadian Adverse Drug Reaction Newsletter*, **6**.

Arnott, S. & Nutt, D. (1994) Successful treatment of fluvoxamine-induced anorgasmia by cyproheptadine. *British Journal of Psychiatry*, **164**, 838–839.

Arya, D.K. (1994) Extrapyramidal symptoms with

selective serotonin re-uptake inhibitors. *British Journal of Psychiatry,* **165**, 728–733.

Baldwin, D. & Johnson, F.N. (1995) Tolerability and safety of citalopram. *Review in Contemporary Pharmacotherapy,* **6**, 315–325.

Baldwin, D. & Rudge, S. (1994) Tolerability of moclobemide. *Reviews in Contemporary Pharmacotherapy,* **5**, 57–65.

Balestrieri, G., Cerudelli, B., Ciaccio, S. & Rizzoni, D. (1992) Hyponatraemia and seizure due to overdose of trazodone. *British Medical Journal,* **304**, 686.

Bass, C. & Kerwin, R. (1989) Rediscovering monoamine oxidase inhibitors. *British Medical Journal,* **298**, 345–346.

Bazire, S. (1996) *The Psychotropic Drug Directory,* Quay Books, Salisbury, UK.

Beasley, C.M., Jr, Dornseif, B.E. & Bosomworth, J.C. *et al.* (1991) Fluoxetine and suicide: a meta-analysis of controlled trials of treatment for depression. *British Medical Journal,* **303**, 685–692.

Benfield, P.B. & Ward, A. (1986) Fluvoxamine: a review of its pharmacodynamic and pharmacokinetic properties and therapeutic efficacy in depressive illness. *Drugs,* **32**, 313–334.

Bergeron, R. & Blier, P. (1994) Cisapride for the treatment of nausea produced by selective serotonin re-uptake inhibitors. *American Journal of Psychiatry,* **151**, 1084–1086.

Blackwell, B., Marley, E., Price, J. & Taylor, D. (1967) Hypertensive interactions between monoamine oxidase inhibitors and foodstuffs. *British Journal of Psychiatry,* **113**, 349–365.

Bourgeois, J.A. (1996) Two cases of hair loss after sertraline use. *Journal of Clinical Psychopharmacology,* **16**, 91–92.

Briggs, G.G., Samson, J.H., Ambrose, P.J. & Schroeder, D.H. (1993) Excretion of bupropion in breast milk. *Annals of Pharmacotherapy,* **27**, 431–433.

Brogden, R.N., Heel, R.C., Speight, T.M. & Avery, G.S. (1981) Trazodone: a review of its pharmacological properties and therapeutic use in depression and anxiety. *Drugs,* **21**, 401–429.

Buist, A. & Janson, H. (1995) Effect of exposure to dothiepin and nordothiaden in breast milk on child development. *British Journal of Psychiatry,* **167**, 370–373.

Caley, C.F. & Weber, S.S. (1993) Paroxetine: a selective serotonin reuptake inhibiting antidepressant. *The Annals of Pharmacotherapy,* **27**, 1212–1221.

Cassidy, S.L. & Henry, J.A. (1987) Fatal toxicity of antidepressant drugs in overdose. *British Medical Journal,* **295**, 1021–1024.

Centurrino, F., Baldessarini, R.J. & Frankenberg,

F.R. *et al.* (1996) Serum levels of clozapine and norclozapine in patients treated with selective serotonin reuptake inhibitors. *American Journal of Pyschiatry,* **153**, 820–822.

Chand, S., Crome, P. & Dawling, S. (1981) One hundred cases of acute intoxication with mianserin hydrochloride. *Pharmacopsychiatria,* **14**, 15–17.

Charney, D.S., Heninger, G.R. & Sternberg, D.E. (1984) The effect of mianserin on alpha$_2$ adrenergic receptor function in depressed patients. *British Journal of Psychiatry,* **144**, 407–416.

Chatterjee, A. & Tosyali, M.C. (1995) Thrombocytopenia and delirium associated with tranylcypromine overdose. *Journal of Clinical Psychopharmacology,* **15**, 143–144.

Ciraulo, D.A., Shader, R.I., Greenblatt, D.J. & Creehan, W. (eds) (1995) *Drug Interactions in Psychiatry,* 2nd edn. Williams & Wilkins, Baltimore.

Committee on Safety of Medicines (1985) Adverse reactions to antidepressants. *British Medical Journal,* **291**, 1638.

Committee on Safety of Medicines (1994) Antidepressant-induced hyponatraemia. *Current Problems,* **20**, 5–6.

Consumers' Association (1993) Selective serotonin re-uptake inhibitors for depression? *Drug and Therapeutics Bulletin,* **31**, 57–59.

Coulter, D.M. & Pillaus, P.I. (1995) Hypertension with moclobemide. *Lancet,* **346**, 1032.

Danjou, P. & Hackett, D. (1995) Safety and tolerance profile of venlaFax:ine. *International Journal of Psychopharmacology,* **10** (Suppl. 2), 15–20.

Davidson, J. & Turnbull, C. (1982) Loss of appetite and weight associated with the monoamine oxidase inhibitor isocarboxazid. *Journal of Clinical Psychopharmacology,* **2**, 263–266.

Davies, R. & Wilde, M. (1996) Mirtazapine: a review of its pharmacology and therapeutic potential in the management of major depression. *CNS Drugs,* **5**, 389–402.

Dencker, S.J. & Hopfner Petersen, H.E. (1989) *Side-effect profile of citalopram and reference antidepressants in depression.* Paper presented at the 22nd Norwegian Congress on Psychiatry, Reykjavik, 10–13 August 1988, 31–42.

Dilsaver, S.C. & Greden, J.F. (1984) Antidepressant-induced activation (hypomania and mania): mechanism and theoretical significance. *Brain Research,* **319**, 29–40.

Dollery, C. (1991) *Therapeutic Drugs.* Churchill Livingstone, Edinburgh.

Duffy, J.D. (1994) Neurogenic stuttering and lateralized motor deficits induced by tranylcypromine. *Behavioural Neurology,* **7**, 171–174.

Duncan, D. & Taylor, D. (1995a) Which is the

safest antidepressant to use in epilepsy? *Psychiatric Bulletin*, **19**, 355–356.

Duncan, D. & Taylor, D. (1995b) Which antidepressants are safe to use in breast-feeding mothers? *Psychiatric Bulletin*, **19**, 549–550.

Einbinder, E. (1995) Fluoxetine withdrawal? *American Journal of Psychiatry*, **152**, 1235.

Ellingrod, V.L. & Perry, P.J. (1994) VenlaFax:ine: a heterocyclic antidepressant. *American Journal of Hospital Pharmacy*, **51**, 3033–3046.

Edwards, J.G. & Glen-Bott, M. (1983) Mianserin and convulsive seizures. *British Journal of Clinical Pharmacology*, **15**, 299S–311S.

Evans, D.L., Davidson, J. & Raft, D. (1982) Early and late side effects of phenelzine. *Journal of Clinical Psychopharmacology*, **2**, 208–210.

Farah, A. & Lauer, T.E. (1996) Possible venlaFax:ine withdrawal syndrome. *American Journal of Psychiatry*, **153**, 576.

Freeman, H. (1993) Moclobemide. *Lancet*, **342**, 1528–1532.

Fitton, A., Faulds, D. & Goa, K.L. (1992) Moclobemide: a review of its pharmacological properties and therapeutic use in depressive illness. *Drugs*, **43**, 561–596.

Gillman, P.K. (1995) Possible serotonin syndrome with moclobemide and pethidine. *Medical Journal of Australia*, **162**, 554.

Goldstein, D.M. & Goldberg, R.L. (1986) Monoamine oxidase inhibitor-induced speech blockage. *Journal of Clinical Psychiatry*, **47**, 604.

Grimsley, S.R. & Jann, M.W. (1992) Paroxetine, sertraline and fluvoxamine: new selective serotonin re-uptake inhibitors. *Clinical Pharmacy*, **11**, 930–957.

Hawley, C. & Smith, V. (1994) Sexual dysfunction and clomipramine: review of 'Effects of antidepressants on sexual function'. *Medical Dialogue*, no. 421.

Hayes, P.E. & Kristoff, C.A. (1986) Adverse reactions to five new antidepressants. *Clinical Pharmacy*, **5**, 471–480 .

Heisler, M.A., Guidry, J.R. & Arnecke, B. (1996) Serotonin syndrome induced by administration of venlaFax:ine and phenelzine. *Annals of Pharmacotherapy*, **30**, 84.

Hoes, M.J.A.J.M. & Zeijpveld, J.H.B. (1996) First report of mirtazapine overdoses. *International Clinical Psychopharmacology*, **11**, 147.

Hyttel, J. (1994) Pharmacological characterization of selective serotonin re-uptake inhibitors (SSRIs). *International Clinical Psychopharmacology*, **9** (Suppl. 1), 19–26.

Isenberg, K.E. (1990) Excretion of fluoxetine in human breast milk. *Journal of Clinical Psychiatry*, **51**, 169.

Jacobson, J.N. (1987) Anorgasmia caused by an MAOI. *American Journal of Psychiatry*, **144**, 527.

Klysner, R., Larsen, J.K., Sørensen, P. *et al.* (1995) Toxic interaction of venlafaxine and isocarboxazid. *Lancet*, **346**, 1298–1299.

Kragh-Sorensen, P. (1982) Antidepressants: cardiovascular effects in elderly patients. *Acta Pharmacologica et Toxicologica*, **53**, 138.

Krishnan, K.R.-R. (1995) Monoamine oxidase inhibitors. In: *The American Psychiatric Press Textbook of Psychopharmacology* (eds A. F. Schatzberg & C. B. Nemeroff). American Psychiatric Press, Inc., Washington, DC.

Lader, M.H. (1996) Tolerability and safety: essentials in antidepressant pharmacotherapy. *Journal of Clinical Psychiatry*, **57** (Suppl. 2), 39–44.

Laird, L.K. & Benfield, W.H. (1995) Mood disorders. I: Major depressive disorders. In: *Applied Therapeutics* (eds L.L. Young & M.A. Koda-Kimble), 6th edn. Applied Therapeutics Inc., Vancouver, W/A. The Clinical Use of Drugs.

Lauerma, H. (1996) Successful treatment of citalopram-induced anorgasmia by cyproheptadine. *Acta Psychiatrica Scandinavica*, **93**, 69–70.

Lazowick, A.L. & Levin, G.M. (1995) Potential withdrawal syndrome associated with SSRI discontinuation. *Annals of Pharmacotherapy*, **29**, 1284–1285.

Lecable, P., Letzelter, J.-M., Lichtblau, E. *et al.* (1995) An open-label study of the clinical acceptability of venlaFax:ine for depression. *Primary Care Psychiatry*, **1**, 119–125.

Lee, A. & Donaldson, S. (1996) Drug use in pregnancy (4) Psychiatric and neurological disorders: Part 1. *Pharmaceutical Journal*, **254**, 87–91.

Leiter, F.L., Nierenberg, A.A., Sanders, K.M. & Stem T.A. (1995) Discontinuation reactions following sertraline. *Biological Psychiatry*, **38**, 694–695.

Lejoyeux, M., Ades, J., Mourad, I., Solomon, J. & Dilsaver, S. (1996) Antidepressant withdrawal syndrome. *CNS Drugs*, **5**, 278–292.

Lichtenwalner, M.R., Tully, R.G. & Cohn, R.D. & Pinder, R.D. (1995) Two fatalities involving phenelzine. *Journal of Analytical Toxicology*, **19**, 265–266.

Lundbeck (1995) *Citalopram: Summary of clinical tolerability. Data on file. Report 001.* Copenhagen: Lundbeck Ltd.

Matheson, I., Pande, H. & Alertsen, A.R. (1985) Respiratory depression caused by N-desmethyldoxepin in breast milk. *Lancet*, **2**, 1124.

McEvoy, G.K. (ed.) (1995) *AHFS 95 Drug Information.* American Society of Health System Pharmacists, Bethesda, Maryland.

Miller, L.J. (1991) Clinical strategies for the use of psychotropic drugs during pregnancy. *Psychiatric Medicine*, **9**, 275–297.

Montgomery, S.A. (1992) Suicide and antidepressants. *Drugs*, **43** (Suppl. 2), 24–31.

Monti, J.M. (1989) Effect of a reversible monoamine oxidase-A inhibitor (moclobemide) on sleep of depressed patients. *British Journal of Psychiatry*, **155** (Suppl. 6), 61–65.

Myrenfors, P.G., Eriksson, T., Sandsteat, C.S. & Sjöberg, F. (1993) Moclobemide overdose. *Journal of Internal Medicine*, **233**, 113–115.

Neuvonen, P.J., Pojhola-Sintonen, S., Tacke, U. & Vuori, E. (1993) Five fatal cases of serotonin syndrome after moclobemide–citalopram or moclobemide–clomipramine overdoses. *Lancet*, **342**, 1419.

North West Regional Drug Information Service (1995) Can SSRIs affect driving ability? *Materia Medica*, November.

Nefazadone (1996) Nefazodone: adverse drug reaction profile. Canadian Adverse.

Otani, K., Tanaka, O., Kaneko, S. *et al.* (1994) Mechanisms of the development of trazodone withdrawal symptoms. *International Clinical Psychopharmacology*, **9**, 131–133.

Östrom, M., Eriksson, A., Thorson, J. & Spigset, O. (1996) Fatal overdose with citalopram. *Lancet*, **348**, 1345–1346.

Pande, A.C. & Sayler, M.E. (1993) Adverse events and treatment discontinuations in fluoxetine clinical trials. *International Clinical Psychopharmacology*, **8**, 267–269.

Pare, C.M.B. (1985) The present status of monoamine oxidase inhibitors. *British Journal of Psychiatry*, **146**, 576–584.

Pastuszak, A., Schick-Boschetto, B., Zuber, C. *et al.* (1993) Pregnancy outcome following first-trimester exposure to fluoxetine (Prozac). *Journal of the American Medical Association*, **269**, 2246–2248.

Peet, M. & Behagel, H. (1978) Mianserin: a decade of scientific development. *British Journal of Clinical Pharmacology*, **5**, 55–95.

Philipp, M., Kohnen, R. & Benkert, O. (1993) A comparison study of moclobemide and doxepin in major depression with special reference to effects on sexual function. *International Clinical Psychopharmacology*, **7**, 149–153.

Pinder, R.M. (1990) The toxicity of antidepressants in overdose: incidence and mechanism. *International Review of Psychiatry*, **2**, 213–227.

Pons, G., Schoerlin, M. & Tam, Y.K. (1990) Moclobemide excretion in human breast milk. *British Journal of Clinical Pharmacology*, **29**, 27–31.

Poulson, E.A. & Robson, J.M. (1964) Effect of phenelzine and some related compounds in pregnancy. *Journal of Endocrinology*, **30**, 205–215.

Power, B.M., Hackett L.P., Dusci L.J. & Ilett, K.F. (1995) Antidepressant toxicity and the need for identification and concentration monitoring in overdose. *Clinical Pharmacokinetics*, **29**, 154–171.

Preskorn, S.H. (1995) Comparison of the tolerability of bupropion, fluoxetine, imipramine, nefazodone, paroxetine, sertraline and venlaFax:ine. *Journal of Clinical Psychiatry*, **56** (Suppl. 6), 12–21.

Purcell, P. & Ghurye, R. (1995) Trazodone and spontaneous orgasms in an elderly postmenopausal woman: a case report. *Journal of Clinical Psychopharmacology*, **15**, 293–295.

Rabkin, J., Quitkin, F., Harrison, W. *et al.* (1984) Adverse reactions to monoamine oxidase inhibitors. Part 1: a comparative study. *Journal of Clinical Psychopharmacology*, **4**, 270–278.

Ray, W.A. (1992) Psychotropic drugs and injuries among the elderly: a review. *Journal of Clinical Psychopharmacology*, **12**, 386–396.

Reynolds, J.E.F. (ed.) (1996) *Martindale: The Extra Pharmacopoeia*, 31st edn. Royal Pharmaceutical Society of Great Britain, London.

Robinson, G.E., Stewart, D.E. & Flak, K. (1996) The rational use of psychotropic drugs in pregnancy and postpartum. *Canadian Journal of Psychiatry*, **31**, 183–190.

Robinson, D.S., Roberts, D.L., Smith, J.M. *et al.* (1996) The safety profile of nefazodone. *Journal of Clinical Psychiatry*, **57** (Suppl., 2), 31–38.

Rowan, J.J. (1976) Excretion of drugs in milk. *Pharmaceutical Journal*, **217**, 184.

Rudorfer, M.V. & Potter, W.Z. (1989) Antidepressants: a comparative review of the clinical pharmacology and therapeutic use of the 'newer' vs. the 'older' drugs. *Drugs*, **37**, 713–738.

Russel, J.L. (1996) Relatively low doses of cisapride in the treatment of nausea in patients treated with venlaFax:ine for treatment refractory depression. *Journal of Clinical Psychopharmacology*, **16**, 35–57.

Seifritz, E., Hatzinger, M., Miller, M.J., Hemmeter, U. & Holsboer-Traschler, E. (1995) Hair loss associated with fluoxetine but not with citalopram. *Canadian Journal of Psychiatry*, **40**, 362.

Shrivastava, R.K., Cohn, C., Crowder, J. *et al.* (1994) Long term safety and clinical acceptability of venlaFax:ine and imipramine in outpatients with major depression. *Journal of Clinical Psychopharmacology*, **14**, 322–329.

Shulman, K.I., Walker, S.E., MacKenzie, S. & Knowles, S. (1989) Dietary restriction, tyramine and the use of monoamine oxidase inhibitors. *Journal of Clinical Psychopharmacology*, **9**, 397–402.

Skowron, D.M. & Stimmel, G.L. (1992) Antidepressants and the risk of seizures. *Pharmacotherapy*, **12**, 18–22.

Steiger, A., Holsboer, F., Gerken, A. *et al.* (1987) Results of an open clinical trial of brofaromine (CGP 11305 A), a competitive, selective and short-acting inhibitor of MAO-A in major endogenous depression. *Pharmacopsychiatry*, **20**, 262–269.

Stimmel, G.L. & Dopheide, J.A. (1996) Psychotropic-induced reductions in seizure threshold. *CNS Drugs*, **1**, 37–50.

Stoukides, J.A. & Stoukides, C.A. (1991) Extrapyramidal symptoms upon discontinuation of fluoxerine. *American Journal of Psychiatry*, **148**, 1263 (letter).

Sullivan, E.A. & Shulman, K.I. (1984) Diet and monoamine oxidase inhibitors: a re-examination. *Canadian Journal of Psychiatry*, **29**, 707–711.

Taylor, D. (1995) Selective serotonin reuptake inhibitors and tricyclic antidepressants in combination: interactions and therapeutic uses. *British Journal of Psychiatry*, **167**, 575–580.

Taylor, D. & Lader, M. (1996) Editorial: the cytochrome enzymes. *British Journal of Psychiatry*, **168**, 529–532.

Taylor, D., Reveley, A. & Faivre, F. (1995) Clozapine induced hypotension treated with moclobemide and Bovril. *British Journal of Psychiatry*, **167**, 409–410.

Thomas, A. & Verbalis, J.G. (1995) Hyponatraemia and the syndrome of inappropriate secretion of antidiuretic hormone associated with drug therapy in psychiatric patients. *CNS Drugs*, **4**, 357–369.

Thompson, J.W., Jr, Ware, M.R. & Blashfield, R.K. (1990) Psychotropic medication and priapism: a comprehensive review. *Journal of Clinical Psychiatry*, **51**, 430–433.

Thornton, S.L. & Resch, D.S. (1995) SIADH associated with sertraline therapy. *American Journal of Psychiatry*, **152**, 809.

Tiller, J.W.G. (1990) Antidepressants, alcohol and psychomotor performance. *Acta Psychiatrica Scandinavica*, (Suppl. 360), 13–17.

Tyrer, P. (1984) Clinical effects of abrupt withdrawal from tricyclic antidepressants and monoamine oxidase inhibitors after long-term treatment. *Journal of Affective Disorders*, **6**, 1–7.

Wagner, W., Plekkenpol, B., Gray, T.E. & Vlaskamph, Esser, H. (1992) Review of fluvoxamine safety data base. *Drugs*, **43** (Suppl. 2), 48–54.

Warrington, S.J., Padgham, C. & Lader, M. (1989) *The Cardiovascular Effects of Antidepressants*. Psychological Medicine Monograph Supplement 16. Cambridge University Press, Cambridge.

Wedin, G.P., Oderda, G.M., Klein-Schwartz, W. & Gorman, R.L. (1986) Relative toxicity of cyclic antidepressants. *Annals of Emergency Medicine*, **15**, 797–804.

Williams, D.R., Peel, W.J. & Coe, P. (1995) Fibreoptic tracheal intubations: severe trismus due to monoamine oxidase inhibitor. *British Journal of Intensive Care*, September, 256–261.

Winston, F. & McCann, M.L. (1972) Antidepressant drugs and excessive weight gain. *British Journal of Psychiatry*, **120**, 693–739.

Woo, O.F., Vredenburg, M., Freitas, P. & Olson, K.R. (1995) Seizures after venlaFax:ine overdose: a case report. *Journal of Toxicology—Clinical Toxicology*, **33**, 349–550.

Zimmer, R., Gieschke, R., Fischbach, R. & Gasic, S. (1990) Interaction studies with moclobemide. *Acta Psychiatrica Scandinavica*, (Suppl. 360), 84–86.

Zisook, S. (1984) Side effects of isocarboxazid. *Journal of Clinical Psychiatry*, **45**, 53–58.

11 Efficacy of treatments for resistant depression

PHILIP J. COWEN

About 20–30% of patients with major depression fail to respond to treatment with a single antidepressant drug given in adequate dosage for an appropriate period of time. At this point there are many possible ways to pursue pharmacological treatment, but few controlled trials to help choose between the various options. In addition, with some exceptions, there are few clinical predictors to help match patients to an appropriate treatment.

Reports of different pharmacological treatments in resistant depression continue to abound (Table 11.1), showing the need for improved management of these disorders. Below, a number of the better studied of these interventions are outlined, together with the current evidence for their efficacy, particularly

Table 11.1 Some treatments for resistant depression.

Treatment	Evidence from controlled trials	Evidence from open studies	Comment
MAOI (non-selective)	++	++	Requires adequate dose
Antipsychotic drugs	++	++	For depressive psychosis
Lithium addition	++	++	Augments wide range of antidepressant drugs. Caution with SSRIs
Triiodothyronine	++	++	Potential cardiovascular problems
Tryptophan (with MAOI or TCA)	0	+	Monitoring for Eosinophilia Myalgia Syndrome needed
TCA* + SSRI†	0	+	Monitoring of plasma TCA levels advisable
Psychostimulants	0	+	Tolerance and dependence possible
Pindolol + SSRIs	0	+	Irritability can occur early in treatment
ECT‡	0	++	High relapse rates after successful treatment

++, Compelling; +, quite good; 0, absent.
* Tricyclic antidepressant.
† Selective serotonin re-uptake inhibitor.
‡ Electroconvulsive therapy.

from blind and placebo-controlled studies. It should be noted that many studies report response rates over a short period of follow-up (6–8 weeks). From the clinical point of view, however, information about progress over several months is more useful.

Another factor worth consideration is the way in which studies assess the clinical response to treatment. For example, a 50% decline in score on the Hamilton Rating Scale for Depression (HRSD) will often be regarded a positive outcome, but patients with high pretreatment HRSD scores can meet this criterion while still retaining significant symptomatology.

Changing the antidepressant

Switching to newer antidepressants

If a patient does not respond to one antidepressant drug, it is comparatively simple to try a preparation with different pharmacological properties. Most of the published studies of this manoeuvre treat patients in an open, sequential way with a newer class of antidepressant; clearly this cannot control for the placebo effect or the possibility of spontaneous remission. With the exception of monoamine oxidase inhibitors, there is, in fact, suprisingly little published evidence that this procedure is really effective, although clinically it appears to be widely used.

For example, in a study by Beasley *et al.* (1990), 35 patients who had shown minimal response to adequate tricyclic antidepressant (TCA) treatment in placebo-controlled trials were treated openly with the selective serotonin re-uptake inhibitor (SSRI), fluoxetine. After 6 weeks of treatment, just over half the patients had responded as judged by a decrease in HRSD scores of at least 50%. However, using the more exacting criteria of a final HRSD score of less than 7, only 17% of the subjects achieved full remission.

The study of Nolen *et al.* (1988a), however, provide less support for the role of SSRIs in TCA-resistant depression. These authors studied 68 depressed patients who had failed to respond to a minimum dose of 150 mg imipramine for 4 weeks. Patients were then randomly allocated to treatment with either the SSRI, fluvoxamine or the selective noradrenaline re-uptake inhibitor, oxprotiline. While about 25% of the patients randomized to oxprotiline responded (as judged by a 50% decrease in HRSD score), none of 35 patients allocated to fluvoxamine met this response criteria.

There appear to be few useful clinical predictors of response to SSRIs in TCA non-responders. It is fairly well established, however, that where a depressive disorder occurs in the setting of an obsessional illness, treatment with an SSRI or clomipramine is likely to be more effective than other antidepressants (Goodman *et al.*, 1992).

There are numerous other small studies which show that patients who fail to respond to TCAs may benefit when switched openly to other kinds of antidepressant drugs such as trazodone or bupropion. A recent study with venlafaxine is of interest because of the numbers of subjects involved, the careful documentation of treatment resistance and the length of follow-up (Nierenberg *et al.*, 1994).

A series of 84 patients with major depression who were highly treatment-resistant (failure respond to at least three adequate trials of antidepressant therapy) were treated with venlafaxine up to 450 mg daily. After 12 weeks of treatment, about one third of the subjects were responders (as judged by a 50% decrease in HRSD ratings). However, only about half the patients maintained this response for the next 3 months. Venlafaxine may therefore be of sustained benefit in a minority of highly treatment-resistant patients.

Switching to monoamine oxidase inhibitors

There is rather better evidence that non-selective irreversible monoamine oxidase inhibitors (MAOIs) are effective in patients resistant to TCAs and other antidepressants. In a continuation of the investigation described above, Nolen *et al.* (1988b) studied 21 patients who had failed to respond to treatment with imipramine, fluvoxamine or oxprotiline. The subjects were randomly allocated to double-blind treatment with nomifensine, a dopamine and noradrenline re-uptake inhibitor, or the MAOI, tranylcypromine. Of the 11 patients receiving tranylcypromine, five responded with a 50% decrease in HRSD score. Only one of the nomifensine-treated subjects showed a similar response. In a subsequent cross-over, five of eight non-responders to nomifensine responded to tranylcypromine. Eight of the 10 patients who responded to tranylcypromine maintained their response for at least 6 months. Tranylcypromine was associated with several adverse effects. About half the subjects experienced dizziness mainly due to postural hypotension, while about a third had headaches and insomnia.

There is also evidence that patients with certain clinical features may have a preferential response to MAOIs. For example, in a series of placebo-controlled trials, the Columbia group have established that patients with features of atypical depression have a significantly higher response rate to phenelzine (about 70%) than imipramine (about 45%) (Quitkin *et al.*, 1989). In a recent study of such patients, 46 subjects who had failed to respond to imipramine were switched under double-blind conditions to phenelzine. After 6 weeks, 31 were 'much improved' or 'very much improved' on Clinical Global Impression (CGI) ratings (McGrath *et al.*, 1993).

Bipolar depressed patients with features of anergia, hypersomnia and hyperphagia may also respond better to MAOIs than TCAs. For example, in a double-blind study in out-patients suffering from this syndrome, Himmelhoch *et al.* (1991) found 'moderate' or 'marked improvement' on the CGI in 21 of 28 subjects given tranylcypromine but in only 10 of 28 treated with imipramine.

Recently, reversible, selective type-A MAOIs have become available. These drugs have the great advantage relative to conventional MAOIs in that they do not cause hypertensive reactions with tyramine-containing foods. In a comparative trial of 93 depressed in-patients who had failed to respond to two adequate courses of antidepressant drug treatment, Volz *et al.* (1994) found that the reversible type A-MAO inhibitor brofaromine (150 mg daily) produced a similar rate of clinical remission (74%) to that seen with tranylcypromine (72%) defined by a 50% decline in HRSD ratings. In this study, however, the dose of tranylcypromine (up to 30 mg daily) was less than that usually given to depressed in-patients; for example, Nolen *et al.* (1988b) used up to 100 mg daily.

The reversible type-A MAOI moclobemide is more widely available than brofaromine. However, there are no studies indicating its usefulness in resistant depression and a little evidence to the contrary (Nolen *et al.*, 1994). For example, the author studied eight out-patients with major depression who had failed to respond to at least one course of a TCA and one course of a SSRI (at therapeutic doses) with lithium augmentation. Subsequently they failed to respond to moclobemide, 600 mg daily for at least 6 weeks. Moclobemide was discontinued and treatment with conventional MAOIs started (tranylcypromine, 3 subjects; isocarboxazid, 3 subjects; phenelzine, 2 subjects). Over the next 8 weeks, five of the eight patients were clinically improved as determined by a fall in HRSD scores of at least 50%. Treatment was well tolerated, although two subjects required the addition of trazodone (50 mg) for insomnia. Three patients had histories of previous response to conventional MAOIs; two of these were responders.

Adding another drug (augmentation strategies)

A problem in switching antidepressant preparations is that withdrawal of the first compound may not be straightforward. Patients may have gained some small benefit from the treatment, for example in terms of improved sleep or reduced tension, and this will be lost. In addition, if the first medication is stopped quickly, withdrawal symptoms may result. On the other hand, gradual tapering of the dose makes the changeover in medication rather protracted, which may not be easily tolerated by a depressed and despairing patient.

For this reason, in patients unresponsive to first-line medication it may be more appropriate to add a second compound to the primary antidepressant, in the hope of producing an additive or even synergistic effect. The major disadvantage of this procedure is that that the risk of adverse effects through drug interaction is increased.

Antipsychotic drugs

Naturalistic studies have shown that patients with depressive psychosis have low response rates to treatment with TCAs alone but may respond well when antipsychotic drugs are combined with a TCA. In a double-blind, random allocation study of 51 in-patients with depressive psychosis, Spiker *et al.* (1985) found that the response rate (final HRSD < 7) to amitriptyline alone was 41%, while that to perphenazine alone was 19%. However, patients receiving combined treatment with these drugs had a significantly higher response rate (78%) than either of the other two groups.

Most of the reports of the drug treatment of depressive psychosis have involved TCAs. However, in an open study Rothschild *et al.* (1993) found that the combination of fluoxetine (up to 40 mg daily) and perphenazine (up to 35 mg daily) produced a 73% response rate (reduction in HRSD rating of at least 50%) in 30 patients with DSM-III-R depressive psychosis.

From this, it appears that a combination of SSRIs and antipsychotic drugs may be effective in depressive psychosis. However, the response criterion was less exacting than that employed by Spiker *et al.* (1985) and the majority of the patients (87%) required 40 mg of fluoxetine. In addition, 14 patients developed tremor and two experienced akathisia. SSRIs can themselves cause extrapyramidal movement disorders and may potentiate the extrapyramidal effects of antipsychotic drugs through both pharmacodynamic and pharmacokinetic interactions (see Young & Cowen, 1994).

Lithium

Lithium given alone has modest antidepressant properties in patients with bipolar disorder but other depressed patients show little response (see Price, 1989). There is now, however, good evidence from uncontrolled and controlled trials that lithium added to ineffective antidepressant treatment can produce useful clinical improvement in patients with major depression. Whether this effect of lithium is a true potentiation (augmentation) of the primary antidepressant compound or represents simply an additive antidepressant effect of its own is debatable. However, naturalistic studies suggest equivalent rates of response to lithium addition in unipolar and bipolar patients (Price *et al.*, 1989; Nierenberg *et al.*, 1990).

Uncontrolled trials have reported that lithium addition is followed by a rapid onset of antidepressant effect (within 48 h) in a high proportion of subjects (60–70%) (de Montigny *et al.*, 1983). Double-blind, placebo-controlled trials

Table 11.2 Placebo-controlled trials* of lithium addition in patients unresponsive to initial antidepressant drug treatment.

Authors	Patients	Design	Response/non-response	
Heninger *et al.* (1983)	RDC unipolar major depression	Double-blind placebo cross-over (12 days)	Lithium	5/8
			Placebo	0/7
Zusky *et al.* (1988)	DSM-III unipolar major depression	Double-blind placebo control, parallel group (14 days)	Lithium	3/8
			Placebo	2/8
Joffe *et al.* (1993a)	RDC unipolar major depression	Double-blind placebo control, parallel group (14 days)	Lithium	9/17
			Placebo	3/16
Stein & Bernadt (1993)	RDC major depression	Double-blind placebo/ low dose† control, parallel group (6 weeks)	Lithium	15/34
			Placebo	6/34
Katona *et al.* (1995)	DSM-III-R major depression	Double-blind placebo control, parallel group (6 weeks)	Lithium	15/29
			Placebo	8/32
Overall response rate			Lithium	62/130 (48%)
			Placebo	25/131 (19%)

* At least 12 days' duration.
† 250 mg lithium daily.

confirm that lithium is effective but show a more gradual onset of action over 2–3 weeks in about 40–50% of depressed patients (Table 11.2). For example, Katona *et al.* (1995) studied 62 patients with major depression who failed to respond to 6 weeks' treatment with lofepramine or fluoxetine. Subjects were randomly allocated to either lithium or placebo for a further 6 weeks. Taking the response criterion as a final HRSD score <10, 15/29 lithium-treated patients were responders compared to 8/32 on placebo. To obtain this result, however, patients with lithium levels <0.4 mmol L^{-1} were excluded.

Lithium appears to be effective in improving antidepressant response when added to different kinds of primary antidepressant treatment, including TCAs, SSRIs, MAOIs and bupropion (Johnson, 1991). Caution is needed when using lithium together with SSRIs because both treatments combine to potentiate brain 5-HT function leading to a risk of 5-HT neurotoxicity (see Young & Cowen, 1994). This combination, however, does not seem to have greater therapeutic efficacy than other lithium-antidepressant combinations, despite the marked increase in brain 5-HT function that it produces (Fontaine *et al.*, 1991; Katona *et al.*, 1995)

A long-term follow-up (mean interval of 29 months) of 66 resistant depressed patients who had received lithium addition treatment showed that 48% were essentially free from significant depressive symptoms (Nierenberg *et al.*, 1990). The only clear predictor of outcome was the acute therapeutic response to lithium addition; that is, if a patient had showed a good initial response they were likely to remain well over the follow-up period. Interestingly, this positive outcome was independent of the length of time for which lithium treatment was continued. Demographic and clinical factors such as age, sex, the presence of melancholic depression, dysthmia, hospitalization and suicide attempts were not useful response predictors.

There have been few comparisons of lithium augmentation with other treatments of resistant depression. However, Dinan and Barry (1989) randomly allocated 30 severely depressed patients who had failed to respond to 150 mg TCA treatment for 4 weeks to either bilateral electroconvulsive therapy (ECT; 6 treatments over 3 weeks) or lithium addition. Of the 15 patients who received lithium, 10 responded (final HRSD rating of <11). The response rate of the ECT-treated patients (11/15) was not different. The lithium addition group included two psychotically depressed patients who did not respond. In this context, it is worth noting that Price *et al.* (1983) reported useful clinical improvement following lithium addition in five out of six patients with depressive psychosis who had failed to respond to combined treatment with desipramine and an antipsychotic drug.

Triiodothyronine

Several open studies have indicated that the addition of triiodothyronine to ineffective TCA treatment can bring about useful clinical response, and this has been supported in three of four controlled studies (Table 11.3). In the most recent investigation, Joffe *et al.* (1993a) studied 50 out-patients with unipolar, non-psychotic major depression. They had failed to respond to 5 weeks' treatment with a TCA (daily dose 2.5 mg kg^{-1}) after which they were randomly allocated to double-blind addition of lithium carbonate, triiodothyronine

Table 11.3 Controlled trials of triiodothyronine (T$_3$) in TCA-resistant depression.

Authors	Patients	Design	Result
Goodwin *et al.* (1982)	In-patients; unipolar depression, 4; bipolar depression, 8	Double-blind addition	8/12 responded
Gitlin *et al.* (1987)	16 out-patients, unipolar major depression	Double-blind placebo controlled cross-over	T$_3$ = placebo
Joffe & Singer (1991)	38 out-patients, non-psychotic unipolar major depression	Double-blind, comparison of T$_3$ and T$_4$	T$_3$ response (9/17) > T$_4$ response (4/21)
Joffe *et al.* (1993a)	50 out-patients, non-psychotic unipolar major depression	Double-blind, placebo-controlled lithium comparison	T$_3$ response (10/17) = lithium (9/17) > placebo (3/16)

(37.5 µg daily) or placebo for 2 weeks. At the end of treatment, 10 of 17 patients treated with triiodothyronine had responded (50% reduction in HRSD with final HRSD score <10). A similar response rate (nine of 17 patients) was noted in patients receiving lithium, while only three of 16 subjects responded to placebo.

Joffe *et al.* (1993b) found few predictors of response to augmentation with triiodothyronine or lithium. Non-responders to lithium appeared to have more severe weight loss and sleep disturbance, while these factors did not distinguish triiodothyronine responders from non-responders. Pre-treatment thyroid function also failed to predict response to triiodothyronine.

Taken together, the data suggest that addition of triiodothyronine is a useful means of augmenting TCA treatment in depressed patients. Interestingly, while triiodothyronine appears to be effective in this respect, thyroxine is probably not. For example, Joffe and Singer (1991) reported that the response rate of TCA-resistant patients to triiodothyronine (nine of 17) was significantly greater than that of thyroxine (four of 21). There are at present no comparative data to show that triiodothyronine can augment the action of other classes of antidepressant drugs.

Precursors

Studies in both experimental animals and humans suggest that it is possible to increase brain 5-HT function by administering precursors such as 5-hydroxytryptophan (5-HTP) and tryptophan (TRP) (see Cowen, 1994). There is evidence from controlled trials that the addition of TRP can improve the therapeutic effect of MAOI treatment. It is also possible that TRP can enhance the efficacy of clomipramine (see Chalmers & Cowen, 1990). However, there are no controlled trials to indicate that TRP can reliably produce therapeutic benefit in patients who have failed to respond to MAOI or TCAs. Nevertheless, the use of TRP has been recommended to supplement the 5-HTP-potentiating effects of lithium–MAOI and lithium–clomipramine combinations (Barker *et al.*, 1987; Hale *et al.*, 1987).

TRP has been associated with the development of the Eosinophilia Myalgia Syndrome (EMS), a severe connective tissue disease that can have a fatal outcome. Subsequent studies have shown that EMS is almost certainly caused by a contaminant that occurred in the production of TRP from a single manufacturing source (Slutsker *et al.*, 1990). It is of interest that when TRP was withdrawn in the UK, several patients whose severe refractory depression had responded to a combination of lithium, phenelzine and TRP relapsed on TRP discontinuation, despite being maintained on lithium–MAOI treatment (Ferrier *et al.*, 1990). This suggests that in some patients TRP was exerting an antidepressant effect.

In the UK it remains possible to prescribe TRP, in combination with other antidepressant drugs, for patients with chronic treatment-resistant depression. It should be noted, however, that the combination of TRP with MAOIs can lead to 5-HT neurotoxicity, so caution is needed. In addition, TRP given with SSRIs can also result in 5-HT toxicity, so this combination is not recommended (Sternbach, 1991; Young & Cowen, 1994).

5-HTP given as a sole treatment does not appear to have a useful role in resistant depression (Nolen *et al.*, 1988b). On the basis of an open case series, Kline and Sachs (1980) reported that the addition of 5-HTP to MAOI treatment produced benefit in 11 of 25 non-responders. However, this report does not appear to have been followed up.

Combination of TCA and MAOI

The combination of TCAs and MAOIs has been in use since the 1960s when the efficacy of this regime was strongly advocated by leading authorities. Although the combination of MAOI and TCAs is reported to be hazardous, the risks of significant interaction can be minimized if reasonable precautions are taken. These include avoiding imipramine and clomipramine, and starting the drugs together at low dose or adding the MAOI cautiously to established TCA treatment (see Chalmers & Cowen, 1990).

In patients not selected for treatment resistance the combination of MAOIs and TCAs does not appear to confer additional therapeutic benefit over either drug used alone (Chalmers & Cowen, 1990). In one controlled study (Davidson *et al.*, 1978) 17 in-patients who had not responded to TCA treatment were randomly allocated to ECT or treatment with phenelzine and amitriptyline. The outcome judged by decrease in HRSD ratings favoured ECT. However, about half this group of patients suffered from depressive psychosis and in such patients ECT (or antidepressants and antipsychotic drugs in combination) would usually be preferred.

An open study by Sethna (1974) of 12 depressed patients who had failed to respond to either TCAs or MAOIs given separately (or ECT in 10 cases) suggested useful clinical effects of MAOI–TCA combination. At follow-up periods of 7–24 months, nine subjects were reported to be without significant depressive symptomatology. Most of these subjects had chronic non-melancholic depression with prominent anxiety symptoms.

In addition to these series, case reports continue to appear where it seems well documented that a patient has failed to respond to either a TCA or a MAOI given alone but achieves a useful clinical response when both drugs are used together (Tyrer & Murphy, 1990). Therefore, although controlled evidence is lacking, it seems likely that individual patients with refractory depression are helped by MAOI–TCA combinations. In general, the adverse effects of the combination are no worse than with either drug alone, although weight gain and postural hypotension may be more troublesome. Conversely, if a MAOI is given with a TCA such as amitriptyline or trimipramine, MAOI-induced insomnia may be prevented.

There is less information about the combination of other antidepressants with MAOIs. Trazodone is fairly commonly used to treat MAOI-induced insomnia and is generally well tolerated (Nierenberg & Keck, 1989). There are also case series in which patients with refractory depression have been treated with a combination of the reversible MAOI-A, moclobemide, and SSRIs such as fluvoxamine. Thus far, this combination has been reported safe and, in some patients, therapeutically effective (see Ebert *et al.*, 1995). The combination of fluvoxamine and moclobemide has also been reported to be safe in healthy volunteers (Dingemanse, 1993).

Despite these reports, it is well established that conventional MAOIs are contraindicated in combination with SSRIs because of the risk of fatal 5-HT toxicity (Sternbach, 1991; Young & Cowen, 1994). Furthermore, there are case reports of fatal adverse reactions following moclobemide–SSRI overdose (see Young & Cowen, 1995). At present, therefore, the combination of SSRI and moclobemide should be used with extreme caution, if it is used at all.

Combination of TCA and SSRI

Some open case series have suggested that combining TCA and SSRI treatment may be helpful in refractory depression. For example, in a retrospective chart review, Weilburg *et al.* (1989) reported a positive response (defined as improvement noted by both patient and clinician) in 22 of 25 depressed out-patients when fluoxetine was added to ongoing TCA treatment. Of further five patients taking trazodone, four also improved. This study does not, of course, clarify whether or not the improvement was due to the fluoxetine alone or the combination of fluoxetine with the TCA. However, in eight patients the therapeutic response was lost when the TCA was withdrawn and restored when it was recommenced.

Subsequently, Weilburg *et al.* (1991) in a similar study found resolution of depression in 13 of 20 out-patients in whom nortriptyline or desipramine were added to ineffective fluoxetine treatment. One patient worsened, with severe agitation. Finally, Seth *et al.* (1992) reported remarkable improvement in eight elderly patients with chronic refractory depression who received SSRI–TCA combination (usually sertraline and nortriptyline). Some patients received concomitant lithium treatment.

The only prospective study of TCA–SSRI treatment was carried out by Fava *et al.* (1994) who treated 41 depressed out-patients who had failed to achieve a 50% reduction in HRSD scores in response to a standard dose of fluoxetine (20 mg daily). Subjects were randomly allocated to three different groups: (a) high-dose fluoxetine (40–60 mg daily), (b) the addition of desipramine (25–50 mg daily), or (c) lithium. Taking response as a final HRSD score (at 5 weeks) of <7, the most effective treatment was high-dose fluoxetine (53% response rate) while lithium and desipramine augmentation appeared of similar efficacy (response rates of 29% and 25%, respectively). However, the plasma levels of lithium obtained in this study were low and probably subtherapeutic.

Taken together, the evidence for the efficacy of TCA–SSRI combinations is not compelling. In addition, there are numerous case reports of adverse reactions with agitation and, rarely, seizures. These reactions are generally associated with marked elevations in plasma TCA levels because SSRIs are potent inhibitors of the cytochrome P450 system by which TCAs are metabolized. While some SSRIs—for example, citalopram and sertraline—may be less likely to produce this effect, plasma TCA monitoring is advisable if combination treatment is used (see Taylor, 1995). Another option may be to use treatment with a single drug such as clomipramine or venlafaxine which produces potent 5-HT and noradrenaline re-uptake inhibition.

Other pharmacological treatments

Treatments listed under this heading have some limited evidence for efficacy in refractory depression. In addition, a number of them—for example, cortisol suppression or pindolol—have an interesting experimental rationale for their use.

Carbamazepine

The main indication for carbamazepine is in the acute management of mania and the prophylaxis of bipolar disorder. In general, the acute antidepressant effects of carbamazepine are not striking. However, Ballenger and Post (1980) described an antidepressant effect of carbamazepine in 4 of 13 bipolar depressed patients, 3 of whom had been unresponsive to lithium.

Subsequently, in a double-blind, cross-over study, Post et al. (1986) found a good clinical response (decrease of at least 2 points on the Bunney–Hamburg scale) to a 4-week course of carbamazepine in 12 of 35 depressed patients. In this study, good response was seen in 10 of 24 bipolar depressives, and two of 11 unipolar depressives. However, most of the patients did not relapse upon subsequent placebo-controlled discontinuation of carbamazepine, questioning the specificity of the treatment effect. In addition, how far the patients studied were, in fact, refractory to conventional treatment is not clear from the authors' description.

In a further blind study, Kramlinger and Post (1989) found that the combination of lithium and carbamazepine produced good clinical improvement (decrease of at least 2 points on the Bunney–Hamburg scale) in eight of 15 patients (13 bipolars) who had failed to respond to carbamazepine alone. Taken together, these data suggest that carbamazepine may be worth trying in bipolar patients with resistant depression, perhaps in combination with lithium. If the latter combination is used, it is worth noting that coadministration of lithium and carbamazepine has been reported to cause neurotoxicity despite the presence of normal plasma concentrations.

Psychostimulants

The widespread use of psychostimulants as the sole treatment for depression has been superseded by antidepressants that are not associated with the development of tolerance or abuse. It is possible, however, that psychostimulants such as amphetamine and methylphenidate may retain a place in the treatment of resistant depression, usually in combination with other antidepressants. For example, Wager and Klein (1988) reported benefit in partial responders to TCAs following the addition of amphetamine in daily doses of 5–20 mg daily. Potential problems of this approach include troublesome hypertensive reactions as well as tolerance to the therapeutic effect.

There is also a small clinical literature on combination treatment with psychostimulant and MAOIs in refractory depression. This combination is normally contraindicated because of the risk of hypertensive crisis. However, in some patients its use appears safe and apparently useful. For example, Fawcett *et al.* (1991) reported that 10 of 32 severely depressed patients, who had failed multiple treatment trials, were 'improved' or 'much improved' for at least 6 months on the combination of MAOI with psychostimulant (pemoline or dexamphetamine). Similarly, Feighner *et al.* (1985) found similar levels of improvement in nine of 16 severely depressed and treatment-resistant patients who received dexamphetamine or methylphenidate in combination with a MAOI (and usually a TCA as well).

Improvements of this nature in such severely ill patients are worth noting. However, it must be emphasized that the combination of psychostimulants and MAOIs is potentially hazardous and should be used with very close monitoring. Serious adverse reactions were not noted in the case series above; however, some patients discontinued treatment for adverse effects including impotence, hypertension, orthostatic hypotension and shakiness.

Adrenal steroid suppression

There is growing interest in the possible role of excessive glucocorticoid secretion in the pathophysiology of depression (Dinan, 1994). Ghadirian *et al.* (1995) studied 20 depressed in-patients (nine with psychotic symptoms) who had failed to respond to at least two trials of antidepressant drug treatment. They were withdrawn from other psychotropic medication and then treated with one or more steroid suppressive drugs (aminoglutethamide, metyrapone, and ketaconazole) for a period of 8 weeks.

Of the 20 patients, 11 were responders (>50% decrease on HRSD scores) and two were partial responders (20–50% HRSD decrease). Patients with psychotic depression faired less well. In responders, improvement was maintained for several months even though steroid suppressive treatment had been discontinued. Side-effects were mild and included light-headedness, headache, nausea and fatigue. The use of steroid-suppressing drugs offers an interesting new avenue for the treatment of resistant depression but clearly controlled trials are needed.

α_2-adrenoceptor antagonists

In laboratory experiments, many different kinds of antidepressant treatment, including TCAs and MAOIs, produce a down-regulation of β-adrenoceptors or the associated noradrenaline-sensitive adenylate cyclase (Vetulani *et al.*, 1976). The speed of the TCA-induced down-regulation can be increased by α_2-adrenoceptor blockade, perhaps because reduction in presynaptic α_2-adrenoceptor function increases noradrenaline outflow (Crews *et al.*, 1981).

These laboratory findings have led to suggestions that combining an α_2-adrenoceptor antagonist with a TCA might speed the onset of antidepressant action or, more speculatively, lead to increased therapeutic benefit in TCA-resistant patients. However, two open studies have failed to confirm the latter possibility (Charney *et al.*, 1986; Schmauss *et al.*, 1988). There is, however, a small case series in which the α_2-adrenoceptor antagonist, idazoxan, given as a sole treatment, produced an effective antidepressant response of several months duration in two resistant bipolar depressed patients. A third patient with resistant unipolar depression showed an initial response but relapsed after a number of weeks (Osman *et al.*, 1990).

Pindolol

Repeated administration of a number of antidepressant drugs, particularly SSRIs and MAOIs, desensitizes inhibitory 5-HT_{1A} autoreceptors on 5-HT cell bodies. It has been suggested that this effect contributes to the antidepressant effect of such drugs by freeing 5-HT cell bodies from feedback control and thereby facilitating the release of 5-HT from nerve terminals (Blier & de Montigny, 1994).

Based on this idea, Artigas *et al.* (1994) proposed that the addition of a 5-HT_{1A} receptor antagonist to the medication of patients who had not responded to conventional antidepressants, particularly SSRIs, might produce a therapeutic effect. Because there are at present no selective 5-HT_{1A} receptor antagonists available for clinical use, these authors employed pindolol, a β-adrenoceptor antagonist with 5-HT_{1A} receptor antagonist properties.

Pindolol (2.5 mg three times daily) was added to the drug treatment of seven patients with major depression who had been resistant to multiple medication trials. Five subjects were currently taking an SSRI (four paroxetine and one fluvoxamine) while one received imipramine and one phenelzine. All subjects showed a decrease in HRSD score of at least 50% after a week of pindolol addition and in five, HRSD scores were less than 8, indicating full remission (Artigas *et al.*, 1994).

Subsequently, Blier and Bergeron (1995) reported on the addition of pindolol (2.5 mg three times daily) to 18 patients with major depression who had failed to respond to treatment at least with antidepressant together with the addition of another treatment, usually lithium. Pindolol (2.5 mg three times daily) was added to paroxetine (eight subjects), sertraline (five subjects), fluoxetine (three subjects), and moclobemide (two subjects). Overall, pindolol produced a significant improvement in depressive symptoms after 1 week. By 2 weeks, all the patients except those on sertraline had a HRSD score of 10 or less showing a very good clinical improvement. Interestingly, none of the sertraline-treated patients responded. It is not clear whether or not this may represent a chance finding.

Pindolol addition in the latter study was generally well tolerated. However, two patients had to stop taking pindolol in the first 3 days because of irritability. Furthermore, one patient who responded to the addition of pindolol to paroxetine developed mania 5 weeks later.

Electroconvulsive therapy

Among the indications for ECT is that of failure to respond to adequate antidepressant drug treatment. Trials of ECT typically report high response rates for ECT (about 80%), but patients unresponsive to drug treatment are not usually considered as a separate group.

Prudic *et al.* (1990) studied the effect of previous antidepressant drug treatment on the response of 53 patients who received bilateral ECT. They found that amongst those who had received adequate pharmacotherapy (a TCA in a dose of at least 200 mg daily for at least 4 weeks), the response rate to ECT (defined as a 60% reduction in HRSD score) was 50%. In contrast, the response rate of patients who had not received adequate drug treatment was significantly greater (86%). The presence of medication resistance therefore decreases the likelihood that a patient will respond to ECT. Nevertheless, about half of such subjects are likely to experience significant improvement.

Another point that needs to be considered is the outcome after ECT. Some limited data suggest that even where ECT is has been therapeutically successful, pretreatment medication resistance can be associated with a high subsequent relapse rate. Sackheim *et al.* (1990) followed 58 patients who responded to ECT and found that 1 year post-treatment, 50% had relapsed, meeting the research diagnostic criteria (RDC) criteria for major depression. The relapse rate in patients who had received adequate drug treatment prior to ECT was significantly higher in those who had not (64% compared to 32%). The relapse rate after ECT was only weakly influenced by whether or not patients received adequate antidepressant drug treatment post-ECT.

Psychosurgery

Chronic, severe and intractable depression is regarded by some as an indication for psychosurgery (see Gelder *et al.*, 1996). There are no controlled trials of this procedure and they would, of course, be extremely difficult to carry out. Poynton *et al.* (1995) described a cohort of 23 severely ill, treatment-resistant patients, 16 of whom had major depression and five of whom had bipolar disorder. They underwent stereotactic subcaudate tractotomy and were followed up prospectively. At 6 months postoperatively the mean HRSD score had fallen from 17.9 to 9.7. After 1 year of follow-up, 13 of the patients had shown either a very good or good response, with the remainder experiencing intermediate benefit or no change. The HRSD scores at 6 months correlated with global outcome, suggesting that at 6 months the pattern of response may be established. No serious physical sequelae of the operation were reported. However, detailed neuropsychological testing showed changes in the pattern of cognitive function. For example, there were improvements in some tests requiring speed and attention but deterioration on others, such as the Stroop task, which depend on intact frontal lobe function.

References

Artigas, F., Perez, V. & Alvarez, E. (1994) Pindolol induces a rapid improvement of depressed patients treated with serotonin reuptake inhibitors. *Archives of General Psychiatry*, **51**, 248–251.

Ballenger, J.C. & Post, R.M. (1980) Carbamazepine in manic depressive illness: a new treatment. *American Journal of Psychiatry*, **137**, 782–790.

Barker, W.A., Scott, J. & Eccelston, D. (1987) The Newcastle Chronic Depression Study: results of a treatment regime. *International Clinical Psychopharmacology*, **2**, 261–272.

Beasley, C.M., Sayler, M.E. & Cunningham, G.E. et al. (1990) Fluoxetine in tricyclic refractory major depressive disorder. *Journal of Affective Disorders*, **20**, 193–200.

Blier, P. & Bergeron, R. (1995) Effectiveness of pindolol with selected antidepressant drugs in the treatment of major depression. *Journal of Clinical Psychopharmacology*, **15**, 217–222.

Blier, P. & de Montigny, C. (1994) Current advances

and trends in the treatment of depression. *Trends in Pharmacological Sciences*, **15**, 220–226.

Chalmers, J.S. & Cowen, P.J. (1990) Drug treatment of tricyclic resistant depression. *International Review of Psychiatry*, **2**, 239–248.

Charney, D.S., Price, L.H. & Heninger, G.R. (1986) Desipramine–yohimbine combination for refractory depression. *Archives of General Psychiatry*, **43**, 1155–1161.

Cowen, P.J. (1994) The effect of tryptophan on brain 5-HT function: a review. *Human Psychopharmacology*, **9**, 371–376.

Crews, F.T., Steven, M.P. & Goodwin, F.K. (1981) Acceleration of beta-receptor desensitisation in combined administration of antidepressant and phenoxybenzamine. *Nature*, **290**, 787–789.

Davidson, J., McLeod, M., Law-Yone, B. & Linnoila, M. (1978) A comparison of electroconvulsive therapy and combined phenelzine-amitriptyline in refractory depression. *Archives of General Psychiatry*, **35**, 639–642.

Dinan, T.G. (1994) Glucocorticoids and the genesis of depressive illness: a psychobiological model. *British Journal of Psychiatry*, **164**, 365–371.

Dinan, T. & Barry, S. (1989) A comparison of electroconvulsive therapy with a lithium and tricyclic combination among depressed tricyclic non-responders. *Acta Psychiatrica Scandinavica*, **80**, 97–100.

Dingemanse, J. (1993) An update of recent moclobemide interaction data. *International Clinical Psychopharmacology*, **7**, 167–180.

Ebert, D., Albert, R., May, A., Stosiek, I. & Kaschka, W. (1995) Combined SSRI–RIMA treatment in refractory depression: safety data and efficacy. *Psychopharmacology*, **119**, 342–344.

Fava, M., Rosenbaum, J.F., McGrath, P.J., Stewart, J.W., Amsterdam, J.D. & Quitkin, F.M. (1994) Lithium and tricyclic augmentation of fluoxetine treatment for major depression: a double blind controlled study. *American Journal of Psychiatry*, **151**, 1372–1374.

Fawcett, J., Kravitz, H.M., Zajecka, J.M. & Schaff, M.R. (1991) CNS stimulant potentiation of monoamine oxidase inhibitors in treatment-refractory depression. *Journal of Clinical Psychopharmacology*, **11**, 127–132.

Feighner, J.P., Herbstein, J. & Damlouji, N. (1985) Combined MAO, TCA, and direct stimulant therapy of treatment-resistant depression. *Journal of Clinical Psychiatry*, **46**, 206–209.

Ferrier, I.N., Eccleston, D., Moore, P.G. & Wood, K.A. (1990) Relapse in chronic depressives on withdrawal of L-tryptophan. *Lancet*, **336**, 380–381.

Fontaine, R., Ontiveros, A., Elie, R. & Vezina, M. (1991) Lithium carbonate augmentation of desipramine and fluoxetine in refractory depression. *Biological Psychiatry*, **29**, 946–948.

Gelder, M.G., Gath, D.H., Mayou, R.M. & Cowen, P.J. (1996) *Oxford Textbook of Psychiatry*. Oxford University Press, Oxford.

Ghadirian, A.M., Engelsmann, F. & Dhar, V. *et al.* (1995) The psychotropic effects of inhibitors of steroid biosynthesis in depressed patients refractory to treatment. *Biological Psychiatry*, **37**, 369–375.

Gitlin, M.J., Weiner, H. & Fairbanks, L. (1987) Failure of T_3 to potentiate tricyclic antidepressant response. *Journal of Affective Disorders*, **13**, 267–272.

Goodman, W.K., McDougle, C.J. & Price, L.H. (1992) Pharmacotherapy of Obsessive Compulsive Disorder. *Journal of Clinical Psychiatry*, **53** (4 Suppl.), 29–37.

Goodwin, F.K., Prange, A.J. & Post, R.M. (1982) Potentiation of antidepressant effects by L-triiodothyronine in tricyclic non-responders. *American Journal of Psychiatry*, **139**, 34–38.

Hale, A.S., Procter, A.W. & Bridges, P.K. (1987) Clomipramine, tryptophan and lithium in combination for resistant endogenous depression: 7 case studies. *British Journal of Psychiatry*, **151**, 213–217.

Heninger, G.R., Charney, D.S. & Sternberg, D.E. (1983) Lithium carbonate augmentation of antidepressant treatment. *Archives of General Psychiatry*, **40**, 1335–1342.

Himmelhoch, J.M., Thase, M.E., Mallinger, A.G. & Houck, P. (1991) Tranylcypromine vs. imipramine in anergic bipolar depression. *American Journal of Psychiatry*, **148**, 910–916.

Joffe, R.T. & Singer, W. (1991) Thyroid hormone potentiation of antidepressants. In: *Advances in Neuropsychiatry and Psychopharmacology*. Vol. 2: *Refractory Depression* (ed. J. D. Amsterdam), pp. 185–189. Raven Press, New York.

Joffe, R.T., Singer, W., Levitt, A.J. & MacDonald, C. (1993a) A placebo-controlled comparison of lithium and triiodothyronine augmentation of tricyclic antidepressants in unipolar refractory depression. *Archives of General Psychiatry*, **50**, 387–393.

Joffe, R.T., Levitt, A.J., Bagby, R.M., MacDonald, C. & Singer, W. (1993b) Predictors of response to lithium and triiodothyronine: augmentation of antidepressants in tricyclic non-responders. *British Journal of Psychiatry*, **163**, 574–578.

Johnson, F.N. (1991) Lithium augmentation therapy for depression. *Reviews in Contemporary Pharmacotherapy*, **2**, 3–52.

Katona, C.L.E., Abou-Saleh, M.T. & Harrison, D.A. et al. (1995) Placebo-controlled trial of lithium augmentation of fluoxetine and lofepramine. *British Journal of Psychiatry*, **116**, 80–86.

Kline, N. & Sachs, W. (1980) Treatment of depression with an MAO inhibitor followed by 5-HTP: an unfinished research project. *Acta Psychiatrica Scandinavica*, **280**, 233–241.

Kramlinger, K.G. & Post, R.M. (1989) The addition of lithium to carbamazepine: antidepressant efficacy in treatment resistant depression. *Archives of General Psychiatry*, **46**, 794–800.

McGrath, P.J., Stewart, J.W. & Nunes, E.V. (1993) A double blind cross-over trial of imipramine and phenelzine for outpatients with treatment-refractory depression. *American Journal of Psychiatry*, **150**, 118–123.

de Montigny, C., Cournoyer, G. & Morissette, R. et al. (1983) Lithium carbonate addition in tricyclic antidepressant-resistant unipolar depression: correlations of the neurobiological actions of tricyclic antidepressant drugs and lithium ion on the serotonin system. *Archives of General Psychiatry*, **40**, 1327–1334.

Nierenberg, A.A. & Keck, P.E. (1989) Management of monoamine oxidase inhibitor-associated insomnia with trazodone. *Journal of Clinical Psychopharmacology*, **9**, 45–54.

Nierenberg, A.A., Price, L.H., Charney, D.S. & Heninger, G.R. (1990) After lithium augmentation: a retrospective follow-up of patients with antidepressant-refractory depression. *Journal of Affective Disorders*, **18**, 167–175.

Nierenberg, A.A., Feighner, J.P., Rudolph, R., Cole, J.O. & Sullivan, J. (1994) Venlafaxine for treatment-resistant unipolar depression. *Journal of Clinical Psychopharmacology*, **14**, 419–423.

Nolen, W.A., Van de Putte, J.J. & Dijken, W.A. et al. (1988a) Treatment strategy in depression. 1. Non-tricyclic and selective reuptake inhibitors in resistant depression: a double blind partial cross-over study on the effects of oxprotiline and fluvoxamine. *Acta Psychiatrica Scandinavica*, **78**, 668–675.

Nolen, W.A., Van de Putte, J.J. & Dijken, W.A. et al. (1988b) Treatment strategy in depression. 2. MAO inhibitors in depression resistant to cyclic antidepressants: two controlled cross-over studies with tranylcypromine vs. L-5-hydroxytryptophan and nomifensine. *Acta Psychiatrica Scandinavica*, **78**, 676–683.

Nolen, W.A., Hoencamp, E., Haffmans, P.M.J. & Bouvy, P.F. (1994) Classical and selective monoamine oxidase inhibitors in refractory major depression. In: *Refractory Depression: Current Strategies and Future Directions* (eds W.A. Nolen, J. Zohar, S.P. Roose & J.D. Amsterdam), pp. 59–68. John Wiley & Sons Ltd, Chichester.

Osman, O.T., Rudorfer, M.V. & Potter, W.Z. (1990) Idazoxan: a selective α_2-antagonist and effective sustained antidepressant in two bipolar depressed patients. *Archives of General Psychiatry*, **46**, 958–959.

Post, R.M., Uhde, T.W., Roy-Byrne, P.P. & Joffe, R.T. (1986) Antidepressant effects of carbamazepine. *American Journal of Psychiatry*, **143**, 29–34.

Poynton, A.M., Kartsounis, L.D. & Bridges, P.K. (1995) A prospective clinical study of stereotactic subcaudate tractotomy. *Psychological Medicine*, **25**, 763–770.

Price, L.H. (1989) Lithium augmentation in tricyclic resistant depression. In: *Treatment of Tricyclic-resistant Depression* (ed. I. L. Extin), pp. 51–79. American Psychiatric Press, Washington, DC.

Price, L.H., Conwell, Y. & Nelson, J.C. (1989) Lithium augmentation and combined neuroleptic-tricyclic treatment in delusional depression. *American Journal of Psychiatry*, **140**, 318–322.

Prudic, J., Sackeim, H.A. & Devanand, D.P. (1990) Medication resistance and clinical response to electroconvulsive therapy. *Psychiatry Research*, **31**, 287–296.

Quitkin, F.M., McGrath, P.J. & Stewart, J.W. et al. (1989) Phenelzine and imipramine in mood reactive depressives. *Archives of General Psychiatry*, **46**, 787–793.

Rothschild, A.J., Samson, J.A., Bessette, M.P. & Carter-Campbell, J.T. (1993) Efficacy of the combination of fluoxetine and perphenazine in the treatment of psychotic depression. *Journal of Clinical Psychiatry*, **54**, 338–342.

Sackeim, H.A., Prudic, J. & Devanand, D.P. et al. (1990) The impact of medication resistance and continuation of pharmacotherapy on relapse following response to electroconvulsive therapy in major depression. *Journal of Clinical Psychopharmacology*, **10**, 96–104.

Schmauss, M., Laakman, G. & Dieterle, D. (1988) Effects of α_2-receptor blockade in addition to tricyclic antidepressants in therapy resistant depression. *Journal of Clinical Psychopharmacology*, **8**, 108–111.

Seth, R., Jennings, A.L., Bindman, J., Phillips, J. & Bergmann, K. (1992) Combination treatment with noradrenaline and serotonin reuptake inhibitors in resistant depression. *British Journal of Psychiatry*, **161**, 562–565.

Sethna, E.R. (1974) A study of refractory cases in depressive illness and their response to combined antidepressant treatment. *British Journal of Psychiatry*, **124**, 265–272.

Slutsker, L., Hoesly, F.C., Miller, L., Williams, P., Watson, J.C. & Flemming, D.W. (1990) Eosinophilia-myalgia Syndrome associated with exposure to tryptophan from a single manufacturer. *Journal of the American Medical Association*, **264**, 213–217.

Spiker, D.G., Weiss, J.C. & Dealy, R.S. (1985) The pharmacological treatment of delusional depression. *American Journal of Psychiatry*, **142**, 430–436.

Stein, G. & Bernadt, M. (1993) Lithium augmentation therapy in tricyclic resistant depression: a controlled trial using lithium in lower than normal doses. *British Journal of Psychiatry*, **162**, 634–640.

Sternbach, H. (1991) The serotonin syndrome. *American Journal of Psychiatry*, **148**, 705–713.

Taylor, D. (1995) Selective serotonin reuptake inhibitors and tricyclic antidepressants in combination: interactions and therapeutic uses. *British Journal of Psychiatry*, **167**, 575–580.

Tyrer, P. & Murphy, S. (1990) Efficacy of combined antidepressant therapy in resistant neurotic disorder. *British Journal of Psychiatry*, **156**, 115–118.

Vetulani, J., Stawarz, R.J., Dingell, J.V. & Sulser, P. (1976) A possible common mechanism of action of antidepressant treatments: reduction in sensitivity of noradrenergic cyclic ANP generating system in the rat limbic forebrain. *Archives of Pharmacology*, **293**, 109–114.

Volz, H.-P., Faltus, F., Magyar, I. & Moller, H.-J. (1994) Brofaromine in treatment-resistant depressed patients: a comparative trial vs. tranylcypromine. *Journal of Affective Disorders*, **30**, 209–217.

Wager, S.G. & Klein, D.F. (1988) Treatment refractory patients: affective disorders. *Psychopharmacology Bulletin*, **24**, 69–74.

Weilburg, J.B., Rosenbaum, J.F., Biderman, J., Sachs, G.S., Pollack, M.H. & Kelly, K. (1989) Fluoxetine added to non-MAOI antidepressants converts non-responders to responders: a preliminary report. *Journal of Clinical Psychiatry*, **50**, 447–449.

Weilburg, J.B., Rosenbaum, J.F., Meltzer-Brody, S. & Shushtari, J. (1991) Tricyclic augmentation of fluoxetine. *Annals of Clinical Psychiatry*, **3**, 209–213.

Young, A.H. & Cowen, P.J. (1994) Antidepressant drugs. In: *Side-effects of Drugs Annual 17* (eds J.K. Aronson & C.J. van Boxtel), pp. 16–25. Elsevier, Amsterdam.

Young, A.H. & Cowen, P.J. (1995) Antidepressant drugs. In: *Side-effects of Drugs Annual 18* (eds J.K. Aronson & C.J. van Boxtel), pp. 14–24. Elsevier, Amsterdam.

Zusky, P.M., Biderman, J. & Rosenbaum, J.F. (1988) Adjunct low dose lithium carbonate in treatment-resistant depression: a placebo controlled study. *Journal of Clinical Psychopharmacology*, **8**, 120–124.

12 The efficacy of electroconvulsive therapy

ALLAN I. F. SCOTT

The focus of this chapter is research evidence for the efficacy of electroconvulsive therapy (ECT) in the treatment of depressive illness, but it must be acknowledged at the outset that the clinical use of ECT is heavily influenced by more than pharmacology. Pippard (1992) found a 12-fold difference in the rate of ECT usage between health districts in the South of England. Hermann *et al.* (1995) found a variation of 0.4 to 81.2 patients per 10 000 population among 317 metropolitan areas of the USA; in approximately one-third of these areas no use of ECT was reported in 1988–89. ECT may simply not be available in some parts of the world. Other non-pharmacological factors that affect usage include psychiatric education and training, individual/community prejudice, and legal restraints. Some critics of ECT have suggested that it causes actual brain damage, but recent prospective brain-imaging studies have found no evidence of any structural brain changes after single or repeated courses of ECT (Devanand *et al.*, 1994; Scott, 1995). The conditions necessary to produce the death of neurones after continuous cerebral seizure activity are in no way approached during modified ECT (Devanand *et al.*, 1994).

Early trials

After the introduction of ECT by Cerletti in Rome in 1938, a substantial number of studies of theoretical interest were conducted (see Fink, 1979; Crow & Johnstone, 1986), but uncertainty over diagnosis, heterogeneity of diagnosis, non-random allocation and non-blind assessment of clinical outcome meant that the vast majority were of uncertain relevance to contemporary practice and of no more than historical interest.

Important comparisons with antidepressant drug treatment

It was the introduction of the tricyclic antidepressants and monoamine oxidase inhibitors (MAOIs) that led to a more thorough and methodologically sound assessment of the effectiveness of ECT in the treatment of depressive illness.

Table 12.1 shows the findings from two large-scale, multicentre, random allocation comparisons of ECT with tricyclic and MAOI antidepressant drug treatment and placebo. The study by Greenblatt *et al.* (1964) was conducted among in-patients at three state hospitals around Boston in the USA and the study by the Medical Research Council (MRC; 1965) was conducted among in-patients at 30 hospitals in three regions of England. There were differences between the two studies in entry criteria and the period of assessment, but the results were broadly similar. ECT was associated with the greatest likelihood of marked improvement or symptom resolution. The MRC trial also concluded that ECT had a faster onset of antidepressant effect than imipramine, but the statistical assessment in support of this statement was not provided.

Both studies were carried out more than 30 years ago. Greenblatt and colleagues (1964) reported that depression occurred in the context of manic-depression, involutional melancholia, or schizoaffective disorder in 65% of the patients randomized; 18% suffered a psychoneurotic depressive reaction; and in 16% the depressive diagnoses were mixed. The MRC study randomized patients whose depressed mood was observable to an examiner and accompanied by one of the following features: guilt, sleep disturbance, hypochondriasis, psychomotor retardation or agitation; 43% of patients were rated as severely ill by clinicians at the outset of treatment. A major criticism of the MRC study is that some imipramine-treated patients might have responded better to a higher dose or longer period of treatment; a similar criticism has been made for the dose of phenelzine. Both studies were largely random-allocation, although the placebo arm of the study by Greenblatt and colleagues was added during the second year. Neither patients nor raters could distinguish who was treated with active antidepressant drug or placebo, but both patients and raters knew who was treated by ECT. Crow and Johnstone (1986) have argued that neither study eliminated the possibility that some aspect of treatment other than the induction of the convulsion was responsible for the therapeutic effect.

The other two studies in Table 12.1 have been included because they assessed the antidepressant effect attributable to the convulsion itself by the inclusion of a simulated ECT condition; they also measured the change in depressive symptoms among ECT-treated patients and compared this to the change among imipramine-treated patients. Robin and Harris (1962) reported that two bilateral ECTs combined with placebo tablets led to a greater reduction in Hamilton Rating Scale Depression (HRSD) score than imipramine plus simulated ECT after only 1 week. Unfortunately, neither the depression ratings nor significance test was reported. The dose of imipramine was not stated and the very poor clinical outcome among patients treated by drug plus simulated ECT suggested that this may have been too low. The trial was reported only in summary, and this left considerable methodological uncertainty about

Table 12.1 Important random allocation studies that compared the efficacy of ECT with antidepressant drug treatment.

Authors	Number of patients randomized	Definition of depression	Treatment	Clinical improvement	Significance test	Clinical outcome (%)	Significance test
Robin and Harris (1962)	31 (no details given)	Depression diagnosed by two clinicians	Six twice-weekly bilateral ECTs plus placebo tablets	ECT produced greater reduction in HRSD* score after first week	Not stated	Marked improvement	Not stated
			Imipramine (?dose) plus simulated ECT			66	
						6	
Greenblatt et al. (1964)	281 (mean age, 46 years; 68% female)	Symptomatically severe depression regardless of specific diagnostic category in the absence of organic brain syndrome, alcoholism or drug addiction	Nine or more bilateral ECTs	No data reported		Markedly improved at 8 weeks	Chi-square
			Imipramine, 200–250 mg			76	*P* < 0.01
			Phenelzine, 60–75 mg			49	*P* < 0.01
			Isocarboxazid, 40–50 mg			50	*P* < 0.001
			Placebo tablets			28	*P* < 0.01
						46	

Study	Patients	Diagnosis	Treatment	Result		None or slight symptoms at 4 weeks	
Medical Research Council (1965)	269 (40–69 years; 70% female; in-patients for at least 4 weeks)	Primary depression of less than 18 months' duration and no adequate treatment in previous 6 months. No physical contra-indication to any of the treatments	Four to eight ECTs Imipramine 200 mg Phenelzine, 60 mg	Imipramine 'a slower action than ECT'	Not stated	71 52 30 39	Not stated†
Gangadhar et al. (1982)	32 (22–66 years; 56% female; status not stated)	ICD-9 (WHO, 1978) 296.1 and 296.3, primary affective disorder (Feighner et al., 1972), endogenous depression (Abrams et al., 1979)	Six bilateral ECTs and placebo tablets Simulated ECT, and imipramine (75 mg 1 week then 150 mg 2 weeks)	Change in HRSD score 68% 53%	Not stated, $P < 0.05$	Change in HRSD score after 6 weeks 88 92	Not stated, NSS

* Hamilton Rating Scale for Depression (Hamilton, 1960).

† The difference between ECT and imipramine was just over twice its standard error and the differences between ECT and phenelzine and placebo were three to four times their standard errors.

its significance. The study by Gangadhar *et al.* (1982) was the only methodo-logically sound study in the ECT literature that compared the rates of the antidepressant effects of ECT and a tricyclic antidepressant, although there might now be some concern that the dose of imipramine was increased too slowly. The reduction in HRSD score was clearly and significantly greater among patients treated by six bilateral ECTs over 2 weeks, although no difference was seen from 4 weeks on; by 4 weeks, ECT-treated patients had received eight bilateral treatments and drug-treated patients had been prescribed 75 mg imipramine for the first week, then 150 mg imipramine for another 3 weeks.

In conclusion, the clinical efficacy of ECT in the treatment of depressive illness that requires in-patient treatment was clearly established in two large random-allocation, multicentre trials. These also suggested that the clinical efficacy of ECT was greater than that of imipramine over 4–8 weeks, but this finding must now be treated with caution because more drug-treated patients might have recovered if higher doses had been allowed.

One of the suggested indications for the use of ECT is that it works more quickly than antidepressant drug treatment, and it is disappointing to note that this topic has not received the research attention that it merits; there is preliminary evidence that the rate of onset of antidepressant effect is greater for bilateral ECT given three times a week than moderate doses of imipramine during the first 2 weeks of treatment.

Recent comparisons of real and simulated ECT

Table 12.2 shows the six trials that have been designed specifically to assess the role of electrically induced cerebral seizure activity in the therapeutic effi-cacy of ECT in depressive illness. Each involved the random allocation of at least 25 depressed patients and included reliable outcome measures that were made by raters reported to be unaware of which patients had been treated with real as opposed to simulated ECT. In the three largest studies, almost all the patients had been withdrawn from concomitant antidepressant drug treat-ment. Every study found that real ECT was superior to simulated ECT in at least one major outcome measure, although in one study the difference was not statistically significant (Lambourn & Gill, 1978). The overall conclusion from these studies was that they disprove the suggestion that some non-con-vulsive aspect of ECT such as the therapeutic attention is entirely responsible for the observed antidepressant effect, and they confirm the findings of semi-nal studies of the mode of action of ECT that the induction of cerebral seizure activity contributes to the therapeutic effect. Nevertheless, some of these stud-ies did arouse considerable controversy at the time (see Crow & Johnstone, 1986). The present author would contrast the debate about the finding that depressed patients improved during a course of simulated ECT with the tacit acceptance of the observation that 39% of depressed patients in the MRC trial recovered on placebo tablets alone (so-called spontaneous recovery). Clearly, factors unrelated to the induction of cerebral seizure activity contribute to the clinical improvement seen in depressed patients treated with ECT in the same way that non-pharmacological factors contribute to the clinical improvement seen in depressed patients admitted to hospital and treated with antidepressant drugs.

The first five studies in Table 12.2 have been subjected to detailed methodological criticism by Crow and Johnstone (1986). Eight patients dropped out of the study by Freeman and colleagues for reasons other than rapid clinical improvement, and how these dropouts were treated in the statistical analysis had a considerable bearing on the findings. The study also included depression rating scales that showed a significant advantage in favour of real ECT after two treatments, but Crow and Johnstone were sceptical that a significant clinical difference could appear so early in a course of ECT; they concluded that the result of the study was not nearly as firm as suggested. It was shown subsequently that substantial improvement can occur early in a course of ECT (Rodger *et al.*, 1994), which would lend credibility to the findings based on depression rating scales.

The clinical improvement observed by Lambourn and Gill among patients treated with real ECT was the least of the studies listed in Table 12.2; it was the only study to use a low-dose, brief-pulse electrical stimulation in combination with unilateral electrode placement; Sackeim *et al.* (1987) later showed that a low-dose technique with a higher electrical dose was therapeutically inferior to low-dose treatment with bilateral ECT and associated with a poor clinical response by the end of a course of treatment (Table 12.3).

The clinical description of patients for inclusion in the Northwick Park ECT trial was rigorous and the vast majority of patients (89%) completed the trial. The degree of clinical improvement observed among patients treated with simulated ECT was the greatest of the studies in Table 12.2, and Crow and Johnstone suggested that the relatively small and well-staffed research ward in which the patients were nursed may have contributed to the non-specific therapeutic effects through increased medical and nursing attention.

No information was provided by West (1981) about the procedures for randomization and clinical assessment without knowledge of treatment grouping in what was reported as a single-author study. Crow and Johnstone believed that this diminished the weight that could be attributed to the findings.

The Leicester trial (Brandon *et al.*, 1984) was the largest ever random-allocation comparison of simulated and real ECT in the treatment of depressive illness. Crow and Johnstone have rightly noted that the initial sample was diagnostically wider than that of the Northwick Park trial, although the meth-

Table 12.2 Studies that compared real ECT and simulated ECT— that is, induction of anaesthesia and muscle relaxation, but without the passage of any electricity. The author has expressed, where possible, clinical improvement as percentage change in rating scale scores after six treatments to allow comparison among studies.

Authors	Number of patients randomized	Definition of depression	Drug treatment during ECT	Electrical dose	Treatment	Clinical improvement (%)	Significance test
Freeman et al. (1978)	40 in-patients (20–70 years)	Primary depressive illness, HRSD* score >15	Antidepressant and benzodiazepine	Not known Maximum output high	Bilateral	Patients treated by simulated ECT for first two treatments needed 1.2 more treatments	Student's two-sample t-test, $P < 0.05$
Lambourn and Gill (1978)	32 in- and out-patients (36–68 years)	Depressive psychosis diagnosed by consultant	Benzodiazepine only	Not known Maximum output low	Right unilateral Simulated	HRSD 52 43	Wilcoxon signed rank test, NSS
Johnstone et al. (1980)	70 in-patients (30–69 years)	Depressive illness (MRC, 1965) Primary depressive illness (Feighner et al. 1972). Endogenous depression (Carney et al., 1965).	Benzodiazepine only	Not known Maximum output high	Bilateral Simulated	HRSD 68 56	Analysis of variance after eight ECTs, $P < 0.01$
West (1981)	25 in-patients (mean age, 52 years)	Primary depression (Feighner et al., 1972)	Antidepressant and benzodiazepine	Not known Maximum output high	Bilateral Simulated	BDI† 59 8	Not stated, $P < 0.002$

						HRSD*	
Brandon et al. (1984)	97 in-patients (mean age, 54 years)	Present State Examination:‡ neurotic and endogenous depression	Benzodiazepine only	Not known Maximum output high	Bilateral	60%§	Analysis of variance after 8 ECTs, $P = 0.0001$
					Simulated	23%§	
						MADRS¶	Analysis of variance
Gregory et al. (1985)	69 in-patients (all under 65 years)	Depressive illness (MRC, 1965) of more than 1 month's duration	Benzodiazepine only (n = 64) and other (n = 5)	Not known Maximum output high	Bilateral	73%‖	$P < 0.005$
					Right unilateral	71%‖	$P < 0.005$
					Simulated	34%‖	

* Hamilton Rating Scale for Depression (Hamilton, 1960).
† Beck Depression Inventory (Beck et al., 1961).
‡ Wing et al. (1974).
§ Interpolated from HRSD scores after four and eight treatments.
¶ Montgomery and Asberg Depression Rating Scale (Montgomery & Asberg, 1979).
‖ Twenty-five patients received fewer than six treatments and ratings after six treatments were available for only 34 patients. MADRS scores were also significantly less after four unilateral ($P < 0.01$) and four bilateral ($P < 0.001$) compared with simulated ECT ($n = 58$).

Table 12.3 Important studies of the effect of electrical dose on the clinical effectiveness of ECT in depressive illness. The author has expressed clinical improvement as percentage change in HRSD score after six treatments to allow comparison among studies.

Author	Number of patients randomized	Definition of depression	Treatment	Electrical dose	Clinical improvement (%)	Significance test	Clinical outcome (%)	Significance test
Robin and De Tissera (1982)	63 in-patients (20–70 years)	Primary depression diagnosed by consultant	Bilateral	Chopped-sine wave (450–900 mC).	79	Kruskal–Wallis analysis of variance, $P < 0.02$	Course completed by six treatments 83	Kruskal–Wallis analysis of variance on total number of treatments, $P < 0.01$
			Bilateral	Low-energy pulse (27–52 mC).	52		41	
			Bilateral	High-energy pulse (185–275 mC).	83		66	
Sackeim *et al.* (1987)	52 in-patients (mean age, 61 years)	Research Diagnostic Criteria (Spitzer *et al.*, 1978), primary major depressive disorder: HRSD score >18	Bilateral	Threshold	55	Student's *t*-test, $P = 0.02$	Clinical response by end of course* 70	Chi-square, $P = 0.002$
			Right unilateral	Threshold	34		28	

Study	Patients	Diagnosis	Electrode placement	Stimulus dose		Statistical analysis	Clinical response by end of course	Statistical test
Abrams et al. (1991)	38 in-patients (all men; mean age, 61 years)	DSM-III: major depression, melancholic subtype, HRSD score >15	Bilateral	378 mC	79	Repeated measures analysis of variance, NSS	78	Chi-square, NSS
			Right unilateral	378 mC	68		65	
Sackeim et al. (1993)	100 in-patients (mean age, 56 years)	Research Diagnostic Criteria: primary major depressive disorder, HRSD score > 18	Right unilateral	Threshold	31	Newman–Keuls comparison of covariate-adjusted group means	Clinical response by end of course* 17	Chi-square
			Right unilateral	2.5 × threshold	59	$P = 0.01$	43	$P = 0.05$
			Bilateral	Threshold	65	$P < 0.05$	65	$P = 0.001$
			Bilateral	2.5 × threshold	72	$P < 0.001$	63	$P = 0.001$

* Defined as at least 60% reduction in HRSD scores and with a final score of less than 17%.

odology was sound. The clinical improvement observed among those treated by real bilateral ECT was similar to that observed in the Northwick Park trial, but the difference in clinical improvement between those treated with six simulated and six bilateral ECT was three times greater in the Leicester trial than that observed in the Northwick Park trial; as noted above, greater clinical improvement was seen among patients treated with simulated ECT at Northwick Park for reasons speculated upon above.

The Nottingham ECT study (Gregory *et al.*, 1985) used inclusion criteria similar to the MRC study, although the age range was extended to include patients younger than 40 years and an additional entry criterion was stipulated that the index episode of depression had lasted for at least 4 weeks. Unfortunately, the results cannot be directly compared with the earlier study, which did not report change in total rating scale scores during the course of ECT. Twenty-five patients (36% of the total sample) were withdrawn before they had received six treatments. Sufficient data from earlier in the course of treatment were reported to confirm that clinical improvement in those treated with ECT was significantly greater than among those treated with simulated ECT after only four treatments. The effect size of the difference between clinical improvement in bilateral and simulated ECT was much closer to that observed in the Leicester study than that observed in the Northwick Park study. The clinical improvement observed after six right unilateral ECTs with a high-output ECT machine was greater than that observed by Lambourn and Gill (1978), when treatment was given with a low-output ECT machine; the importance of electrical dose in determining the clinical effectiveness of unilateral ECT will be discussed in detail below.

In conclusion, the role of the electrically induced convulsion in the therapeutic efficacy of ECT was established by these six random-allocation comparisons of simulated and real ECT in which the clinical improvement observed among patients treated with real ECT was always greater than that observed among patients treatment with simulated ECT; the only study in which the greater improvement was not statistically significant used a technique of unilateral ECT that has subsequently been shown to be inadequate. The first five of these studies have been subject to detailed methodological scrutiny by Crow and Johnstone (1986) and, writing 10 years later, the criticisms of greatest pertinence remain the uncertainty to what extent the assessments of outcome were made without knowledge of treatment in the study by West, and the importance in the statistical handling of early withdrawals from treatment and its impact upon the effect size.

Duration of clinical effect

Early reports of the use of ECT in depressive illness noted that relapse was sometimes a problem and this was later quantified in studies conducted with the then newly introduced tricyclic antidepressants. Seager and Bird (1962) observed that 11 of 16 patients (69%) who had been successfully treated for depression by ECT relapsed within 6 months while prescribed placebo tablets in contrast to patients prescribed imipramine, of whom only two out of 12 (17%) relapsed. An important study by Barton *et al.* (1973) monitored the progress of 50 patients who had suffered a primary depressive illness that had been successfully treated with ECT; no treatment for depression was offered during follow-up, although hypnotics were prescribed. Twenty-three patients (46% of the sample) relapsed without treatment within 12 weeks, and 16 of those who relapsed (70%) did so within 2 weeks of the end of the course of ECT.

The Northwick Park, Leicester and Nottingham ECT studies all included assessment in the 6 months after ECT, although treatment was then open for all patients. No significant advantage was found for ECT-treated patients. Crow and Johnstone (1986) concluded that the effects of the induced convulsion were of limited duration.

A distinction is now made between symptomatic remission and actual recovery from the index episode of depressive illness. Among patients who are symptom-free after treatment with ECT, as many will be in potentially temporary remission as fully recovered and continuation antidepressant drug treatment ought to be standard (Royal College of Psychiatrists Special Committee on ECT 1995). ECT is just like any other pharmacological treatment for depressive illness in this regard.

Selection of depressed patients for ECT

There have been many attempts to correlate clinical features, physiological measures, or personality characteristics with successful outcome after ECT (Fink, 1979). Early studies often included patients suffering from schizophrenia and neurotic conditions as well as patients suffering from depressive illness and many of the putative correlates with recovery were simply characteristics of depressed patients as opposed to schizophrenic or neurotic patients. None of the studies has ever included a comparison group of patients who received no treatment at all to investigate the possibility that a putative correlate of a good outcome was actually a correlate of the likelihood of spontaneous recovery. Crow and Johnstone (1986) have argued that only the inclusion of a group of patients treated by simulated ECT will answer the potential objection that any correlate of a good outcome is simply a correlate of a good outcome to any physical treatment for depressive illness. A combined analysis of the Leicester and Northwick Park trials found that depressed patients with either retardation or delusions accounted for most of the difference in clinical improvement between the patients treated by real and simulated ECT. The difference in clinical improvement between real and simulated ECT in depressed patients without retardation or delusions was not statistically significant (Buchan *et al.*, 1992).

This finding stimulated a further analysis of the results from the Nottingham trial (O'Leary *et al.*, 1995), with different results. There was a marked and statistically significant difference in clinical improvement among depressed patients without psychomotor retardation or delusions between real and simulated ECT. The paper also contained a useful comparison of percentage improvement in different categories of depressed patients among the Leicester, Northwick Park and Nottingham trials. The major difference among the three trials was the extent of the clinical improvement in patients treated with simulated ECT at Northwick Park; possible reasons have already been discussed above. The average percentage change in HDRS score was 57%, whereas it was 30% in the Leicester trial and 38% in the Nottingham trial. O'Leary and colleagues suggested that the different patterns of improvement with simulated and real ECT among the trials might also be explained by differences in the study samples in factors such as the length of stay in hospital before ECT, previous failure of the index episode to respond to antidepressant drug treatment, and a past history of a good response to ECT. They noted that about three-quarters of the patients treated with simulated ECT in the Leicester and Nottingham trials had failed to improve with antidepressant drug treatment; a comparison figure for the Northwick Park trial was not available. This was an important observation, and it is unfortunate that no definition of antidepressant drug failure was provided in either the Leicester or Nottingham trials.

In conclusion, there was general agreement among the trials that in moderate to severe depressive illness that required in-patient treatment, patients with delusions, agitation or retardation improved substantially after real bilateral ECT and this improvement was greater than that seen after simulated ECT. This is part of the evidence in support of the recommendation that the best predictor of recovery after ECT is the presence and number of the typical features of depressive illness itself (Scott, 1989). It has not been established that any one symptom or sign of depressive illness identifies depressed patients who will improve substantially with real as opposed to simulated ECT; it may be that other clinical factors such as the length of the index episode, earlier treatment resistance during the index illness, and a past history of good ECT response also influence the likelihood of recovery.

The dexamethosone suppression test renewed interest in potential biological predictors of recovery. There were early promising reports of an association between non-suppression before treatment and early normalization during a course of ECT with a good clinical outcome, but later studies found no association between non-suppression and either immediate outcome or outcome 6 months after ECT (Scott, 1989). In summary, there are no established physiological measures or tests that are superior to clinical criteria in the selection of depressed patients for whom ECT would be an effective treatment.

ECT in the elderly

In the author's experience, 30% of contemporary depressed patients treated by ECT are older than 65 years, and it is disappointing to note the lack of research data pertaining to the elderly depressed patient. It is clear that the vast majority of depressed patients included in the studies of real and simulated ECT were under the age of 70 years (see Table 12.2). Benbow (1989) reviewed the use of ECT in the treatment of depressive illness in old age and concluded that the elderly respond to ECT at least as well as younger people. She also noted that the small number of studies that had considered which clinical features might correlate with a good response to ECT found that it was the classical cluster of so-called endogenous features that were associated with a good outcome; however, psychic anxiety was not necessarily the unfavourable feature as suggested in the early literature on the prediction of ECT response. The largest retrospective review of elderly depressed patients treated by ECT was not included in her review; Kramer (1987) described the clinical outcome of 50 elderly depressed patients, 22 of whom were at least 75 years old. Kramer himself noted that retrospective case reports were somewhat limited, but concluded that ECT was safe and very effective in the elderly patients he described. Physical illness is more prevalent in elderly depressed patients and the safe practice of ECT is described elsewhere (Royal College of Psychiatrists Special Committee on ECT, 1995).

ECT in young people

There are no randomized comparative studies of the use of ECT in depressed adolescents or children, and this section is included because of a recent debate about the use of ECT in depressed young people. The literature consists of case reports and descriptive studies that began to appear in the early years after the introduction of ECT, and these have been reviewed by Tomb (1991). The efficacy and potential role of ECT in the management of depressive illness in young people cannot be established from these reports; ECT had been given safely in most cases, but there were also a few reports of prolonged seizures. It has been suggested that ECT should only be considered for young people when other treatments have failed, and specific guidance has been given about consent and the second opinions in those depressed people under the age of 16 years (Royal College of Psychiatrists Special Committee on ECT, 1995). The present author would draw attention to the warning that young people may have low seizure thresholds and that young people ought to be treated with the most up-to-date ECT machines that allow treatment with low electrical doses.

Electrical dose and clinical efficacy

The electrical stimulation produced by contemporary ECT machines differs from that of traditional ECT machines, both in the waveform of the stimulation and in the intensity of electrical energy. Moreover, the amount of electrical energy supplied by contemporary ECT machines is preset by the treating doctor (hence the term 'constant current'), whereas it is the voltage applied to the head that was standard in traditional ECT machines (hence the term 'constant voltage'); the electrical charge delivered by traditional machines therefore varies inversely with the impedance between the electrodes. Constant-voltage ECT machines usually delivered a sine wave or modified sine wave stimulation and contemporary constant-current ECT machines deliver electrical stimulation in the form of a train of brief square-wave pulses that induce cerebral seizure activity more efficiently (see Royal College of Psychiatrists Special Committee on ECT, 1995).

The ECT literature does contain reports that early constant-current ECT machines were not as effective as traditional constant-voltage ECT machines and also that some depressed patients who failed to recover with brief-pulse stimulation subsequently went on to recover after treatment with constant-voltage ECT, although treatments were often complicated by a switch from unilateral to bilateral electrode placement (see Scott *et al.*, 1992). A few prospective studies have found no difference in therapeutic efficacy between sine-wave and brief-pulse stimulation (see Scott *et al.*, 1992), although Andrade *et al.* (1988) found that more patients recovered when treated with sine-wave stimulation. The treatments also differed, however, in another important aspect in that the electrical dose delivered with sine-wave stimulation was substantially higher than that with brief-pulse stimulation.

All of the studies listed in Table 12.2 used a constant-voltage ECT machine, thus the actual dose of electrical energy delivered to patients was not known. One of the few early studies that included any attempt to quantify the actual doses of electrical energy delivered was conducted by Robin and DeTissera (1982).[1] Although the average length of the convulsions were almost identical

---

[1] Charge = current × effective duration of current flow.
In brief-pulse current, charge (milliCoulombs) = current (amperes) × pulse width (milliseconds) × frequency (Hz) × stimulus duration (seconds).

in each of the three treatment groups, the patients treated with low-energy pulses had the slowest rate of improvement and the poorest final outcome (see Table 12.3). The authors suggested that the amount of electrical energy influenced the therapeutic outcome of ECT; they speculated that the induction of a convulsion was necessary to produce a therapeutic effect with ECT, but that the convulsion itself need not necessarily produce the therapeutic effect itself.

Robin and DeTissera also suggested that the convulsive threshold may have a bearing on the outcome of ECT. Sackeim *et al.* (1987) developed an empirical titration method to establish the minimum amount of electrical energy to induce a convulsion of defined minimum length at the outset of a course of treatment. Electrical stimulation consisted of a standard current of 800 mAmp delivered in 1.5 ms square-wave pulses, and the dose was adjusted firstly by frequency and then by length of stimulation. Their study was novel in that the electrical charge delivered was adjusted for each patient to just exceed the threshold, defined empirically at the start of a course of treatment. When the minimum electrical dose necessary to produce generalized cerebral seizure activity was used (so-called threshold dosing), bilateral ECT led to a greater rate of clinical improvement after six treatments and significantly greater likelihood of recovery by the end of a course of treatment. The treatment groups did not differ in the average length of convulsion or cerebral seizure activity measured by single-channel electroencephalogram, and the authors suggested this challenged the claim that the induction of generalized cerebral seizure activity was sufficient in itself for the antidepressant effect of ECT.

Their next study tested the hypothesis that for both unilateral and bilateral electrode placements, a higher electrical dose leads to more rapid clinical improvement (Sackeim *et al.*, 1993). The hypothesis was supported for both electrode placements (see Table 12.3), and confirmed the weak antidepressant effect of threshold right unilateral ECT. The likelihood of recovery after right unilateral ECT with a stimulation 2.5 times threshold was greater than that seen in right unilateral ECT with threshold stimulation. The likelihood of recovery after high-dose right unilateral ECT was not significantly different to that after either of the bilateral treatments, but the final HRSD score 1 week after completion of treatment was significantly higher than after either of the bilateral treatments. This suggested that even high-dose right unilateral ECT may not be as efficacious as bilateral ECT. Detailed cognitive assessments were also carried out that showed that patients treated with the higher dose of unilateral treatment took nearly twice as long to become fully orientated than did patients treated with threshold unilateral treatment. Patients treated with either of the bilateral treatments took twice as long again to become fully orientated. In general, electrode placement had a more pronounced and persistent effect on cognition than dosage; these findings were important because they confirmed that unilateral ECT has an advantage over bilateral ECT by minimizing adverse cognitive effects.

The work of Sackeim and colleagues has stimulated interest in the value of the routine empirical titration of the seizure threshold at the outset of treatment, particularly for unilateral ECT. The need for such a procedure has been questioned by Abrams (1992), who argued that a fixed high-dose stimulus with unilateral electrode placement optimized the risk-benefit balance for ECT. He cited his own earlier study that found no significant difference between bilateral and right unilateral ECT when both were given with a fixed high-dose stimulus (see Table 12.3). Although there were no statistically significant differences between bilateral and right unilateral ECT, the rate of improvement and likelihood of recovery by the end of a course of treatment were both greater for bilateral ECT, and these differences may have become statistically significant if a larger sample of patients had been recruited.

Sackeim *et al.* (1993) have also argued that it is desirable to adjust the electrical dose for each patient to take account of their seizure threshold to minimize adverse cognitive effects. Their later study showed that the adverse cognitive effects that were dose-related were related not to the absolute dose administered but the extent to which the dose exceeded the seizure threshold. They also noted that the initial seizure threshold varied widely and that some patients have very low thresholds; a high fixed dose in such patients might lead to marked adverse cognitive effects that were disproportionate to the therapeutic benefit. It was important to note that Abrams *et al.* (1991) did not assess the extent of adverse cognitive effects after fixed high-dose stimulation.

ECT after a failure to respond to antidepressant drug treatment

This is a topic of considerable contemporary interest, particularly in clinical settings where ECT is not available to patients as a first choice treatment for depressive illness. The MRC clinical trial of treatment of depressive illness reported, albeit only as a summary, that half the patients who had failed to recover with imipramine subsequently recovered when treated by ECT. This contrasted with the 71% recovery rate among patients who were treated with ECT as a first treatment. A salient criticism of this and other similar studies is that the dose and/or duration of antidepressant drug treatment were inadequate to reliably categorize illnesses as resistant to antidepressant drug treatment. Prudic *et al.* (1990) prospectively categorized 53 depressed patients with major depression of endogenous subtype into those who had and had not received an adequate trial of an antidepressant drug; the minimum requirement to meet the definition of an adequate antidepressant trial was the equivalent of imipramine 200 mg for 4 weeks in nonpsychotic depressive illness. Applying their criteria for response as described in Table 12.3, they found that 86% of patients who had not received an adequate course of an antidepressant drug for the index episode went on to recover, whereas only 50% of the patients who had received an adequate trial before bilateral ECT went on to recover. There were, however, other differences between the two groups of patients: the group who had failed to respond to an antidepressant drug was on average younger, had a lower prevalence of psychosis, and had been depressed twice as long; the authors reported that none of these was found to be statistically significant predictor of improvement in depression rating scores in regression analyses.

In contrast, Kindler *et al.* (1991) found no statistically significant difference in the likelihood of recovery after a course of bilateral ECT between patients who had or had not received an adequate trial of an antidepressant drug. Those who did not recover after a course of ECT were more depressed at the outset of the course of ECT and had been depressed longer before ECT. Although these two studies used the same definition of recovery after ECT, they were not directly comparable because they used a different scale to rate the intensity of pharmacological treatment before ECT.

In conclusion, the available literature confirms the clinical impression that patients who have already failed to recover with antidepressant drug treatment can subsequently recover when treated with bilateral ECT, but that the likelihood of recovery may be less than among the generality of depressed patients treated with ECT. It has not been shown conclusively that this association is the result of treatment resistance itself rather than another related factor: for example, that patients who have already received another form of treatment before ECT have been depressed longer than patients who are offered ECT as a first treatment.

Prescription of ECT and its antidepressant effect

In the UK, bilateral ECT is usually given twice weekly, whereas in the USA it is usually given three times a week. Until recently, the factors that influence the onset and rate of the antidepressant effect of ECT have been little studied, although the available evidence has been reviewed elsewhere (Scott & Whalley, 1993).

It was once claimed that there is a delay in the onset of any antidepressant effect, although it has now been recognized that marked clinical improvement can occur after only three bilateral treatments (Rodger *et al.*, 1994). Gangadhar *et al.* (1993) compared the clinical improvement in depressed patients of melancholic subtype who were randomly allocated to thrice-weekly bilateral ECT or twice-weekly bilateral ECT plus one simulated ECT each week. Patients treated with real ECT twice weekly improved just as quickly as patients treated thrice weekly, although it must be noted that stimulation was given with a constant-voltage ECT machine that presumably delivered a high electrical dose. In contrast, Lerer *et al.* (1995) found that thrice-weekly bilateral ECT with brief-pulse stimulation about 1.5 times the seizure threshold led to a more rapid antidepressant effect after 2 weeks. Adverse cognitive effects were more marked in the group treated thrice weekly, and there was also a cumulative impairment in some aspects of cognition later in the course of treatment. The authors concluded that twice-weekly bilateral ECT was preferred for routine clinical practice unless the need for rapid clinical improvement was pressing.

Depressive illness which does not respond to ECT

This topic arises in two ways in clinic practice. The first concerns at what stage to abandon a course of ECT if no clinical improvement occurs. The second concerns treatment-resistant depressive illness, when an earlier course of ECT was recorded as producing no improvement. Only a few guiding principles can be given because of the lack of appropriate research. First, a depressive illness ought not to be considered as resistant to ECT until the patient has received bilateral ECT. Price and McAllister (1986) showed clearly that depressed patients who failed to improve with brief-pulse unilateral ECT may subsequently recover when treated by bilateral ECT; it is regrettable that treatment was complicated from a switch to brief-pulse stimulation to sine-wave stimulation. Neverthless, this finding was compatible with later research that suggested that even high-dose unilateral ECT may not be as efficacious as bilateral ECT. Second, ECT needs to be properly administered; that is, it must be confirmed that a generalized tonic clonic convulsion was observed after each stimulation. The use of the cuff technique and electroencephalogram have definite advantages in this respect. Third, there is the actual number of properly administered treatments. The Royal College of Psychiatrists noted that in the past it had been suggested that no more than eight properly administered treatments be given in the absence of any clinical improvement, although the American Psychiatric Association (1990) advised that the need for more treatments be re-assessed after 6–10 treatments. Devanand *et al.* (1991) found that most patients who do not improve with typical courses of bilateral ECT have previously failed to improve with antidepressant drug treatment; they suggested that 15 or more bilateral treatments with a dose of electricity 150% above the seizure threshold may be necessary. In contrast, Abrams (1992) believed that if no substantial antidepressant effect had been observed in a case of typical depressive illness after 12 treatments, then it was prudent to withhold further treatment for several days in order to observe the patient.

Practical issues

The following practical issues arise from the studies which have been reviewed in this chapter.

1   The best indicators of the likelihood of recovery from depressive illness after ECT are the number and severity of symptoms and signs of depressive illness itself.

2   Whether or not ECT can bring about clinical improvement in certain types of depressive illness that could not have been achieved by other means is yet to be clearly established. If one symptom or sign of depressive illness alone can be expected to discriminate between patients who improve with real ECT and not with simulated ECT, then the presence of depressive delusions is the most promising candidate. Patients with visible psychomotor change also improve significantly more with real as opposed to simulated ECT, but there is no consensus about whether these impairments can identify those patients who will improve specifically with ECT. The lack of consensus may be because clinical features other than signs and symptoms of depressive illness are related to likelihood of recovery—for example, the length of the index episode, an earlier failure to improve with antidepressant drug treatment, and a past history of a good response to ECT.

3   All the published comparisons of antidepressant drug treatment and ECT in the treatment of depressive illness can be criticized because the upper doses allowed were less than recommended today, leading to the criticism that more drug-treated patients might have recovered if higher doses had been used. There is preliminary evidence that thrice-weekly bilateral ECT leads to a greater clinical improvement in the first 2 weeks of treatment than a moderate dose of imipramine.

4   A common contemporary indication for ECT in depressive illness is an earlier failure to improve with antidepressant drug treatment, and it is disappointing to note the lack of methodologically sound research on this topic. There is clear evidence that patients who have not recovered after 200 mg of imipramine over 4 weeks can recover if treated subsequently with bilateral ECT. The extent to which a failure to improve with antidepressant drug treatment influences the likelihood of recovery after ECT is unresolved, but it seems likely that the rate of recovery is less than that seen among patients who receive ECT as a first choice treatment. It has not been clearly established that treatment resistance itself reduces the likelihood of recovery rather than the length of the index episode, and there is also debate about the actual definition of treatment resistance.

5   The importance of induced cerebral seizure activity in contributing to the therapeutic efficacy has been clearly established in studies that have compared the antidepressant effect of real vs. simulated ECT. It is also now

generally accepted that although cerebral seizure activity itself is a necessary prerequisite for maximum therapeutic efficacy, it is not sufficient in itself to guarantee this. The electrical dose used to induce cerebral seizure activity influences the rate of antidepressant effect in both unilateral and bilateral ECT and is critical in determining the final outcome after a course of unilateral ECT. There is still an unresolved debate about how this research evidence should influence the routine clinical practice of ECT. Most critics advocate stimulus dosing where the electrical dosage is adjusted for each patient to take account of that individual patient's seizure threshold. Fixed high-dose stimulation has also been advocated. The debate will be resolved if it is shown that stimulus dosing leads to fewer or less marked adverse cognitive effects than fixed high-dose stimulation. Techniques of empirical dose titration have been illustrated elsewhere (Royal College of Psychiatrists Special Committee on ECT 1995).

6   While unilateral electrode placement has a clearly established advantage over bilateral placement in that it causes less cognitive impairment, it is yet to be established that a technique of unilateral ECT is as effective as bilateral ECT in terms of clinical improvement by the end of a course of treatment. If the minimization of adverse cognitive effects is an important consideration for an individual patient, high-dose unilateral ECT may be prescribed initially; a switch to bilateral ECT may be indicated later in the course of treatment if clinical improvement is slight or slow.

7   Bilateral ECT with brief-pulse stimulation can be given twice weekly without any cumulative cognitive impairment and can be recommended as an appropriate frequency in routine clinical practice. If a rapid onset of antidepressant effect is of paramount importance, the frequency of ECT can be increased to thrice weekly at least in the early stage of treatment.

8   About 30% of contemporary depressed patients treated by ECT are elderly and it is disappointing that little specific research has been conducted in this group. The minimization of adverse cognitive effects is clearly a pertinent issue and the advantages and disadvantages of twice- and thrice-weekly bilateral ECT have not been investigated in the elderly.

9   Continuation antidepressant drug treatment is essential after recovery with ECT to lessen the substantial likelihood of relapse in the early weeks and months after successful treatment. A common contemporary indication for ECT is an earlier failure to improve with antidepressant drug treatment and the appropriate pharmacological management of the continuation phase in patients who subsequently respond to ECT has not been adequately researched.

References

Abrams, R., Swartz, C.M. & Vedak, C. (1991) Antidepressant effects of high-dose right unilateral electroconvulsive therapy. *Archives of General Psychiatry*, **48**, 746–748.

Abrams, R. (1992) *Electroconvulsive Therapy*, 2nd edn. Oxford University Press, Oxford.

Abrams, R., Taylor, M.A. & Hayman, N. *et al.* (1979) Unipolar mania revisited. *Journal of Affective Disorders*, **1**, 59–68.

American Psychiatric Association (1990) *Clinical Guidelines for the Practice of ECT*. American Psychiatric Association, Washington, DC.

Andrade, C., Gangadhar, B.N., Subbakrishna, D.K. *et al.* (1988) A double-blind comparison of sinusoidal wave and brief-pulse electroconvulsive therapy in endogenous depression. *Convulsive Therapy*, **4**, 297–305.

Barton, J.L., Mehta, S. & Snaith, R.P. (1973) The prophylactic value of extra ECT in depressive illness. *Acta Psychiatrica Scandinavica*, **49**, 386–392.

Beck, A.T., Ward, C.H., Mendelson, M. *et al.* (1961) An inventory for measuring depression. *Archives of General Psychiatry*, **4**, 561–571.

Benbow, S.M. (1989) The role of electroconvulsive therapy in the treatment of depressive illness in old age. *British Journal of Psychiatry*, **155**, 147–152.

Brandon, S., Cowley, P., McDonald, C. *et al.* (1984) Electroconvulsive therapy: results in depressive illness from the Leicestershire trial. *British Medical Journal*, **288**, 22–25.

Buchan, H., Johnstone, E.C., McPherson, K. *et al.* (1992) Who benefits from electroconvulsive therapy? Combined results of the Leicester and Northwick Park trials. *British Journal of Psychiatry*, **160**, 355–359.

Carney, M.W.P., Roth, M. & Garside, R.F. (1965) The diagnosis of depressive syndromes and the prediction of ECT response. *British Journal of Psychiatry*, **111**, 659–674.

Crow, T.J. & Johnstone, E.C. (1986) Controlled trials of electroconvulsive therapy. *New York Academy of Sciences*, **462**, 12–29.

Devanand, D.P., Dwork, A.J., Hutchinson, E.R. *et al.* (1994) Does ECT alter brain structure? *American Journal of Psychiatry*, **151**, 957–970.

Devanand, D.P., Sackeim, H.A. & Prudic, J. (1991) Electroconvulsive therapy in the treatment-resistant patient. *Psychiatric Clinics of North America*, **15**, 905–923.

Feighner, J.P., Robins, E., Guze, S.B. *et al.* (1972) Diagnosic criteria for use in psychiatric research. *Archives of General Psychiatry*, **26**, 57–63.

Fink, M. (1979) *Convulsive Therapy: Theory and Practice*. Raven Press, New York.

Freeman, C.P.L., Basson, J.V. & Crighton, A. (1978) Double-blind controlled trial of electroconvulsive therapy and simulated ECT in depressive illness. *Lancet*, **i**, 738–740.

Gangadhar, B.N., Kapur, R.L. & Kalyanasundaram, S. (1982) Comparison of electroconvulsive therapy with imipramine in endogenous depression: a double-blind study. *British Journal of Psychiatry*, **141**, 367–371.

Gangadhar, B.N., Janakiramaiah, N., Subbakrishna, D.K. *et al.* (1993) Twice vs. thrice weekly ECT in melancholia: a double-blind prospective comparison. *Journal of Affective Disorders*, **27**, 273–278.

Greenblatt, M., Grosser, G.H. & Wechsler, H. (1964) Differential response of hospitalized depressed patients to somatic therapy. *American Journal of Psychiatry*, **120**, 935–943.

Gregory, S., Shawcross, C.R. & Gill, D. (1985) The Nottingham electroconvulsive therapy study: a double-blind comparison of bilateral, unilateral and simulated ECT in depressive illness. *British Journal of Psychiatry*, **146**, 520–524.

Hamilton, M. (1960) A rating scale for depression. *Journal of Neurology, Neurosurgery and Psychiatry*, **23**, 56–62.

Hermann, R.C., Dorwart, R.A., Hoover, C.W. *et al.* (1995) Variation in ECT use in the United States. *American Journal of Psychiatry*, **152**, 869–875.

Johnstone, E.C., Deakin, J.F.W., Lawler, P. *et al.* (1980) The Northwick Park electroconvulsive therapy trial. *Lancet*, **ii**, 317–320.

Kindler, S., Shapira, B., Hadjez, J. *et al.* (1991) Factors influencing response to bilateral electroconvulsive therapy in major depression. *Convulsive Therapy*, **7**, 245–254.

Kramer, B.A. (1987) Electroconvulsive therapy use in geriatric depression. *The Journal of Nervous and Mental Disease*, **175**, 233–235.

Lambourn, J. & Gill, D. (1978) A controlled comparison of simulated and real ECT. *British Journal of Psychiatry*, **133**, 514–519.

Lerer, B., Shapira, B., Calev, A. *et al.* (1995) Antidepressant and cognitive effects of twice- vs. three-times-weekly ECT. *American Journal of Psychiatry*, **152**, 564–570.

Medical Research Council (1965) Clinical trial of the treatment of depressive illness. *British Medical Journal*, **i**, 881–886.

Montgomery, S.A. & Asberg, M. (1979) A new depression scale designed to be sensitive to change.

British Journal of Psychiatry, **134**, 382–389.

O'Leary, D., Gill, D., Gregory, S. *et al.* (1995) Which depressed patients respond to ECT? The Nottingham results. *Journal of Affective Disorders*, **33**, 245–250.

Pippard, J. (1992) Audit of electroconvulsive treatment in two National Health Service Regions. *British Journal of Psychiatry*, **160**, 621–637.

Price, T.R.P. & McAllister, W. (1986) Response of depressed patients to sequential unilateral non-dominant brief-pulse and bilateral sinusoidal ECT. *Journal of Clinical Psychiatry*, **47**, 182–186.

Prudic, J., Sackeim, H.A. & Devanand, D.P. (1990) Medication resistance and clinical response to electroconvulsive therapy. *Psychiatry Research*, **31**, 287–296.

Robin, A. & DeTissera, S. (1982) A double-blind controlled comparison of the therapeutic effects of low and high energy electroconvulsive therapies. *British Journal of Psychiatry*, **141**, 357–366.

Robin, A.A. & Harris, J.A. (1962) A controlled trial of imipramine and electroplexy. *Journal of Mental Science*, **108**, 217–219.

Rodger, C.R., Scott, A.I.F. & Whalley, L.J. (1994) Is there a delay in the onset of the antidepressant effect of electroconvulsive therapy? *British Journal of Psychiatry*, **164**, 106–109.

Royal College of Psychiatrists Special Committee on ECT (1995) *The ECT Handbook*. Royal College of Psychiatrists, London.

Sackeim, H.A., Decina, P., Canzler, M. *et al.* (1987) Effects of electrode placement on the efficacy of titrated, low-dose ECT. *American Journal of Psychiatry*, **144**, 1449–1455.

Sackeim, H.A., Prudic, J., Devanand, D.P. *et al.* (1993) Effects of stimulus intensity and electrode placement on the efficacy and cognitive effects of electroconvulsive therapy. *New England Journal of Medicine*, **328**, 839–846.

Scott, A.I.F. (1989) Which depressed patients will respond to electroconvulsive therapy? The search for biological predictors of recovery. *British Journal of Psychiatry*, **154**, 8–17.

Scott, A.I.F. (1995) Does ECT alter brain structure? *American Journal of Psychiatry*, **152**, 1403.

Scott, A.I.F. & Whalley, L.J. (1993) The onset and rate of the antidepressant effect of electroconvulsive therapy: a neglected topic of research. *British Journal of Psychiatry*, **162**, 725–732.

Scott, A.I.F., Rodger, C.R., Stocks, R.H. *et al.* (1992) Is old-fashioned electroconvulsive therapy more efficacious? A randomised comparative study of bilateral brief-pulse and bilateral sine-wave treatments. *British Journal of Psychiatry*, **160**, 360–364.

Seager, C.P. & Bird, R.L. (1962) Imipramine with electrical treatment in depression: a controlled trial. *Journal of Mental Science*, **108**, 704–707.

Spitzer, R.L., Endicott, J. & Robins, E. (1978) Research diagnostic criteria: rationale and reliability. *Archives of General Psychiatry*, **35**, 773–782.

Tomb, D.A. (1991) Other organic treatments. In: *Child and Adolescent Psychiatry: A Comprehensive Textbook* (ed. M. Lewis), pp. 914–917. Williams & Wilkins, London.

West, E.D. (1981) Electroconvulsive therapy in depression: a double-blind controlled trial. *British Medical Journal*, **282**, 355–357.

Wing, J.K., Cooper, J.E. & Sartorius, N. (1974) *The Measurement and Classification of Psychiatric Symptoms*. Cambridge University Press, Cambridge.

World Health Organization (1978) *Mental Disorders: Glossary and Guide to their Classification in Accordance with the Ninth Revision of the International Classification of Diseases*. World Health Organization, Geneva.

13 Lithium and other drug treatments for recurrent affective disorder

JOHN COOKSON

Mood stabilizers are drugs which are used in the prophylaxis of recurrent affective disorders. They include lithium, certain anticonvulsants—particularly carbamazepine and valproate—antipsychotic drugs and monoamine re-uptake inhibitors (MARIs) and, on a less scientific basis, calcium antagonists, monoamine oxidase inhibitors and thyroid hormone. The main mood stabilizers are best known for their acute antimanic properties, but some have antidepressant actions. Their prophylactic use is primarily in bipolar disorder, but some are used also in unipolar recurrent depression. As described in Chapter 9, antidepressants are used in the prophylaxis of unipolar affective disorders.

Classification

The distinguishing feature of bipolar disorder is a history of an episode of mania or hypomania. Kraepelin's concept of manic-depressive illness was too broad, and in 1957 Leonard proposed a distinction between bipolar patients (those with a history of mania) and unipolar depressives (Leonard, 1979). Some patients with recurrent depression have hypomanic episodes (not requiring hospitalization), especially on recovery from depression, and these were described as BP-II; those with a history of mania, as BP-I (Dunner *et al.*, 1976b). Unipolar mania accounts for 5–10% of bipolar disorder but has not been established as being different in any way from BP-I disorder. Because of the different combinations of severity of manic and depressive episodes, Angst (1985) proposed four categories: MD (in which both manic and depressive episodes are severe enough to require hospitalization), Md, mD (BP-II) and md (cyclothymia). Unipolar depressives with a family history of mania are sometimes called BP-III or pseudo-unipolar. Kukopulos *et al.* (1985) has used the sequence of mood changes to distinguish patients in whom mania is followed by depression, followed by a well interval (MDI), from those with depression followed by mania (DMI), those with a continuously circular pattern (CC) and those with completely separate affective swings.

Table 13.1 Diagnostic criteria for mania.

	Criteria
A	Distinct period of elation or irritability
B	Three of the following:
	over-activity,
	increased talkativeness or pressure of speech,
	flight of ideas or racing thoughts,
	inflated self-esteem or grandiosity (which may be delusional),
	decreased need for sleep,
	distractibility,
	indiscreet behaviour with poor judgement (sexual, financial, etc.)
C	Marked impairment in occupational or social function

Diagnostic criteria

The manic syndrome is one of the most clearly defined in psychiatry. Table 13.1 shows the inclusion criteria for the diagnosis according to DSM-IV (American Psychiatric Association, 1994).

Natural history of bipolar disorder

Mania is very rare before puberty and it is doubtful if it ever occurs before the age of 9 years. The peak age of first hospitalization is in the late teens, the median in the mid-20s, and the mean age of first hospitalization about the age of 26 years. There have often been earlier affective episodes sufficient to cause some impairment or to receive treatment outside hospital. There is a slight secondary peak of onset amongst women aged 45–50 and first episodes of mania continue to be seen in late life. An onset over the age of 60 is more likely to be associated with organic brain disease (Stone, 1989).

Number and duration of episodes

The great majority of patients have more than one episode, confirming the view that bipolar disorder is a recurrent illness. The duration of manic episodes in the pretreatment era was usually 3–12 months with a mean of 6 months. These times are usually much shortened by treatment (Bebbington & Ramana, 1995. In an individual, the episode duration tends to be stable through the course of the illness but the onset may become more rapid in later episodes (Post *et al.*, 1981).

Frequency of episodes

The interval from one episode to the next tends to decrease during the first five episodes. For instance, in Kraepelin's series the average time between the first and second episode was 5 years and between the fifth and sixth, 2 years. However, in an individual there is great variability in the length between episodes, and a tendency for episodes to be clustered at particular times in the patient's life (Cutler & Post, 1982); for instance, when they have difficulties coping with children, or when relationships are ending. It is possible that antidepressant treatments increase the tendency to switch from depression to mania, and have altered the natural course of the illness towards more frequent episodes. The work of Angst (1985) is cited in support of this; he found an increase in the incidence of manic switches, when the era before treatment was compared with that after the introduction of electroconvulsive therapy (ECT) and antidepressant drugs.

Rapid cycling. If the patient has four or more affective episodes in a year, they are said to be in a phase of rapid cycling. This can occur at the onset of illness but is much more common later in its course. It is also commoner in females. Antidepressant medication (particularly tricyclic antidepressants) can increase the frequency of cycling, and withdrawal of antidepressants can restore normal cycling in such patients (Wehr & Goodwin, 1979). Some cases of rapid cycling are associated with clinical or subclinical hypothyroidism, although a causal relationship has not been proved; lithium treatment might contribute to this occurring (Bauer *et al.*, 1990). Rare cases exist—about 20 in the world literature—of patients who oscillate from mania to depression and back again every 48 h (ultra-rapid cycling) (Dirlich *et al.*, 1981). Recently, ultradian cycling has been described in otherwise typical bipolar patients; mood change in such patients occur in a matter of minutes or hours and resemble the changes in borderline personalities (Kramlinger & Post, 1996).

Outcome

Death by suicide occurs in about 15–20% of cases (Black *et al.*, 1987) and a proportion of patients become socially and economically disadvantaged. In a Canadian study, patients lost 11% of their productive time in the 15–20 years after their index admission (Bland & Orn, 1982). There can be a considerable social and economic burden on the family (Fadden *et al.*, 1987).

Life events

A prospective study showed an increased rate of life events in the month before mania, but the proportion of patients so affected was small (Hunt *et al.*, 1992). It has been suggested that the first episode is more likely to be triggered by life events than later episodes (Sclare & Creed, 1987). This view is in keeping with the suggestion that a process of 'kindling' occurs, facilitating the development of subsequent episodes (see below), and Post (1992b) has re-viewed the possible biochemical substrates for the progressive effects of stress in recurrent affective disorders. Insomnia or sleep deprivation has been sug-gested to be an important factor that may trigger a manic episode (Wehr *et al.*, 1987). This may be relevant to the observation that flying overnight from west to east is more likely to lead to mania than travel in the opposite direction (Jauhar & Weller, 1982). A short course of sedative antipsychotic may be help-ful in bipolar patients with transient sleep disturbance to reduce the risk of developing mania. It is sensible for patients to keep a regular structure to their daily activities and exercise, as this may help to entrain their biological rhythms.

Marriage

Manic symptoms tend to be destructive to existing relationships. Although marriages often survive individual episodes of mania, the divorce rate in bi-polar disorder is very high—57% in one series, whereas it was 8% in unipolar depressive patients (Brodie & Leff, 1971). Very few of the spouses of bipolar patients have seen the patient during a manic episode prior to marriage. Fortunately, effective treatment often improves the quality of the marriage.

Alcohol and drug abuse in recurrent affective disorder

Some patients increase and some decrease alcohol or drug abuse when manic or depressed rather than euthymic (Bernadt & Murray, 1986). Alcohol and stimulants such as amphetamine and cocaine are used by patients to restore hypomania during a dysphoric phase, or to heighten existing states of elation (Gawin & Kleber, 1986).

These drugs can alter the course of bipolar disorder by triggering mania; they diminish impulse control and impair judgement and are serious risk factors for suicide. Therefore the recognition and treatment of alcohol or drug abuse in recurrent affective patients is a matter of urgency. Cannabis has been associated with an increase in psychotic symptoms in mania (Harding & Knight, 1973), and with the induction of mania (Rottanberg *et al.*, 1982).

Lithium

Lithium is the best-investigated drug for the treatment of mania and the prophylaxis of bipolar and unipolar affective illness.

Placebo-controlled studies of bipolar disorder

There have been four placebo-controlled studies of lithium in mania which used a crossover design. These were conducted in Denmark by Schou *et al.* (1954) and later in double-blind designs in England by Maggs (1963), and in the USA (Goodwin *et al.*, 1969; Stokes *et al.*, 1971). In a total of 116 patients on lithium, there was an overall response rate of 78%, much greater than on placebo. Lithium usually has a few days' delay in its onset, requires 2–3 weeks to approach a full effect on mania, and may take longer. The study of valproate by Bowden *et al.* (1994; see below) used lithium as a comparator in addition to placebo.

Controlled studies of lithium prophylaxis for bipolar affective disorder

There have been 10 major double-blind comparative trials of lithium vs. placebo in the prophylaxis of bipolar patients. Three types of design have been used. Two studies used *double-blind discontinuation*, patients already on lithium being assigned randomly either to continue on lithium or to switch to placebo. In the study by Baastrup *et al.* (1970), 55% of patients who switched to placebo, and none of those continued on lithium, relapsed within 5 months. About half of the relapses were manic and half depressive. However, this design is weakened by the occurrence of lithium withdrawal mania (see below). One study used a *crossover design* which also involved a lithium withdrawal phase (Cundall *et al.*, 1972).

A *prospective design* was used by Coppen *et al.* (1971) in the UK and by Prien *et al.* (1973) in the USA and in five other studies. Overall, in 204 patients on lithium prospectively, about 35% relapsed in the study period (which varied from 4 months to 3 years), compared to about 80% of 221 patients on placebo (see Goodwin & Jamison, 1990). In these studies the efficacy of lithium was more apparent for manic than for depressive relapses. However, retrospective mirror-image studies, designed to clarify this, suggested that the efficacy in preventing depression may even be greater than that in preventing mania (Poole *et al.*, 1978). Lithium improves both the severity and frequency of episodes. Usually it also stabilizes the mood between major episodes.

Placebo-controlled studies of lithium in the prophylaxis of unipolar depression

The prospective studies of lithium in the prophylaxis of unipolar depression are limited by the broader concept of unipolar depression and by the relatively short follow-up periods which in some cases blur the distinction between the re-emergence of the index episode and true prophylaxis. Two of the above prospective trials included unipolar depressives and found no difference in the efficacy of lithium compared to that in bipolar patients (Coppen *et al.*, 1971; Prien *et al.*, 1973). Prien *et al.* (1984) found imipramine superior to lithium in the prophylaxis of the most severe depressive episodes, and of equal efficacy for moderately severe depression. Other prospective double-blind comparative trials have found lithium superior to imipramine and to placebo (Kane *et al.*, 1982), equivalent to amitriptyline (Glen *et al.*, 1984), and superior to maprotiline or mianserin (see Coppen & Abou-Saleh, 1983). In a non-blind randomized controlled trial, fluvoxamine was superior to lithium in preventing recurrences (Franchini *et al.*, 1994).

Predicting response to lithium

Patients with typical bipolar disorder and complete recovery between episodes are more likely to benefit (Grof *et al.*, 1993). A family history of bipolar disorder is so strongly associated with prophylactic efficacy as to question whether 'secondary' bipolar disorder ever responds to lithium; indeed, neurological signs predict a poor response (Himmelhoch *et al.*, 1980). Patients whose first episode was manic rather than depressive do better on lithium (Prien *et al.*, 1984), and the MDI pattern predicts a better response than the DMI pattern (Faedda *et al.*, 1991). It is thought that a good response to lithium in acute mania or depression predicts prophylactic efficacy. Manic patients who respond tend to be classical manics rather than mixed or schizoaffective (Himmelhoch *et al.*, 1976; Swann *et al.*, 1986). Elated-grandiose manics showed a better response than destructive-paranoid manics in one study (Murphy & Beigel, 1974), but not in another (Swann *et al.*, 1986). Dysphoric manics were less likely to improve (Post *et al.*, 1989). Patients with a rapid-cycling phase of illness are often less responsive to lithium (Dunner & Fieve, 1974). Other factors mitigating strongly against prophylactic efficacy are poor adherence to treatment, and drug abuse.

In the prophylaxis of unipolar depressive disorder, a good response to lithium is predicted by a family history of mania or of response to lithium, stable premorbid personality, low neuroticism, and good interepisode functioning (Coppen & Abou-Saleh, 1983).

Mode of action

Lithium has numerous effects on biological systems, especially at high concentrations. It is unclear which of these are relevant to its therapeutic effects (see Wood & Goodwin, 1987).

Ionic mechanisms

As the smallest alkaline cation, lithium can substitute for sodium, potassium, calcium and magnesium in several ways. It penetrates cells via sodium and other channels, but is extruded less efficiently than sodium by the sodium–potassium active transport system and other transporters. Thus the cell to plasma ratio for lithium (about 0.5 in red blood cells) is much higher than that for sodium. Within the cell, lithium can interact with systems that normally involve other cautions, including transmitter release and second messenger systems.

Second messenger systems: adenylate cyclase

Many neurotransmitters and hormones (e.g. antidiuretic hormone (vasopressin) (ADH) at V2 receptors, dopamine at D1 receptors and noradrenaline at beta receptors) interact with receptors that use cyclic-AMP as the second messenger. Lithium is known to inhibit cyclic AMP production in these systems. In humans, therapeutic levels of lithium have been shown to inhibit the glucagon-induced rise in plasma c-AMP (Waller *et al.*, 1984). The inhibition by lithium of ADH-linked adenylate cyclase (Dousa, 1974) is thought to contribute to the polyuria and polydipsia (nephrogenic diabetes insipidus) which is a side-effect. Goitre and hypothyroidism are due in part to interference with the action of thyroid-stimulating hormone (TSH, thyrotrophin) at its receptors in the thyroid (Wolff *et al.*, 1970).

Phosphoinositide turnover

This second messenger system involves the formation of inositol phosphates which control intracellular-free calcium levels. The phosphoinositide cycle provides the second messengers for several neurotransmitter systems including thyrotrophin releasing hormone (TRH) in the pituitary, acetylcholine at muscarinic M-1 receptors, noradrenaline at alpha$_1$, and 5-hydroxytryptamine (5-HT) at 5-HT$_{2A}$ receptors. Lithium inhibits inositol monophosphatase (Berridge, 1984; Hokin, 1993) and has an inhibitory or stabilizing effect on responses (for instance, to acetylcholine). The fact that lithium preferentially inhibits phosphatidyl inositol turnover in activated neural systems (Belmaker *et al.*, 1996) may explain its mood stabilizing properties.

Effects on 5-HT

Lithium can potentiate both the uptake of L-tryptophan (Das Chargas Rodrigues & Zwicker, 1985) and its conversion to 5-hydroxytryptophan

(Rastoge & Singhal, 1977), the precursor of 5-HT. It can also potentiate the release of 5-HT (Sharp *et al.*, 1991) and can potentiate 5-HT$_{1A}$-mediated responses (Goodwin *et al.*, 1986); for instance, in man the rise in prolactin levels induced by L-tryptophan (McCance-Katz *et al.*, 1992) but not that induced by d-fenfluramine is potentiated by lithium (Shapira *et al.*, 1992).

Receptor up-regulation

Lithium can block the development of dopamine receptor super-sensitivity that normally occurs during prolonged treatment with dopamine-blocking (antipsychotic) drugs (Klawans & Weiner, 1976). It has been suggested that lithium might reduce the development of tardive dyskinesia in bipolar patients on antipsychotic drugs. Although in two studies tardive dyskinesia was more common in patients who had a briefer exposure to lithium, in a third study the opposite was found (Dinan & Kohen, 1989).

Side-effects

Lithium has actions on many bodily systems, even at therapeutic doses. These are important, as some require intervention and several contribute to non-compliance. The majority of patients on lithium experience at least one side-effect, depending on the doses used (Vestergaard *et al.*, 1980). All patients should be informed about side-effects and signs of toxicity.

Thyroid

Lithium tends to reduce thyroid function. The most sensitive laboratory index, increased TSH, occurs in 23% of patients (Transbol *et al.*, 1978). Thyroid enlargement (goitre) develops in about 5% (Myers *et al.*, 1985), and clinical hypothyroidism in between 5% and 10% of patients, depending upon the dose and duration of treatment (Yassa *et al.*, 1988). Patients with pre-existing thyroid antibodies or a family history of thyroid disease are at greater risk of developing hypothyroidism (Lazarus *et al.*, 1981), and lithium treatment can increase antibody levels (Calabrese *et al.*, 1985; Myers *et al.*, 1985).

Kidney

Polyuria and excessive thirst with polydipsia are noted by about one third of patients on lithium. The condition is usually reversible, but after long-term treatment it is not always so (Bucht *et al.*, 1980). Giving lithium once daily, as opposed to divided doses, was associated with lower daily urine volumes in some studies, although others found no difference (Bowen *et al.*, 1991). For patients in whom a reduction in dose is not appropriate in order to avoid polyuria, the loop diuretic frusemide or amiloride, with or without potassium supplements, may be helpful. In 1977, Hestbech *et al.* reported histological changes in patients on lithium including glomerular damage, interstitial fibrosis and tubular atrophy (focal interstitial nephropathy). However, similar findings were later made in patients who had received no lithium treatment. Much further work has shown that during long-term treatment with lithium, monitored at therapeutic doses, no deterioration occurs in glomerular filtration rate in the vast majority of patients. However, occasional cases of chronic renal failure have been reported and attributed by nephrologists to lithium, even in patients whose lithium levels have been monitored carefully; this is thought to be a rare idiosyncratic reaction to lithium (Waller & Edwards, 1989). Episodes of lithium toxicity may produce renal damage with reduced glomerular filtration rates (Johnson, G., 1984).

Central nervous system

A fine tremor of the hands occurs in about 25% of patients, and is similar to that in anxiety (Gelenberg & Jefferson, 1995). It can be worsened by tricyclic antidepressants. Beta-blockers such as propanolol (starting at 10 mg twice daily) reduce this and are probably best taken intermittently (Montastruc *et al.*, 1994). Lithium can increase extra-pyramidal (parkinsonian) side-effects in patients on antipsychotic drugs (Tyrer *et al.*, 1980), and can itself produce cog-wheel rigidity in a small minority of patients (Asnis *et al.*, 1979). In contrast to neuroleptic-induced parkinsonism, this does not improve with anticholinergic drugs. Cerebellar tremor and incoordination are signs of toxicity, as are more severe forms of fine tremor and parkinsonism.

Mental and cognitive effects

There is some objective evidence of an effect of therapeutic levels of lithium upon memory (Kocsis *et al.*, 1993) but not all studies show this (Kolk *et al.*, 1993). Memory problems are frequently affirmed by patients interviewed about possible side-effects. The use of ECT in patients on lithium has been associated with acute organic brain syndrome or prolonged confusional states, but a retrospective case-control study did not find a higher frequency of adverse effects of ECT in patients on lithium (Jha *et al.*, 1996). The possible effect of lithium upon creativity was explored by Schou (1979), who interviewed 24 successful artists and professionals taking lithium. Some did not want to continue lithium because of this effect, but the majority, although missing some hypomanic swings, considered that their long-term productivity and creativity were higher under lithium treatment. Only six thought they were diminished. In therapeutic doses, lithium does not impair psychomotor coordination and is not a bar to driving private motor vehicles, although a diagnosis of manic-depressive illness excludes patients from driving certain public service vehicles (Cookson, 1989) and after an admission for mania, the patient may not drive for 6–12 months according to the UK Driver and Vehicle Licensing Agency.

Cardiovascular effects

Lithium can produce benign reversible T-wave flattening or inversion, a pattern similar to that with hypokalaemia. Cardiac dysrhythmias are rare with therapeutic doses, especially in younger patients but sinus node arrhythmius have been described (sick sinus syndrome) (Mitchell & MacKenzie, 1982). Caution should be exercised in using lithium in patients with cardiac failure and the elderly. The mortality rate among patients on lithium is similar to that of manic-depressives before lithium was introduced (Norton & Whalley, 1984).

Skin

Lithium can produce or exacerbate acne (Kanzaki, 1991) and psoriasis (Abel, 1992). Tetracyclines should be used with caution because of their possible interaction with lithium, but retinoids can be used. Hair loss and altered texture may also occur in about 12% of patients (Llau *et al.*, 1995), and there may be golden discoloration of the distal nail plates.

Parathyroid, bones and teeth

Lithium produces mild increases in parathyroid hormone level and serum calcium (Fitzpatrick & Spiegel, 1988) and Stancer and Forbath (1989) reported clinical hyperparathyroidism in patients on lithium. No long-term effects on bone have been found in animals or man (Birch *et al.*, 1982), although it is unknown whether this applies to the growing bones of children. There is no evidence of a direct effect of lithium upon the teeth, but dry mouth or increased consumption of sweet drinks will lead to caries.

Metabolic effects and weight gain

About 25% of patients gain more than 10 pounds in weight. The mechanism is unknown and an attempt to replicate the weight gain in volunteers was unsuccessful (Chen & Silverstone, 1990). Although increased consumption of sweet drinks is cited, an increase in food intake and altered metabolism are also possible. Lithium produces subtle alterations in glucose and insulin metabolism, and may occasionally worsen control of diabetes. Fluid retention and oedema may occur especially with higher doses. Lithium may antagonize aldosterone and increase angiotensin levels (Stewart *et al.*, 1988).

Gastro-intestinal system

About one third of patients experience mild abdominal discomfort, some-times with loose motions during the first few weeks of treatment, especially with higher doses (Schou *et al.*, 1970; Bone *et al.*, 1980; Vestergaard *et al.*, 1980). By using divided doses, these side-effects can usually be avoided. Sometimes a slow-release preparation is tolerated better, but occasionally these them-selves irritate the lower bowel. Severe or persistent diarrhoea suggests toxicity.

Sexual function

Impairment of sexual drive, arousal and ejaculation have been attributed to lithium, but are thought to be rare (Blay *et al.*, 1982). The luteinizing hormone (LH) response to the releasing hormone LHRH is potentiated by lithium treat-ment (Hunter *et al.*, 1989), similarly to the potentiation of the TSH response to TRH (Lombardi *et al.*, 1993).

Neuromuscular junction

Lithium reduces acetylcholine release and impairs neuromuscular transmis-sion. Normally, the safety factor in neuromuscular transmission is sufficient to overcome these effects. Lithium potentiates neuromuscular blocking agents, including succinylcholine (Diamond & Brown, 1987), and exacerbates myasthenia gravis.

Respiratory effects

Lithium can produce respiratory depression in patients with chronic obstruc-tive airways disease, especially at toxic blood levels (Lawler & Cove-Smith, 1986).

Blood and bone marrow

Lithium produces a benign reversible leucocytosis (Prakash, 1987), probably by an effect on marrow growth factors.

Contraindications

There are no absolute contraindications to lithium treatment but caution is required in people with renal failure, heart failure, recent myocardial infarction, electrolyte imbalance, the elderly and in patients who are unreliable in taking medication or prone to dehydration.

Pregnancy

In the first trimester, lithium carries a risk of cardiac malformations, such as Ebstein's anomaly, in the fetus. Recent cohort studies suggest the risk of major congenital abnormalities may be 4–12%, whereas it is 2–4% in women taking other drugs not known to be teratogenic (Kallen & Tandberg, 1983; Jacobson *et al.*, 1992; Cohen *et al.*, 1994). Screening tests, including high-resolution ultrasound and echocardiography examination of the fetus at 16–18 weeks' gestation, are advisable in women exposed to lithium. The anticonvulsants carbamazepine and valproate in early pregnancy are associated with brain and neural tube developmental defects in about 1% of births (Rosa, 1991). Because of the possible developmental effects upon the child, pregnancy (in bipolar patients) should if possible be managed without psychotropic drugs. Antipsychotics are probably the safest, if antimanic medication is needed) when pregnancy is planned; there is a risk of transient extrapyramidal side-effects in the neonate if these are continued.

Symptoms of lithium toxicity

Clinical features

Lithium toxicity is indicated by the development of three groups of symptoms—gastro-intestinal, motor (especially cerebellar) and cerebral (Table 14.2). Nausea and diarrhoea progress to vomiting and incontinence. Marked fine tremor progresses to a coarse (cerebellar or parkinsonian) tremor, giddiness, cerebellar ataxia and slurred speech, and to gross incoordination with choreiform movements and muscular twitching (myoclonus), upper motor neurone signs (spasticity and extensor plantar reflexes), electroencephalogram (EEG) abnormalities and seizures (Reed *et al.*, 1989). In mild toxicity there is impairment of concentration but this deteriorates into drowsiness and disorientation, and in more severe toxicity there is marked apathy and impaired consciousness leading to coma (Gadallah *et al.*, 1988). A Creutzfeldt–Jakob-like syndrome with characteristic EEG changes, myoclonus and cognitive deterioration has been described, and was in these cases reversible (Smith & Kocen, 1988). Patients who have recovered from acute lithium toxicity can be left with permanent cerebellar signs (Schou, 1984; Adityanjee, 1989).

Table 13.2 Symptoms of lithium toxicity.

	Symptom		
Severity	Gastro-intestinal	Motor	Cerebral
Mild	Nausea Diarrhoea	Severe fine tremor	Poor concentration
Moderate	Vomiting	Coarse tremor Cerebellar ataxia Slurred speech	Drowsiness Disorientation
Severe	Vomiting Incontinence	Choreiform/parkinsonian movement General muscle twitching (myoclonus) Spasticityn and cerebellar dysfunction EEG abnormalities and seizures	Apathy Coma

Practical aspects of lithium treatment

A physical examination and tests of the blood and urine should, if possible, precede drug treatment or take place soon after the patient is sedated in order to elucidate any intercurrent physical illness, especially infection, and any causes of secondary mania (e.g. drugs), and to determine baseline renal, hepatic and thyroid function.

Selection of patients

Maintenance treatment should be considered after a second major episode of bipolar disorder or a third episode of unipolar disorder, especially if the interval between episodes was less than 5 years. Because the intervals between the first and second episodes tend to be longer than between subsequent episodes, maintenance treatment should only be used after a first episode if the dangers of a subsequent episode are thought to justify it—for instance, if the episode was severe and disruptive, had a relatively sudden onset and was not precipitated by external factors; if the person's job is very sensitive; or there is a suicide risk.

Lithium blood levels and monitoring

The narrow gap or overlap between therapeutic and toxic blood levels of lithium necessitates careful monitoring of lithium levels, usually based on samples taken 12h after the last dose. The pharmacokinetics of lithium involve rapid absorption, with a peak at 4h followed by distribution in body fluids and slow penetration of the intracellular space and brain. Elimination is largely by the kidney, and the plasma half-life varies from 7 to 20 h in physically healthy individuals but is longer in the elderly or physically unwell. Thornhill and Field (1982) found it to range from 15 to 55 h in euthymic psychiatric patients. Thus, on a regular dose, steady-state blood levels would be reached after a period of between 2 and 9 days. Many of the features of toxicity may reflect high intracellular rather than extracelluar levels; hence, in assessing toxicity and efficacy, clinical judgement rather than blood levels should be paramount. Recent studies have indicated that blood levels lower than those formerly used are sufficient in prophylaxis (Coppen *et al.*, 1983). Thus, efficacy was preserved until levels were below 0.6 mE L^{-1}. For some patients, lower levels than this would suffice, although Gelenberg *et al.* (1989) found that a group with levels of 0.8–1.0 mE L^{-1} had a better outcome than a group with levels of 0.4–0.6 mE L^{-1}. In the elderly, a level of 0.5 mE L^{-1} is recommended (Hardy *et al.*, 1987). Recommendations vary about monitoring lithium, renal and thyroid function tests, but even in the most stable patient these tests should be performed at least once a year, and during less stable phases lithium levels should be done frequently. The development of hypothyroidism is often signalled by weight gain and lethargy and should be distinguished from depression. Treatment with L-thyroxine is usually straightforward. The occurrence of thyrotoxicosis during lithium treatment has also been described, and there may be a rebound exacerbation when lithium is discontinued.

Antidepressants and lithium

Depression occurring during lithium treatment can be treated with MARIs. In patients with BP-I disorder, the course of antidepressant treatment should be gradually discontinued as the depression improves, in order to reduce the risk of triggering a manic episode (Quitkin *et al.*, 1985), and to avoid the induction of rapid cycling (Wehr & Goodwin, 1979, 1987). For patients with a predominantly depressive pattern of bipolar disorder (BP-II), the combination of lithium and a MARI may be more effective in preventing depression than either drug alone (Shapiro *et al.*, 1989). Kane *et al.* (1982) found lithium more effective than imipramine or placebo in preventing depressive recurrences in BP-II patients. There is some evidence that selective serotonin reuptake inhibitors (SSRIs) such as paroxetine are less likely to trigger mania than tricyclic antidepressants (Montgomery & Roberts, 1994); however, some individuals with bipolar disorder are readily switched into mania by SSRIs.

Toxicity

Diagnosis. Lithium toxicity should be assumed in patients on lithium with vomiting or severe nausea, cerebellar signs or disorientation. Other evidence of likely toxicity includes poor concentration, muscle twitching, tremor, dysthymia, ataxia and hyperreflexia; convulsions and renal failure are serious signs of advanced toxicity. Lithium treatment should be stopped immediately, and serum lithium, urea and electrolyte levels measured. However, the severity of toxicity bears little relationship to serum lithium levels (Hansen & Amdisen, 1978), and neurotoxicity can occur with serum levels in the usual therapeutic range (West & Meltzer, 1979). Diagnosis should be based upon clinical judgement and not upon the blood level. Lithium should only be restarted (at an adjusted dose) when the patient's condition has improved, or an alternative cause of the symptoms has been found.

Treatment. Often, cessation of lithium and provision of adequate salt and fluids, included saline infusions, will suffice. In patients with high serum levels (greater than $3 \, \text{mEL}^{-1}$) or coma, haemodialysis can speed the removal of lithium and reduce the risk of permanent neurological damage (Johnson, G., 1984).

Outcome. Patients who survive episodes of lithium toxicity will often make a full recovery. However, a proportion have persistent renal or neurological damage with cerebellar symptoms, spasticity and cognitive impairment. This outcome is more likely if patients are continued on lithium, while showing signs of toxicity or during intercurrent physical illnesses (Schou, 1984). Patients with persistent neurological damage had also shown more advanced signs of toxicity (Hansen & Amdisen, 1978). The signs of toxicity develop gradually over several days during continued lithium treatment and, in some cases, continue to develop for days after treatment is stopped. Serum lithium levels can also continue to rise after treatment is stopped, probably through release of lithium from intracellular stores (Sellers *et al.*, 1982).

Factors predisposing to lithium toxicity. Conditions of salt depletion (diarrhoea, vomiting, excessive sweating during fever or in hot climates) can lead to lithium retention. Drugs which reduce the renal excretion of lithium include thiazide diuretics but not frusemide or amiloride, (Alexander & Perry, 1987), certain non-steroidal anti-inflammatory drugs (ibuprofen, indomethacin, piroxicam, naproxen and phenylbutazone (Imbs *et al.*, 1987) but not aspirin, paracetamol or sulindac), and certain antibiotics (erythromycin, metronidazole and probably tetracyclines). These drugs should be avoided if possible. If they must be used, the dose of lithium should be reduced and blood levels monitored. In patients with serious intercurrent illnesses, especially infections, lithium should be stopped or reduced in dose, and carefully monitored until the patient's condition is stable. Gastroenteritis is particularly liable to lead to toxicity. In the elderly, renal function is decreased, lower doses are required, and toxicity can develop more readily (Stone, 1989).

Lithium–neuroleptic combination

Combinations of high levels of lithium with high doses of antipsychotics including haloperidol have been associated with severe neurological symptoms, hyperthermia, impaired consciousness and irreversible brain damage (Cohen & Cohen, 1974; Loudon & Waring, 1976). The conditions reported resemble both lithium toxicity and neuroleptic malignant syndrome. Antipsychotic drugs can increase intracellular lithium levels, suggesting a possible mechanism for this interaction (Von Knorring, 1990). Subsequent series have demonstrated the safety of combining haloperidol (up to 30 mg per day) with lithium at levels of up to 1 mE L^{-1} (see Johnson *et al.*, 1990). In practice, when combining lithium with antipsychotics, the blood levels should generally be maintained below 1 mE L^{-1}, staff should be advised to observe and report the development of neurological symptoms, and lithium should be temporarily discontinued if they develop. The combination of antipsychotics and lithium in bipolar patients can also lead to troublesome somnambulism requiring reduction of doses (Charney *et al.*, 1979).

Withdrawal of lithium

Symptoms of anxiety, irritability and emotional lability can occur following sudden discontinuation of lithium (King & Hullin, 1983). In a double-blind placebo-controlled crossover study, sudden cessation of lithium in bipolar patients led to the development of mania 2–3 weeks later in seven out of 14 patients (Mander & Loudon, 1988).

A review of all published studies suggested that half the bipolar patients who discontinued lithium had a recurrence within 5 months, usually of mania (Suppes *et al.*, 1991). In occasional patients, discontinuation of lithium leads to recurrent affective swings which cannot be controlled by the reintroduction of lithium (Post *et al.*, 1990). Discontinuation of lithium should therefore be gradual. Patients whose mood has been stable are less likely to relapse on stopping lithium than those who have continued to show mild mood swings ('metastable'). Lithium may be reduced at the rate of one quarter to one eighth of the original dose every 2 months, to minimize the risk of precipitating withdrawal mania; further studies are needed to clarify this. There are no clear guidelines for deciding when to advise patients to stop lithium, but if they have relapses in spite of good adherence to treatment and satisfactory blood levels, or if they have remained well on lithium for 3–4 years, the benefits and risks of continuing lithium should be reviewed. The possible occurrence of lithium withdrawal should be part of the information given to patients on lithium. It has been estimated that to balance the risk of mania arising from abrupt discontinuation, a first-episode manic patient would need to continue on lithium for a minimum of 2 years (Goodwin, 1994).

Natural outcome on lithium

Dickson and Kendell (1986) reported a threefold increase in admissions for mania in Edinburgh during the period 1970–81 when the use of lithium increased. This highlights the difficulty of delivering an effective treatment to a community. A large proportion of patients at risk do not seek treatment, and many who do, adhere poorly to lithium. In addition, there is the risk of withdrawal mania in those who stop treatment too abruptly—for instance, when feeling no need for it during a mild upswing of mood.

A naturalistic follow-up in the USA found no difference in outcome over 18 months between bipolar patients discharged on or off lithium (Harrow *et al.*, 1990). However, these patients were not randomly assigned. Under circumstances where steps are taken to encourage and check adherence, relapse rates and affective morbidity on lithium, as low as those in controlled trials, can be achieved (McCreadie & Morrison, 1985; Coppen & Abou-Saleh, 1988). This is part of the rationale for specialist lithium or affective disorder clinics. A case record study of 827 manic-depressive or schizoaffective patients treated with lithium for more than 6 months showed that mortality was reduced to that of the general population (Müller-Oerlinghausen *et al.*, 1992). A similar finding was reported by Coppen *et al.* (1991).

Adherence to treatment

In the UK the use of lithium is only about 0.8 per 1000 population, even in centres with active lithium clinics (McCreadie & Morrison, 1985); about half the patients who commenced on lithium discontinued it within 1 year, but a quarter remained on it for over 10 years. The patients who are less likely to adhere tend to be younger, male and to have had fewer previous episodes of illness. The reasons they give for stopping are: drug side-effects, missing periods of elation, feeling well and in no need of treatment, feeling depressed or less productive, or not wanting to depend on medication. The side-effects most often given as reasons for non-adherence are excessive thirst and polyuria, tremor, memory impairment and weight gain. In order to increase adherence, the doctor should take side-effects seriously, keep lithium levels as low as possible, educate the patients and their families about their illness and the use of lithium, and discuss adherence with the patient. For non-adherent patients, the regular contact provided by counselling or psychotherapy can be useful and has been shown to improve compliance and affective morbidity (Glick *et al.*, 1985). It may be helpful to plot a 'life chart' with the patient (Squillace *et al.*, 1984).

Alternatives to lithium in prophylaxis

Even in favourable clinical trials, lithium prophylaxis was unsuccessful in over 30% of patients. More recent studies put the average failure rate much higher and alternative treatments are clearly needed (Prien & Gelenberg, 1989; Post, 1990).

Carbamazepine

The mood-stabilizing effect of carbamazepine was first recognized in epilepsy. Japanese psychiatrists were the first to report that carbamazepine improved acute mania, even in patients who were resistant to other drugs (Okuma *et al.*, 1973, 1981). Ballenger and Post (1980) independently studied carbamazepine in bipolar disorder; these authors had developed the theory that affective illness might involve a 'kindling' process in limbic brain areas, such as they had found with cocaine-induced behavioural changes in animals.

There have only been small placebo-controlled studies to confirm the antimanic efficacy of carbamazepine, but studies comparing carbamazepine with antipsychotic drugs or lithium show it approximately as effective as lithium with about 60% of patients doing well (Post, 1990). There is some delay in its action, but less so than with lithium. In one controlled study of treatment-resistant depression, about one third of patients showed some acute antidepressant response over 3–4 weeks (Post *et al.*, 1986).

Controlled studies of carbamazepine prophylaxis

The first controlled studies of the use of carbamazepine in the prophylaxis of bipolar disorder were those of Okuma *et al.* (1981) and Post *et al.* (1983). The drug has now been shown to be superior to placebo in one cross-over study (Post *et al.*, 1983), and to be of similar efficacy to lithium in at least five studies of bipolar disorder (Coxhead *et al.*, 1992; Simhandl *et al.*, 1993). Approximately 65% of bipolar patients appeared to show a good response (Post, 1992a). The trials of carbamazepine have been reviewed critically (Prien & Gelenberg, 1989) and a meta-analysis concluded that further controlled studies are needed to define its efficacy and place in clinical practice (Dardennes *et al.*, 1995). Silverstone and Romans (1996) suggest that carbamazepine may have been less effective than lithium in unipolar depressive disorder in the study by Watkins *et al.* (1987).

Mechanism of action

An 'antikindling' effect may underlie some of the actions of carbamazepine. However, the pharmacological mechanism of action in acute mania is unknown. Carbamazepine potentiates central 5-HT transmission in normal subjects, as judged by the prolactin response to L-tryptophan (Elphick *et al.*, 1990). It reduces L-type calcium channel activation by depolarization, and may block the excitatory transmitter glutamate at its receptors (Post *et al.*, 1994).

Side-effects

The commonest side-effects of carbamazepine are nausea, dizziness, ataxia and diplopia. A maculopapular itchy rash develops within 2 weeks in up to 15% of patients and requires great caution and usually cessation of the drug. More serious idiosyncratic side-effects include agranulocytosis, aplastic anaemia and Stevens–Johnson syndrome; these contraindicate further treatment with carbamazepine. Carbamazepine regularly lowers the white cell count by a pharmacological effect on the marrow: a moderate leukopenia occurs in 1–2% of patients (Tohen *et al.*, 1995). Agranulocytosis and aplastic anaemia can develop suddenly, and occur in about eight patients per million treated. Hyponatremia and water intoxication can occur through potentiation of ADH and can lead to malaise, confusion and fits.

Pharmacokinetics and drug interactions

Carbamazepine induces liver enzymes, resulting in the lowering not only of its own blood levels after 3 weeks of treatment, but also increasing the metabolism of other drugs, including haloperidol and oral contraceptives (Ketter *et al.*, 1991). Its own plasma half-life may fall from 48 h to 7 h during long-term treatment. On the other hand, the blood level of carbamazepine is increased by drugs including erythromycin, verapamil, dextropropoxyphene and cimetidine. Thyroid hormone metabolism is increased and blood levels lowered; particularly in combination with lithium, carbamazepine may precipitate hypothyroidism.

Practical aspects of carbamazepine treatment

Selection of patients

Patients who respond to carbamazepine differ somewhat from those responding to lithium, and a history of non-response to lithium does not reduce the chances of responding to carbamazepine. Patients with a history of dysphoric mania, or mixed states, can benefit from carbamazepine. Patients with no family history of mania may have a greater chance of responding to carbamazepine (Post *et al.*, 1987). Patients with bipolar disorder secondary to brain damage can also benefit. In contrast to lithium, rapid-cycling patients benefit as much from carbamazepine as do other bipolar patients. In longer-term use in some patients, there may be partial loss of efficacy by the third year of treatment, although it is not clear to what extent poor adherence to medication is responsible. More recent findings, however, have questioned the efficacy of carbamazepine in some bipolar patients resistant to lithium (Calabrese *et al.*, 1995).

Dosage

The recommended starting dose is 100 mg twice daily, increasing at weekly intervals up to 400 mg twice daily. Gradual introduction of the drug is thought to reduce the incidence of side-effects, including nausea, rashes and blood dyscrasias. Patients should be warned of side-effects, and advised particularly to report any rashes, fevers or severe sore throats, which may herald agranulocytosis and require immediate discontinuation of the drug.

Blood tests

Serum levels are sometimes helpful in monitoring carbamazepine therapy but, as in epilepsy, clinical judgement is generally more useful in deciding on dose changes. No clear relationship between blood level and antimanic effect was found by Post *et al.* (1987) or in prophylaxis by Simhandl *et al.* (1993). A range of $15–30\,\mu\text{mol}\,\text{L}^{-1}$ ($5–10\,\text{mg}\,\text{L}^{-1}$) is generally cited in epilepsy. The differential blood count and electrolyte levels should be monitored in the first few weeks. Hyponatremia requires a reduction of dose or discontinuation. Carbamazepine should be stopped immediately if the total white cell count is less than 3000 per cubic millimetre or the neutrophil count is less than 1500.

Lithium and carbamazepine combination

Many patients who fail to improve when taking carbamazepine alone do so when lithium is added (Kramlinger & Post, 1989). Some patients appear to benefit more from the combination than from either drug alone, although combination may—as with neuroleptics—increase the risk of lithium neurotoxicity (Shukla *et al.*, 1984).

Valproate

Valproate is also effective in a proportion of manic patients including non-responders to antipsychotic drugs and lithium. Patients who respond to valproate do not necessarily respond to carbamazepine and vice versa. In the first large parallel-group placebo-controlled study (which included only patients who were unresponsive to, or intolerant of, lithium), 10 of 17 patients on valproate improved compared to only 3 of 19 on placebo (Pope *et al.*, 1991). Most of the improvement occurred within 1–4 days of achieving therapeutic levels. Bowden *et al.* (1994) compared valproate (as divalproex) to lithium or placebo in a 3-week parallel-group double-blind study of 179 patients, half of whom had been unresponsive to lithium previously. The proportion of patients showing 50% improvement was greater for valproate (48%) and lithium (49%) than for placebo (25%). Valproate was as effective in rapid-cycling manics as in other manic patients and equally effective in the patients previously judged responders or non-responders to lithium. Subsequent analyses indicate that patients with mixed affective states may benefit more from valproate than from lithium. Few patients in the study had a return to normal functioning within 3 weeks, and the place of valproate in routine practice seems likely—as in the case of lithium—to be as an adjunct to antipsychotic drugs, perhaps particularly in those manic patients with a significant mixture of depressive symptoms, and as prophylaxis.

Valproate in prophylaxis

Valproate has been studied less methodically in prophylaxis but it may be useful in those who are resistant to lithium or carbamazepine (McElroy *et al.*, 1992). The drug is effective in a large proportion of patients during the rapid-cycling periods of their illness; in one study the efficacy against mania appeared greater than against depression (Calabrese & Delucchi, 1990). Gerner and Stanton (1992), reviewing the world literature, observed a 54% response rate in 375 patients. Some clinicians consider that valproate may be more effective than lithium in preventing recurrences of depression or mixed states in bipolar patients, and that elderly patients may tolerate valproate better than lithium.

Mechanism of action

The drug is thought to increase the function of the inhibitory transmitter gamma-amino-butyric acid (GABA); there is little direct evidence for increased GABA levels but GABA-B receptors may be up-regulated by valproate. The drug may also enhance central serotonin activity, and may reduce adrenocorticotrophin (ACTH) and cortisol levels (Maes & Calabrese, 1994).

Side-effects

Mild side-effects which are dose-dependent include nausea, vomiting and stomach cramps: these can be managed by reducing the dose of valproate. Lethargy, hair-thinning, elevated liver function tests and thrombocytopaenia are also dose dependent and can be managed by dose reduction. Serious idiosyncratic reactions to valproate which contraindicate further treatment with valproate include liver failure, pancreatitis and agranulocytosis. A fetal valproate syndrome has also been described with cardiac and other congenital abnormalities, and with jitteriness and seizures in the neonate (Thisted & Ebbeson, 1993).

Practical aspects of treatment with valproate

Selection of patients

Patients who do not respond to lithium or carbamazepine, or who cannot tolerate them, should be tried on valproate. Those who have responded to valproate during mania may benefit, and include those with mixed affective disorders. The drug should be avoided during pregnancy.

Dosage

The starting dose is 200 mg two to three times daily, rising by 200 mg at 3-day intervals, to 2000 mg daily according to clinical response. The drug has a plasma half-life of 8–20 h, which may be prolonged by cimetidine.

Blood test monitoring

The recommended plasma concentration is in the range of 50–150 mg L^{-1}. Liver function levels should be monitored before treatment and periodically during the first 6 months.

Combination

Some patients benefit from the combination of lithium and valproate, having not responded to either drug alone (Mitchell *et al.*, 1994).

Lamotrigine

Lamotrigine is an anticonvulsant with beneficial effects on mood in epilepsy. An open study in 85 bipolar patients gave encouraging results both in bipolar depression and in mania (Cookson *et al.*, 1996; Walden *et al.*, 1996), and controlled studies are underway. It is generally well tolerated, without weight gain or cognitive impairment and probably without teratogenic risk. However, up to 10% of patients develop a rash which is potentially serious. The risk of serious allergic reactions may be reduced by increasing the dose slowly in steps of 25 mg per week to an average of 150 mg per day. Higher doses are required in patients on carbamazepine, and lower in patients on valproate because of the effects of these drugs on hepatic oxidase enzymes which metabolise the drug.

Mechanism of action

Lamotrigine blocks fast sodium channels, thereby reducing the size of action potentials in nerve fibres. It has also profound effects reducing calcium currents. These actions are thought to reduce the release of neurotransmitters, especially the excitatory transmitter glutamate which is released at cortical projections in the limbic areas of the ventral striatum, an area which also receives an inhibitory input from the mesolimbic dopamine pathway.

Antipsychotic drugs in prophylaxis

Because of sedative effects and long-term neurological side-effects, antipsychotic drugs should be avoided if possible for long-term use in bipolar patients. However, for those who have frequently recurring episodes, and either do not benefit from, or do not adhere to, oral medication, depot formulations of antipsychotic drugs can provide a period of stability (Lowe & Batchelor, 1990). Two studies of bipolar patients using a mirror-image design found that during depot treatment, there were less manic episodes (White *et al.*, 1993), or less manic and depressive episodes (Littlejohn *et al.*, 1994). It has been suggested that patients with bipolar disorder are particularly susceptible to developing tardive dyskinesia (Hamra *et al.*, 1983). Other authors have found a prevalence (about 20%) similar to that among patients with chronic schizophrenia (Hunt & Silverstone, 1991). However, tardive dyskinesia may be more preventable in bipolar patients since a wider range of alternative treatments are available than for schizophrenia. In practice, the combination of an antipsychotic drug with lithium is very common for the treatment of mania, and the majority of manic patients are discharged on antipsychotic medication (Licht *et al.*, 1984) and remain on it after 6 months (Keck *et al.*, 1996). The development of new antipsychotics with less propensity to cause tardive dyskinesia is important for bipolar patients.

Mechanism of action

Antipsychotics are primarily antagonists at dopamine D_2 receptors, and to varying extents at alpha$_1$ adrenoceptors. These actions, within the limbic system probably underlie their antimanic properties (Cookson *et al.*, 1981, 1985) and their effects on hormone levels in mania (Cookson, 1985).

Atypical antipsychotics in bipolar disorder

Maintenance treatment with clozapine may be of value in some cases of bipolar illness resistant to other treatments including other antipsychotics (Zarate *et al.*, 1995). Weekly blood count monitoring is required because of the risk of agranulocytosis.

Risperidone, which combines potent dopamine receptor blockade with blockade of $5\text{-}HT_2$ receptors has not been investigated in controlled trials in bipolar disorder. However, the serotonin antagonist methysergide exacerbates mania (Coppen *et al.*, 1969), and treatment with risperidone has been associated with the onset of mania in some bipolar schizoaffective patients (Dwight *et al.*, 1994).

Other drugs as mood stabilizers

The calcium channel blocker verapamil has been found effective in acute mania, although few controlled studies have been conducted (Dinan *et al.*, 1988; Hoschl & Kozeny, 1989). In a double-blind comparison, verapamil in doses of 40–120 mg three times daily was less effective in mania than lithium (Walton *et al.*, 1996). Nifedipine and diltiazem have also been reported to have antimanic effects. Pazzaglia *et al.* (1993) have described mood-stabilizing effects of nimodipine (a dihydropiperidine, which has greater liquid solubility) in a group of bipolar patients during phases of ultradian cycling, when there is also evidence of low cerebral metabolism in brain scans. It is of theoretical interest that the cholinesterase inhibitor physostigmine has antimanic properties; however, its side-effects preclude clinical use (Janowsky *et al.*, 1973). Likewise, the addition of lecithin (a precursor of acetyl choline) may potentiate other antimanic medication, but its value in clinical practice is doubtful. L-tryptophan may have antimanic properties (Prange *et al.*, 1974) but placebo-controlled trials have not consistently supported this. The use of clonidine in neuroleptic-resistant mania has been reported but placebo controlled studies have not confirmed its value (Janicak *et al.*, 1989).

Adjunctive thyroid hormone

There is evidence from placebo-controlled studies that L-thyroxine or tri-iodothyronine in replacement doses can potentiate the antidepressant effect of monoamine re-uptake inhibitors in patients with resistant depression. However, in long-term prophylaxis this treatment eventually loses efficacy (Wehr *et al.*, 1988). High-dose thyroid hormone treatment has also been advocated for resistant bipolar patients, especially rapid-cyclers, but prospective placebo-controlled studies are required to establish this as an effective treatment (Bauer & Whybrow, 1990).

Conclusion

Recurrent affective disorder carries a poor prognosis in terms of frequency of recurrences, divorce, physical illness and suicide. It is also compatible with periods of successful leadership, productivity and creativity (Andreason, 1987; Jamison, 1995; Post, 1996). Treatment with mood stabilizers can reduce the frequency and severity of recurrences, minimizes the disruption of personal function, and reduces the mortality and suicide risk. Sufferers from this condition should be educated concerning the nature of their condition and the treatments available, and should be encouraged to choose effective treatment and to use it to best advantage.

References

Abel, E.A. (1992) Diagnosis of drug-induced psoriasis. *Seminars in Dermatology*, **11**, 269–274.

Adityanjee (1989) The syndrome of irreversible lithium-effectuated neurotoxicity. *Pharmaco-psychiatry*, **22**, 81–83.

Alexander, B. & Perry, P.J. (1987) Diuretics. In: *Lithium Combination Treatment* (ed. F.N. Johnson), pp. 177–200. Karger, Basel.

American Psychiatric Association (1994) *Diagnostic and Statistical Manual of Mental Disorders*, 4th edn. American Psychiatric Association; Washington, DC.

Andreasen, N.C. (1987) Creativity and mental illness: prevalence rates in writers and their first-degree relatives. *American Journal of Psychiatry*, **144**, 1288–1292.

Angst, J. (1985) Switch from depression to mania: a record study over decades between 1920 and 1982. *Psychopathology*, **18**, 140–155.

Asnis, G.M., Asnis, D., Dunner, D.L. & Fieve, R.R. (1979) Cogwheel rigidity during chronic lithium therapy. *American Journal of Psychiatry*, **136**, 1225–1226.

Baastrup, P.C., Poulsen, J.C. Schou, M., Thomsen, K. & Amdisen, A. (1970) Prophylactic lithium: double-blind discontinuation in manic-depressive and recurrent-depressive disorder. *Lancet*, **ii**, 326–330.

Ballenger, J.C. & Post, R.M. (1980) Carbamazepine in manic depressive illness. a new treatment. *American Journal of Psychiatry*, **137**, 782–790.

Bauer, M.S. & Whybrow, P.C. (1990) Rapid-cycling bipolar affective disorder. II. Treatment of refractory rapid-cycling with high dose levothyroxine: a preliminary study. *Archives of General Psychiatry*, **47**, 435–440.

Bauer, M.S., Whybrow, P.C. & Winokur, A. (1990) Rapid-cycling bipolar affective disorder. Association with Grade I hypothyroidism. *Archives of General Psychiatry*, **47**, 427–432.

Bebbington, P. & Ramana, R. (1995). The epidemiology of bipolar affective disorder. *Social Psy-*

chiatry and Psychiatric Epidemiology, **30**, 279–292.

Belmaker, R.H., Berdusky, Y., Agam, G., Levine, J. & Kofman, O. (1996) How does lithium work in manic depression? Clinical and psychological correlates of the inositol theory. *Annual Review of Medicine*, **47**, 47–56.

Bernadt, M.W. & Murray, R.M. (1986) Psychiatric disorder, drinking and alcoholism. *British Journal of Psychiatry*, **148**, 393–400.

Berridge, M. (1984) Inositol triphosphate and diaglycerol as second messengers. *Biochemical Journal*, **220**, 345–360.

Birch, N.J., Horsman, A. & Hullin, R.P. (1982) Lithium, bone and body weight studies in long-term lithium-treated patients and in the rat. *Neuropsychobiology*, **8**, 86–92.

Black, D.W., Winokur, G. & Nasrallah, M.A. (1987) Suicide in sub-types of major affective disorder: a comparison with general population suicide mortality. *Archives of General Psychiatry*, **44**, 878–880.

Bland, R.C. & Orn, H. (1982) Course and outcome of affective disorders. *Canadian Journal of Psychiatry*, **27**, 573–578.

Blay, S.L., Toledo Ferraz, M.P. & Calil, H.M. (1982) Lithium-induced male sexual impairment: two case reports. *Journal of Clinical Psychiatry*, **43**, 497–498.

Bone, S., Rose, S.P., Dunner, D.L. & Fieve, R.R. (1980) Incidence of side effects in patients on long-term lithium therapy. *Amerian Journal of Psychiatry*, **137**, 103–104.

Bowden, C.L., Brugger, A.M., Swann, A.C. *et al.* (1994) Efficacy of Divalproex vs. lithium and placebo in the treatment of mania. *Journal of the American Medical Association*, **271**, 918–924.

Bowen, R.C., Grof, P. & Grof, E. (1991) Less frequent lithium administration and lower urine volume. *American Journal of Psychiatry*, **148**, 189–192.

Brodie, H.K.H. & Leff, M.J. (1971) Bipolar depression: a comparative study of patient characteristics. *American Journal of Psychiatry*, **127**, 1086–1090.

Bucht, G., Wahlin, A., Wentzel, T. & Wimblad, B. (1980) Renal function and morphology in long-term lithium and combined lithium–neuroleptic treatment. *Acta Medica Scandinavica*, **208**, 381–385.

Calabrese, J.R. & Delucchi, G.A. (1990) Spectrum of efficacy of valproate in 55 patients with rapid-cycling bipolar disorder. *American Journal of Psychiatry*, **147**, 431–434.

Calabrese, J.R., Gulledge, A.D., Hahn, K. *et al.* (1985) Autoimmune thyroiditis in manic-depressive patients treated with lithium. *American Journal of Psychiatry*, **142**, 1318–1321.

Calabrese, J.R., Bowden, C., & Woyshville, M.J. (1995) Lithium and anticonvulsants in the treatment of bipolar discords. In: *Psychopharmacology: The Fourth Generation of Progress* (eds F.E. Bloom & D.J. Kupfer), pp. 1099–1111. Raven Press, New York.

Charney, D.S., Kales, A., Soldatos, C. & Nelson, J.C. (1979) Somnambulistic-like episode, secondary to contained lithium-neuroleptic treatment. *British Journal of Psychiatry*, **135**, 418–424.

Chen, Y. & Silverstone, T. (1990) Lithium and weight gain. *International Clinical Psychopharmacology*, **5**, 217–225.

Cohen, W.J. & Cohen, N.H. (1974) Lithium carbonate, haloperidol, and irreversible brain damage. *Journal of the American Medical Association*, **230**, 1283–1287.

Cohen, L.S., Friedman, J.M., Jefferson, J.W. *et al.* (1994) A reevaluation of risk of in utero exposure to lithium. *Journal of American Medical Association*, **271**, 146–150.

Cookson, J.C. (1989) Manic-depressive illness and driving. *Travel Medicine International*, **7**, 105–108.

Cookson, J.C., Silvestone, T. & Wells, B. (1981) A double-blind comparative clinical trial of pimozide and chlorpromazine in mania: a test of the dopamine hypothesis. *Acta Psychiatrica Scandinavica*, **64**, 381–397.

Cookson, J.C., Silverstone, T., Williams, S. & Besser G.M. (1985) Plasma corticol levels in mania: associated clinical ratings and change during treatment with haloperidol. *British Journal of Psychiatry*, **146**, 498–502.

Cookson, J.C., Kundu, S., Anderson, J. *et al.* (1996) Lamotrigine in treatment-refractory bipolar disorder. *Journal of Psychopharmacology*, **10** (Suppl. 3) A39.

Coppen, A. & Abou-Saleh, M.T. (1983) Lithium in prophylaxis of unipolar depression: a review. *Journal of the Royal Society of Medicine*, **76**, 297–301.

Coppen, A. & Abou-Saleh, M.T. (1988) Lithium therapy: from clinical trials to practical management. *Acta Psychiatrica Scandinavica*, **78**, 754–762.

Coppen, A., Prange, A.J., Whybrow, P.C., Noguera, R. & Paez, J.M. (1969) Methysergide in mania: a controlled trial. *Lancet*, **2**, 338–340.

Coppen, A., Noguera, R., Bailey, J. *et al.* (1971) Prophylactic lithium in affective disorders: controlled trial. *Lancet*, **ii**, 275–279.

Coppen, A., Abou-Saleh, M.T., Milln, P., Bailey, J. & Wood, M.K. (1983) Decreasing lithium dosage reduces morbidity and side-effects during prophylaxis. *Journal of Affective Disorders*, **5**, 353–362.

Coppen, A., Standish-Barry, H., Bailey, J. *et al.* (1991) Does lithium reduce the mortality of recurrent mood disorders? *Journal of Affective Disorders*, **23**, 1–7.

Coxhead, N., Silverstone, T. & Cookson, J.C. (1992) Carbamazepine versus lithium in the prophylaxis of bipolar affective disorder. *Acta Psychiatrica Scandinavica*, **85**, 114–118.

Cundall, R.L., Brooks, P.W. & Murray, L.G. (1972) A controlled evaluation of lithium prophylaxis in affective disorders. *Psychological Medicine*, **2**, 308–311.

Cutler, N.R. & Post, R.M. (1982) Life course of illness in untreated manic-depressive patients. *Comprehensive Psychiatry*, **23**, 101–115.

Dardennes, R., Even, C., Bange, F. *et al.* (1995) Comparison of carbamazepine and lithium in the prophylaxis of bipolar disorder: a meta-analysis. *British Journal of Psychiatry*, **166**, 378–381.

Das Chargas Rodrigues, F. & Zwicker, A.P. (1985) Chronic lithium prevents REM sleep-deprivation-induced increased responsiveness to apomorphine. *Journal of Pharmaceutics and Pharmacology*, **37**, 210–211.

Diamond, B.I. & Brown, R.L. (1987) Anaesthetic agents and associated medications. In: *Lithium Combination Treatment* (ed. F. N. Johnson), pp. 217–232. Karger, Basel.

Dickson, W.E. & Kendell, R.E. (1986) Does maintenance lithium therapy prevent recurrences of mania under ordinary clinical conditions? *Psychological Medicine*, **16**, 521–530.

Dinan, T.G. & Kohen, D. (1989) Tardive dyskinesia in bipolar affective disorder: relationship to lithium therapy. *British Journal of Psychiatry*, **15**, 55–57.

Dinan, T.G., Silverstone, T. & Cookson, J.C. (1988) Cortisol, prolactin and growth hormone levels with clinical ratings in manic patients treated with verapamil. *International Clinical Psychopharmacology*, **3**, 151–156.

Dirlich, G., Kammerloher, A., Schulz, H. *et al.* (1981) Temporal coordination of rest–activity cycle: body temperature, urinary free cortisol and mood in a patient with 48-hour unipolar depressive cycles in clinical and time-cue-free environments. *Biological Psychiatry*, **16**, 163–179.

Dousa, T.P. (1974) Interaction of lithium with vasopressin-sensitive cyclic AMP system of human renal medulla. *Endocrinology*, **95**, 1359–1366.

Dunner, D.L. & Fieve, R.R. (1974) Clinical factors in lithium prophylaxis failure. *Archives of General Psychiatry*, **30**, 229–233.

Dunner, D.L., Gershon, E.S. & Goodwin, F.K. (1976b) Heritable factors in the severity of affective illness. *Biological Psychiatry*, **11**, 31–42.

Dwight, M.M., Kech, P.E., Stanton, S.P., Strakowski, S.M. & McElroy, S.L. (1994) Antidepressant activity and mania associated with risperidone treatment of schizo-affective disorder. *Lancet*, **344**, 554–555.

Elphick, M., Yang, J.D. & Cowen, P.H. (1990) Effects of carbamazepine on dopamine and serotonin-mediated neuroendocrine responses. *Archives of General Psychiatry*, **47**, 135–143.

Fadden, G., Bebbington, P. & Kuipers, L. (1987) Caring and its burdens: a study of spouses of depressed patients. *British Journal of Psychiatry*, **151**, 660–667.

Faedda, G.L., Baldessarini, R.J., Tohen, M., Strakowski, S.M. & Waternaux, C. (1991) Episode sequence in bipolar disorder and response to lithium treatment. *American Journal of Psychiatry*, **148**, 1237–1239.

Fitzpatrick, L.A. & Spiegel, A.M. (1988) Normal regulation of parathyroid hormone secretion. In: *Lithium and the Endocrine System* (ed. F. N. Johnson), pp. 194–201. Karger, Basel.

Franchini, L., Gasperini, M. & Smeraldi, E. (1994) A 24-month follow-up study of unipolar subjects: a comparison between lithium and fluvoxamine. *Journal of Affective Disorders*, **32**, 225–231.

Gadallah, M.F., Feinstein, E.I. & Massry, S.G. (1988) Lithium intoxication: clinical course and therapeutic considerations. *Mineral Electrolyte Metabolism*, **14**, 146–149.

Gawin, F.H. & Kleber, H.D. (1986) Abstinence symptomatology and psychiatric diagnosis in cocaine abusers. *Archives of General Psychiatry* **43**, 107–113.

Gelenberg, A.J. & Jefferson, J.W. (1995) Lithium tremor. *Journal of Clinical Psychiatry*, **56**, 283–287.

Gelenberg, A.J., Kane, J.M., Keller, M.B. *et al.* (1989) Comparison of standard and low serum levels of lithium for maintenance treatment of bipolar disorder. *New England Journal of Medicine*, **321**, 1489–1493.

Gerner, R.H. & Stanton A. (1992) Algorithm for patient management of acute manic states: lithium, valproate or carbamazepine? *Journal of Clinical Psychopharmacology*, **12** (Suppl.), 57–63.

Glen, A.I.M., Johnson, A.L. & Shephered, M. (1984) Continuation therapy with lithium and amitriptyline in unipolar depressive illness: a randomised double-blind controlled trial. *Psychological Medicine*, **14**, 37–50.

Glick, I.D., Clarkin, J.F., Spencer, J.H. *et al.* (1985) A controlled evaluation of inpatient family intervention: Preliminary results of the six-month follow-up. *Archives of General Psychiatry*, **42**, 882–886.

Goodwin, F.K. & Jamison, K.R. (1990) *Manic-Depressive Illness*. Oxford University Press, Oxford.

Goodwin, F.K., Murphy, D.C. & Bunney, W.F. (1969) Lithium carbonate treatment in depression and mania: a longitudinal double-blind study. *Archives of General Psychiatry*, **21**, 486–496.

Goodwin, G.M. (1994) Recurrence of mania after lithium withdrawal: implications for the use of lithium in the treatment of bipolar affective disorder. *British Journal of Psychiatry*, **164**, 149–152.

Goodwin, G.M., De Souza, R.J., Wood, A.J. & Green, A.R. (1986) The enhancement by lithium of the 5-HT$_{1A}$-mediated serotonin syndrome in the rat: evidence for a post-synaptic mechanism. *Psychopharmacology*, **90**, 488–493.

Grof, P., Alda, M., Grof, E., Fox, D. & Cameron, P. (1993) The challenge of predicting response to stabilising lithium treatment. *British Journal of Psychiatry*, **163** (Suppl. 21), 16–19.

Hamra, B., Nasrallah, H., Clancy, J. & Finn, R. (1983) Psychiatric diagnosis and risk for tardive dyskinesia. *Archives of General Psychiatry*, **40**, 346–347.

Hansen, H.E. & Amdisen, A. (1978) Lithium intoxication (Report of 23 cases and a review of 100 cases from the literature). *Quarterly Journal of Medicine*, **47**, 123–144.

Harding, T. & Knight, F. (1973) Marijuana-modified mania. *Archives of General Psychiatry*, **29**, 635–637.

Hardy, B.G., Shulman, K.I., Mackenzie, S.E., Kutcher, S.P. & Silverberg, J.D. (1987) Pharmacokinetics of lithium in the elderly. *Journal of Clinical Psychopharmacology*, **7**, 153–158.

Harrow, M., Goldberg, J.F., Grossman, L.S. & Meltzer, H.Y. (1990) Outcome in manic disorder: a naturalistic follow-up study. *Archives of General Psychiatry*, **47**, 665–671.

Hestbech, J., Hansen, H.E., Amdisen, A. & Olsen, S. (1977) Chronic renal lesions following long-term treatment with lithium. *Kidney International*, **12**, 205–213.

Himmelhoch, J.M., Mulla, D., Neil, J.F., Detre, T.P. & Kupfer, D.J. (1976) Incidence and significance of mixed affective states in a bipolar population. *Archives of General Psychiatry*, **33**, 1062–1066.

Himmelhoch, J.M., Neil, J.F., May, S.J., Fuchs, C.Z. & Licata, S.M. (1980) Age, dementia, dyskinesias, and lithium response. *American Journal of Psychiatry*, **137**, 941–945.

Hokin, L.E. (1993) Lithium increases accumulation of second messenger inositol 1,4,5-trisphosphate in brain cortex slices in species ranging from mouse to monkey. *Advanced Enzyme Regulation*, **33**, 299–312.

Hoschl, C. & Kozeny, J. (1989) Verapamil in affective disorders: a controlled, double-blind study. *Biological Psychiatry*, **25**, 128–140.

Hunt, N. & Silverstone, T. (1991) Tardive dyskinesia in bipolar affective disorder: a catchment area study. *International Clinical Psychopharmacology*, **6**, 45–50.

Hunt, N., Bruce-Jones, W. & Silverstone, T. (1992) Life events in bipolar affective disorder. *Journal of Affective Disorders*, **25**, 13–20.

Hunter, R., Christie, J.E., Whalley, L.J. *et al.* (1989) Luteinizing hormone responses to luteinizing hormone release hormone (LHRH) in acute mania and the effects of lithium on LHRH and thyrotropin releasing hormone tests in volunteers. *Psychological Medicine*, **19**, 69–77.

Imbs, J.L., Danion, J.M., Schmidt, M., Welsch, M. & Singer, L. (1987) Non-steroidal anti-inflammatory drugs. In: *Lithium Combination Treatment* (ed. F. N. Johnson), pp. 201–216. Karger, Basel.

Jacobson, S.J., Jones, K., Johnson, K. *et al.* (1992) Prospective multi-centre study of pregnancy outcome after lithium exposure during first trimester. *Lancet*, **339**, 530–533.

Jamison, K.R. (1989) Mood disorders and seasonal patterns in British writers and artists. *Psychiatry*, **52**, 125–134.

Jamison, K.R. (1995) *An Unquiet Mind*. Picador, London.

Janicak, P.G., Sharma, R.P., Easton, M., Comaty, J.E. & Davis, J.M. (1989) A double-blind, placebo controlled trial of clonidine in the treatment of acute mania. *Psychopharmacology Bulletin*, **25**, 243–245.

Janowsky, D.S., El-Yousef, M.K., Davis, J.M. & Sekerke, H.J. (1973) Parasympathetic suppression of manic symptoms by physostigmine. *Archives of General Psychiatry*, **28**, 542–547.

Jauhar, P. & Weller, M.P.I. (1982) Psychiatric morbidity and time zone changes: a study of patients from Heathrow Airport. *British Journal of Psychiatry*, **140**, 231–235.

Jha, A.K., Stein, G.S. & Fenwick, P. (1996) Negative interaction between lithium and electroconvulsion therapy: a case-controlled study. *British Journal of Psychiatry*, **168**, 241–243.

Johnson, D.A.W., Lowe, M.R. & Batchelor, D.H. (1990) Combined lithium-neuroleptic therapy for manic-depressive illness. *Human Psychopharmacology*, **5** (Suppl.), 262–297.

Johnson, F.N. (1984) *The History of Lithium Therapy*. Macmillan, London.

Johnson, G. (1984) Lithium. *Medical Journal of Australia*, **141**, 595–601.

Johnson, G.F.S., Hunt, G.E., Duggin, G.G., Hoovalt, J.S. & Tiller, D.J. (1990) Renal function and lithium treatment: initial and follow-up tests in manic depressive patients. *Journal of Affective Disorders*, 6, 249–263.

Kallen, B. & Tandberg, A. (1983) Lithium and pregnancy: a cohort study on manic-depressive women. *Acta Psychiatrica Scandinavica*, 68, 134–139.

Kane, J.M., Quitkin, F.M., Rifkin, A., Ramos-Lorenzi, J.R., Nayak, D.P. & Howard, A. (1982) Lithium carbonate and imipramine in the prophylaxis of unipolar and bipolar II illness. *Archives of General Psychiatry*, 39, 1065–1069.

Kanzaki, T. (1991) Acneiform eruption induced by lithium carbonate. *Journal of Dermatology*, 18, 481–483.

Keck, P.E., McElroy, S.L., Strakowski, S.M., Balistrem, T.M., Kizer, D.L. & West, S.L. (1996) Factors associated with maintenance anti-psychotic treatment of patients with bipolar disorder. *Journal of Clinical Psychiatry*, 57, 147–151.

Ketter, T.A., Post, R.M. & Worthington, K. (1991) Principles of clinically important drug interactions with carbamazepine: part 1. *Journal of Clinical Psychopharmacology*, 11, 198–203.

King, J.R. & Hullin, R.P. (1983) Withdrawal symptoms from lithium: four case reports and a questionnaire study. *British Journal of Psychiatry*, 143, 30–35.

Klawans, H.L. & Weiner, W.J. (1976) The pharmacology of choreatic movements. *Progress in Neurobiology*, 6, 49–80.

Kocsis, J.H., Shaw, E.D., Stokes, P.E. et al. (1993) Neuropsychological effects of lithium discontinuation. *Journal of Clinical Psychopharmacology*, 13, 268–275.

Kolk, A., Kathmann, N. & Greil, W. (1993) No short-term changes of cognitive performance and mood after single doses of two different lithium retard preparations. *Pharmacopsychiatry*, 26, 235–239.

Kramlinger, K.G. & Post, R.M. (1989) Adding lithium carbonate to carbamazepine: anti-manic efficacy in treatment-resistant mania. *Acta Psychiatrica Scandinavica*, 79, 378–385.

Kramlinger K.G. & Post, R.M. (1996) Ultra-rapid and ultradian cycling in bipolar affective illness. *British Journal of Psychiatry*, 168, 314–323.

Kukopulos, A., Minnai, G. & Muller-Oerlinghausen, B. (1985) The influence of mania and depression on the pharmocokinetics of lithium: a longitudinal single-case study. *Journal of Affective Disorders*, 8, 159–166.

Lawler, P.G., & Cove-Smith, J.R. (1986). Acute respiratory failure following lithium intoxication. *Anaesthesia*, 41, 623–627.

Lazarus, J.H., John R., Bennie EH, Chalmers, RJ, Crockett, G. (1981) Lithium therapy and thyroid function: a long-term study. *Psychological Medicine*, 11, 85–92.

Leonard, K. (1979) *The Classification of Endogenous Psychoses* (ed. E. Robins; trans. R. Berman). Irvington Publishers, New York.

Licht, R.W., Gouliea, G., Vesterfaarl P., Dybbro, J., Lumd, H. & Merubdet, L. (1994) Treatment of manic episodes in Scandinavia: the use of neuroleptic drugs in a clinical routine setting. *Journal of Affective Disorders*, 32, 179–185.

Littlejohn, R., Leslie, F. & Cookson, J.C. (1994) Depot anti-psychotics in the prophylaxis of bipolar disorder. *British Journal of Psychiatry*, 65, 827–829.

Llau, M.E., Viraben, R. & Montastruc, J.L. (1995) Drug-induced alopecia: review of literature. *Therapie*, 50, 145–150.

Lombardi, G., Panza, N., Biondi, B. et al. (1993) Effects of lithium treatment on hypothalamic-pituitary-thyroid axis: a longitudinal study. *Journal of Endocrinological Investigations*, 16, 259–263.

Loudon, J.B. & Waring, H. (1976) Toxic reactions to lithium and haloperidol. Lancet, ii, 1088.

Lowe, M.R. & Batchelor, D.H. (1990) Lithium and neuroleptics in the management of manic-depressive psychosis. *Human Psychopharmacology*, 5, 267–274.

Maes, M. & Calabrese, J.R. (1994) Mechanisms of action of valproate in affective disorders. In: *Anti-convulsants in Mood Disorder* (eds R. T. Joffe & J. R. Calabrese) pp. 93–110. Marcel Dekker, New York.

Maggs, R. (1963) Treatment of manic illness with lithium carbonate. *British Journal of Psychiatry*, 109, 56–65.

Mander, A.J. & Loudon, J.B. (1988) Rapid recurrence of mania following abrupt discontinuation of lithium. Lancet, ii, 15–17.

McCance-Katz, E., Price, L.H., Charney, D.S. & Heninger, G.R. (1992) Serotonergic function during lithium augmentation of refractory depression. *Psychopharmacology-Berlin*, 108, 93–97.

McCreadie, R.G. & Morrison D.P. (1985) The impact of lithium in South-West Scotland: *British Journal of Psychiatry*, 146, 70–74.

McElroy, S.L., Keck, P.E. Pope, H.G. et al. (1992) Valproate in the treatment of bipolar disorder: literature review and clinical guidelines. *Journal of Clinical Pharmocology*, 12, 42S–52S.

Mitchell, J.E. & MacKenzie, T.B. (1982) Cardiac effects of lithium therapy in man: a review. *Journal of Clinical Psychiatry*, 43, 47–51.

Mitchel, P., Withers, K., Jacobs, G. et al. (1994) Combining lithium and sodium valproate for bipolar disorder. *Australian and New Zealand Journal of Psychiatry*, 28: 141–143.

Montastruc, J.L., Llau, M.E., Rascol, O. & Senard, J.M. (1994) Drug-induced parkinsonism: a review. *Fundamentals of Clinical Pharmacology*, **8**, 293–306.

Montgomery, S.A. & Roberts, A. (1994) SSRIs: well tolerated treatment for depression. *Human Psychopharmacology*, **9**, S7–S10.

Müller-Oerlinghausen, B., Ahren, B., Grof, E. *et al.* (1992) The effects of long-term lithium treatment on the mortality of patients with manic-depressive and schizo-affective illness. *Acta Psychiatrica Scandinavica*, **86**, 218–222.

Murphy, D.L. & Beigel, A. (1974) Depression, elation, and lithium carbonate responses in manic patient sub-groups. *Archives of General Psychiatry*, **31**, 643–648.

Myers, D.H. Carter, R.A., Burns, B.H., Armond, A., Hussein, S.B. Chengapa, V.K. (1985) A prospective study of the effects of lithium on thyroid function and on the prevalance of thyroid antibodies. *Psychological Medicine*, **15**, 55–61.

Norton, B. Whalley, L.J. (1984) Mortality of a lithium-treated population. *British Journal of Psychiatry*, **145**, 277–282.

Okuma, T., Kishimoto, A., Inoue, K. *et al.* (1973) Anti-manic and prophylactic effects of carbamazepine (Tegretol) on manic depressive psychosis: a preliminary report. *Folia Psychiatrica Neurology Japan*, **27**, 283–297.

Okuma, T., Inanaga, K., Otsuki, S. *et al.* (1981) A preliminary double-blind study of carbamazepine in prophylaxis of manic-depressive illness. *Psychopharmacology*, **73**, 95–96.

Pazzaglia, P.J., Post, R.M., Ketter, T.A. *et al.* (1993) Preliminary controlled trial of nimodipine in ultra-rapid cycling affective dysregulation. *Psychiatry Research*, **49**, 257–272.

Pope, H.G., McElroy, S.L., Keck, P.E. & Hudson, J.I. (1991) Valporate in the treatment of acute mania: a placebo-controlled study. *Archives of General Psychiatry*, **48**, 62–68.

Post, F. (1996) Verbal creativity, depression and alcoholism: an investigation of one hundred American and British writers. *British Journal of Psychiatry*, **168**, 545–555.

Post, R.M. (1990) Prophylaxis of bipolar disorders. *International Review of Psychiatry*, **2**, 227–320.

Post, R.M. (1992a). Anticonvulsants and novel drugs. In: *Handbook of Affective Disorders* (ed. E.S. Paykel), pp. 387–417. Churchill Livingstone, Edinburgh.

Post, R.M. (1992b) Transduction of psychosocial stress into the neurobiology of recurrent affective disorder. *American Journal of Psychiatry*, **149**, 999–1010.

Post, R.M., Ballenger, J.C., Rey, A.C. & Bunney, W.E. Jr (1981) Slow and rapid onset of manic episodes: implications for underlying biology. *Psychiatry Research*, **4**, 229–237.

Post, R.M., Uhde, T.W., Ballenger J.C. & Squillace, K.M. (1983) Prophylactic efficacy of carbamazepine in manic-depressive illness. *American Journal of Psychiatry*, **140**, 1602–1604.

Post, R.M., Uhde, T.W., Roy-Byrne, P.P. & Joffe, R.T. (1986) Antidepressant effects of carbamazepine. *American Journal of Psychiatry*, **143**, 29–34.

Post, R.M., Uhde, T.W., Roy-Byrne, P.P. & Joffe, R.T. (1987) Correlates of antimanic responses to carbamazepine. *Psychiatry Research*, **21**, 71–84.

Post, R.M., Rubinow D.R., Uhde, T.W. (1989) Dysphoric mania: clinical and biological correlates. *Archives of General Psychiatry*, **46**, 353–358.

Post, R.M., Leverich, G.S., Rosoff, A.S. & Altshuler, L.L. (1990) Carbamazepine prophylaxis in refractory affective disorders: a focus on long-term follow-up. *Journal of Clinical Psychopharmacology*, **20**, 318–327.

Post, R.M., Weiss, S.R.B., Chuang, D.M. & Ketter, T.A. (1994) Mechanism of action of carbamazepine in seizure and affective disorders. In: *Anticonvulsants in Mood-Disorders* (ed. R.T. Joff & J.R. Calabrese), pp. 43–92. Marcel Dekker, New York.

Prakash, R. (1987) Blood. In: *Depression and Mania: Modern Lithium Therapy* (ed. F. N. Johnson), pp. 218–220. IRL Press, New York.

Prange, A.J., Wilson, I.C., Lynn, C.W., Alltop, L.B. & Stikeleather, R.A. (1974) L-tryptophan in mania: contribution to a permissive hypothesis of affective disorders. *Archives of General Psychiatry*, **30**, 56–62.

Prien, R.F. & Gelenberg, A.J. (1989) Alternatives to lithium for preventive treatment of bipolar disorder. *American Journal of Psychiatry*, **146**, 840–848.

Prien, R.F., Caffey, E.M. Jr & Klett, C.J. (1973) Prophylactic efficacy of lithium carbonate in manic-depressive illness. *Archives of General Psychiatry*, **28**, 337–341.

Prien, R.F., Kupfer, D.J., Mansky, P.A. *et al.* (1984) Drug therapy in the prevention of recurrences in unipolar and bipolar affective disorder: report of the NIMH Collaborative Study Group comparing lithium carbonate, imipramine and a lithium carbonate–imipramine combination. *Archives of General Psychiatry*, **41**, 1096–1104.

Quitkin, F.M., Kane, J., Rifkin, A., Ramos-Lorenzi, J.R. & Mayak, D.V. (1985) Prophylactic lithium carbonate with and without imipramine for bipolar 1 patients: a double-blind study. *Archives of General Psychiatry*, **38**, 902–907.

Rastoge, R.B. & Singhal, R.L. (1977) Lithium modification of behavioural activity and brain biogenic amines in developing hyperthyroid rats. *Journal of Pharmacology and Experimental Therapeutics*, **201**, 92–102.

Reed, S.M., Wise, M.G. & Timmerman, I. (1989) Choreoathetosis: a sign of lithium toxicity. *Journal of Neuropsychiatry and Clinical Neurosciences*, **1**, 57–60.

Rosa, F.W. (1991) Spina bifida in infants of women treated with carbamazepine during pregnancy. *New England Journal of Medicine*, **324**, 674–677.

Rottanberg, D., Robins, A.H., Ben-Arie, O., Teggan, A. & Elk, R. (1982) Cannabis-associated psychosis with manic features. *Lancet*, **ii**, 1364–1366.

Schou, M. (1979) Artistic productivity and lithium prophylaxis in manic-depressive illness. *British Journal of Psychiatry*, **135**, 97–103.

Schou, M. (1984) Long-lasting neurological sequelae after lithium intoxication. *Acta Psychiatrica Scandinavica*, **70**, 594–602.

Schou, M., Juel-Neilson, N., Stromgren, E. & Voldby, H. (1954) The treatment of manic psychoses by administration of lithium salts. *Journal of Neurology, Neurosurgery and Psychiatry*, **17**, 250–260.

Schou, M., Baastrup, P.C., Grof P., Weis, P. Angst, J. (1970) Pharmacological and clinical problems of lithium prophylaxis. *British Journal of Psychiatry*, **116**, 615–619.

Sclare, P. & Creed, F. (1987) Life events and the onset of mania. *British Journal of Psychiatry*, **156**, 508–514.

Sellers, J., Tyrer, P., Whiteley, A., Banks, D.C. & Barer, D.H. (1982) Neurotoxic effects of lithium with delayed rise in serum lithium levels. *British Journal of Psychiatry*, **140**, 623–625.

Shapira, B., Yagmur, M.J., Gropp, C., Newman, M. & Lerer, B. (1992) Effect of clomipramine and lithium on fenfluramine-induced hormone release in major depression. *Biological Psychiatry*, **31**, 975–983.

Shapiro, D.R., Quitkin, F.M. & Fleiss, J.L. (1989). Response to maintenance therapy in bipolar illness: effect of index episode. *Archives of General Psychiatry*, **46**, 401–405.

Sharp, T., Bramwell, S.R., Lambert, P. & Grahame-Smith, D.G. (1991) Effect of short- and long-term administration of lithium on the release of endogenous 5-HT in the hippocampus of the rat *in vivo* and *in vitro*. *Neuropharmacology*, **3**, 977–984.

Shukla, S., Godwin, C.D., Long, L.E.B. & Miller, M.G. (1984) Lithium-carbamazepine neurotoxicity and risk factors. *American Journal of Psychiatry*, **141**, 1604–1606.

Silverstone, T. & Romans, S. (1996) Long term treat-

ment of bipolar disorder. *Drugs*, **51**, 367–382.

Simhandl, C., Denk, E. & Thau, K. (1993) The comparative efficacy of carbamazepine low and high serum level and lithium carbonate in the prophylaxis of affective disorders. *Journal of Affective Disorders*, **28**, 221–231.

Smith, S.J.M. & Kocen, R.S. (1998) A Creutzfeldt–Jakob like syndrome due to lithium toxicity. *Journal of Neurology, Neurosurgery and Psychiatry*, **51**, 120–123.

Stancer, H.C. & Forbath, N. (1989) Hyperparathyroidism, hypothyroidism, and impaired renal function after 10 to 20 years of lithium treatment. *Archives of Internal Medicine*, **149**, 1042–1045.

Stewart, P.M., Atherden, S.M., Stewart, S.E., Whalley, L., Edwards, C.R.E & Padfield, P.L. (1988) Lithium carbonate: a competitive aldosterone antagonist? *British Journal of Psychiatry*, **153**, 205–207.

Stokes, P.E., Shamoian, C.A., Stoll, P.M. & Patton, M.J. (1971) Efficacy of lithium as acute treatment of manic-depressive illness. Lancet, **i**, 1319–1325.

Stone, K. (1989) Mania in the elderly. *British Journal of Psychiatry*, **155**, 220–224.

Suppes, T., Baldessarini, R.J., Faedda, G.L. & Tohen, M. (1991) Risk of recurrence following discontinuation of lithium treatment in bipolar disorder. *Archives of General Psychiatry*, **48**, 1082–1088.

Swann, A.C., Secunda, S.K., Katz, M.M. *et al.* (1986) Lithium treatment of mania: clinical characteristics, specificity of symptom change, and outcome. *Psychiatry Research*, **18**, 127–141.

Thisted, E. & Ebbesen, F. (1993) Malformations, withdrawal manifestations and hypoglycaemia after exposure to valproate *in utero*. *Archives of Disease in Childhood*, **69**, 288–291.

Thornhill, D.P. & Field, S.P. (1982) Distribution of lithium elimination in a selected population of psychiatric patients. *European Journal of Clinical Phamacology*, **21**, 351–354.

Tohen, M., Castillo, J., Baldessarini, R.J., *et al.* (1995) Blood dyscrasias with carbamazepine and valproate: a pharmacoepidemiological study of 2,228 patients at risk. *American Journal of Psychiatry*, **152**, 413–418.

Transbol, I., Christiansen, C. & Baastrup, P.C. (1978) Endocrine effects of lithium: I. Hypothyroidism, its prevalence in long-term treated patients. *Acta Endocrinology*, **87**, 759–767.

Tyrer, P., Alexander, M.S., Regan, A. & Lee, I. (1980) An extrapyramidal syndrome after lithium therapy. *British Journal of Psychiatry*, **136**, 191–194.

Vestergaard, P., Amdisen, A. & Schou, M. (1980) Clinically significant side effects of lithium treatment: a survey of 237 patients in long-term treatment. *Acta Psychiatrica Scandinavica*, **62**, 193–200.

Von Knorring, L. (1990) Possible mechanisms for the presumed interaction between lithium and neuroleptics. *Human Psychopharmacology*, **5**, 287–292.

Walden, J., Von Wegerer, J., Beger, M. & Grunze, H. (1996) Efficacy of antiepileptic drugs in the treatment of psychiatric diseases. *EEG Labor*, **18**, 32–47.

Waller, D.G. & Edwards, J.G. (1989) Lithium and the kidney: an update. *Psychological Medicine*, **19**, 825–831.

Waller, D.G., Albano, J.D.M., Millar, J.G.B. & Polak, A. (1987) AMP responses to parathyroid hormone and glucagon during lithium treatment. *Clinical Science*, **66**, 557-559.

Walton, S.A. Berk, M. & Brook, S. (1996) Superiority of lithium over verapamil in mania: a controlled trial. *European Psychiatry*, **11** (suppl. 4), 294S.

Watkins, S.E., Callendar, K., Thomas, DR *et al.* (1987) The effect of carbamazepine and lithium on remission from affective illness. *British Journal of Psychiatry*, **150**, 180–182.

Wehr, T.A. & Goodwin, F.K. (1979) Rapid cycling in manic-depressives induced by tricyclic antidepressants. *Archives of General Psychiatry*, **36**, 555–559.

Wehr, T.A. & Goodwin, F.K. (1987) Can antidepressants cause mania and worsen the course of affective illness? *American Journal of Psychiatry*, **144**, 1403–1411.

Wehr, T.A., Sack, D.A. & Rosenthal, N.E. (1987) Sleep reduction as a final common pathway in the genesis of mania. *American Journal of Psychiatry*, **144**, 201–204.

Wehr, R.A., Sack, D.A., Rosenthal, N.E. & Cowdry R.W. (1988) Rapid cycling affective disorder: contributing factors and treatment responses in 51 patients. *American Journal of Psychiatry*, **145**, 179–184.

West, A.P. & Meltzer, H.Y. (1979) Paradoxical lithium neurotoxicity: a report of five cases and a hypothesis about risk for neurotoxicity. *American Journal of Psychiatry*, **136**, 963–966.

White, E., Cheung, P. & Silverstone, T. (1993) Depot antipsychotics in bipolar affective disorder. *International Clinical Psychopharmacologist*, **8**, 119–122.

Wolff, J., Berens. S.C. & Jones, A.B. (1970) Inhibition of thyrotropin-stimulated adenyl cyclase activity of beef thyroid membranes by low concentration of lithium ion. *Biochemical and Biophysical Research Communications*, **39**, 77–82.

Wood, A.J. & Goodwin, G.M. (1987) A review of the biochemical and neuropharmacological actions of lithium. *Psychological Medicine*, **17**, 579–600.

Yassa, R., Saunders, A., Nastase, C. & Camille, Y. (1988) Lithium induced thyroid disorders: a prevalence study. *Journal of Clinical Psychiatry*, **49**, 14–16.

Zarate, C.A., Tohen, M., Banov, M.D. *et al.* (1995) Is clozapine a mood stabilizer? *Journal of Clinical Psychiatry*, **56**, 108–112.

14 The management of depression in general practice

SCOTT WEICH AND ANTHONY MANN

Thirty years ago the first substantial study of psychiatric morbidity in primary care was published by Shepherd *et al.* (1966). A one-in-eight sample of patients attending 46 general practices in London were assessed. Of the 15 000 patients at risk, one in seven were consulting for a psychiatric condition (largely, depression and anxiety). The authors' recommendation was not to call for more psychiatrists, but to strengthen the primary care team to deal with these conditions, which most of the collaborating general practitioners (GPs) regarded as their own problem. It is surprising, therefore, that in the UK and the USA, only in the last few years, has there been a general acceptance by health service planners, psychiatrists and primary care personnel that neurotic disorders do constitute a significant burden to the individual sufferer, the general practice and the public purse. With this acceptance comes exciting possibilities for improvement for all three should effective treatments be introduced in primary care.

The intervening 30 years have seen the publication of the results of a programme of research that has defined more precisely the type and extent of psychiatric morbidity seen by GPs and, more recently, begun the evaluation of strategies for better detection and treatment. This work has been greatly facilitated by the creation of standard measures: the General Health Questionnaire (Goldberg & Williams, 1988) and the Clinical Interview Schedule (Goldberg *et al.*, 1970; Lewis *et al.*, 1992) which were specifically created for case-finding among primary care patients. Eighty to ninety per cent of patients with mental disorders that present to GPs suffer from depression, anxiety or a mixture of the two states. Only a minority of patients present their distress in psychological terms, the majority through a process of somatization (Goldberg & Bridges, 1988). Patients are likely to present at times of social stress and also when physically ill. The GP's picture, therefore, is a complicated one and difficult to unravel in the brief consultations in the surgery.

Goldberg and Huxley (1992) have constructed a hierarchical model to show the relationship of this primary care morbidity to that seen in secondary care. Using existing prevalence data, they indicated that only about 50% of the morbidity is, in fact, detected in primary care and, of the detected, only about 5–10% is referred for specialist help. A large volume of psychiatric activity, therefore, happens outside the scope of the psychiatric services, approximately three patients consulting seen in primary care at a point in time, with a diagnosable psychiatric disorder, for any one being seen in all components of the psychiatric services combined at that time.

Over the 30 years, a well-rehearsed response to this demonstration of the scale of primary care psychiatry has been that the disorders seen there are relatively mild and self-limiting. GPs were stated to be responsible for patients with socioeconomic problems and the 'worried well', in contrast to the work of the community psychiatrist (Bennett, 1973). These prejudices have been overcome with the demonstration of the severity of many cases of depression among the spectrum of disorders seen in primary care. Some 5–10% suffer from a major depressive disorder (Blacker & Clare, 1987) and the recent World Health Organization (WHO) multicentre study indicated that 10.4% can be classed as having a current depression using ICD-10 World Health Organization (WHO) criteria, with a further 2% with dysthymia (Ustun *et al.*, 1995). The outcome for the patients is not as good as might be imagined. Only a minority recover quickly; the majority of sufferers will tend to have a fluctuating course and approximately one-fifth become chronic, unremittant cases and high users of primary care (Mann *et al.*, 1981). Finally, the cost to the economy of this primary care morbidity through disability days and the cost to the health service through frequent consultation and prescription have been shown to be considerable (Croft-Jefferys & Wilkinson, 1989).

Recognition now of the potential for benefit for the public health and the individual patient has led to recent activity. In the UK and other European countries, a campaign to defeat depression has been launched by the Royal Colleges of Psychiatrists and General Practitioners (Paykel & Priest, 1992). A series of research initiatives has been funded with the aim to improve detection and treatment in primary care under the general rubric *Strengthening the Primary Care Team*. Also, the changes in the structure of the National Health Service in the UK has placed more pressure on psychiatrists at a local level to collaborate more closely with their GP colleagues, thereby restoring psychiatric attention to the common disorders in general practice, often through setting up liaison consultations in the surgery.

This chapter will first discuss the evidence that increasing detection of depression in primary care is of value and second, the status of management in primary care and the research studies that are underway to improve the situation.

Does detection of depression in general practice influence outcome?

Rates of detection of depression in primary care vary greatly in different parts of the world (Ustun *et al.*, 1995). Although detection rates of 75% and above have been reported in one or two centres (von Korff *et al.*, 1987; Ustun *et al.*, 1995), most studies of routine primary care attenders in Western Europe and North America have reported that primary care physicians fail to recognize around one-half of prevalent cases of depression (Marks *et al.*, 1979; Freeling *et al.*, 1985; Blacker & Clare, 1987; Ormel *et al.*, 1991; Goldberg & Huxley, 1992; Paykel & Priest, 1992; Ustun *et al.*, 1995). Since even the 'best' GPs appear to miss a large proportion of the cases that pass through their surgeries (primarily because patients choose to report somatic rather than psychological complaints) (Goldberg & Bridges, 1988; Goldberg & Huxley, 1992), it is important to consider whether detection of depression in primary care makes any difference to patient outcome before advocating changes in clinical practice (Paykel & Priest, 1992).

Evidence concerning the consequences of GP recognition of depression comes from two sources: naturalistic outcome studies and randomized trials. In The Netherlands, Ormel and his colleagues (1990) found that recognition was associated with a reduction in psychiatric symptoms and social disability at follow-up 14 months later among 179 'new' cases of psychiatric disorder (patients who had not received a psychiatric diagnosis in the 12 months prior to the index consultation), irrespective of diagnosis. These authors also reported an association between recognition and a briefer mean duration of index episode for new cases of anxiety but not depression (Ormel *et al.*, 1991). The effects of recognition on outcome did not appear to be confounded by previously reported associations between recognition and greater initial severity and shorter duration of the index episode of psychiatric disorder (Freeling *et al.*, 1985), though the beneficial effects of recognition were found to be greatest for patients with the least severe disorders (Ormel *et al.*, 1990). A weaker positive association between recognition and (better) outcome was also observed 3 years after the index consultation (Ormel *et al.*, 1993). While recognition was associated with a greater likelihood of receiving a mental health intervention (most commonly psychotropic medication), this did not explain (i.e. confound) the association between recognition and outcome at 14 months (Ormel *et al.*, 1990).

Randomized controlled trials in which GPs were given information about the mental state of patients with previously unrecognized psychiatric disorder have produced contradictory results. While two early studies found that informing GPs about the presence of 'unrecognized' psychiatric morbidity (as detected by a screening questionnaire) was associated with higher rates of recovery at 1 (Zung *et al.*, 1983) and 3 months (Johnstone & Goldberg, 1976), and briefer overall episode duration (Johnstone & Goldberg, 1976), subsequent studies have failed to replicate these results (Hoeper *et al.*, 1984; Shapiro *et al.*, 1987). In an excellent review of this literature, Goldberg and Huxley (1992) concluded that feeding back the results of a psychiatric assessment alone was of little use in the absence of advice about patient management, a conclusion echoed elsewhere (Paykel & Priest, 1992; Wright, 1994; Lewis, 1992). Two recent randomized trials in this area support this interpretation. Dowrick and Buchan (1995) found no association between disclosure of Beck Depression Inventory (BDI) score and outcome among cases of depression not recognized by GPs. In a naturalistic arm of this study, unrecognized cases of depression had lower BDI scores at the outset than patients whose depression was 'spontaneously' recognized by their GP, and this difference *increased* during the 12-month study period. In a randomized study of consecutive attenders, Lewis *et al.* (1996) found that while providing GPs with details of subjects' General Health Questionnaire (GHQ) score had little effect on outcome, feedback of a more detailed computerized psychiatric assessment based on the Revised Clinical Interview Schedule was associated with a modest improvement in outcome at 6 weeks and 3 months, though not at 6 months.

GPs tend to detect the more severe cases of depression while overlooking those cases most likely to remit spontaneously, a fact which limits the capacity of randomized trials of disclosure of GHQ or BDI scores to detect an improvement in outcome for previously undetected cases compared with no treatment. Taken together, these findings confirm the view of Goldberg and Huxley that detection of depression *per se* has at best a modest effect on outcome, and none at all in the absence of advice or training on the management of depression (Goldberg & Huxley, 1992). Indeed, it may be that the 'often haphazard and inadequate' treatment of patients with conspicuous psychiatric morbidity in primary care first described by Shepherd *et al.* in 1966, and confirmed elsewhere by others (Ormel *et al.*, 1991; Katon *et al.*, 1992), is of greater significance in explaining the persistently high prevalence of depression in both the community and primary care, despite the availability of treatments of proven effectiveness (Brugha, 1995). The detection of depression by GPs is a necessary but not sufficient precursor to adequate treatment, and the imperative must surely be to provide GPs and patients with information about the nature and treatment of depression through a combination of professional and public education (Katon *et al.*, 1992).

Treatment strategies in primary care

Any account of management in primary care has to take into account the specifics of the situation—brief consultations in busy surgeries, patients with depression of varying levels of severity which is usually part of a complex clinical picture with a concurrent physical illness or marked social stresses. Patients in primary care do not necessarily see themselves as 'psychiatric', and indeed may be afraid of receiving treatment for a mental illness, whether it be medication or a psychological treatment. Negotiation of treatment and monitoring of compliance and prognosis is therefore necessary but, in day-to-day practice, often hard to achieve.

The GP needs to decide whether *antidepressant medication* should be prescribed and, if so, how to ensure compliance. In addition, or instead, a *psychological treatment* or a *social intervention* to ameliorate the patient's circumstances may be appropriate. Here, the GP has to consider how this is best achieved in the surgery or the locality, given the enormous variation of availability of skilled personnel to deliver this approach. In the background will be the need to consider whether any current physical illness or its treatment is promoting or maintaining the depression or whether the treatment for depression could be medically risky. Finally, he/she will have to decide whether a *specialist referral* is now appropriate and, in particular, to be alert to the potential for suicide. Specific management approaches under these areas will be discussed more fully below.

The GP, therefore, is the linchpin to the approach to management of depression in primary care. Several initiatives are in progress to make this management as sophisticated as possible and to improve the confidence of the GP. Increased input concerning the diagnosis and treatment of mental illnesses into the postgraduate programmes is being promoted by a network of regional GP fellows, trained and supported by a senior GP funded for this purpose by the Department of Health and the Mental Health Foundation. Guidelines for treatment have been prepared as part of the 'Defeat Depression' campaign, both for older and younger adults (Paykel & Priest, 1992; Effective Health Care, 1993; Katona *et al.*, 1995). Computerized treatment algorithms have been devised that will allow the GP on his/her own surgery computer to access specialist help quickly (Lewis *et al.*, 1988). Facilitation (a process whereby a professional in certain areas is attached to a practice to introduce changes in that practice over a short period) is another approach. Facilitation has been successful in introducing better practice for assessing cardiovascular risk (Armstrong, 1992). It is now being evaluated for its impact upon the detection and management of anxiety and depression by means of a randomized controlled trial conducted in 18 London practices. Early results suggest that detection at least is improved as the result of facilitation (Bashir, personal communication).

There is, however, a risk. GPs, already under pressure after contractual changes, may resent bombardment by well-intentioned guidelines or visitors from outside the practice. It is, perhaps, not adequately recognized that GPs themselves are not a homogeneous group in their attitude to treatment of depression. The Depression Attitude Questionnaire was recently applied to a random sample of GPs who were part of the Medical Research Council's Research Framework (Botega *et al.*, 1992). Their responses, when subject to cluster analysis, suggested three groupings: those who had interest and sympathy for their depressed patients and wanted to personally do more, along the psychotherapeutic lines; those with a more strictly medical/organic view of depression who wanted clear-cut lines of physical treatment; those who found depressed patients very heavy-going and wished the treatment to be conducted by others. Any strategies from outside to improve management in general practice should, therefore, take account of this variation. An approach suitable for one GP is likely to irritate another GP. It is also clear that guidelines and protocols must be developed in partnership with the GP, allowing individual variations in attitude and local resources. The burden of detection and care can also be shared by practice nurses and health visitors who work regularly in the practice and/or by specialists, such as counsellors or psychologists who may be employed by the practice for this purpose. This *multidisciplinary teamwork* in primary care will be discussed later.

Physical treatments

This section will not rehearse the evidence that antidepressant medication helps patients with depression, nor discuss which antidepressant should be preferred. These are discussed elsewhere in this book (Chapters 9 and 10). This section will focus on the evidence that depressed patients seen in primary care can benefit from medication, but also discuss obstacles to effective prescribing.

The vast majority of studies of efficacy of antidepressants have been conducted on out-patient samples with mild to moderately severe depression. A meta-analysis published by the US Department of Health and Human Services (1993) in *Clinical Practice Guidelines*: *Depression in Primary Care* pointed to the efficacy of antidepressant medication over placebo and anxiolytic for cases of major depression. They also reported on a subanalysis of seven studies that took place in primary care, where they showed a drug efficacy of 57.8% compared with placebo of 35.6%—the latter being higher than the studies in in-patient settings. In the UK, some specific studies have shown the superiority of amitriptyline (median dose, 125 mg) over placebo, when taken for a 6-week period by patients who meet research criteria for depression with a minimal Hamilton Rating Scale for Depression (HRSD) score of 6 (Hollyman *et al.*, 1988). Subsequent research has focused on comparative studies between the various forms of antidepressants for use in primary care. The meta-analyses of research in these settings would suggest equal benefit between tricyclic antidepressants (TCAs) and selective serotonin re-uptake inhibitors (SSRIs), but with a tendency for lower dropout from the SSRI group (Song *et al.*, 1993). Prescription needs to be continued for at least 4–6 months (Effective Health Care, 1993; Old Age Depression Interest Group, 1993).

While it is, therefore, established that antidepressants are useful for depression that meets a particular severity criterion on the HRSD, it is not at all clear how effective they are for the group of patients with mild to moderate depression who are commonly seen in primary care (Paykel *et al.*, 1988). There seems to be a tendency for a small dose to be given to a 'little' depression. To answer this question, the Medical Research Council is currently funding a study taking place in 20 practices, in which antidepressant medication is being compared, for benefit among patients with mild depression, with problem-solving—a psychological approach conducted by practice nurses (Mynors-Wallis *et al.*, 1995).

The evidence remains that antidepressant medication is beneficial in primary care for those with a depression of moderate severity. However, in actual practice, dosages are often prescribed at subtherapeutic levels and compliance is poor: less than 60% of patients actually maintaining treatment for more than 3 weeks (Johnson, 1981). A recent survey of 80 000 prescriptions conducted by Donaghue and Tylee (1996) shows the mean dose for tricyclic prescription is currently 56 mg per day, but there is a huge range between GPs on the length of time for which these are prescribed. In contrast, the dosage for the newer antidepressants and the SSRIs are usually at the therapeutic level. It seems that the concern of GPs and complaints by the patients about side-effects to TCAs are a major factor in explaining this deficiency. Both may be overcome if the predominance of tricyclic medication yields to SSRIs in prescription frequency in general practice. The latter have fewer side-effects and a narrower dose range. Thus, this change will probably result in more patients receiving antidepressant medication in an effective range of treatment, despite lack of evidence for superiority of the SSRIs over TCAs in conditions of full dosage and maximal compliance.

However, the medication itself is not the complete story for difficulties in effective use of pharmacotherapy in general practice. A study reported from South Wales compared a sample of GPs and psychiatrists for their attitudes to depression and their treatment strategies (Kerr *et al.*, 1995). There were predictable differences in attitude to depression between psychiatrists and GPs, but it was clear that there was a worrying difference between GPs and psychiatrists in their use of antidepressant medication. Approximately 50% of the GPs were reported as prescribing less than the recommended dosage of antidepressant medication and 40% for less than 4 months—the recommended continuation time. This group of GPs were compared with their colleagues, who claimed to treat in full doses for longer time, for their beliefs. The low prescribers tended to have a strong belief in the value of psychotherapy and much less conviction about the biochemical basis of depression. Patients, too, are reluctant to take antidepressant medication, particularly the older patients, associating these drugs with a potential for addiction. Explanation of the pre-scription and why it is necessary, with follow-up and support, would seem mandatory after prescription. This is hard to deliver in a busy general prac-tice where many patients can get 'lost'. Here is a possible role for the practice nurse who can work with GPs as part of the multidisciplinary effort (Wilkinson *et al.*, 1993). The reluctance to take antidepressant medication by older pa-tients was clearly demonstrated in a recent study, in which a community nurse acted as a case manager for depression in primary care. Only a third of the prescriptions for antidepressant medication were accepted by the study popu-lation drawn from a community sample of people over 65 (Blanchard *et al.*, 1995).

Therefore, although antidepressant medication is clearly effective for mod-erate to severe depression, the attitude of some GPs and patients makes them unwilling or uncertain participants in this form of treatment. For this reason, psychological treatments are often more popular and will now be considered.

Psychological treatments

Like social interventions (see below), evaluation of psychological interven-tions for depression in primary care has been hampered by a lack of clarity and specificity in the treatments which have been studied (King *et al.*, 1994). Though we have distinguished between 'social' and 'psychological' interven-tions for the purposes of this chapter on the grounds that the former usually includes practical assistance in modifying the social environment (e.g. help in securing benefits or re-housing), this distinction is somewhat artificial, since social work also comprises 'psychological' activities such as providing 'support by encouragement and listening, [and] help to understand feelings' (Scott & Freeman, 1992).

Despite the recent vogue for 'counselling' (Corney, 1992; Sibbald *et al.*, 1993), there is little evidence about the effectiveness of psychological inter-ventions in primary care, a state of affairs which reflects the combined diffi-culties associated with evaluating psychological treatments in general and conducting large trials in general practice (Brewin & Bradley, 1989; Greenberg, 1991; Tognoni *et al.*, 1991; King *et al.*, 1994). Among published trials, several psychological interventions have been found to be superior to placebo (no treatment) in the management of major depression in primary care, though there is no evidence that any are more or less effective than treatment with a TCA at a dose equivalent to amitriptyline 150mg daily, at least within the first 3 or 4 months of commencing treatment.

Two studies have considered the outcome of psychological interventions for general practice patients suffering from a range of non-psychotic psychiatric disorders. Brodaty and Andrews (1983) found no difference in outcome between patients with non-psychotic psychiatric morbidity of at least 6 months' duration (defined as a persistently elevated GHQ score) who received eight weekly half-hour sessions of 'problem-oriented' psychodynamic psychotherapy compared with those who saw their GP for a similar amount of time, and those who received 'standard GP care', even after adjusting for baseline differences between groups. In addition to its non-randomized design, interpretation of the findings from this study were hindered further by a high dropout rate and a failure to analyse the results on an intention-to-treat basis. Gournay and Brooking (1994) compared the outcome for patients with 'non-psychotic psychiatric problems' randomized to immediate intervention from a community psychiatric nurse (CPN), a waiting list control group or continuing standard GP care. All three groups were found to have improved significantly on a wide variety of psychiatric and social measures at 6 months, though no differences in outcome were found between groups. Though the work of the 11 CPNs involved in the study was not prescribed (or described), the majority 'saw "counselling" as central to their role'.

In a randomized controlled trial, Teasdale *et al.* (1984) found that general practice patients with RDC major depression (Spitzer *et al.*, 1978) who received an average of 15h of cognitive therapy from a clinical psychologist in addition to standard GP care recovered more rapidly than patients who received standard GP care alone, though the difference in outcome between these groups disappeared within 3 months of the cessation of cognitive therapy. This study was limited by small numbers, a relatively high dropout rate in the cognitive therapy group and a decision to analyse results only for subjects who accepted the intervention. As described above, Scott *et al.* (1992) found no difference in outcome at 16 weeks for patients who received an average of 10 sessions of cognitive-behaviour therapy from a clinical psychologist compared with those who received either standard GP care or amitriptyline from a psychiatrist. The dropout rate was higher, and overall satisfaction lower, in the cognitive therapy than in the group allocated to social work intervention. More recently, Mynors-Wallis *et al.* (1995) reported the results of a randomized controlled trial of six fortnightly sessions of brief 'problem-solving treatment', delivered by a psychiatrist or a GP, compared with amitriptyline (150mg daily) and a drug placebo for primary care patients with major depression. Though superior to placebo, no difference in outcome was found between problem-solving and amitriptyline at 6 or 12 weeks. Patients in the problem-solving group reported high levels of satisfaction, and were less likely to drop out of treatment than subjects in either of the other groups.

Social treatments

Although both socioeconomic adversity, such as poverty, poor housing and unemployment (Platt *et al.*, 1990; Goldberg & Huxley, 1992; Blazer *et al.*, 1994; Meltzer *et al.*, 1995) and difficulty in interpersonal relationships (Brown & Harris, 1978; Brown *et al.*, 1986) are common among depressed subjects, being both causes and consequences of this disorder (Brown & Harris, 1978; Brown *et al.*, 1986; Warr, 1987; Bruce *et al.*, 1991; Brown & Moran, 1994; Weich *et al.*, 1997), there have been few studies of specific social interventions in depression in primary care or elsewhere. While it seems likely that social interventions may be part of standard GP care (the control condition in many trials in primary care), there have been few attempts to evaluate individual components of such care. Indeed, in all primary care trials of social interventions (of which we are aware) the experimental condition has been allocation to treatment by an individual from a specific discipline (e.g. social worker, health visitor or practice nurse), rather to any one type of social intervention (Corney, 1984; Johnstone & Shepley, 1986; Corney & Murray, 1989; Goldberg & Huxley, 1992; Scott & Freeman, 1992; Wilkinson, 1992).

The most detailed study of this nature was a randomized controlled trial by Corney (1984) of allocation to a social worker for women with acute depression. Though no overall difference was found in clinical or social outcome for subjects (women aged 18–45) allocated to a social worker attached to a GP compared with GP management alone, subgroup analyses revealed a benefit from social work treatment for women with 'acute-on-chronic' depression with major marital difficulties. Though analyses were based on small numbers, this group were described as having more social problems at outset, and were both more likely to accept the social work treatment and to receive practical help than other subjects. In a review of this and other social intervention studies, Corney and Murray argued that intervention by a social worker is likely to be of greatest benefit to those with the most long-standing and severe depressive illnesses, on the grounds that 'early intervention may be harmful, the social worker interfering with the client's own abilities to cope, or affecting the support received from informal sources' (Corney & Murray, 1989).

This view was challenged in a more recent trial where social work intervention was compared with standard GP care, cognitive-behaviour therapy from a clinical psychologist and antidepressant medication prescribed by a psychiatrist among patients in primary care recruited when they were 'about to start treatment for a depressive illness' (Scott & Freeman, 1992). Though criticized for failing to adequately describe the social work intervention, the artificiality of the psychiatrist arm of the study (restricted to prescription and advice on matters related to pharmacotherapy), and a randomization procedure which led to significant intergroup baseline differences in depression severity (Scott *et al.*, 1994), this study found a high rate of overall recovery, but few differences in outcome between groups. The best outcome was found in the social work group, though this group included the highest proportion of women, and had the lowest mean severity of depression at baseline. No attempt was made to adjust for these potential sources of confounding. The other notable finding was that subjects who received the social work intervention were significantly more satisfied with their treatment than other study participants.

Multidisciplinary teamwork

The GP refers only a minority of patients for specialist care. However, the attachment of mental health professionals to work in collaboration in the practice is occurring, but not in a uniform manner. In a survey of general practices in six district health authorities, it has been shown that 48% had direct links with the CPN; 41% with a social worker; 17% with a counsellor; 15% with a psychologist; and 16% with a psychiatrist (Sibbald *et al.*, 1993). These attachments, however, were not evenly spread. Some practices had three or four such attachments, while a substantial minority had none at all. There have been no published evaluations as yet of the outcome for patients with depression from practices working with such links compared to those where the GP works alone.

Of particular relevance for the treatment of depression among these specialist attachments are the CPNs and counsellors. The move away from hospitals has meant a shift of caseload for CPNs from psychotic patients to those with depression and anxiety, as they receive referrals directly from GPs. However, the rarity of CPNs means that one is normally linked to five practices; thus, any one CPN can only come into contact with a minority of patients with depression. Further, one recent study indicated that CPNs working with neurotic patients produced no extra benefit to an ordinary outpatient referral (Gournay & Brooking, 1994). Counsellors are usually referred patients with a wide variety of social and relationship difficulties of which the core symptom of the patient is depression. The counsellors' approaches to treatment are enormously varied, depending on training received. It has been reported that counselling is very popular with patients (Anderson & Hasler, 1979) and can reduce prescription rates of psychotropic medication (Waydenfield & Waydenfield, 1980). However, only one properly conducted randomized controlled trial has been carried out; the results of this are awaited. Until these are published, it can only be noted that counsellors have been an important growth area in primary care, perhaps reflecting a public demand for psychological rather than pharmacological help for states of depression and anxiety.

Most general practices employ nurses, either to work in the surgery or in the community. These nurses will come into contact with many patients at risk for depression: the physically ill, the elderly, new mothers, etc. Potentially, therefore, these nurses could contribute to the management of depressed patients being treated by the GP. A role is already established for nurses to run clinics in general practice for sufferers from chronic diseases such as asthma, hypertension and diabetes. Nurses could run a support clinic for patients with depression, allowing time for education of patient and family, monitoring compliance to antidepressants and the detection of social factors that might be maintaining depression. A group of practice nurses has been recently trained to assess depression and to use a structured manual to follow up such patients, working as an adjunct to the GP. After a successful pilot (Wilkinson *et al.*, 1993), this role was evaluated by means of a randomized controlled trial (GP treatment alone vs. GP and nurse working together) in 20 practices (Mann *et al.* submitted). Five hundred and seventy patients with conspicuous depression, the majority suffering from a major depression, were recruited. The outcome of the study confirmed the feasibility and popularity of the nurse clinics, but no added benefit in outcome could be detected. It seemed that the presence of these practice nurses, who were trained to assess and then discuss the depressed patient with the GP as part of the intervention arm, had an important effect upon the GP who changed practice for the patients in the control arm that he/she was seeing alone. As a result, all participants in the trial benefited from a high prescription rate of antidepressants (74%) with excellent compliance (79%). Perhaps having a practice nurse interested in and available to help in the care of depressed patients increases the assurance of GPs in their own treatment.

Multidisciplinary teamwork in primary care is still in its infancy, but it is likely that patients with depression will benefit from the extra time for assessment and monitoring that nurses could carry out. In theory, the specific skills of attached professionals should improve the addition of specific interventions and the outcome for depressed patients. However, evaluative studies of this work is awaited. A demonstration of a lack of specificity of approach by attached workers is worrying. During a survey of 40 practices in South London, R. Corney (personal communication) asked the professionals attached to these practices what types of therapy they offered. The responses from the CPNs, counsellors and psychologists indicated that all three groups interchangeably offered psychodynamic therapies, stress management, cognitive behaviour therapy and anxiety management. Only one activity seemed to be job-specific: that of giving depot injections by the nurses. Much more research is required if the continuation of this range of attachments is justified. At the moment, although the GP may believe that something different is being delivered by a counsellor or a psychologist to a depressed patient, it may be that they are receiving similar, unspecified intervention from both groups.

The primary–secondary care interface

As was highlighted earlier in this chapter, the nature and scale of the burden of psychiatric morbidity in primary care has been documented with increasing precision in the 30 years following the seminal study by Shepherd *et al.* (1966). It has been estimated recently that each of the 30 000 GPs in Britain sees 300–600 anxious and depressed patients each year, a number far beyond the capacity of the 2000 consultant psychiatrists and 5000 CPNs, even if they spent all of their time in primary care (Lloyd & Jenkins, 1995). In view of the large numbers of specialist mental health care professionals working in primary care settings (Kendrick *et al.*, 1993), substantial concerns have also been expressed about the care of patients with chronic psychotic illnesses, and it is likely that secondary care personnel will come under increasing pressure to devote more time to this group (Gournay & Brooking, 1994; Lloyd & Jenkins, 1995). While there is some evidence that shifting psychiatric out-patient clinics into general practice reduces demand on secondary care services (Tyrer *et al.*, 1984), evaluation of a service in which the secondary care team was based in primary care suggested that GPs referred patients they might otherwise have managed themselves (Jackson *et al.*, 1993). There is therefore a clear need to strengthen the primary care team through the introduction of specialist knowledge on the detection, diagnosis and management of the common mental disorders, anxiety and depression, in ways which do not involve diverting scarce secondary care personnel away from patients with severe mental illness.

We have already highlighted two experimental interventions designed to strengthen the primary care team, namely the introduction of *mental health facilitators* and training for *practice nurses* in the assessment and support of depressed patients. Other ways in which it has been suggested that this might be achieved are through specific training packages for GPs (Gask, 1992), the development and dissemination of clinical practice guidelines (including guidelines on the indications for referral to secondary care) (Effective Health Care, 1993), and through the use of information technology (Lewis, 1992).

There has been a proliferation of clinical guidelines in many western countries across a range of specialities (Haines & Feder, 1992), including psychiatry (Effective Health Care, 1993; Paykel & Priest, 1992; US Department of Health & Human Services, 1993). There is consistent evidence that consensus statements based on expert opinion and disseminated through publication in journals have little impact on clinician behaviour (Grol, 1990). Instead, guidelines are most likely to be acted upon if those who are to use them participate in their development (North of England Study of Standards & Performance in General Practice, 1992), and if doctors are given patient-specific reminders about treatment at the time of consultation (Haines & Feder, 1992; Grimshaw & Russell, 1993). Computer-based clinical decision support systems are capable of combining patient information with treatment guidelines to produce patient-specific prompts (Johnston *et al.*, 1994). The application of this technology in psychiatry has been limited by the difficulty of obtaining standardized clinical data on which to base these guidelines, given the extreme variability in doctors' clinical assessments. It has now been demonstrated that self-administered computerized assessments of common mental disorder are reliable, unbiased and valid, and are acceptable and easy to use for patients within primary care (Lewis *et al.*, 1988; Lewis, 1992; Lewis, 1994).

Though GPs vary greatly in their rates of referral to secondary care services (Creed *et al.*, 1990; Fertig *et al.*, 1993), comparisons of such rates are notoriously difficult to interpret (Marinker *et al.*, 1988; Roland, 1992). Despite knowledge about the characteristics of both patients and doctors which are associated with psychiatric referral (see Goldberg & Huxley, 1992), there is limited empirical evidence on which to base guidelines for appropriate psychiatric referral, or that such guidelines would reduce referral rates substantially (Russell & Grimshaw, 1992; Fertig *et al.*, 1993). While risk to self or others is likely to remain an absolute indication for referral, other indications are a matter for local negotiation between stakeholders at the primary–secondary interface, including GPs, psychiatrists and all those responsible for planning and purchasing mental health services.

Conclusions

'Undertreatment', or perhaps more correctly 'unmet need for treatment', is probably the single most important issue in the management of depression in general practice (Brugha, 1995). We would argue that it is necessary to move beyond the study of case recognition to consider both physician (e.g. unwillingness to prescribe antidepressants at high enough doses for long enough) and patient (non-compliance with treatment) variables associated with treatment adherence and clinical outcome. One area which has not yet been explored fully is the effect of patient attitudes on the outcome of depression in general practice (Katon *et al.*, 1992); depressed patients frequently elect not to consult their GP at all, while those who do rarely present psychological complaints. This may be the result of misconceptions about (among other things) the nature of depression, the ability (or willingness) of their GP to help, and the likelihood of being offered physical rather than psychological treatment (or vice versa). We simply do not know enough about patient preferences, or how these influence consultation behaviour or compliance with treatment.

A second unresolved issue concerns the effectiveness of alternatives to pharmacological interventions, either alone or in combination with physical interventions. Clear conclusions have been hampered by, first, the lack of specificity in the treatments which have been evaluated, second, general difficulties associated with evaluating psychological treatments (including subject motivation; Brewin & Bradley, 1989) and the difficulty of distinguishing between effects attributable to the intervention and those which are due to the therapist), and finally the problems associated with undertaking large-scale trials in general practice (especially non-participation by GPs who initially agree to recruit patients; Tognoni *et al.*, 1991). Though there have been a few trials of specific therapies (e.g. cognitive therapy and problem-solving therapy), most studies have evaluated the outcome for patients referred to professionals from a particular discipline (e.g. social worker or CPN). Indeed, we are not aware of any evaluations of specific *social* interventions in primary care (e.g. debt counselling or befriending).

Despite the very significant and exciting developments in the primary care of psychiatric disorder which have taken place in the 30 years since the study by Shepherd and colleagues (Shepherd *et al.*, 1966), there is little evidence of any substantial reduction in the prevalence of depression, either in primary care settings or in the community (Brugha, 1995). The heaviest burden rests on the shoulders of GPs (Goldberg & Huxley, 1992; Shah, 1992), perhaps even more now than in 1966. As a direct result of changes in the delivery of specialist psychiatrist services, secondary care staff are now occupied almost exclusively with the care of patients with the most severe psychiatric disorders, which commonly means the psychotic disorders. It is ironic that community psychiatrists should have so little time to devote to those illnesses which are most prevalent in, and costly to, the community.

It is of the utmost importance that psychiatrists should not abandon their vital role in the primary care of depression. Psychiatrists are the one group best placed to ensure that only treatments of proven effectiveness (i.e. those which are 'evidence-based') are implemented in primary care settings. As medical colleagues, GPs are naturally inclined to look to psychiatrists for advice in this area. Should this leadership not be forthcoming, the vacuum is likely to be filled by more vocal advocates of interventions, such as counselling, which have yet to be shown to work.

References

Anderson, S. & Hasler, J. (1979) Counselling in general practice. *Journal of the Royal College of General Practitioners,* **29**, 352–356.

Armstrong, E. (1992) Facilitators in primary care. *International Review of Psychiatry,* **4**, 339–342.

Bennett, D.H. (1973) Community mental health services in Britain. *American Journal of Psychiatry,* **130**, 1065–1070.

Blacker, C.V.R. & Clare, A.W. (1987) Depressive disorder in primary care. *British Journal of Psy-*

chiatry, **150**, 737–751.

Blanchard, M.R., Waterreus, A. & Mann, A.H. (1995) The effect of primary care nurse intervention upon older people screened as depressed. *International Journal of Geriatric Psychiatry,* **10**, 289–298.

Blazer, D.G., Kessler, R.C., McGonagle, K.A. & Swartz, M.S. (1994) The prevalence and distribution of major depression in a national community sample: the National Comorbidity Survey. *American Journal of Psychiatry,* **151**, 979–986.

Botega, N., Mann, A., Blizard, R. & Wilkinson, G. (1992) General practitioners and depression: first use of the Depression Attitude Questionnaire. *International Journal of Methods in Psychiatric Research,* **2**, 169–180.

Brewin, C.R. & Bradley, C. (1989) Patient preferences and randomised controlled trials. *British Medical Journal,* **299**, 313–315.

Brodaty, H. & Andrews, G. (1983) Brief psychotherapy in family practice. *British Journal of Psychiatry,* **143**, 11–19.

Brown, G.W. & Harris, T. (1978) *Social Origins of Depression.* Tavistock, London.

Brown, G.W. & Moran, P. (1994) Clinical and psychosocial origins of chronic depressive episodes. I: A community survey. *British Journal of Psychiatry,* **165**, 447–456.

Brown, G.W., Andrews, B., Harris, T., Adler, Z. & Bridge, L. (1986) Social support, self-esteem and depression. *Psychological Medicine,* **16**, 813–831.

Bruce, M.L., Takeuchi, D.T. & Leaf, P.J. (1991) Poverty and psychiatric status. *Archives of General Psychiatry,* **48**, 470–474.

Brugha, T.S. (1995) Depression undertreatment: lost cohorts, lost opportunities? *Psychological Medicine,* **25**, 3–6.

Corney, R. (1992) The effectiveness of counselling in general practice. *International Review of Psychiatry,* **4**, 331–337.

Corney, R.H. (1984) The effectiveness of attached social workers in the management of depressed female patients in general practice. *Psychological Medicine,* Supplement **6**, 1–47.

Corney, R. & Murray, J. (1989) The evaluation of social interventions. In: *The Scope of Epidemiological Psychiatry* (eds P. Williams, G. Wilkinson & K. Rawnsley), pp. 343–354. Routledge, London.

Creed, F., Gowrisunkur, J., Russell, E. & Kincey, J. (1990) General practitioner referral rates to district psychiatry and psychology services. *British Journal of General Practice,* **40**, 450–454.

Croft-Jefferys, C. & Wilkinson, G. (1989) Estimated costs of neurotic disorder in UK general practice. *Psychological Medicine,* **19**, 549–558.

Donaghue, J.M. & Tylee, A. (1996) The treatment of depression: prescribing patterns of antidepressants in primary care in the UK. *British Journal of Psychiatry,* **168**, 164–168.

Dowrick, C. & Buchan, I. (1995) Twelve month outcome of depression in general practice: does detection or disclosure make a difference? *British Medical Journal,* **311**, 1274–1276.

Effective Health Care (1993) The treatment of depression in primary care. *Effective Health Care Bulletin,* **5**, 1–12.

Fertig, A., Roland, M., King, H. & Moore, T. (1993) Understanding variation in rates of referral among general practitioners: are inappropriate referrals important and would guidelines help to reduce rates? *British Medical Journal,* **307**, 1467–1470.

Freeling, P., Rao, B.M., Paykel, E.S., Sireling, L.I. & Burton, R.H. (1985) Unrecognised depression in general practice. *British Medical Journal,* **290**, 1880–1883.

Gask, L. (1992) Training general practitioners to detect and manage emotional disorders. *International Review Journal of Psychiatry,* **4**, 293–300.

Goldberg, D. & Huxley, P. (1992) *Common Mental Disorders: A Biopsychosocial Approach.* Routledge, London.

Goldberg, D.P. & Bridges, K. (1988) Somatic presentation of psychiatric illness in primary care setting. *Journal of Psychosomatic Research,* **32**, 137–144.

Goldberg, D.P. & Williams, P. (1988) *The User's Guide to the General Health Questionnaire.* NFER-Nelson, Windsor.

Goldberg, D.P., Cooper, B., Eastwood, M.R., Kedward, H.B. & Shepherd, M. (1970) A standardised psychiatric interview for use in community surveys. *British Journal of Preventive and Social Medicine,* **24**, 18–23.

Gournay, K. & Brooking, J. (1994) Community psychiatric nurses in primary health care. *British Journal of Psychiatry,* **165**, 231–238.

Greenberg, G. (1991) Clinical trials in general practice. *British Medical Journal,* **303**, 940.

Grimshaw, J.M. & Russell, I.T. (1993) Effect of guidelines on medical practice: a systematic review of rigorous evaluations. *Lancet,* **342**, 1317–1322.

Grol, R. (1990) National standard setting for quality of care in general practice: attitudes of general practitioners and response to a set of standards. *British Journal of General Practice,* **40**, 361–364.

Haines, A. & Feder, G. (1992) Guidance on guidelines. *British Medical Journal,* **305**, 785–786.

Hoeper, E., Nycz, G., Kessler, L., Burke, J. & Pierce,

W. (1984) The usefulness of screening for mental illness. *Lancet*, **i**, 33–35.

Hollyman, J.A., Freeling, P., Paykel, E.S., Bhat, A. & Sedgwick, P. (1988) Double-blind placebo-controlled trial of amitriptyline among depressed patients in general practice. *Journal of the Royal College of General Practitioners*, **38**, 393–397.

Jackson, G., Gater, R., Goldberg, D., Loftus, L. & Taylor, H. (1993) A new community mental health team based in primary care: a description of the service and its effects on service use in the first year. *British Journal of Psychiatry*, **162**, 375–384.

Johnson, D.A.W. (1981) Treatment compliance in general practice. *Acta Psychiatrica Scandinavica*, **63** (Suppl. 209), 447–453.

Johnston, M.E., Langton, K.B., Haynes, R.B. *et al.* (1994) Effects of computer-based clinical decision support systems on clinician performance and patient outcome. *Annals of Internal Medicine*, **120**, 135–142.

Johnstone, A. & Goldberg, D. (1976) Psychiatric screening in general practice: a controlled trial. *Lancet*, **i**, 605–608.

Johnstone, A. & Shepley, M. (1986) The outcome of hidden neurotic illness treated in general practice. *Journal of the Royal College of General Practitioners*, **36**, 413–415.

Katon, W., von Korff, M., Lin, E., Bush, T. & Ormel, J. (1992) Adequacy and duration of antidepressant treatment in primary care. *Medical Care*, **30**, 67–76.

Katona, C., Freeling, P., Hinchcliffe, K., Blanchard, M. & Wright, A. (On behalf of the Consensus Group of the Royal Colleges of General Practitoners & Psychiatrists) (1995) Recognition and management of depression in late life in general practice: consensus statement. *Primary Care Psychiatry*, **1**, 107–113.

Kendrick, T., Sibbald, B., Addington-Hall, J., Brennerman, D. & Freeling, P. (1993) Distribution of mental health professionals working on site in English and Welsh general practices. *British Medical Journal*, **307**, 544–546.

Kerr, M., Blizard, R. & Mann, A. (1995) General practitioners and psychiatrists: comparison of attitudes to depression using the Depression Attitude Questionnaire. *British Journal of General Practice*, **45**, 89–92.

King, M., Broster, G., Lloyd, M. & Horder, J. (1994) Controlled trials in the evaluation of counselling in general practice. *British Journal of General Practice*, **44**, 229–232.

Lewis, G. (1992) Computers in primary care. *International Review of Psychiatry*, **4**, 307–310.

Lewis, G. (1994) Assessing psychiatric disorder with a human interviewer or a computer. *Journal of Epidemiology and Community Health*, **48**, 207–210.

Lewis, G., Pelosi, A.J., Glover, E. *et al.* (1988) The development of a computerised assessment for minor psychiatric disorder. *Psychological Medicine*, **18**, 737–745.

Lewis, G., Pelosi, A.J., Araya, R. & Dunn, G. (1992) Measuring psychiatric disorder in the community: a standardised assessment for use by lay interviewers. *Psychological Medicine*, **22**, 465–486.

Lewis, G., Sharp, D., Bartholomew, J. & Pelosi, A.J. (1996) Computerised assessment of common mental disorders in primary care: effect on clinical outcome. *Family Practice*, **13**, 120–126.

Lloyd, K. & Jenkins, R. (1995) The economics of depression in primary care: Department of Health initiatives. *British Journal of Psychiatry*, **27** (Suppl.), 60–62.

Mann, A., Jenkins, R., Cutting, J. & Cowen, P. (1981) The 12 month outcome of patients with neurotic illness in general practice. *Psychological Medicine*, **11**, 839–847.

Marinker, M., Wilkin, D. & Metcalfe, D.H. (1988) Referral to hospital: can we do better? *British Medical Journal*, **297**, 461–464.

Marks, J.N., Goldberg, D.P. & Hillier, V.F. (1979) Determinants of the ability of general practitioners to detect psychiatric illness. *Psychological Medicine*, **9**, 337–353.

Meltzer, H., Gill, B. & Petticrew, M. (1995) *OPCS Surveys of Psychiatric Morbidity in Great Britain. Report no. 1. The prevalence of psychiatric morbidity among adults aged 16–64 living in private households in Great Britain.* HMSO, London.

Mynors-Wallis, L.M., Gath, D.H., Lloyd-Thomas, A.R. & Tomlinson, D. (1995) Randomised controlled trial comparing problem solving treatment with amitriptyline and placebo for major depression in primary care. *British Medical Journal*, **310**, 441–445.

North of England Study of Standards and Performance in General Practice (1992) Medical Audit in General Practice. 1: Effect on doctors' clinical behaviour for common childhood conditions. *British Medical Journal*, **304**, 1480–1484.

Old Age Depression Interest Group (1993) How long should the elderly take anti-depressants? A double-blind placebo-controlled study of continuation/prophylaxis therapy with dothiepin. *British Journal of Psychiatry*, **162**, 175–182.

Ormel, J., van den Brink, W., Koeter, M.W.J. *et al.* (1990) Recognition, management and outcome of psychological disorders in primary care: a naturalistic follow-up study. *Psychological Medicine*, **20**, 909–923.

Ormel, J., Koeter, M.W.J., van den Brink, W. & van de Willige, G. (1991) Recognition, management and course of anxiety and depression in general practice. *Archives of General Psychiatry*, **48**, 700–706.

Ormel, J., Oldehinkel, T., Brilman, E. & van den Brink, W. (1993) Outcome of depression and anxiety in primary care: a three-wave $3\frac{1}{2}$-year study of psychopathology and disability. *Archives of General Psychiatry*, **50**, 759–766.

Paykel, E.S. & Priest, R.G. (1992) Recognition and management of depression in general practice: consensus statement. *British Medical Journal*, **305**, 1198–1202.

Paykel, E.S., Hollyman, J.A., Freeling, P. & Sedgewick, P. (1988) Predictors of therapeutic benefit from amitriptyline in mild depression: a general practice placebo controlled trial. *Journal of Affective Disorders*, **14**, 83–95.

Platt, S., Martin, C. & Hunt, S. (1990) The mental health of women with children living in deprived areas of Great Britain: the role of living conditions, poverty and unemployment. In: *The Public Health Impact of Mental Disorder* (eds D. Goldberg & D. Tantam), pp. 124–135. Hogrefe and Huber, Toronto.

Roland, M. (1992) Measuring appropriateness of hospital referrals. In: *Hospital Referrals* (eds M. Roland & A. Coulter), pp. 137–149. Oxford University Press, Oxford.

Russell, I. & Grimshaw, J. (1992) The effectiveness of referral guidelines: a review of the methods and findings of published evaluations. In: *Hospital Referrals* (eds M. Roland and A. Coulter), pp. 179–211. Oxford University Press, Oxford.

Scott, A.I.F. & Freeman, C.P.L. (1992) Edinburgh primary care depression study: treatment outcome, patient satisfaction and cost after 16 weeks. *British Medical Journal*, **304**, 883–887.

Scott, J., Moon, C.A.L., Blacker, C.V.R. & Thomas, J.M. (1994) A.I.F. Scott & C.P.L. Freeman's 'Edinburgh Primary Care Depression Study'. *British Journal of Psychiatry*, **164**, 410–415.

Shah, A. (1992) The burden of psychiatric disorder in primary care. *International Review of Psychiatry*, **4**, 243–250.

Shapiro, S., German, P., Skinner, E. *et al.* (1987) An experiment to change detection and management of mental morbidity in primary care. *Medical Care*, **25**, 327–339.

Shepherd, M., Cooper, B., Brown, A.C. & Kalton, G. (1966) *Psychiatric Disorders in General Practice*. First edn. Oxford University Press, Oxford.

Sibbald, B., Addington-Hall, J., Brenneman, D. & Freeling, P. (1993) Counsellors in English and Welsh general practices: their nature and distribution. *British Medical Journal*, **306**, 29–33.

Song, F., Freemantle, N., Sheldon, T.A. *et al.* (1993) Selective serotonin reuptake inhibitors: meta-analysis of efficacy and acceptability. *British Medical Journal*, **306**, 683–687.

Teasdale, J.D., Fennell, M.J.V., Hibbert, G.A. & Amies, P.L. (1984) Cognitive therapy for major depressive disorder in primary care. *British Journal of Psychiatry*, **144**, 400–406.

Tognoni, G., Alli, C., Bettelli, G. *et al.* (1991) Randomised clinical trials in general practice: lessons from a failure. *British Medical Journal*, **303**, 969–971.

Tyrer, P., Sievewright, N. & Wollerton, P. (1984) General practice psychiatric clinics: impact on psychiatric services. *British Journal of Psychiatry*, **145**, 15–19.

US Department of Health and Human Services (1993) *Depression in Primary Care*. Vol. 2: *Treatment of Major Depression*. Agency for Health Care Policy and Research, Rockville, Maryland.

Ustun, T.B. & Sartorius, N. (eds) (1995) *Mental Illness in General Health Care*. John Wiley & Sons, Chichester.

von Korff, M., Shapiro, S., Burke, J.D. *et al.* (1987) Anxiety and depression in a primary care clinic. *Archives of General Psychiatry*, **44**, 152–156.

Warr, P. (1987) *Work, Unemployment and Mental Health*. Oxford Science Publications, Oxford.

Waydenfield, D. & Waydenfield, S.W. (1980) Counselling in general practice. *Journal of the Royal College of General Practitioners*, **30**, 671–677.

Weich, S., Churchill, R., Lewis, G. & Mann, A. (1997) Do socio-economic risk factors predict the incidence and maintenance of psychiatric disorder in primary care? *Psychological Medicine*, **27**, 73–80.

Wilkinson, G. (1992) The role of the practice nurse in the management of depression. *International Review of Psychiatry*, **4**, 311–316.

Wilkinson, G., Allen, P., Marshall, E., Walker, J., Brown, W. & Mann, A.H. (1993) The role of the practice nurse in depression in general practice: treatment adherence to antidepressant medication. *Psychological Medicine*, **23**, 229–237.

Wright, A.F. (1994) Should general practitioners be testing for depression? *British Journal of General Practice*, **44**, 132–135.

Zung, W.W.K., Magill, M., Moore, J.T. & George, D.T. (1983) Recognition and treatment of depression in a family medical practice. *Journal of Clinical Psychiatry*, **44**, 3–6.

15 The management of depression in the community

GERALDINE STRATHDEE AND
KAMALDEEP BHUI

The development of community psychiatric services in Britain has been shaped by two fundamental and consistent themes. The first being that the traditional service systems dominated by large institutions should be replaced with a more balanced and flexible range of alternative services. Second, these new services should be directed towards meeting individual needs (Hunter & Wistow, 1987). Many factors have led to rudimental changes in the nature of service provision. These include the increasing body of evidence which strongly suggests an influence of social and environmental factors in improving patient and carer outcomes, the changing preferences of the majority of patients for community-based treatment and the growing concern with the economics of priority in the health service.

The components of a comprehensive community mental health service system

While the old institutional model often provided for both the health and social care needs of its inhabitants, community-based services must develop a comprehensive and integrated range of service components. There is an international consensus on the essential elements and these are set out in the Health of the Nation Key Area Handbook (1994) and the Spectrum of Care (Health of The Nations, 1996).

Internationally, the method of developing and delivering such a comprehensive range of services is through the establishment of community mental health teams (CMHTs). Such teams are responsible for populations ranging from 45 000 in the UK to 100 000 in parts of Europe. This chapter will therefore examine the deployment of CMHTs in assessing patients with depression. It will also explore the influences such teams can have on the planning and development of the service components essential for the effective treatment of individuals with depression.

Table 15.1 The structural components of a comprehensive mental health service.

Identification and needs assessment systems
Range of hospital and community beds
Case management and assertive outreach
Day care, rehabilitation, education and work
Crisis response
Assessment and consultation
Carer and community education and support
Primary care liaison
Community agency liaison
User involvement and advocacy

Community mental health teams

CMHTs have their origin in the American Community Mental Health Centre programme of the 1960s. The teams were mandated to provide services which could respond to the needs of the severely mentally ill (SMI). However, when located in community mental health centres, the focus of work shifted to 'the worried well' resulting in the neglect of those with severe mental illness (Sayce *et al.*, 1991). Perhaps exacerbated by the strength of its primary care infra-structure where the vast majority of mental health morbidity presents, CMHTs in Britain have followed a similar pathway. A Sainsbury Centre study has identified over 300 CMHTs practising across England, comprised of at least four members from two or more disciplines, with a caseload of individuals with mental health disorders largely residing in the community (Oynett *et al.*, 1994). In 1994 focus on the work, organization, service development ap-proaches and management styles in British teams formed the subject of inten-sive studies by a number of national agencies (Audit Commission, 1994; 3rd Quinquennial Community Psychiatric Survey; White, 1994; Health of The Nations, 1994; Mental Health Foundation, 1994; Ritchie, 1994).

All the reviews comment on how variable the targeting of the SMI by the CMHTs appears to be. In some instances, less than 10% of the caseload of community psychiatric nurses working with the SMI in community services were people with either manic-depressive disorders or schizophrenia.

A strategic approach

A strategic approach to the planning and implementation of services and working practices is essential if a CMHT is to effectively focus its work on the most vulnerable patients with the most complex needs. Primarily these include patients with major depression and schizophrenia. Those with mod-erate degrees of depression not responding to management by primary care physicians, and patients presenting with somatic problems repeatedly to their general practitioners (GPs) also need to be regarded as a priority. A large number of those with less severe depression remain unseen by specialist services mainly because of resource limitations, atypical presentations or inability to benefit from the existing style of service delivery. Women with young children, and ethnic minorities, for example, fail to optimally benefit and are discussed in more detail below. Yet GPs (primary care physicians) report that they are unable to influence the illness episodes of many patients who are ineligible for care by secondary specialist services. This has resulted in the increased use of counselling and alternative therapies which are purchased by GPs. This occurs in the absence of an effective and financially viable role for the secondary specialist mental health services. These specialist services have focused largely on those suffering from severe depressive disorders with overt suicidality and behavioural disturbance. Yet, such service providers identify the independent deployment of counselling and psychotherapy services in primary care as detrimental to the provision of existing secondary services and as being of questionable long-term benefit. A comprehensive strategy must therefore aim to reach those groups not served by current services.

Any strategy should be informed by an understanding of the theoretical evaluation, research and practice findings in community care programmes. It is equally important to have information detailing where, and by what adaptations, such international findings can inform good practice suited to unique local service requirements and patients with special needs. Such an evaluation must take account of the limitations inherent in well-funded 'model' programmes and harness transportable pragmatic working practices (Test & Scott, 1990; Audit Commission, 1994; Wood, 1996). Table 15.2 outlines the key elements such a strategy should embrace.

First, a system for the assessment and recognition of the needs of patients with severe, moderate and mild depression is necessary. Second, a network of service structural components developed to take account of the research evidence and with a clear understanding of the outcomes they aim to achieve. Third, specific attention should be given to the availabilty of a range of effective therapeutic interventions. Such interventions must address the wider

Table 15.2 A strategy for the effective deployment of CMHTs.

Knowledge of the epidemology of the local area
Strategy for the identification of those with depression
Development of the structural components
Use of effective interventions
Effective organization and management of the CHMT
Planning for staff skill mix, training and support

needs (including basic social requirements) of those with depression and should have demonstrated improvements in health and social outcomes. This assumes that those delivering these interventions are trained to do so in an optimal manner. Next, explicit and effective organizational and management techniques must be used within the CMHT to thoroughly address the service demands within the allocated budgets. Fundamentally, this will involve clear interdisciplinary procedural guidelines as well as mutually understood, respected and agreed roles. Finally, an analysis of the skill mix of the CMHT staff and the range of effective interventions held by the team must be carried out. These skills and interventions should meet the needs of the target population. There should be structured opportunity for continuing skill attainment and refinement through personal training development programmes for all staff. Burnout amongst community teams drastically reduces the momentum of long-term strategic plans. Preventive management strategies should be employed to lessen the possibility of an eventual manpower crisis.

Table 15.3 The range of needs of those with mental health disorders.

Needs and effective interventions	The long-term mentally ill	Common primary care conditions
Case identification and case register recall	+++	+
Crisis intervention in the community and at home	+++	+
Medication	+++	+
Respite and crisis community beds	+++	+
Family education and support	+++	++
Marital/sexual counselling	+	+++
Behavioural/cognitive therapies	+	+++
Supportive counselling	++	+++
Case management and assertive outreach	+++	+
Physical care	+++	+++
Social skills and stress management	+++	+++
Day care	+++	+
Welfare benefits advice	++	++
Housing	++	++
Legal advice	+	+
Support group/self-help group	++	+++
Information and education about illness and services	+++	+++

Table 15.3 illustrates the similarities between the specific potential unmet needs of those with severe affective disorders (manic-depressive disorder or major unipolar depression), and those of patients with more common forms of depression and neurotic disorders, although differences in degree and profile remain. Such a body of needs cannot be met by any single agency, but alliances between health, social services, housing and the voluntary sector

can succeed in providing a comprehensive, complementary and cost-efficient service framework.

Identification and assessment

In order to plan strategically, a community team must first assess the full extent of the potential demands upon them. As a starting point the CMHT must develop, over a 2–5 year timetable, a detailed profile of the number and needs of all individuals with the most severe disorders in the defined locality. In the context of affective disorders these include those with bipolar and unipolar depression, a history of suicide attempts, repeated deliberate self harm and previous violent acts. Special emphasis should be placed on those with clearly defined comorbid conditions which are undermining to their capacity for optimal work with providers and place them at higher risk of suicide on the basis of empirical epidemiological and clinical findings.

In Britain, the Office of Population and Census National Morbidity survey produced surprising findings suggesting a wider variation in the prevalence of psychosis in the UK than had previously been identified (OPCS, 1995). This varies from 0.2% in affluent areas to 0.9% in more deprived areas. Overall about 14% of adults had some sort of neurotic health problem as measured by the CIS-R. Depressive ideas were present amongst 5–14% of cases with 71 respondents per thousand reporting mixed anxiety and depressive states. It clearly demonstrates that one in seven of the population suffer from a neurotic disorder, most often depression. By using locally applied epidemiological techniques, teams can estimate the expected number of individuals with depression for their area and at least plan with some reliability.

GPs are responsible for treating the bulk of psychiatric disorders. Up to a third of GP attendees may have psychosocial problems but approximately half of these may not be detected (Goldberg & Huxley, 1992; Wright, 1993). Depression and anxiety states form 90% of the mental illness caseload of GPs, with 5% reaching DSM-III-R caseness and 10% having impaired functioning because of depressive symptoms (Paykel & Priest, 1992). Of those with major psychiatric morbidity, only a proportion will be in contact with the specialist services. In their long-term follow-up of a cohort of Maudsley patients with depression, Lee and Murray (1988) found that over 50% had lost contact with mental health services. Between 25 and 40% may be in contact only with their GP, social services, the housing agencies, police, local churches or user groups. A fundamental building block in establishing an effective team is the development of an identification or case finding component of the service. The establishment of regular liaisons with all other agencies who may be serving the needs of the SMI in the community is essential. Table 15.4 indicates the likely contact points of people with mental health disorders.

Table 15.4 Identifying people with mental health disorders: contact sources.

Mental health service contacts
   Out-patient and domiciliary visit records
   CPN case-load and depot clinic patients
   Mental Health Act and in-patient audit data
   Crisis attenders, e.g. A/E attenders
   CPA, Supervision register, S.117 (in GB)
   Residents of long-stay institutions

Primary care team contacts
   Practice register diagnoses
   Repeat psychotropic drug prescriptions of antipsychotics and antidepressants
   Frequent emergency and other consultations
   Hostel/group home/sheltered residence populations
   CMHT attenders and health visitor contacts

Social service contacts
   Area social worker case-loads
   Care management clients
   Housing department clients causing concern

Voluntary sector and other agency contacts
   Residents of sheltered accommodation
   Individuals in distress presenting to churches
   Individuals causing local police officers concern
   Imprisoned and homeless people
   Probation officer case-loads
   Drop-in and other casual facility users
   User groups

Many services in Britain have used the implementation of the Care Programme Approach (CPA) as a vehicle to audit how the number of SMI in contact with the service compares with that expected from the epidemiological data.

Needs assessment for rational service planning

Having identified individuals with depression, the next step is to introduce a system of needs assessment. Table 15.5 indicates the full range of needs of people with mental health disorders. If an assessment fails to include attention to the social as well as clinical needs, then long-term outcomes are demonstrably poorer (Craig *et al.*, 1994). Scales commonly used include the Hospital Anxiety and Depression Scale (HADS), the Beck Depression Inventory, the Montgomery Asperg Depression rating scale and the Zung self-rating scale. We refer those interested in a more detailed and comprehensive list of scales and their specific application to examine Freeman and Tyrer, 1989.

In Britain, the basis for an agreed interagency definition of the service priority group and categories for needs assessement has been formed by services in which local health and social services colleagues have integrated

Table 15.5 Effective interventions for people with depression.

Housing with adequate support
Welfare benefits and financial advice
Rehabilitation, practical skills and support
Work and education
Physical and dental care
Medication and psychoeducational programmes
Behavioural-cognitive therapy for psychotic symptoms
Cognitive analytic therapy
Identification and development of coping strategies
Crisis prevention and relapse prevention
Family problem-solving therapy
Counselling
Formal psychoanalytic psychotherapy
Complementary practitioners
Spiritual/religious support

the CPA and Care Management. The routine collection of a clinical data set and care planning assessment and review is vital. When this has been incorporated into the CMHT culture it can ensure that service developments are based on the aggregated needs of patients and can inform the case for resources It also facilitates multiagency co-ordination of service planning and delivery. In sum, it is vital at a national level for the mental health agenda (Kingdon, 1994).

Case management and assertive outreach services

The central task of the CMHT is to establish systems which ensure a continuing focus on the severely mentally ill and provide effective packages of care. In many areas, traditional 'stand-alone' and tertiary rehabilitation services are being decreased in size or replaced by the CMHT. A range of methods are employed by the CMHT in order to ensure that they continue to prioritize the severely mentally ill. They may have an agreed case-mix for each team member's caseload, or use a small number of dedicated case managers. In areas with high levels of morbidity, small separate teams of case managers providing an assertive outreach function are regarded as the most effective way of maintaining a continued focus on the most vulnerable client group (Ford *et al.*, 1996)

Case management as a service (or at least a technique) is essential to combine all the necessary service elements into one coherent package of care. In practice, case management for the long-term mentally ill has developed into a range of approaches that can be described along 12 different axes (Thornicroft, 1990). These techniques aim to ensure that patients receive consistent and continuing services for as long as is necessary. Several studies have compared a number of models of case management offering acute home-based care with hospital care (Stein & Test, 1980; Hoult & Reynolds, 1984; Muijen *et al.*, 1992). Despite differences in the models and evaluative methodologies used, these and several other studies confirm a decrease in hospital admissions, improvement in clinical outcomes, social functioning and greater patient satisfaction from acute home-orientated care. However, CMHTs cannot regard case management as a panacea for treating people with depression. The lesson to be learned from the USA is that 'in many settings the response to the lack of basic services for clients has been to let them eat case management' (Goldman & Taube, 1988).

Case management is only effective where those practising employ effective intervention techniques, and where the system is supported by an adequate resource infrastructure. The failure to engage patients in the experimental programme poses a major and enduring barrier to treatment, despite intensive case management (Lehman *et al.*, 1993). The most likely time for readmission and suicide attempts occurs within the first 4–6 weeks after discharge. Thus keyworker follow-up work is more likely to be successful if it is intense during this vulnerable period.

Home care is the preferred treatment in cases where family dynamics have a major role, preserving the patient's autonomy is paramount, and hospitalization would be deleterious (Soreff, 1983). Dean and Gadd (1990) have demonstrated that the location of treatment in a home treatment study was significantly influenced by the social characteristics of the patients, i.e. marital state, age (especially in men), ethnicity, living conditions and by characteristics of the referral (occurring out of hours, assessment taking place at hospital or police station). A home-based treatment system can help patients to break the vicious cycle of social isolation and establish supportive social contacts (Thornicroft & Breakey, 1991).

Hospital and community beds

People with schizophrenia account for 60% of all in-patient bed use in British mental health units. Those with severe depression make up the majority of the remainder. The context of the current funding distribution means that in some areas as little as 10% (and on average only 25%) of the total mental health budget is available to community work. It is therefore essential that the use of expensive hospital beds by CMHTs is critically examined and of high quality and based on sound therapeutic reasons. A great deal of controversy has surrounded the optimal number, use and management of acute mental health beds. The evidence points to the need for a broad range of initiatives to address the problems. For example, some services have required additional acute beds to deliver safe care (Mental Health Task Force, 1994).

Lelliott and Wing's (1994) study of the new long-stay found that 61% of patients were considered to be inappropriately placed in hospital beds, 47% required a community-based residential setting, and of these over half were in hospital because no suitable community placement was available. Several analyses of acute bed unit use indicate that 30–70% of those in the beds are 'revolving door regulars', well known to services. A significant proportion had been readmitted within 3 months of discharge due to a lack of high support community accommodation and effective discharge planning mechanisms.

The success of community-based services is crucially related to the nature and availability of accommodation with appropriate levels of support, whether provided in individual's homes, by local authorities or by independent sector providers. CMHTs must have a wide range of hospital and community beds available to them. These should range from responsive and community-sensitive secure facilities for mentally disordered offenders, through to acute hospital beds. Twenty-four-hour staffed units in hospital hostels and community places for the new long-stay, especially those with mild to moderate challenging behaviours need to be provided. Finally, a range of community beds from crisis diversion, quarter- and half-way hostels and respite facilities through to residential and supported permanent accommodation are also vital (Strathdee, 1996). CMHTs are ideally placed to play a lead in ensuring the planning of such facilities if they are able to present concrete local data on the numbers and needs of their patients and the number and range of bed provision needed.

CMHTs and bed management

In addition to planning and ensuring the development of an adequate number and range of beds, community teams have used a range of techniques to prevent unnecessary and inappropriate acute bed use. The organization of their service on a defined sector basis facilitates comprehensive case identification, needs assessment and effective interagency planning. In a study where the CMHTs' senior and experienced clinicians carried out initial assessments in the patient's home instead of hospital out-patient clinic sites, admission was reduced by 50–70% (Burns *et al.*, 1993). Gate-keeping (i.e. being involved in the decision to admit a patient) by senior doctors and nurses can assist junior staff who may be less experienced in risk assessment and the deployment of safe alternatives to admission. Consistent research findings demonstrate that integrated hospital and community services are essential to maximize the use of resources. Unless community teams have control over their own hospital beds, both bed use and length of stay are significantly increased.

Crisis response services

Individuals with depression are vulnerable to environmental stressors which can exacerbate symptoms and foster relapse. Successful CMHTs must aim to provide support and help for the client and their family members/carers during the crisis, while maintaining the client's status as a functioning community member. Studies of users, carers and GPs produce almost interchangeable findings. All want crisis services to be accessible from a single telephone call or face-to-face contact. They would value services providing crisis diversion facilities as a viable alternative to hospitalization on a 24-hour, 7-day basis (Phelan *et al.*, 1995). Such services need to be manned by experienced and known mental health professionals. However, on a national scale this type of service is provided by a very limited number of teams (Johnson & Thornicroft, 1995).

Day care and rehabilitation programmes

In a comprehensive review, Holloway (1988) defines several possible functions of the day hospital. It can provide an alternative to hospital admission when acutely ill (a model well elaborated by Creed (1995)), support, supervision and monitoring during the transition between hospital and home. It is usually a source of long-term structure and support for those with long-term difficulties and a site for brief intensive therapy for those who require short-term focused rehabilitation. Finally, it can offer an information, training and communication resource. Wood (1994), as the occupational therapist responsible for the development of day-care services for a CMHT, stresses the importance of user consultation and the establishment of formal liaison with other local providers of work, education and day care. In one service, model employment specialists are part of the community mental health centre team, providing their services in the community team site. Emphasis is placed on client preferences, rapid job finding, continuous assessment, competitive employment, integrated work settings and follow-along supports (Becker & Drake, 1994). Furthermore, the range of social needs differ little between those with affective disorders and those with schizophrenia and length of duration of contact with a service helps to re-establish social and family supports.

Assessment and consultation services

Up until the past few decades, the majority of consultation services were conducted in hospital out-patient settings. The evaluation of these services indicated dissatisfaction with communication patterns and clinical and referrer outcomes. Non-attendance rates were shown to be up to 45%. The response of clinicians, uninformed by policy or research considerations, was to work on a sessional basis in primary care centres. The sessional clinics were criticised early on for running a service that could result in psychiatrists serving only 'the worried well', particularly those with depression and anxiety. However, the evidence now refutes this. They generally provide a service to many of those who either did not have a service or who had dropped out of contact with the specialist services. Such isolated groups include women with long-term disorders, young men with schizophrenia, the homeless with psychosis and those with paranoid disorders who feel stigmatised by attendance at a hospital site (Tyrer, 1984).

Primary care and community agency liaison

In Britain where there is a large primary care infrastructure, CMHTs have developed a number of models to establish a system of liaison. In areas where GP fundholders are common some have helped to fund small, integrated and practice-based primary care liaison teams. More commonly, community teams have dedicated specialist workers who act as the single access point and gatekeeper for referrals. Others have evolved a system whereby each member of the team is the 'link worker' for a particular general practice. In nearly all cases the appropriate model is best determined by local circumstance. Liaison is easier in areas where the primary care teams are based in large health centres. Where GP surgeries are widely dispersed (particularly in inner city areas), the establishment of feasible systems becomes far more problematic. Table 15.6 proposes a range of initiatives to improve joint working between primary health care teams and the CMHT (Strathdee & Jenkins, 1995). The measures are based on the successful shared care model developed for other patient groups with longer-term disorders such as diabetes and asthma.

A study examining the effects of a community mental health service on the practice and attitudes of general practitioners indicated that GPs with access to a psychiatric team were significantly more satisfied with the specialist support services. They were also more likely to give high priority to community psychiatric nurses and psychiatric social workers working as part of a primary health care team if they facilitated access to the service (Warner *et al.*, 1993).

Ensuring that specialist mental health workers liaise with primary care services has not always proved easy. Community psychiatric nurses in many community services were the first to develop attachments to particular general practices. Where the nurses have been hospital based and work as members of the secondary care team, 80% of their referrals are from psychiatrists. Thus, individuals with SMI form a considerable proportion of their work-

Table 15.6 Interagency and primary care liaison in the care of individuals with depression.

Communication strategy
 A directory of street boundaries, sector team names, roles and contact numbers
 Booklets describing therapies available
 Named contacts to advise on appropriate referrals

Crisis response
 Single and well-publicized telephone contact access point
 Agreed crisis response time-scales, roles and responsibilities

Assessment and out-patient services
 Agreed referral-appointment interval
 Stated referral criteria for members of the CMHT
 Clear communication with stated objectives of management, predicted
 response, complications and side-effects
 6-monthly review plans for long-term patients
 Clearly stated role of GP and specialist in treatment
 Clarification of prescribing responsibilities

Shared care for individuals with depression
 Set up a joint case register similar to diabetes
 Prioritize the most severely ill
 Agree annual physical care reviews
 Ensure GP verbal/physical/fax input into CPA care planning reviews
 Identify GP/practice nurse role in development of relapse prevention plans
 Agree protocols for group homes/hostels
 Discuss consequences of expensive new psychotropic drugs and ECRs
 Obtain support for appropriate range of beds and community alternatives to hospital admission

---

load. Where nurses, although employed by secondary care services, are attached to particular general practices, the referral pattern shifts, with 80% of their referrals coming directly from the GPs. Caseloads tend to be large and composed of patients with neurotic and adjustments disorders. Although the caseloads of both hospital and primary care-based CPNs remain similar in terms of the number of individuals with schizophrenia, the mean time in contact with psychotic patients amounts to one-third of the time spent with nonpsychotic patients and almost entirely limited to the administration of injections.

Effective interventions for the treatment of depression and common mental health morbidity in primary care

Whatever the structural links between primary and secondary care teams are, the important question is how best to provide effective, evidence-based interventions to the maximum number of patients. A two-pronged approach seems appropriate. First, the skills of the primary care team who already provide the majority of care need to be enhanced and appropriate training given. Second, those with more severe and moderate difficulties will need and benefit from direct care by the CMHT. The community mental health team is particularly helpful in reducing the burden posed by patients with neurotic and psychosocial problems, but can result in de-skilling the general practitioners who end up undertaking less mental health work themselves (Warner *et al.*, 1993). An educational approach therefore seems most likely to lead to overall improved care in the longer term. Table 15.7 illustrates some of the training found to be useful and effective for primary health care staff.

Table 15.7 Developing effective interventions in primary care.

CMHT initiatives
  Provision of a resources directory of all statutory and other mental health resources locally, e.g. day care, dropins, counselling services
  Development of joint good practice protocols for common conditions such as depression
  Employment and supervision of primary care-based counsellors, psychologists, etc.
  Provision training to PHCT
  Provision of updates on new psychotropic medication, therapies and information leaflets, videos, etc.

PHCT initiatives: increased training for:
  Practice nurses
    Recognition and management of depression, stress management
    Mental state assessment
    Administration and review of medication
    Assessment of tardive dyskinesia
    Relapse prevention
    Psychoeducation
  Health visitors
    Recognition and prevention of depression in young mothers/children
    Recognition of depression in the elderly and chronically physically ill
    Problem-solving for mentally ill parents
    Problem-solving for parents of adolescents
  District nurses
    Recognition of depression in the elderly and physically ill
  Receptionists:
    Dealing with difficult patients

Treatment alliance: an essential for effective intervention

One important reason for persistent depressive symptoms is the failure of patients to adhere to the agreed treatment plan. The use of psychotropic medication to treat depressive symptoms has proven effective, particularly if combined with a psychotherapeutic and social problems management approach. Yet up to 50% of patients may not be taking their medication in sufficient amounts. Strategies to establish a dialogue with patients about their objections to certain medication regimens are an essential part of the community management of depression where intensive 'medication' supervision is not available. Poor compliance can be influenced by specific factors related to the medication, the patient, the illness experience or the treatment setting (Fawcett, 1995). Strategies designed to improve the uptake of medication include keeping the regimen simple, tailoring to daily rituals, providing explicit written instructions and implementing drug regimes gradually. Involving the patient in the decision-making process and providing a warm, positive feedback for compliance and attainment of the therapeutic goals also helps to encourage compliance (Churchill, 1985). A fuller account of non-compliance with psychotropic medication is given elsewhere (Frank *et al.*, 1995; Sair *et al.*, 1995).

Risk management

Managing the depressed patient in the community without admission requires a careful assessment and review of suicide risks as well as the risks of each treatment decision. One should consider each of the risk factors associated with suicide as illustrated in Table 15.8.

Table 15.8 Risk factors associated with suicide.

History of depression or schizophrenia
History of alcohol and/or substance misuse
Family history of depression, schizophrenia, DSH, completed suicide
Family history of alcoholism
Previous DSH/suicide attempt
Stressors and capacity to deal with them: intelligence and supports
Comorbidity: physical illness, bereavement, chronic pain
Presence of behaviour disturbance/violence/impulsivity
Level of supervision available if stays at home and providers of supervision
Past range of treatments and response to treatments
Previous compliance with treatment
Expressing suicidal ideas
Objective measures of depression (scales) and suicide intent scales
Are family and supporters in crisis themselves such that admission is necessary?

If adequate supervision can be provided at home by a patient's family and by professionals during home visits, one should explicitly document the risk factors, the potential outcomes, the likelihood of each occurring and the potential severity of each outcome. An explanation as to why the treatment package should effectively contain the community treatment risk also needs to be included. The motivation for the decisions and the stages of reasoning should be made clear instead of continuing to only document the final decisions. Each decision should be allocated a risk time period after which the decision and its consequences are reviewed. A plan may be reviewed every 12 to 24 h initially, depending on the level of risk carried and what can clinically be regarded as a safe risk period. Once some improvement has occurred and the level of despair expressed is less, then the risk periods could be increased. In addition, one should also involve the patient in a crisis plan if it is anticipated that they may experience profound suicidal ideas. Effective communication with the primary care teams could also help prevent a crisis and reduce the risk as they can carry out some of the review visits. Day care may help to relieve relatives and carers and give patients a sense of support. Furthermore, day care services can help assess level of dysfunction and provide occupational and social interventions which may be of specific importance for the individual. Some suicide scales enable the enumeration of risk, otherwise simple scales can be constructed for use by specific teams. An example of risk assessment in the community management of mentally disordered offenders has been well described (Carson, 1993) and could be adapted to improve stategies for the community care of depressed patients. However, any strategy must take account of known epidemiologically associated factors.

Groups with special needs

Women

In all the major epidemiological surveys women have been found to have 1.4–3 times higher rates of depression (Juel-Nielson *et al.*, 1961; Odegaard, 1961; Paykel *et al.*, 1970). This is largely accounted for by unipolar depression as the sex ratio for bipolar disorder is 1:1. Several hypotheses have been advanced to explain these findings (Paykel, 1991). Women may be more likely to seek help when depressed, and research is being carried out into the impact levels of female sex hormones and genetic differences (Watson & Studd, 1990). Social vulnerability, absence of support, low self-esteem and women's general social position are thought to be important factors influencing mild to moderate depression (Brown & Harris, 1978; Brown & Prudo, 1981; Brown *et al.*, 1986; Morris *et al.*, 1991). A final theory suggests that each sex perceives, interacts with and responds to distress in a manner which is depressogenic in women and gives rise to other disorders in men. The latter hypothesis is supported by Winokur *et al.* (1971) who describes a familial 'depressive spectrum disorder' which is manifest as alcoholism and personality disorder in men and depression in women. Furthermore, the diagnostic profile of women presenting to GPs differs from their male counterparts. The nature of the intervention can also differ: specifically, women may be offered benzodiazepines more often, their distress being conceptualized as an anxiety state (Ashton, 1991).

Women developing severe and chronic mental illness are less likely to receive an effective intervention which limits and appropriately ends their illness episode (Perkins & Rowland, 1991). Chronicity of symptoms may therefore be a function of inflexible services structures, as well as a failure to diagnose depression accurately and administer the appropriate treatment. The social needs of women should be addressed in conjunction with social services, housing, child care services, educational establishments, parenting services and relationship counselling to ensure specific provisions are made. A sound infrastructure of flexible and responsive health service delivery must exist if the services are to be fully effective. Home treatments are increasingly demonstrated to be a patient preference. For mothers or women who receive their main source of support from their immediate communities, assessments and treatment are most appropriately delivered at home. This will help to maintain and reinforce already established social support rather than un- dermine and replace long-standing support structures with less flexible, less familiar and rationed statutory equivalents. Women-only services including admission wards are especially valuable when considering the range of services suitable for ethnic minorities or specific religious groups.

Ethnic minorities

Evidence shows that the African and Caribbean populations of Britain have a 3–6 times higher incidence of diagnosed schizophrenia than white people (Harrison *et al.*, 1988; Littlewood & Lipsedge, 1981; Wessley *et al.*, 1991) and a recent study extended this finding to all ethnic minorities (King *et al.*, 1994). By comparison, the rates of depression and anxiety disorders as identified amongst ethnic minority GP attendees and by hospital admissions, appears to be lower than those identified for white attendees (Bebbington *et al.*, 1981; Cochrane, 1977; Birchwood *et al.*, 1992). Gillam *et al.* (1989) demonstrated that Black and Asian people attended their GP as often as the control group, but often attended for physical complaints rather than for specific mental illness. The outcome seems to be somewhat paradoxical, as factors such as social ad- versity, including racism, poor housing and unemployment, which are thought to contribute to higher rates of psychosis are also expected to lead to higher rates of depression (Lloyd, 1993).

Little attention has been given to the systematic identification of de- pression amongst black communities. Worsening suicide rates in the USA, especially amongst young black men, has alerted British psychiatrists to the possibility that black people appear to present when in crisis. Thus, effective interventions may not occur at the early stage of an illness episode or the inter- vention sought by a depressed patient is not that offered by existing health services. Distress experiences may also present differently amongst minorities because of an inherently different sense of self and object relatedness (Bhui *et al.*, 1995); first rank symptoms, for example, are of less diagnostic signifi- cance amongst some communities (Fernando, 1988). Unfamiliar idioms of distress employed by ethnic minorities may remain unrecognized, causing a significant delay in the implementation of therapeutic interventions.

In addition, the suicide rates amongst young Asian women are increasing (Merril *et al.*, 1990; Raleigh *et al.*, 1990). Cultural conflict, hopelessness in the face of social adversity, employment disadvantage and racism have all been put forward as explanations. High levels of morbidity may go undetected partly because an individual's appraisal of symptoms may result in explanatory models and illness behaviour which are unfamiliar to many GPs and psychiatrists (Belliapa, 1991; Krause *et al.*, 1991). Such explanatory models and patterns of help seeking (for example prayer or increased attendance at a temple) will be unique to each culture and are likely to involve the traditional healers and complementary medicine practitioners (Bhopal, 1986; Wilson, 1994). Some cultural groups hold the belief that a certain amount of adversity is inevitable and necessary for healthy spiritual and temporal relationships. Distinguishing such beliefs from depressive ideas will prove difficult for inexperienced and culturally unfamiliar health professionals, although much has been written on somatization of depression in non-western communities (Bal, 1984; Burke, 1986; Leff, 1988). The absence of shared meanings, concepts of self and world views contributes to the emphasis on physical symptoms which are more directly amenable to undistorted translation (Mumford, 1992). It may be that somatization arises through the premature closure of assessments which are limited in their potential depth of communication (Bhui, 1994). Thus existing models of treatment need adaptation and more assessment sessions are necessary to explore the cultural context in which symptoms arise and treatment is to be given. A more detailed account of service adaptations, including the use of interpreters, is dealt with elsewhere (Westermeyer, 1991; Bhui *et al.*, 1995). Culture-specific assessment and treatment strategies should be developed in alliance with patients and their relatives. Most depression scales developed on the basis of symptom profiles are likely to be as insensitive to depression across cultures as clinical assessments. One suggested solution is to employ culture experts or advocates to help with the recognition and diagnosis of symptoms. The use of children and other family members (e.g. parents or siblings) should be discouraged as it is invariably likely to give rise to a distorted version of events and symptom appraisal.

Conclusions

The management of the majority of individuals with depression has taken place in the community setting. The challenge for the future is to determine the most effective ways in which agencies working in the community can liaise and work together. This applies particularly to Community Mental Health Teams and Primary Health Care Teams. Agencies and teams need to examine how best they can acquire and use the effective interventions known to achieve optimal outcomes for the patients they serve.

References

Ashton, H. (1991) Psychotropic prescribing in women. *British Journal of Psychiatry,* **158** (Suppl.), 30–35.

Audit Commission (1994) *Finding a Place: A Review of Mental Health Services for Adults.* HMSO, London.

Bal, S. (1984) *The Symptomatology of Mental Illness amongst Asians in the West Midlands.* BA Dissertation. Department of Economics and Social Sciences, Wolverhampton Polytechnic.

Becker, D. & Drake, R. (1994) Individual Placement and Support: a community mental health center approach to vocational rehabilitation. *Community Mental Health Journal,* **30** (2), 193–206.

Bebbington, P., Hurry, J. & Tennant, C. (1996) Psychiatric disorders in selected immigrant groups in Camberwell. *Social Psychiatry,* **16**, 43–51.

Belliapa, J. (1991) *Illness or distress? Alternative models of Mental Health.* Confederation of Indian Organisations (UK).

Bhopal., R. (1986) The Inter-relationship of Folk, Traditional and Western Medicine within an Asian Community in Britain. *Social Science Medicine,* **22** (no. 1), 99–105.

Bhui, K., Christie, Y. & Bhugra, D. *et al.* (1995) Essential elements in culturally sensitive psychiatric services. *International Journal Social Psychiatry,* **41**(4), 242–256.

Bhui, K. (1994) *Somatic symptoms in Asian patients.* MSc thesis. UMDS, University of London.

Birchwood, M., Cochrane, R. MacMillam, F. *et al.* (1992*).* The influnce of ethnicity and family structure on relaspe in first episode schizophrenia. *British Journal of Psychiatry,* **161**, 783–790.

Brown, G., & Harris, T., (1978) *Social origins of depression. A study of psychiatric disorder in women.* Tavistock, London.

Brown, G., Andrews, B., Harris, T. *et al.* (1986) Social support self esteem and depression. *Psychological Medicine,* **16**, 813–831.

Brown, G. & Prudo, R. (1981) Psychiatric disorder in urban and rural populations: 1. Aetiology of depression. *Psychological Medicine,* **11**, 581–589.

Burke, A. (1986) Racism, Prejudice and Mental Illness. In: *Transcultural Psychiatry* (ed. J. L. Cox). Croom Helm, London.

Carson, D. (1993) *Risk Taking with Mentally Disordered Offenders.* SLE Publications, Southampton.

Cochrane, R. (1977) Mental illness in immigrants to England and Wales: an analysis of mental hospital admissions. *Social Psychiatry,* **12**, 25–35.

Churchill, D.N. (1985) Compliance—how to measure it. *Modern Medicine in Canada,* **40**, 1203–1211.

Craig, T. (1994) *The Homeless Mentally Ill Initiative: An Evaluation.* HMSO, London.

Creed, F. (1995) *Acute day hospital care in Emergency Mental Health Services in the Community,* (eds Phelan, M., Strathdee, G. & Thornicroft, G.) Cambridge University Press, Cambridge.

Dean, C. & Gadd, E. (1990) Home treatment for acute psychiatric illness. *British Medical Journal,* **301** (6759), 1021–1023.

Fawcett, J. (1995) Compliance: definitions and key issues. *Journal of Clinical Psychiatry,* **56** (Suppl. 1), 5–10.

Fernando, S. (1988) *Race, Culture and Psychiatry.* Routledge, London.

Ford, R., Ryan, P., Norton, P., Beadsmore, A., Craig, T & Muijen, M. (1996) Does intensive care management work? Clinical, social and quality of life outcomes from a controlled study. *Journal of Mental Health,* **54**, 361–368.

Frank, E.Kupfer, D. & Siegal, R. (1995) Alliance not compliance: a philosphy of outpatient care. *Journal of Clinical Psychiatry,* **56** (Suppl. 1), 11–17.

Freeman, C. & Tyrer, P. (1989) *Research Methods in Psychiatry.* Royal College of Psychiatrists, London.

Gillam, S., Jarman, B. & White, P. *et al.* (1989) Ethnic differences in consultation rates in urban general practice. *British Medical Journal,* **299**, 953–957.

Goldberg, D. & Huxley, P. (1992) *Common Mental Disorders.* Routledge, London.

Goldman, H. (1981), Defining and outlining the chronically mentally ill. *Hospital and Community Psychiatry,* **32**, 21–27.

Goldman, H. & Taube, C. (1988) High users of outpatients mental health services, II implications for practice and policy. *American Journal of Psychiatry,* **145**, 24–28.

Harrison, G. *et al.* (1988) A prospective study of severe mental disorder in Afro-Caribbean Patients. *Psychological Medicine,* **18**, 643–657.

Health of the Nation (1994) *Key Area Handbook: Mental Illness.* DoH/HMSO London.

Health of the Nation (1996) *Spectrum of Care: Local Services for People with Mental Health Problems.* DoH London.

Holloway, F. (1988) Day Care and Community Support. In: *Community Care in Practice* (eds A. Lavenders & F. Holloway). John Wiley, Chichester.

Hoult, J. & Reynolds, I. (1984) Schizophrenia: a comprehensive trial of community oriented and hospital oriented psychiatric care. *Acta Psychiatrica Scandinavica,* **69**, 359–372.

Hunter, D. & Wistow, G. (1987) Mapping the organisational context. 1 Central departments, boundaries and responsibilities. In: *Community Care in Britain: Variations on a Theme*, pp.18–46. The King Edward Hospital Fund, London.

Johnson, S. & Thornicroft, G. (1995) Service models in emergency psychiatry: An international view. In: *Emergency Mental Health Services in the Community*. CUP, Cambridge.

Juel-Nielson, N., Bille, M. & Flygenring, J. (1961) Frequency of depressive states within geographically delimited populations groups. *Acta Psychiatrica Scandinavica*, **162**, 69–80.

Kingdon, D. (1994) The Care Programme Approach. *Psychiatric Bulletin*, **18** (2), 68–70.

King, M., Coker, E., Leavey, G., Hoare, A. & Johnson-Sabine, E. (1994) Incidence of psychotic illness in London: comparison of ethnic groups. *British Medical Journal*, **309**, 1115–1119.

Krause, I.B. (1989) Sinking heart: a Punjabi communication of distress. *Social Science and Medicine*, **2**, 563–575.

Lee, A.S. & Murray, R.M. (1988) The long term outcome of the Maudsley depressives. *British Journal of Psychiatry*, **153**, 741–751.

Leff, J. (1988) *Psychiatry Around the Globe: A transcultural view*. Gaskell Series. Royal College of Psychiatrists, London.

Lehman, A., Herron, J., Schwartz, R. & Myers, C. (1993) Rehabilitation for adults with severe mental illness and substance use disorders. A clinical trial. *Journal of Nervous and Mental Disorders*, **181** (2), 86–90.

Lelliott, P. & Wing, J. (1994) National audit of new long-stay psychiatric patients. 2. Impact on services. *British Journal of Psychiatry*, **165**, 160–169.

Littlewood, R. & Lipsedge, M. (1988) Psychiatric illness among British Afro-Caribbeans. *British Medical Journal*, **296**, 950–951.

Lloyd, K. (1993) Depression and anxiety amongst Afro-Carribeans general practice attenders in Britain. *International Journal Society of Psychiatry*, **39**, 1–9.

Mental Health Task Force (1994) Mental Health in London: Priorities for Action. London.

Meltzer, D., Hale, A.S. & Malik, S.J. *et al.*(1991) Community care for patients with schizophrenia one year after hospital discharge. *British Medical Journal*, **303**, 1023–1026.

Mental Health Foundation (1994) *Creating Community Care: Report of the Mental Health Foundation Inquiry into the Care for People with Severe Mental Illnesss*. Mental Health Foundation, London.

Merril, J., Owens, J., & Wynne, S. *et al.* (1990) Asian suicides. *British Journal of Psychiatry*, **156**, 748–749.

Morris, R., Woods, R., Davies, K. & Morris, L.

(1991) *British Journal of Psychiatry*, **158** (suppl, 10), 69–74.

Muijen, M., Marks, I., Connolly, J. & Audini, B. (1992) Homebased care and standard hospital care for patients with severe mental illness: a randomised, controlled trial. *British Medical Journal*, **304**, 749–754.

Mumford, D. (1992) Does somatisation explain anything? *Psychiatry in Practice Spring*, **11(1)**, 11–14.

Odegaard, O. (1961) The epidemiology of depressive psychosis. *Acta Psychiatrica Scandinavica*, **162**, 33–38.

OPCS (1995) *The National Psychiatric Morbidity Survey: Household Survey*. HMSO, London.

Onyett, S., Heppleston, T. & Bushnell, D. (1994) *The Organisation and Operation of Community Metal Health Teams in England*. The Sainsbury Centre for Mental Health, London.

Paykel, E., Klerman, G. & Prusoff, B. (1970) Treatment setting and clincial depression. *Archives of General Psychiatry*, **22**, 11–21.

Paykel, E. (1991) Depression in women. *British Journal of Psychiatry*, **158** (suppl.), 22–29.

Paykel, E. & Priest, R. (1992) Recognition and management of depression in General Practice. Consensus statement. *British Medical Journal*, **305**, 1198–1202.

Perkins, R. & Rowland, L. (1991) Sex differences in service usage in long term psychiatric care. Are women adequatly served. *British Journal of Psychiatry*, **158** (suppl. 10), 75–79.

Phelan, M., Strathdee, G. & Thornicroft, G. (eds) (1995) *Emergency Mental Health Services in the Community*, Cambridge University Press, Cambridge.

Raleigh, V., Balusa, L. & Balarajan, R. *et al.* (1990) Suicides amongst immigrants from the Indian sub-continent. *British Journal of Psychiatry*, **156**, 46–50.

Ritchie, J. *et al.* (1994) *The Report of the Inquiry into the Care and Treatment of Christopher Clunis*. NE & SE Thames Regional Health Authorities/ DoH, London.

Sayce, L., Craig, T. & Boardman, A. (1991) The development of community mental health centres in the UK. *Social Psychiatry and Psychiatric Epidemiology*, **26**, 14–20.

Sair, A., Bhui, K. & Strathdee, G. (1997) Compliance or collaboration: the use of psychoeducation in psychiatry. A Brief Review. *Psychiatric Bulletin* (in press).

Soreff, S. (1983) New directions and added dimensions in home psychiatric treatment *American Journal of Psychiatry*, **140** (9), 1213–1216.

Strathdee, G. (1990) The delivery of psychiatric

care. *Journal of the Royal Society of Medicine*, **83**, 222–225.

Strathdee, G. & Jenkins, R. (1995) Contracting for primary care mental health services. In: *Purchasing Mental Health Services* (eds Thornicroft, G. & Strathdee, G.) HMSO,London.

Test, M. & Scott, R. (1990) Theoretical and research bases of community care programmes. In: *Mental Health Care Delivery: Innovations, Impediments and Implementation* (eds Marks, I. & Scott, R. Cambridge University Press, Cambridge.

Test, L. & Stein, M. (1980) Alternative to Hospital Treatment. 1 Conceptual model, treatment program and clinical evaluation. *Archives of General Psychiatry*, **37**, 392–397.

Thornicroft, G. (1990) The concept of case management for the long-term mental illness. *International Review of Psychiatry*, **3**, 125–132.

Thornicroft, G. & Breakey, W. (1991) The COSTAR programme: Improving social networks of the long-team mentally ill. *British Journal of Psychiatry*, **159**, 245–249.

Tyrer, P. (1984) Psychiatric clinics in general practice: an extension of community care. *British Journal of Psychiatry*, **149**, 449–457.

Warner, R., Gater, R., Jackson, M. & Goldberg, D. (1993) Effects of a community mental health service on the practice and attitudes of general practitioners. *British Journal of General Practitioners*, **43** (377), 507–511.

Watson, N. & Studd, J. (1990) Gonadal hormones and depression in women. In: *Current Approaches Series: Prediction and Treatment of Recurrent Depression* (eds J. Cobb & N. Goeting). Duphar Medical Relations, Southampton.

Wessley *et al.* (1991) Schizophrenia and Afro-Caribbeans: a case control study. *British Journal of Psychiatry*, **159**, 795–801.

Westermeyer. (1991) Working with an interpreter in psychiatric assessments. *Journal of Nervous and Mental Diseases*, **178** (12), 745.

Wood, H. (1994) *Community Mental Health Team Manager*, pp. 1–6. Mental Health Foundation, London.

White, E. (1994) *3rd Quinquennial Community Psychiatric Nursing Survey* Manchester University Department of Nursing, Manchester.

Wilson, M. (1994) *Mental Health and Britain's Black Communities*. NHS Management Executive: Mental Health Task Force and Kings Fund Centre.

Winoker, G., Cardoret, R., Dorzab, J. & Baker, M. (1971) Depressive Disease: a genetic study. *Archives of General Psychiatry*, **24**, 135–144.

Wright, A. (1993) *Depression: Recognition and Management in General Practice*. RCGP, London.

16 The management of depression in children and adolescents

ERIC FOMBONNE

Up to the early 1980s, depression in children and adolescents had not been studied since it was considered a very rare occurrence. Most investigators considered that, due to an immature ego and superego development, depression could not occur before the final phases of adolescent development. Over the last 15 years, the picture has changed dramatically and research in epidemiological, clinical, genetic, neurobiological, pharmacological and psychological aspects of childhood depression has blossomed. This chapter starts with a brief overview of background knowledge on the assessment, distribution, risk factors and outcome of affective disorders in young people; it then continues with an up-to-date review of treatment techniques used with children and adolescents suffering from an affective disorder.

Definition, diagnosis, assessment and comorbidity

Definition and diagnosis

Depressive manifestations are often found among children in conjunction with other forms of psychopathology or they may be experienced as part of normal development. It is therefore crucial to differentiate, within the affective phenomena, varying levels of definition and severity.

The first level is that of depression as a symptom. High levels of depressed mood are experienced by over a third of adolescents surveyed in community studies (Petersen et al., 1993); and feelings of sadness and misery are also very common among children and adolescents suffering from other forms of psychopathology, be they emotional or disruptive disorders (Harrington et al., 1996). In several studies comparing clinical samples to community samples, depressed mood has been found to be the individual psychiatric feature or the most predictive of referral status (Achenbach, 1991). The second level is that of a depressive syndrome, which is generally identified in multivariate analysis of symptom scales and questionnaires. This broad construct of negative affect often fails to differentiate specific anxious and depressive dimensions and it is therefore of limited clinical usefulness. The third level of definition is that of depressive disorder, a psychiatrically defined cluster of symptoms persisting over a minimal period of time, associated with substantial impairment in functioning, as defined in current classification schemes.

The use of strict criteria to diagnose depression among children is, however, a recent phenomenon. A few decades ago, unreliable formulations such as 'masked depression' or 'depression equivalent' were used to account for childhood affective disturbances. Attempts to devise diagnostic criteria for children (Weinberg *et al.*, 1973) were shortlived and, by the late 1970s, several studies had shown that major depression could be recognized in children with the same diagnostic criteria as for adults. Along with their adult colleagues, child psychiatrists use the DSM-IV and ICD-10 definitions of affective disorders. In order to account for slight differences in the clinical picture amongst younger subjects, it is noted in the DSM-IV definition of Major Depression that depressed mood in children and adolescents is often substituted with irritable mood. In addition, the duration criterion of depressed mood for the diagnosis of Dysthymic Disorder is set at 1 year in children and adolescents. Otherwise, the criteria and diagnostic subdivisions used in children are the same as that for adults.

Assessment and comorbidity

Symptom checklists, questionnaires and diagnostic interviews are widely used in child psychiatry and are recommended to assess depressive disorders with desirable levels of reliability (see Table 16.1). Assessment procedures often rely on several informants (i.e. parents, teachers and children) and data from these different sources need to be combined in a final formulation. Self-report questionnaires provide a convenient means to assess the severity of depressive symptoms and are suitable to monitor changes over time in patients. They only take a few minutes to complete and the scoring procedures and interpretation of the scores are generally straightforward. However, despite relatively good psychometric properties, these questionnaires have in general too low a specificity and sensitivity to be used for diagnostic purposes. The assessment of affective disorders and of comorbid disorders is therefore best conducted with diagnostic interviews. Irrespective of the particular method used, the diagnostic assessment should involve a detailed interview of both the child and the parents. The level of agreement between children and parents on the reporting of symptoms and on the final diagnosis has been typically variable across studies, with the best agreement being generally found for symptoms involving clear-cut behavioural changes such as weight and appetite loss, psychomotor retardation, suicide attempts and sleeping difficulties. Rules for combining discrepant parent and child reports are being studied, and most professionals currently use a best estimate

Table 16.1 Depression in children and adolescents: most commonly used assessment tools.

Assessment tool	Age range	Main use	Comments	Recommended reference
General psychopathological checklists				
Child Behaviour Checklist	4–18	Epidemiological	Item 103 (Unhappy, sad or depressed)	Achenbach (1991)
Teacher Report Form	4–18	Clinical	Anxious-Depressed Factor	
Youth Self-Report	11–18			
Rutter A2 Scale (parent)	5–15	Epidemiological	1 depression item	Elander and Rutter (1996)
Rutter B2 Scale (teacher)			emotional score	
Strength and Difficulties Questionnaire (parent/teacher/self-report)	5–18	Clinical/ epidemiological	1 depression item emotional score	Goodman (1994)
Scales specific to depression (self-report)				
Children's Depression Inventory	7–15	Clinical	27 items. Revision of the Beck Depression Inventory for children and adolescents	Kovacs (1982)
Depression Self-Rating Scale	Children	Clinical	18 or 21 items	Birleson *et al.* (1987)
Centre for Epidemiological Studies Depression Scale	Adolescents 12+	Epidemiological	20 items (4 positive, 16 depression)	Radloff (1977)
Mood and Feelings Questionnaire	8–16	Epidemiological Clinical	30 items or short version with 13 items (SMFQ)	Angold *et al.* (1995) Wood *et al.* (1995)
Children's Depression Scale	9–16	Clinical	66 items	Tisher & Lang (1983) Lang and Tisher (1987)
Reynolds Child/Adolescent Depression Scale	8–13	Clinical	1 positive affect and 5 depression sub-scores 30 DSM-III-like items	Reynolds (1986)
Depression rating scale (clinical raters)				
Children's Depression Rating-Scale—Revised		Clinical	18 items (15 verbal responses + 3 observational items); downward revision of the Hamilton scale Suitable for treatment studies	Poznanski *et al.* (1984)
Diagnostic interview				
Child and Adolescent Psychiatric Assessment	5–18	Epidemiological Clinical	Diagnostic assessments of affective disorders (DSM-IV and ICD-10) and of comorbid disorders	Hodges (1993)
Child Assessment Schedule				
Schedule for Affective Disorders and Schizophrenia for School-Aged Children				
Diagnostic Interview Schedule for Children				
Diagnostic Interview for Children and Adolescents				
Interview Schedule for Children				

procedure whereby a symptom is considered as present when any informant reports it. Obviously, the weight given to the assessment of individual symptoms varies according to the clinical experience of the investigator, the individual characteristics of the child and his/her family, and also to the severity and pervasiveness of symptoms.

Comorbidity is the rule rather than the exception both in clinical and community samples. Anxiety disorders are the most frequent comorbid diagnoses. Separation anxiety, phobias and generalized anxiety are found in about 40–60% of children and adolescents with depression. Conduct disorders are found in 20–30% of children referred for depression. In older children and adolescents, substance abuse and eating disorders are found with high rates too. The same results have been found in community studies where the comorbidity between affective disorders and other psychiatric disorders was assessed. In most community studies at least 50% of children and adolescents diagnosed with an affective disorder have a comorbid disorder, with several studies showing rates of 10% or less of 'pure' depressive disorder uncomplicated by comorbid problems. The patterns and correlates of comorbidity in community studies have been similar to those found in clinically referred samples.

Epidemiology

Epidemiological estimates for the prevalence of major depression and dysthymia in children and adolescents vary enormously as a function of different sampling frames, case finding techniques, case definition and instrumentation (Fombonne, 1997a). Amongst school-aged, prepubertal children, prevalence rates have been consistently low in community studies. Thus, in the Isle of Wight study (Rutter *et al.*, 1970), the prevalence rate for depression was 0.1% among 10-year-olds. Similar figures have derived from other studies (Fleming & Offord, 1990) and the 6-month or 12-month prevalence rate is not in excess of 1% in this age group. Interestingly, more boys than girls have been found suffering from depression in prepubertal children. By contrast, a preponderance of girls is consistently found in adolescent samples, especially in studies which have focused on mid or late adolescence. By the age of 14 or 15, the adult preponderance of females is found with a typical 2:1 gender ratio. The prevalence rate for adolescent samples is also much higher with, on average, a period prevalence of 3–4% (Fombonne, 1997a).

Besides age and gender, the assessment of risk factors in relation to the development of depression in childhood and adolescence has been somewhat difficult, due to either the small number of cases identified in these community surveys or to the design limitations of these studies. In particular, difficulties arose from the cross-sectional nature of these investigations which do not allow for a proper identification of causal factors. Moreover, due to the high frequency of comorbid disorders, it has been difficult to assess to which extent factors associated with depression were specific risk factors for the development of affective disorders, as opposed to risk factors for other comorbid disorders or non-specific risk indicators of general psychiatric morbidity. Epidemiological studies in various child and adolescent samples have, however, concurred with findings from adult studies in showing a trend towards younger birth cohorts to be at increased risk for affective disorders, with an earlier age of onset for depression for the youths born in the last three decades (Fombonne, 1994, 1998). The reasons for this increased incidence of depression are still poorly understood (Fombonne, 1995).

Outcome studies

Short-term outcome

Among the few studies which have systematically examined the natural history of depression in children and adolescents, the study by Kovacs *et al.* (1984a,b) was the first to point to the strong recurrence risk of depression following a first index episode. These authors followed up children aged 8–13 years, whose first episode consisted of a major depression or a dysthymic disorder, or an adjustment disorder with depressed mood. The average length of the episodes of depression was 7 months for major depression and nearly 4 years for dysthymic disorders. These two groups had a high risk of subsequent episodes, with about a fourth of children with major depression having a relapse within a year, the figures going up to 40% at 2 years and 72% at a 5-year follow-up. Comparable figures were obtained in a follow-up study of children hospitalized for depression with a rate of 45% of readmissions at 2 years (Asarnow *et al.*, 1988). In the first investigation, relapse was associated with an earlier age of onset and the co-occurrence of dysthymic disorder, whereas the pattern of comorbidity did not affect the outcome. Relapse rates in follow-up samples of depressed children and adolescents identified in community surveys have broadly shown similar findings, although the absolute rate of relapses tended to be lower in these unselected samples. Thus, adolescents with unipolar depression were followed up at 1 year by Lewinsohn *et al.* (1993) who found that about one-fifth of them had relapsed within a year, this rate being none the less higher than that for other psychiatric disorders.

Long-term outcomes

Few studies have investigated the consequences of childhood depression in adult life. However, one study provided follow-up data on a group of children referred for psychiatric services with a depression and reassessed on average 18 years later (Harrington *et al.*, 1990, 1991). Depressed children had four times the risk of developing major depression in adulthood as compared to that for non-depressed psychiatric controls. Furthermore, the increased risk seemed to apply only to affective disorders in adult life and not to other psychiatric disorders, suggesting a strong specific continuity between childhood and adult depression which cannot be explained by comorbid disorders. This follow-up study also indicated that the depressed group had increased contact with medical services and increased use of medication in adult life. The social and economical impact of child and adolescent depression have similarly been documented in other studies.

Links with suicidal behaviours

Strong links exist between childhood depression and suicidal behaviours. Thus, depression was found to be the strongest predictor of suicidal ideas, plans and attempts in a large sample of referred adolescents seen at the Maudsley Hospital (Fombonne, 1997b). Findings from follow-up studies in adult life of depressed children also concur in showing an increased risk of suicide mortality which extends into adult life. Thus, two studies with the longest periods of follow-up (Harrington *et al.*, 1990; Rao *et al.*, 1993) provide a rough estimate in the neighbourhood of 4–5% for the cumulative risk of suicidal death in early adult life following an episode of depression in childhood or early adolescence. The strength of the association between depression and completed suicide is most obvious in recent psychological autopsy studies which have been conducted in the last decade (Marttunen *et al.*, 1991; Brent *et al.*, 1993; Shaffer *et al.*, 1996). Thus, in the recent New York study where 120 suicidal deaths under the age of 20 were compared to 147 matched community controls, mood disorders were one of the strongest risk factors. A medium rate of 60% was found for affective disorders with about half of them corresponding to clear-cut episodes of major depression. Thus, depression in children and adolescents predicts suicidal ideas, attempts and completed suicides both in the short and long term.

Family and genetic factors

Controlled studies of first-degree relatives using the family history method have consistently found higher rates of affective disorders among relatives of depressed children than among relatives of psychiatric or normal controls (Livingston *et al.*, 1985; Kutcher & Marton, 1991). When direct assessments of relatives were used, similar findings were obtained. Thus, in a study comparing 48 prepubertal depressed children with anxious and normal controls, Puig-Antich *et al.* (1989a) found higher rates of depression among relatives of the depressed group as well as a high frequency of alcoholism. Familial loading for affective disorders varied according to clinical characteristics of the depression in the proband child, with increased loading for depression with endogenous features and decreased loading for depression associated with conduct disorder. Similarly, the rate of depression among relatives of depressed children was twice as high than that of relatives of non-depressed psychiatric controls matched for non-affective symptoms in the Maudsley study (Harrington *et al.*, 1993), suggesting that the increased familial loading for depressive disorders was indeed specific to depression and not accounted for by associated psychiatric conditions. Studies of offsprings of affectively ill parents have also pointed towards links between adult and childhood or adolescent depression. Thus, Weissman *et al.* (1987) found much higher lifetime rates of depression and other disorders such as substance abuse among offsprings of depressed parents as compared to those of normal controls; a follow-up of these offsprings showed that over half of them had developed a first episode of depression by the end of adolescence (Weissman *et al.*, 1992). Other studies have broadly confirmed these results. There is therefore little doubt that depression runs in families of depressed children and adolescents. Both genetic and environmental mechanisms seem to be implicated in the increased familial loading for affective disorders (Hammen, 1991; Radke-Yarrow *et al.*, 1992); twin and adoption studies would be needed to tease apart the interplay between nature and nurture in the intrafamilial transmission of vulnerability to child and adolescent depression.

Neurobiological studies

Neuroendocrine and sleep studies have been conducted in depressed children and adolescents in order to validate the diagnosis of childhood depression against a biological standard or to demonstrate stable biological dysfunction across the life span. While validating studies have been largely inconclusive due to between-studies variation in subjects' age, diagnostic criteria, levels of severity, treatment setting, and confounding factors such as concurrent suicidality or comorbid conditions, promising results have been reached linking biological markers of adult and childhood, and especially adolescent, depression.

Hypercorticolaemia is less frequently repeated in childhood than in adult depression (Dahl *et al.*, 1989; Puig-Antich *et al.*, 1989b; Kutcher *et al.*, 1991; Goodyer *et al.*, 1996). Studies of the dexamethasone suppression test (DST) have also yielded disappointing and inconsistent results. On average, DST results had a low sensitivity and specificity among samples of children, with slightly better performances in samples of in-patients and with older, adolescent subjects. Similarly, the cortico-releasing hormone (CRH) challenge tests have not shown the blunted ACTH reaction in children, contrary to what is usually observed in adults (Ryan *et al.*, 1992). The explanations for these findings are still uncertain.

The growth hormone (GH) response to insulin-induced hypoglycaemia has been shown to be decreased among prepubertal children compared to neurotic controls, with follow-up evidence that this blunted response was maintained after recovery (Puig-Antich *et al.*, 1984a,b).

Puig-Antich and colleagues. (1984a,b) also found an increased nocturnal secretion of GH among depressed children. However, these findings have not been replicated consistently in other studies, providing an overall mixed picture about the amine hypothesis in the biology of childhood depression.

Studies of sleep abnormalities in children have shown reduced rapid eye movement (REM) latencies in some samples (Emslie *et al.*, 1990) but not in others (Puig-Antich *et al.*, 1982), although abnormalities were found in the subjects of the latter study when they had recovered. In adolescents, more electro-encephalographic (EEG) abnormalities have been found (Lahmeyer *et al.*, 1983; Dahl *et al.*, 1990), especially in suicidal and in-patient subjects. Overall, the findings suggest that EEG changes in depression vary according to both developmental stage and characteristics of the depressive episode.

Pharmacological studies

By contrast to adult depression, studies of antidepressant medications have largely failed to demonstrate efficacy over placebo in controlled trials. A double-blind placebo-controlled study of the efficacy of imipramine was conducted on 53 depressed children by Puig-Antich *et al.* (1987). Of the 38 children who completed the protocol (mean age 9.6 years), there was no difference in the response rate for imipramine and for placebo (56% vs. 68%). A plasma study was conducted for 30 of these children which suggested that response was more likely to occur with higher plasma concentrations of imipramine and desipramine, and with lower severity of depressive symptoms (Ryan *et al.*, 1986). It was therefore concluded that a possible explanation for the failure of this study to show a significant difference was due to the use of too low doses and also possibly because the washout period was not prolonged enough. Information on comorbid disorders was not available in this study. Comorbidity was taken into account in another study comparing imipramine vs. placebo in young depressed children (Hughes *et al.*, 1990). Depression occurring in conjunction with conduct disorder had a better response to placebo than to the active medication; by contrast, depression occurring in isolation or with anxiety disorders showed a better response to imipramine than to placebo. An investigation of the efficacy of nortriptyline was performed in a double-blind placebo-controlled study of 56 12-year-old children with a prolonged depressive disorder (Geller *et al.*, 1992a). In this severely afflicted group, the response was poor in both the active treatment and the placebo groups with no difference between the two. A follow-up study of these patients (Geller *et al.*, 1992b, 1993) suggested that prolonged use of tricyclic medication over a 6-month period was associated with an increased risk of switching to mania, this risk being more pronounced in those children who had a positive family history for affective disorders. Similar negative findings were obtained in one other study of imipramine (Petti & Law, 1982) and in two studies of amitriptyline (Kramer & Feiguine, 1981; Kashani *et al.*, 1984) of limited samples of prepubertal children with depression. The small sample sizes of these studies could explain in themselves the lack of statistically significant difference across groups. Most of these studies reported trends towards improvement in the active treatment conditions, but a similar high response rate in the placebo groups. A recent meta-analysis of 12 randomized controlled trials has been undertaken by Hazell *et al.* (1995) to review the evidence for efficacy of tricyclic medications. Using stringent selection criteria for the studies included in their meta-analysis, these authors showed that the effect size for active drugs across these studies was estimated at 0.35 standard deviation for change scores of depressive symptomatology and that the odds-ratio of response to medication vs. placebo was 1.08, both indicating non-significant benefit over placebo. This lack of demonstrated efficacy raises the issues of possible biological differences underlying childhood depression as compared to the findings in adults. One particularity of these studies is that the placebo response rate has been excessively high, therefore obscuring a possible benefit from the antidepressant in the actively treated groups; comorbid disorders also may have confounded the results of some trials and more attention should certainly be given in the future to diagnostic criteria used to select subjects in these trials. The task ahead in current research programmes is to combine treatment studies with biological, clinical and family history data to identify subgroups of depressed children and adolescents who are likely to be responders to active antidepressant medications.

Controlled studies on the efficacy of selective serotonin re-uptake inhibitors (SSRIs) are fewer. One study assessed the efficacy of fluoxetine in 13–18-year-old adolescents selected on the basis of high depression scores on the Hamilton scale (Simeon *et al.*, 1990). There was a trend for better response in the fluoxetine group which failed to reach statistical significance due to both a small sample size and a period of investigation which did not exceed 8 weeks. However, a more recent study based on a larger sample of 96 children and adolescent out-patients with major depression, aged between 8 and 18, has been completed which indicates a significant improvement in the fluoxetine group over the placebo condition (Emslie *et al.* 1995).

No controlled study of monoamine oxydase inhibitors (MAOIs) has been conducted and there are only anecdotal case reports suggesting their usefulness in depression not responding to tricyclics. However, they are not recommended in children and adolescents, mainly because young subjects were shown to be less compliant with the dietary requirements (Ryan *et al.*, 1988a). The more recent reversible MAOIs have not yet been used in children and adolescents. Other compounds such as maprotiline, mianserin, trazodone, lofepramine and bupropion have not been properly tested. Drug combinations also have been little studied. Lithium augmentation has provided encouraging results although the beneficial effect seems to be less clearcut than with adult non-responders (Ryan *et al.*, 1988b; Strober *et al.*, 1992). MAOI augmentation has been little explored because of the dietary compliance problems already mentioned. Properly controlled studies are still required on this issue.

Based on current evidence and practice, the prediction that a child will respond to antidepressant medication would be enhanced if the depressive symptoms are severe and associated with biological features, if there is evidence for a familial history of affective illnesses and if there are no comorbid, especially disruptive, disorders. The use of SSRIs is likely to increase following the results of the most recent trials and because they are relatively safe in overdose. Child psychiatrists, however, continue to prescribe tricyclic antidepressants since most practitioners have had experience of good response to tricyclic medications in individual cases. More clinical trials on their efficacy are clearly needed and, in light of the methodological problems of available trials, premature conclusions on their lack of effect should be avoided. It is worth noting that clomipramine has shown a beneficial effect in childhood obsessive compulsive disorder (OCD), and it is therefore unclear why these medications would not have also a positive effect in depression.

Care should be taken with prescription of tricyclic antidepressants. Several sudden deaths have been reported in recent years amongst children or adolescents treated with tricyclics (four with desipramine and one with imipramine) (Riddle *et al.*, 1993). These sudden deaths, thought to be cardiac-related, occurred in most instances with drug levels within the therapeutic range. In this context, desipramine is not recommended as a first choice. Baseline electrocardiograms (ECGs) are recommended before starting a tricyclic which might be contraindicated in some instances (PR >0.20 s; QRS >0.11 s). Changes in cardiac parameters during treatment (increase in PR or QRS intervals, heart rate over 130/min, increased blood pressure) call for a reduction of dosage or discontinuation of the drug. Other classical side-effects of tricyclics have been described among children including switching to mania, common side-effects and withdrawal syndromes. Dosage should be gradually increased, with typical starting doses of 1 mg/kg/day being very progressively increased up to 4 mg/kg/day. Dosage will be increased up to the point where clinical benefits become evident, or side-effects are too pronounced or plasma levels are at the upper limit of the therapeutic range. The extent to which plasma levels should be used to monitor a child treated with tricyclics depends upon many factors; levels should, however, be checked in cases of non- or partial response, signs of toxicity, or concerns about compliance. Similarly, the frequency with which repeat ECGs are needed varies with several parameters; it is, however, recommended to repeat an ECG when a stable high dosage has been reached, or before in the advent of any untoward clinical sign. Treatment with SSRIs is easier to monitor owing to fewer cardiotoxic and anticholinergic effects. The prescription and monitoring of SSRIs amongst children follows broadly the same rules as those for adults.

Once a response has been obtained with one antidepressant, it is advised to continue medication for at least a 6-month period which corresponds to the duration of an untreated episode. Medications should subsequently be reduced very progressively. As in adult depression, electroconvulsive therapy (ECT) has been used in children and adolescents with severe unipolar depression or bipolar disorder. There has been little systematic research on the efficacy and long-term effects of ECT in this age group. A review of 32 case reports suggested, nevertheless, improvement in 80% of the cases of depression (Bertagnoli & Borchardt, 1990). ECT is therefore a useful treatment to consider in severe affective disorders resistant to antidepressants (Cizadlo & Wheaton, 1995). Finally, the treatment of bipolar disorders in children and adolescents is similar to that of adults, with lithium and carbamazepine being the first-line medications.

Psychological therapies

Cognitive-behavioural therapy

Children and adolescents with depression have been shown to have negative styles of thinking, low self-esteem and cognitive biases whereby they attribute negative events to internal, global and stable self characteristics. It is unclear whether these features are found as a predisposing characteristic before young subjects experience a first episode of depression, or if they are merely state markers of depression. However, together with impaired social relationships and behavioural changes occurring in a depressive episode, these cognitive features provide natural targets for rational interventions based on cognitive-behavioural therapy (CBT) principles.

Several cognitive-behavioural programmes have now been developed which contain components such as activity scheduling, cognitive restructuring, problem-solving and social skills training in various combinations of 10–20 sessions. Treatment manuals have been available for several of these programmes. The first evaluation studies have been conducted in school settings and among samples of adolescents selected for their high scores on a questionnaire measure. Treatments were often administered in groups. Most of these studies have documented a beneficial effect of intervention when compared to waiting-list or attention placebo controls (Reynolds & Coats, 1986; Stark *et al.*, 1987; Kahn *et al.*, 1990; Lewinsohn *et al.*, 1990; Stark, 1990).

A further step towards the individual treatment of patients diagnosed with depression was achieved by the Manchester's group who devised a treatment package suitable for referred out-patients (Vostanis & Harrington, 1994). This package consists of nine to 10 sessions which, depending on the presenting problems of the child, on his/her developmental and cognitive level, combine interventions focusing on self-reinforcement, emotional recognition, problem-solving skills, social skills training and, for the most able children, cognitive restructuring. Indeed, this package associates different techniques based on behavioural activation, social skill training and more proper cognitive techniques. This time-limited intervention is well accepted by children; it is focused on the here and now of the child's condition, works towards achieving measurable goals and provides some role to the parents as adjunct therapist. In a controlled study of its efficacy, Wood *et al.* (1996) studied 53 children and adolescents with depressive disorders who were randomly assigned to either CBT or relaxation training used under controlled conditions. The post treatment assessment indicated a clear supremacy of CBT over relaxation on overall adjustment and measures of depressive symptomatology. Comorbid conditions were not improved by the intervention, providing some evidence for the specificity of the treatment regarding depressive symptoms. However, follow-up on these children showed high relapse rates in both groups, with the gains of CBT being somewhat lost several months after treatment. Current studies are now exploring the usefulness of more prolonged treatment and of continuation forms of CBT.

Interpersonal psychotherapy

Interpersonal psychotherapy has been modified for use with adolescents (IPT-A; Moreau *et al.*, 1991). This time limited psychotherapy extends over a 12-week period with weekly sessions of 45 min each. The treatment is divided into three phases. In the initial phase a review of depressive symptoms is rigorously conducted and the problem areas are identified with the youngsters. Five problem areas can be the focus of the psychological work and they include: grief, role transitions, interpersonal role disputes, interpersonal deficits and a problem area of single-parent families has been added to account for the higher frequency of single-parent families as a context for modern adolescent development. The middle phase of treatment focuses on two problem areas which have been agreed upon between the therapist and the adolescent as being the areas where improvement is most needed. Then the treatment terminates with closing sessions. A manual is available for this treatment (Mufson *et al.*, 1993). Interpersonal psychotherapy for adolescents (IPT/A) has been systematically investigated and interesting results have been reported on a small sample of 14 depressed adolescents in an open clinical trial conducted during a 12-week period (Mufson *et al.*, 1994). There was a significant decrease in depressive symptoms and a significant improvement over the course of the treatment in social functioning. However, replication of these encouraging results are needed in a controlled study.

Other interventions

Various other kinds of intervention have been used in treating childhood depression. Of these, social skills training has been shown to be superior to therapeutic support group in treating depressed out-patient adolescents in post-treatment measures although no difference persisted at 9 months' follow-up (Fine *et al.*, 1991). It is worth noting that social skills constitute one component of most CBT programmes. When necessary, other interventions focusing on the child will target comorbid disorders but it is out of the scope of this chapter to review them.

Generic counselling has been used in mild forms of depressive symptoms but its efficacy is not demonstrated. An empathic attitude and sessions providing emotional support are probably harmless but current evidence suggests that focused work aiming at behavioural activation, stress reduction, problem-solving, self-monitoring and cognitive restructuring are more efficient in reducing levels of depressive symptoms as compared to more undifferentiated psychological treatments.

Treatment almost inevitably includes a family or parental component. In most cases, parents benefit from advice and counselling on the nature of depressive symptoms and disorders, on providing support to the child in reducing stress and promoting positive mood changes, and in monitoring drugs and suicidal behaviours. Parents can be more directly involved in the individual treatment of the child and they might contribute to the schedule of daily activities, to the diary recording, or to the identification of negative cognitive biases in the natural context of the life of their child. Direct involvement of parents as 'cotherapists' is a common procedure in some phases of CBT with children. Formal family therapy is less often justified unless there are dysfunctional relationships and interactions relevant to the child's depression. One study has compared a group CBT for adolescents with and without a parallel parental group intervention comprising 14 h of psycho educational treatment (Lewinsohn *et al.*, 1990). No difference was found between these two treatment modalities which did equally better than a waiting-list control group. Formal family therapy has not been assessed in childhood depression.

The management of child and adolescent depression

There are strong similarities in the management of childhood depression with that of the rest of the life span. Some differences are now outlined with respect to assessment, treatment setting and treatment choice.

Assessment

Besides the depressive disorder, careful attention should be paid to comorbid disorders which will need to be addressed separately in most cases. Children and adolescents live in families and in group settings, typically a school. Assessment of intrafamilial relationships are therefore a core focus of the initial assessment. The presence of a mental disorder in one parent, parental discord and disharmony, quarrels and violent arguments between family members, scapegoating of the child, emotional, physical and sexual abuse, are all associated risk factors of childhood psychopathology and ought to be detected. Family assessment can also be important in identifying sources of stress in the family life (i.e. a disabled sibling, a recently diagnosed cancer in the parent, loss of a loved grandparent, a recent move or transition to another school, etc.) which might justify specific measures. It is also useful in identifying, in the familial group, members who have a positive and supportive attitude towards the child, with the aim to build on these protective relationships during treatment and in the future. Physical illness in the child can also be a precipitating factor; among biological events, onset of puberty in girls has been consistently associated with increased risk of depressive symptoms, especially amongst early maturers and when puberty occurs with simultaneous social changes such as transition to secondary school. Similarly, school factors are crucial especially as parents are not always aware of their existence. Thus, a child might suffer from a specific learning disorder or from a general learning backwardness that could be further assessed with proper psychometry. Teachers' reports on both academic achievement and behavioural descriptions are also routinely requested as part of the assessment. Bullying in schools and the quality of peer-relationships can exert substantial psychological pressure on children and adolescents which may go unnoticed by adults. The assessment must therefore rely on several informants (subjects, parents, school).

Treatment setting

In the majority of cases, depressed children and adolescents are treated as out-patients. Out-patient management allows to reduce the short- and long-term impact on child and adolescent development of missed learning and social opportunities. In-patient admission is, however, required in subjects with severe suicidal thoughts and cognitions, with biological features which massively interfere with school and family life, or with psychotic symptoms. In-patient treatment may also be useful if remission has not been obtained after a properly conducted psychological treatment, or after non-response to conventional antidepressants. In some instances, admission might also be required to start a biological treatment in circumstances where the familial milieu does not offer the necessary guarantees in terms of managing safely the drug in the home environment, or monitoring side-effects and suicidal ideas. In-patient admission can otherwise be dictated by the treatment needs of comorbid conditions. This might be so when comorbid substance abuse or eating disorder is a concern. A group of children present with affective disorders associated with conduct symptoms or disorders, often arising from a background of psychosocial adversity. In the first instance, social services might play a decisive role in providing a life setting for the youngster from which treatment is more likely to be accepted and beneficial.

Selection of treatment modality

Multimodal treatment is the rule in child disorders. Each treatment package will therefore involve a combination of individual treatment and of contextual intervention addressing the family or school issues, whether or not these are seen as playing a direct causal influence on the depression.

In most forms of mild or moderate depression, the first line treatment consists of psychological therapies. CBT appears to be the most validated intervention in terms of its efficacy to reduce depressive symptoms; IPT-A, social skills training and other forms of time-limited interventions aiming at symptom reduction, behavioural activation and skills learning are also appropriate. There are currently no clearcut guidelines to pick up which of these interventions is most likely to work with which patient. To a large extent, the existing treatment manuals and programmes encompass overlapping components. With a young child, for example, the behavioural activation aspects of CBT will be the most important feature of their treatment whereas a sophisticated mature adolescent might benefit more directly from pure cognitive techniques. The main goal is to tailor the treatment to the individual needs and to the context of the child. Other forms of interventions (i.e. counselling, relaxation) have proved ineffective.

Antidepressants are selected for young subjects with biological features, bipolar depression, or for depression not responding to psychological treatment. Given the lack of evidence in favour of tricyclics and their relative toxicity, SSRIs are a good choice to start medication. Their relative safety in overdose, and their fewer side-effects are particularly suited to teenagers. SSRIs also constitute an acceptable alternative to the treatment of depressions of at least moderate intensity, when no psychological intervention is readily available.

Lack of response to the preceding interventions should lead to a referral to specialist services. With the exception of older adolescents whose treatment follows the same lines as for adults, the effective prescription of other biological treatments are best provided in specialist services. No study has so far been conducted on the efficacy of combined psychological and biological treatment as compared to unimodal treatments in this age group. In practice, most practitioners combine these two approaches when they have chosen a drug treatment, together with other psychosocial measures (parent/family work, school liaison, etc.). It is important to keep in mind that most depressed children and adolescents do recover within 1 year and that relapse rates are high. Even if recovery is under way, there is some value in offering psychological intervention along the principles of CBT to foster the recovery and prevent relapse.

References

Achenbach, T.M. (1991) *Manual for the Child Behaviour Checklist/4–18 and 1991 profile.* Burlington, VT: University of Vermont, Department of Psychiatry.

Angold, A., Costello, E.J., Messer, A., Pickles, A., Winder, F. & Silver, D. (1995) Development of a short questionnaire for use in epidemiological studies of depression in children and adolescents. *International Journal of Methods in Psychiatric Research,* 5, 237–249.

Asarnow, J.R., Goldstein, M.J., Carlson, G.A., Perdue, S., Bates, S. & Keller, J. (1988) Childhood-onset depressive disorders: a follow-up study of rates of rehospitalization and out-of-home placement among child psychiatric inpatients. *Journal of Affective Disorders,* 15, 245–253.

Bertagnoli, M.W. & Borchardt, C.M. (1990) A review of ECT for children and adolescents. *Journal of the American Academy of Child and Adolescent Psychiatry,* 29, 302–307.

Birleson, P., Hudson, I., Buchanan, D.G. & Wolff, S. (1987) Clinical evaluation of a self-rating scale for depressive disorder in childhood (Depression Self-Rating Scale). *Journal of Child Psychol-*

ogy and Psychiatry, 28, 43–60.

Brent, D.A., Perper, J.A., Moritz et al. (1993) Psychiatric risk factors for adolescent suicide: case-control study. *Journal of the American Academy of Child and Adolescent Psychiatry,* 32, 521–529.

Cizadlo, B.C. & Wheaton, A. (1995) Case study: ECT treatment of a young girl with catatonia. *Journal of the American Academy of Child and Adolescent Psychiatry* 34, 332–335. [See also letters to the Editor, *Journal of the American Academy of Child and Adolescent Psychiatry,* 34, 1256–1257.]

Dahl, R., Puig-Antich, J., Ryan et al. (1989) Cortisol secretion in adolescents with major depressive disorder. *Acta Psychiatrica Scandinavica,* 80, 18–26.

Dahl, R., Puig-Antich, J., Ryan, N.D. et al. (1990) EEG sleep in adolescents with major depression: the role of suicidality and inpatient status. *Journal of Affective Disorders,* 19, 63–75.

Elander, J. & Rutter, M. (1996) Use and development of the Rutter parents' and teachers' scales. *International Journal of Methods in Psychiatric Research,* 6, 63–78.

Emslie, G.J., Rush, A.J., Weinberg, W.A.,

Rintelmann, J.W. & Roffward, H.P. (1990) Children with major depression show reduced rapid eye movement latencies. *Archives of General Psychiatry*, **47**, 119–124.

Emslie, G.J., Kowatch, R., Costello, L., Travis, G. & Pierce, L. (1995) *Double-blind study of fluoxetine in depressed children and adolescents*. Symposium at the Annual Conference of the American Academy of Child and Adolescent Psychiatry, October 1995, Toronto.

Fine, S., Forth, A., Gilbert, M. & Haley, G. (1991) Group therapy for adolescent depressive disorder: a comparison of social skills and therapeutic support. *Journal of the American Academy of Child and Adolescent Psychiatry*, **30**, 79–85.

Fleming, J.E. & Offord, D.R. (1990) Epidemiology of childhood depressive disorders: a critical review. *Journal of the American Academy of Child and Adolescent Psychiatry*, **29**, 571–580.

Fombonne, E. (1994) Increased rates of depression: update of epidemiological findings and analytical problems. *Acta Psychiatrica Scandinavica*, **90**, 145–156.

Fombonne, E. (1995) Depressive disorders: time trends and possible explanatory mechanisms. In: *Psychosocial Disorders in Young People: Time trends and their causes* (eds M. Rutter & D. Smith) pp. 544–615. Wiley & Sons, Chichester.

Fombonne, E. (1997a) The epidemiology of child and adolescent depression. *Psychological Medicine* (in preparation).

Fombonne, E. (1997b) Suicidal behaviours in young people: time trends and their correlates. (submitted).

Fombonne, E. (1998) Time trends for affective disorders. In: *Where and When: Influence of historical time and place on aspects of psychopathology* (eds P. Cohen, L. Robins & C. Slomkowski) Lawrence Erlbaum Associates, Mahwah, New Jersey.

Geller, B., Cooper, T., Graham, D.L., Fetner, H.H., Marsteller, F.A. & Wells, J.M. (1992a) Pharmacokinetically designed double-blind placebo-controlled study of nortriptyline in 6–12-year-olds with major depressive disorder. *Journal of the American Academy of Child and Adolescent Psychiatry*, **31**, 34–44.

Geller, B., Fox, L.W., Cooper, T.B. & Garrity, K. (1992b) Baseline and 2- to 3-year follow-up characteristics of placebo-washout responders from the nortriptyline study of depressed 6- to 12-year olds. *Journal of the American Academy of Child and Adolescent Psychiatry*, **31**, 622–628.

Geller, B., Fox, L.W. & Fletcher., M. (1993) Effects of tricyclic antidepressants on switching to mania and on the onset of bipolarity in depressed 6- to 12-year-olds. *Journal of the American Academy of Child and Adolescent Psychiatry*, **31**, 43–50.

Goodman, R. (1994) A modified version of the Rutter Parent Questionnaire including extra items on children's strengths. *Journal of Child Psychology and Psychiatry*, **35**, 1483–1494.

Goodyer, I.U., Herbert, J. & Altham, P.M.E. *et al.* (1996) Adrenal secretion during major depression in 8-to 16-year olds. *Psychological Medicine*, **26**, 245–256.

Hammen, C. (1991) Depression runs in families. In: *The Social Context of Risk and Resilience in Children of Depressed Mothers*. Springer-Verlag, New York.

Harrington, R., Fudge, H., Rutter, M., Pickles, A. & Hill, J. (1990) Adult outcomes of childhood and adolescent depression. I. Psychiatric status. *Archives of General Psychiatry*, **47**, 465–473.

Harrington, R.C., Fudge, H., Rutter, M., Pickles, A. & Hill, J. (1991) Adult outcomes of childhood and adolescent depression: II. Risk for antisocial disorders. *Journal of the American Academy of Child and Adolescent Psychiatry*, **30**, 434–439.

Harrington, R.C., Fudge, H., Rutter, M., Bredenkamp, D., Groothues, C. & Pridham, J. (1993) Child and adult depression: a test of continuities with data from family study. *British Journal of Psychiatry*, **162**, 627–633.

Harrington, R., Rutter, M. & Fombonne, E. (1996) Developmental pathways in depression: multiple meanings, antecedents and endpoints. *Development and Psychopathology*, **8**, 601–616.

Hazell, P., O'Connell, D., Hearthcote, D., Robertson, J. & Henry, D. (1995) Efficacy of tricyclic drugs in treating child and adolescent depression: a meta-analysis. *British Medical Journal*, **310**, 897–901.

Hodges, K. (1993) Structured Interviews for Assessing Children. *Journal of Child Psychology and Psychiatry*, **34** (1), 49–68.

Hughes, C.W., Preskorn, S.H., Weller, E., Hassanein, R. & Tucker, S. (1990) The effect of concomitant disorders in childhood depression on predicting treatment response. *Psychopharmacology Bulletin*, **26**, 235–238.

Kahn, J.S., Kehle, T.J., Jenson, W.R. & Clarke, E. (1990) Comparison of cognitive-behavioural, relaxation, and self-modeling interventions for depression among middle-school students. *School Psychology Review*, **19**, 196–211.

Kashani, J.H., Shekin, W.O. & Reid, J.C. (1984) Amitriptyline in children with major depressive disorder. A double-blind crossover pilot study. *Journal of the American Academy of Child and Adolescent Psychiatry*, **23**, 348–351.

Kovacs, M. (1982) The Children's Depression Inventory. Manuscript. University of Pittsburgh.

Kovacs, M., Feinberg, T.L., Crouse-Novak, M., Paulsuskas, S.L. & Finkelstein, R. (1984a) Depressive disorders in childhood. I. A longitudinal prospective study of characteristics and recovery. *Archives of General Psychiatry*, **41**, 229–237.

Kovacs, M., Feinberg, T.L., Crouse-Novak, M., Paulsuskas, S.L., Pollock, M. & Finkelstein, R. (1984b) Depressive disorders in childhood. II. A longitudinal study of the risk for a subsequent major depression. *Archives of General Psychiatry*, **41**, 643–649.

Kramer, A.D. & Feiguine, R.J. (1981) Clinical effects of amitriptyline in adolescent depression: A pilot study. *Journal of the American Academy of Child Psychology and Psychiatry*, **20**, 636–644.

Kutcher, S. & Marton, P. (1991) Affective disorders in first degree relatives of adolescent onset bipolar, unipolars, and normal controls. *Journal of the American Academy of Child Psychiatry*, **30**, 75–78.

Kutcher, S., Malkin, D., Silverberg, J. *et al.* (1991) Nocturnal cortisol, thyroid stimulating hormone, and growth hormone secretory profiles in depressed adolescents. *Journal of the American Academy of Child Psychiatry*, **30**, 407–414.

Lahmeyer, H.W., Poznanski, E.O. & Bellur, S.N. (1983) EEG sleep in depressed adolescents. *American Journal of Psychiatry*, **140**, 1150–1153.

Lang, M. & Tisher, M. (1987) *Children's Depression Scale Manual* (North American edn). Consulting Psychologists Press, Palo Alto, CA.

Lewinsohn, P.M., Clarke, G.N., Hops, H. & Andrews, J. (1990) Cognitive-behavioural treatment for depressed adolescents. *Behaviour Therapy*, **21**, 385–401.

Lewinsohn, P.M., Hops, H., Roberts, R.E., Seeley, J.R. & Andrews, J.A. (1993) Adolescent psychopathology: I. Prevalence and incidence of depression and other DSM-III-R disorders in high school students. *Journal of Abnormal Psychology*, **102**, 133–144.

Livingston, R., Nugent, H., Rader, L. & Smith, R.G. (1985) Family histories of depressed and severely anxious children. *American Journal of Psychiatry*, **142**, 1497–1499.

Marttunen, M.J., Aro, H.M., Henriksson, M.M. & Lönnqvist, J.K. (1991) Mental disorders in adolescent suicide: DSM-III-R axes I and II diagnoses in suicides among 13- to 19-year-olds in Finland. *Archives of General Psychiatry*, **48**, 834–839.

Moreau, D., Mufson, L., Weissman, M.M. & Klerman, G.L. (1991) Interpersonal psychotherapy for adolescent depression: description of modification and preliminary application. *Journal of the American Academy of Child and Adolescent Psychiatry*, **30**, 642–651.

Mufson, L., Moreau, D., Weissman, M.M. & Klerman, G.L. (1993) *Interpersonal psychotherapy for Depressed Adolescents*. Guilford Press, New York.

Mufson, L., Moreau, D., Weissman, M.M., Wickramaratne, P., Martin, J. & Samoilov, A. (1994) Modification of Interpersonal Psychotherapy with depressed adolescents (IPT-A): Phase I and II studies. *Journal of the American Academy of Child and Adolescent Psychiatry*, **33**, 695–705.

Petersen, A.C., Compas, B., Brooks-Gunn, J., Stemmler, M., Ey, S. & Grant, K. (1993) Depression in adolescence. *American Psychologist*, Feb., 155–168.

Petti, T.A. & Law, W. (1982) III. Imipramine treatment of depressed children: A double-blind pilot study. *Journal of Clinical Psychopharmacology*, **2**, 107–110.

Poznanski, E., Grossman, J.A., Buchsbaum, Y., Banegas, M., Freeman, L. & Gibbons, R. (1984) Preliminary studies of the reliability and validity of the children's depression rating scale. *Journal of the American Academy of Child Psychiatry*, **23**, 191–197.

Puig-Antich, J., Goetz, R. & Hanlon, C. *et al.* (1982) Sleep architecture and REM sleep measures in prepubertal children with major depression: a controlled study. *Archives of General Psychiatry*, **39**, 932–939.

Puig-Antich, J., Novacenko, M.S. & Davies, M. *et al.* (1984a) Growth hormone secretion in prepubertal children with major depression. I. Final report on response to insulin-induced hypoglycemia during a depressive episode. *Archives of General Psychiatry*, **41**, 455–460.

Puig-Antich, J., Goetz, R. & Davies, M. *et al.* (1984b) Growth hormone secretion in prepubertal children with major depression. II. Sleep-related plasma concentrations during a depressive episode. *Archives of General Psychiatry*, **41**, 463–466.

Puig-Antich, J., Novacenko, H., Tabrizi, M.A. *et al.* (1984) Growth hormone secretion in prepubertal major depressive children. III: Response to insulin induced hypoglycemia in a drug-free, fully recovered clinical state. *Archives of General Psychiatry*, **41**, 461–475.

Puig-Antich, J., Perel, J.M., Lupatkin, W. *et al.* (1987) Imipramine in pubertal major depressive disorders. *Archives of General Psychiatry*, **44**, 81–89.

Puig-Antich, J., Goetz, D., Davies, M. *et al.* (1989a) A controlled family history study of prepubertal major depressive disorder. *Archives of General Psychiatry*, **46**, 406–418.

Puig-Antich, J., Dahl, R. & Ryan, N. (1989b) Cortisol secretion in prepubertal children with major depressive disorders. *Archives of General Psychiatry*, **46**, 801–809.

Radke-Yarrow, M., Nottelmann, E., Martinez, P., Fox, M.B. & Belmont, B. (1992) Young children of affectively ill parents: a longitudinal study of psychosocial development. *Journal of the American Academy of Child Psychiatry*, **31**, 68–77.

Radloff, L.S. (1977) The CES-D Scale: A self-report scale for research in the general population. *Applied Psychological Measurement*, **1**, 385–401.

Rao, U., Weissman, M.M., Martin, J.A. & Hammond, R.W. (1993) Childhood depression and risk of suicide: a preliminary report of a longitudinal study. *Journal of the American Academy of Child and Adolescent Psychiatry*, **32**, 1, 21–27.

Reynolds, W.M. (1986) A model for the screening and identification of depressed children and adolescents in school settings. *Professional School Psychology*, **1**, 117–129.

Reynolds, W.M. & Coats, K.I. (1986) A comparison of cognitive-behavioural therapy and relaxation training for the treatment of depression in adolescents. *Journal of Consulting and Clinical Psychology*, **54**, 653–660.

Riddle, M., Geller, B. & Ryan, N. (1993) Another sudden death in a child treated with desipramine. *Journal of the American Academy of Child and Adolescent Psychiatry*, **32**, 792–797.

Rutter, M., Tizard, J. & Whitmore, K. (1970) *Education, health and behaviour*. Longmans, London.

Ryan, N.D., Puig-Antich, J., Cooper, T. *et al.* (1986) Imipramine in adolescent major depression: plasma level and clinical response. *Acta Psychiatrica Scandinavica*, **73**, 275–288.

Ryan, N.D., Puig-Antich, J., Rabinovich, H. *et al.* (1988a) MAOIs in adolescent major depression unresponsive to tricyclic antidepressants. *Journal of the American Academy of Child and Adolescent Psychiatry*, **27**, 755–758.

Ryan, N.D., Meyer, V., Dachille, S., Mazzie, D. & Puig-Antich, J. (1988b) Lithium antidepressant augmentation in TCA-refractory depression in adolescents. *Journal of the American Academy of Child and Adolescent Psychiatry*, **27**, 371–376.

Ryan, N.D., Birmaher, B. & Perel, J. *et al.* (1992) Neuroendocrine response to L-5 hydroxy-tryptophan challenge in prepubertal major depression. *Archives of General Psychiatry*, **49**, 843–851.

Shaffer, D., Gould, M.S., Fisher, P. *et al.* Psychiatric diagnosis in child and adolescent suicide.

Archives of General Psychiatry (in press).

Simeon, J.G., Dinicola, V.E., Ferguson, H.B. & Copping, W. (1990) Adolescent depression: A placebo controlled fluoxetine treatment study and follow-up. *Progress in Neuropsychopharmacology and Biological Psychiatry*, **14**, 791–795.

Stark, K.D., Reynolds, W.M. & Kaslow, N. (1987) A comparison of the relative efficacy of self-control therapy and a behavioural problem-solving therapy for depression in children. *Journal of Abnormal Child Psychology*, **15**, 91–113.

Stark, K.D. (1990) *Childhood Depression: School-based Intervention*. Guilford Press, New York.

Strober, M., Freeman, R., Rigali, J., Schmidt, S. & Diamond, R. (1992) The pharmacotherapy of depressive illness in adolescence: II. Effects of lithium augmentation in nonresponders to imipramine. *Journal of the American Academy of Child and Adolescent Psychiatry*, **31**, 16–20.

Tisher, M. & Lang, M. (1983) The Children's Depression Scale: review and further developments. In: *Affective Disorders in Childhood and Adolescence* (eds D. P. Cantwell & G. A. Carlson) pp. 81–203. MTP Press, Lancaster.

Vostanis, P. & Harrington, R. (1994) Cognitive behavioural treatment of depressive disorder in child psychiatric patients—rationale and description of a treatment package. *European Child and Adolescent Psychiatry*, **3**, 111–123.

Weinberg, W.A., Rutman, J., Sullivan, L., Penick, E.C. & Dietz, S.G. (1973) Depression in children referred to an educational diagnostic center: diagnosis and treatment. *Journal of Pediatrics*, **83**, 1065–1072.

Weissman, M.M., Gammon, D., John, K. *et al.* (1987) Children of depressed parents: increased psychopathology and early onset of major depression. *Archives of General Psychiatry*, **44**, 847–853.

Weissman, M.M., Fendrich, M., Warner, V. & Wickramaratne, P. (1992) Incidence of psychiatric disorder in offspring at high and low risk for depression. *Journal of the American Academy of Child Psychiatry*, **31**, 640–648.

Wood, A., Kroll, L., Moore, A. & Harrington, R.C. (1995) Properties of the mood and feelings questionnaire in adolescent psychiatric outpatients: a research note. *Journal of Child Psychology and Psychiatry*, **36**, 327–334.

Wood, A., Harrington, R.C. & Moore, A. (1996) Controlled trial of a brief cognitive-behavioural intervention in adolescent patients with depressive disorders. *Journal of Child Psychology and Psychiatry*, **37**, 737–746.

17 Depression after childbirth

MAUREEN MARKS AND
R. CHANNI KUMAR

There are some features of childbearing which give depressions occurring in this context unique characteristics. The physiological concomitants of pregnancy and parturition, particularly those which involve the endocrine system, are likely to have an impact on maternal mood. The psychological aspects of pregnancy, parturition and becoming a parent and the difficulties inherent in negotiating these major developmental steps are also likely to be involved in the postnatal mental health of new mothers. In addition, there is the turbulence created in an existing family with the arrival of a new family member and the adjustments which have to be made not only by parents, but also the extended family, for example the newly created grandparents, and by other siblings if the infant is not the first. There is also the inevitable stress of caring for a new infant, the anxieties around feeding and crying, the sleep loss and so on. When a parent does become depressed, the impact of this on the newborn infant must also be considered. Finally, the welfare of both mother and baby has to be taken into account when treatment strategies are developed and sometimes the conflict between the needs of each may be difficult to resolve.

Prevalence and incidence

There is growing evidence to suggest that psychiatric morbidity in women, particularly depression, is closely connected with childbearing (Gater et al., 1989; Bebbington et al., 1991). There is a steep rise in the risk of psychiatric admission for psychotic illness after childbirth (Pugh et al., 1963; Paffenbarger, 1964) to about 25 times prepregnancy levels (Kendell et al., 1987) and, in addition, about 10–15% of women experience non-psychotic depressions soon after childbirth. Depression prevalence rates vary according to criteria employed to establish disorder and the time period covered. Examples of prospective studies using Research Diagnostic Criteria (Spitzer et al., 1978) have included O'Hara et al., 1984 (12%, first 9 weeks), Kumar and Robson, 1984 (15%, first 3 months), Carothers and Murray (1990) (11%, 6th week). Peak onset appears to be in the first 2–6 weeks after delivery (Watson et al., 1984; Cox et al., 1993a).

Several case control studies have compared rates of depression in parturient women with those in non-childbearing women and, in contrast to the psychoses, have found no increased *prevalence* of depressions after childbirth, at least of those severe enough to be categorized as according to Research Diagnostic Criteria (RDC) cases (Cooper *et al.*, 1988; O'Hara *et al.*, 1990; Whiffen & Gotlib, 1993). Cox *et al.* (1993a), however, noted an increase in *incidence* (i.e. new cases) of depression at around 1 month postpartum.

Phenomenology

There is little in terms of clinical presentation and psychiatric history to distinguish postpartum and non-postpartum depressions, apart from the confounding of the normal physical correlates of parturition with depressive symptomatology (e.g. tiredness, sleeping difficulties) and differences in symptom severity. Most postnatal depressions are relatively mild and short-lived (Cox *et al.*, 1993a; Whiffen & Gotlib, 1993) but a significant proportion become severe and intransigent, frequently lasting a year or longer (Cox *et al.*, 1982; Watson *et al.*, 1984) and sometimes requiring admission.

It is important to differentiate between postpartum depressions, which are usually non-psychotic, and postpartum psychoses. The latter are a heterogeneous group of illnesses defined largely by their temporal relationship to parturition (see Brockington & Cox-Roper, 1988) with different aetiolgy, incidence and timing of onset from non-psychotic postpartum depressions (Kendell *et al.*, 1987; Marks *et al.*, 1992a). There is, however, some overlap: 35% of admissions to the Mother and Baby Unit at the Bethlem Hospital are for depressive illnesses, about half of which have psychotic features (Kumar *et al.*, 1995a).

Overall, the risk of maternal suicide in the first postnatal year is low, one sixth of the expected rate (Appleby, 1991). When suicides do occur, the woman is likely to be psychotic (Appleby, 1996).

Identification of women at risk

Psychiatric history

The most important indicator of risk is psychiatric history. There is a threefold increase in the rate of depression after childbirth in women with histories of depression compared to those without (Carothers & Murray, 1990; Marks *et al.*, 1992a; Appleby *et al.*, 1994; Cooper & Murray, 1995). Sub-clinical symptoms of depression and anxiety during the pregnancy are also precursors (Pitt, 1968; Watson *et al.*, 1984; Marks *et al.*, 1992a).

In a meta-analysis of 59 prospective studies which investigated risk factors for postnatal depression, O'Hara and Swain (1996) found that past history of psychopathology produced the largest effect size. They concluded that

> there is a continuity of psychiatric disturbance that extends back many years before a woman's pregnancy, through her pregnancy and into the postpartum period ... the question which remains is the extent to which childbearing *per se* affects the timing or severity of postpartum disturbance (p. 45).

None the less, there is a subgroup of women whose depressions occur only after childbirth (Cooper & Murray, 1995) and it is considered likely that for these women issues connected with childbirth, either physiological (e.g. hormonal) disturbances, or psychological (e.g. difficulties with the mothering role) may be of particular relevance. Future research into this group of women may reveal important differences in aetiology, treatment and outcome.

Psychosocial stress

Caring for a newborn baby requires enormous reserves of energy, as well as commitment and resilience. There is also the need to manage anxieties inherent in the development of a new relationship. This takes its toll on even the most robust of parents but for those with pre-existing psychological fragilities the experience of early parenthood is particularly fraught. The existing evidence suggests that the vulnerability–stress model of depression applies to postpartum illness, as with depressions occurring at other times. Adverse life events and social difficulties (Paykel *et al.*, 1980; O'Hara *et al.*, 1984; Watson *et al.*, 1984; Marks *et al.*, 1992a), poor social support and/or marital problems (Paykel *et al.*, 1980; Kumar & Robson, 1984; O'Hara *et al.*, 1984; Watson *et al.*, 1984; O'Hara & Zekoski, 1988; O'Hara & Swain, 1996) and childcare stressors (Cutrona 1984) have been linked with postpartum depression. However, two retrospective studies of depressed women admitted to hospital within 1 month postpartum found either a marginal effect (Martin *et al.*, 1989) or no effect (Dowlatshahi & Paykel, 1990) of social adversity suggesting that social factors may be of less importance in the more severe postpartum depressions.

Maternal factors

For some women issues concerning childbirth and mothering are more important than social stress *per se*. Such difficulties may stem from the woman's own early experience of parenting and her consequent identification with the mothering role (Ruble *et al.*, 1990; Gotlib *et al.*, 1991) or from more recent problems or changes in her life. Reproductive difficulties such as infertility problems, unplanned pregnancy, a previous termination, miscarriage or stillbirth and obstetric complications (Kumar & Robson, 1984; O'Hara, 1986; Edwards *et al.*, 1994; Yoshida *et al.*, 1997) have all been linked to subsequent postpartum depression. Then there is the inevitable emotional upheaval associated with the transition to parenthood, for example, the change in status from that of employment in the workforce with its daily social contact and financial rewards to the unremarked isolation and strapped financial circumstances of maternity (McIntosh, 1993). The woman's relationship with her partner also inevitably changes and this can cause difficulties (Marks & Lovestone, 1995).

Maternal depression and the family

Impact of infant on mother

Disturbances in the woman's relationship with her infant have also been linked to maternal depressions, although it is difficult to disentangle cause and effect in these cases. Clearly a mother who is depressed or becoming so is likely to have an impact on her infant's mood and behaviour, and also is likely to perceive her infant more negatively. However, there is evidence to suggest that the infant's temperament can influence maternal mood directly. In addition, the mother's perception of an infant may lead to subsequent maternal depression. For example, poor motor scores and high irritability, assessed in the neonate, are predictors of the onset of maternal depression by 8 weeks postpartum (Murray *et al.*, 1996) as is mother's perceived satisfaction with infant feeding (Sanderson *et al.*, 1996).

Not all mothers feel immediately after delivery that they love their babies and sometimes feelings of affection and attachment emerge slowly over days or weeks. However, many mothers who are depressed also express concerns about their relationship with their infant. These may include feelings of inadequacy and guilt for not coping well as a mother, excessive worries about the infant's physical health, fears that they may harm the infant in some way or persisting feelings of either indifference or dislike for their baby (Margison, 1982; Kumar, 1997).

Impact of mother on infant

There is an increasing body of evidence that maternal depression may sometimes have long-term adverse impact on the psychological development of the new child (Cogill *et al.*, 1986; Murray, 1992; Sharp *et al.*, 1995) especially if the depression occurs during the infant's first year (Sharp *et al.*, 1995). These effects are thought to be related to the way depressed mothers interact with their infants. Depressed mothers have been shown to be distracted and preoccupied, expressionless and unstimulating, or irritable and intrusive. The form, content and emotional tone of their speech with the infants is also different. They focus on their infants less and they tend to be more critical and hostile (Murray *et al.*, 1993). There can be disturbances in the quality of mothers' reactions to cues from their infants, for example their synchrony and contingency with them, and these disturbances can result in patterns of behaviour in the infant which mirror the mother (Field *et al.*, 1988). Such disturbances may lead to impairments in the infants' memory and learning processes (Singer & Fagan, 1992) and to the development of insecure attachment patterns (Ainsworth *et al.*, 1978).

There may also be more disturbing consequences. A New Zealand study (Mitchell *et al.*, 1992) found that mothers of infants who had cot deaths were three times more likely to have been depressed at 1 month postpartum than other mothers. In this study, depression had been assessed prospectively. The Edinburgh Postnatal Depression Scale had been administered by health visitors, at 4 weeks postpartum, to all mothers in a number of districts who had delivered during the year of the study. Forty-seven per cent of mothers whose infants subsequently had cot deaths scored as cases of depression at this time, compared to 16% of control mothers. Cot death mothers were also more likely to have been treated for depression in the past and also more likely to have a family history of *postnatal* depression than control mothers. A more recent British study has replicated the New Zealand findings (Sanderson *et al.*, 1996). Sociodemographic and medical data were collected from all mothers who delivered in Sheffield during 1988–93, at birth and at 1 month postpartum, including scores on the Edinburgh Postnatal Depression Scale (EPDS). There were subsequently 42 cases of unexpected infant death. The relative risk of sudden infant death was found to be almost four times greater among women with high scores on the EPDS compared to the low-scoring group.

Explanations of these effects are highly speculative at present but are likely to invoke at the very least certain characteristic features of the depressed mother–infant relationship. It may be, for example, that depressed mothers are less attuned to their infants' state of health and well-being, and less able to respond appropriately to any changes in the infant (Mitchell *et al.*, 1992).

Fathers and the marital relationship

There is no increase in the prevalence of depression in fathers following childbirth (Kendell *et al.*, 1976; Ballard *et al.*, 1994), although men may have more subclinical depressive symptoms during the first few weeks after their wives have had a baby (Ballard & Davies, 1996).

Fathers, however, influence and are influenced by their partners' depressions. Brown *et al.* (1990a, 1990b) have demonstrated the importance of the quality of close personal relationships, particularly the marital relationship, in the occurrence of, and recovery from, depressions in women with children.

For women suffering from postpartum depression, both the onset and course are influenced by the woman's relationship with her partner. Maternal perceptions of poor marital support or marital problems have been linked to enhanced rates of postpartum depression in community samples (Kumar & Robson, 1984; Watson *et al.*, 1984; Boyce *et al.*, 1991) and the marital relationship has also been implicated in the more severe depressions. For example, women without partners are more likely to be admitted to psychiatric hospital after delivery (Kendell *et al.*, 1987). Women with histories of severe depression are more likely to have a reoccurrence of illness after childbirth if they have partners who are uncommunicative (Marks *et al.*, 1992b). Conversely, partners who express appreciation of their wives appear to protect women at risk from postpartum relapse (Marks *et al.*, 1996).

Men whose wives experience psychiatric illness after childbirth have enhanced rates of depression (Harvey & McGrath, 1988; Lovestone & Kumar, 1993). Lovestone and Kumar showed that partners of women admitted to a psychiatric mother and baby unit were more likely to be depressed than either partners of women admitted outside the postpartum period or control partners of postpartum women who are well. The men whose wives had been admitted were also more likely to have had a depression in the past than the other men.

These data suggest there may be couples who are at risk of maternal depression. In these couples, if the mother is depressed then the father is also likely to have some mood disturbance. Treatment strategies involving both parents, for example marital or family therapy may be of benefit. At present there has been no study of the efficacy of this kind of help.

Management

Treatments are those used for depressions generally and have been covered in detail in other chapters. However, an important but difficult aspect in the management of maternal depression is that decisions about treatment have to take into account both the mother's and her infant's well-being. These include judgements about immediate risk of harm to the infant and also long-term ones concerning the mother's ability as a parent which have to be balanced with the problems which might result from over-intrusive care and which may impair the mother's natural and healthy relationship with her infant.

Another difficulty concerns the reluctance of mothers who are depressed to recognize that this is so, and then to feel it is safe to seek help for their condition. Many mothers feel they are not coping, that they have failed as mothers, and sometimes fear that should their mental state become public they could lose care of their child. These concerns, as well as more general fears about 'going mad' and being stigmatized, mean that women are often reluctant to have contact with psychiatric services. Offers of care therefore need to take into account the acceptability of the form of care delivery to the mother.

Strategies of treatment are also influenced by the fact that peripartum women have close contact with obstetric, health visitor and primary care services. This means that detection of cases and delivery of care are increasingly being carried out at a primary care level, and that there is more psychiatric liaison with these groups in the provision of care to postnatally depressed women.

Psychiatric services

Most postnatal depressions are mild and self-limiting and treatment can probably be limited to supportive counselling (Holden *et al.*, 1989). However, about one-third (Oates, 1989) may require more active intervention, either pharmacological and/or psychological. A very small proportion (1 in a 1000 of all parturient women) may require in-patient admission. Thus, as for depressions occurring outside the postnatal period, most mothers can be cared for in the community with regular General Practitioner (GP) and health visitor contact. A variety of services have been developed for those mothers whose illnesses are more severe. These include psychiatric out-patient contact, day hospital care, and in-patient mother and baby units.

Psychiatric referral

Parturient women are in repeated contact with obstetric services, and one way of targeting women who are depressed or at risk of becoming so is via these services. For example, at King's College Hospital, London, there is an obstetric–psychiatric liaison service which provides a psychiatric service to perinatal women identified at antenatal booking as having histories of mental disorder. Under this scheme, patients with histories, or current, significant psychiatric illness (screened by midwives at antenatal booking) are offered an appointment with a psychiatrist and are then monitored by the psychiatrist at regular intervals during the pregnancy and postpartum. However, many women are reluctant to accept this kind of psychiatric contact and take-up rates are low—about one-quarter of women referred do not attend their initial psychiatrist appointment and a further quarter of those who do, fail to attend later appointments (Appleby *et al.*, 1989).

Mother and baby units

One response to the requirements of severely or psychotically depressed new mothers has been the joint hospitalization of both mother and baby, either to general psychiatric admission wards or to specialized Mother and Baby Units. A preference for joint admission is based on the assumption that mother–infant separation is damaging to the burgeoning mother–infant relationship and may have deleterious consequences for the child's development (Bowlby, 1980). It is thought, too, that the infant's presence may facilitate improvement in the mother's mental state and may even hasten her discharge. Few argue with the benefits of keeping mother and child together, but there are difficulties inherent in admitting them to what tend these days to be geographically centralized services located some distance from the woman's home. The mother and infant become separated from the woman's partner and other siblings, visiting may be difficult for the family, and after discharge the nursing couple must not only adjust to doing without the intensive support that in-patient admission offers but also become reintegrated into their family and community. For the most severely ill mothers, especially those who do not have adequate family support, joint admission may be the best option. However, intensive programmes of community care for postnatally ill mothers which have been developed as an adjunct, or sometimes as an alternative, to admission are also effective (Oates, 1988), as is community care in combination with day hospital support (Cox *et al.*, 1993b).

Antidepressant medication

As long as the mother is not breastfeeding, indications for the use of antidepressant medication in the treatment of depressions occurring postnatally are similar to those applying to depressions occurring at other times. There appears to be no study which has compared the relative efficacy of different antidepressants for this condition.

If the mother is breastfeeding, drug treatment must involve the possibility of hazard to the developing infant. Inevitably, therefore, there is considerable caution around the issue of prescribing psychotropic medication to breast-feeding mothers, with the result that knowledge about the transfer of drugs to the infant through breastmilk and the possible impact on the infant is limited.

Most of the evidence currently available on antidepressant medication and breastfeeding concerns the tricyclic antidepressants (TCAs) although there are a few case studies of selective serotonin re-uptake inhibitors (SSRIs). Essentially, the data suggest that these drugs and their principal metabolites pass freely into breast milk and that milk:plasma ratios are generally around unity. Reports of drug or drug metabolites detected in infant plasma or serum have been rare (TCAs, 3 instances; SSRIs, 1 instance) as have reports of any adverse effects in infants (doxepin, 1 instance; fluoxetine, 1 instance) (see Buist *et al.*, 1990; Yoshida & Kumar, 1996; for reviews).

Thus, the dose ingested by infants appears to be minimal and reports of harm rare. However, the total numbers of studies and subjects studied are very small (*n* = 44 for tricyclic compounds, *n* = 5 for SSRIs) and observations of infants have not always been systematic. In light of the present state of knowlege, there seems to be no reason to prevent a mother who is taking tricyclic antidepressants from breastfeeding if she wishes to, with the possible exception of doxepin. Less is known about the SSRI group of drugs, but if they are particularly indicated and provided that the infants are carefully monitored, breastfeeding should not be prohibited. Pre-term, immature infants should not be exposed to psychotropic drugs, and the baby should always be monitored for any adverse effects and healthy before allowing a medicated mother to breastfeed.

Hormones

There has long been the idea that postpartum depression may be linked to physiological changes occurring during and immediately after pregnancy. This view, largely anecdotal and until recently untested, has lead to various proponents of sex steroids as either prophylaxis or treatment for postnatal depression.

There are very large changes in steroids over the course of pregnancy and parturition. For example, cortisol, prolactin and testosterone levels increase. Progesterone and oestrogen reach plasma levels of 100–200 times prepregnancy levels and then drop steeply immediately after delivery, returning to prepregnancy values within days. Changes in the levels of some of these hormones have been linked to alterations in mood, although the evidence is scanty and sometimes conflicting. For example, there is evidence that physiological doses of oestrogen may improve mood (Sherwin & Gelfand, 1985; Ditkoff *et al.*, 1991) and that doses of progesterone may depress it (Magos *et al.*, 1986; Sherwin, 1991); that reductions in levels of either oestrogen (see Wieck, 1989, 1996) or progesterone (see Harris, 1996) may depress mood.

The mechanism for effects such as these is thought to be related to an impact of steroid hormones on neuronal neurotransmitter systems. More precise description of their action will not be covered here except to say that interactions with various neurotransmitter systems have been implicated. These include dopaminergic and serotonergic function. (Interested readers are referred to Wieck, 1996, for a summary of this research.) There is some evidence that increased sensitivity of the dopamine system may predispose women at risk of depression because of their histories of psychiatric illness, to a depressive relapse after childbirth (Wieck *et al.*, 1991; McIvor *et al.*, 1996) and Wieck *et al.* (1991) have suggested that rapid falls in oestrogen at parturition may over-sensitize the dopamine systems of women who are already at risk. Further evidence for a link with oestrogen comes from its successful use as an antidepressant in postnatally depressed women. In a double-blind, placebo-controlled trial, Gregoire *et al.* (1996) administered oestradiol patches to women suffering from postnatal depression and found that women in the active group showed significantly enhanced mood within 1 month of treatment. This study needs to be replicated and the mechanism of action of oestrogen to be elucidated.

Evidence for the efficacy of other hormonal treatments, for example the use of natural progesterone (Dalton, 1980) is at present mostly anecdotal and properly controlled studies have yet to be undertaken.

Social and psychological treatments

Health visitor support

Health visitors have become increasingly involved in the detection of postnatal depression and in caring for women identified as depressed (see Holden, 1996), either in support groups (Pitts, 1995; Romaine, 1995) or individually. Holden *et al.* (1989) demonstrated that weekly counselling sessions by trained health visitors is a successful treatment for postnatal depression. Women identified as having a postnatal depression were allocated to a control or treatment group. Women in the treatment group received eight consecutive weekly visits from the health visitors. After 3 months, 69% of women in the treatment group had recovered compared to 38% of the controls. This mode of care was popular with patients: 92% of the women identified as depressed agreed to participate and of those who did so, 91% completed the trial.

Psychotherapy

In a randomized controlled trial, Cooper and Murray (1997) assessed the benefits of different psychotherapies. An unselected sample of depressed women, with infants aged between 8 and 18 weeks, were randomly allocated to either non-directive counselling, cognitive behaviour therapy, psychodynamic psychotherapy or to a control condition which received routine primary care. Sessions were carried out at home and lasted about an hour. The mean number of sessions was eight (range, five to ten). Mothers and infants were followed up at intervals after treatment ended. All therapy conditions were associated both with improved maternal mood and with mothers reporting improvements in their relationships with their infants. There were no differences between treatments. While treatment had no direct impact on any of the infant measures taken, early remission in the mother was associated with security of attachment in the infant. These data highlight the importance of early detection and treatment of maternal depressions, not only for the mother but also her infant. They confirm that the more quickly a mother's depression is curtailed, the less likely it will have lasting negative effects on her infant.

Combination of pharmacological and psychological treatments

Appleby *et al.* (1997) assessed the benefits of combining antidepressant medication with brief counselling for the treatment of women depressed at 6–8 weeks after delivery. In a randomized controlled treatment trial, depressed women received either fluoxetine or placebo with either one or six sessions of cognitive behavioural counselling. Fluoxetine and counselling each produced improvements in maternal mood but there was no additional advantage from receiving both forms of treatment together. The authors suggest that the choice of treatment therefore could be left up to individual women.

Peer group support

Many women find it easier to seek help from non-professionals such as can be obtained from self-help support groups developed and run by their peers. In Britain such organizations exist locally (for example, Newpin in London) and at a national level (for example, National Childbirth Trust; Association for Postnatal Mental Illness). Help provided includes befriending, where a member, usually a woman who has herself suffered postnatal depression, is introduced to the depressed women and becomes available to her for help and support as required.

Prevention

Where possible, prevention is preferable to treatment, and programmes aimed at doing so have been developed for women identified during pregnancy as being at risk.

Antidepressant medication

In an open clinical trial, Wisner and Wheeler (1994) tested the efficacy of antidepressant medication administered during the postpartum period to prevent a recurrence of postpartum depression in women who had at least one previous postpartum episode that met DSM-III-R (American Psychiatric Association, 1987) criteria for non-bipolar major depression without psychotic features. Twenty-three women took part in the study, 15 of whom chose medication. Patients were given the antidepressant medication that had been effective for their previous episode, or nortriptyline, within 24h after delivery. They were then monitored for 3 months and their psychiatric outcome during this follow-up period was compared with the eight women who elected to be monitored without medication. Only 7% of women who received medication had a recurrence of depression (DSM-III-R criteria) whereas 63% of untreated women became depressed. While this study needs replication in a randomized, placebo-controlled trial, the findings suggest that for women who have had a previous, severe postpartum depression, judiciously administered antidepressant medication may be of prophylactic benefit.

Antenatal and postnatal support groups

These have been shown to be effective but unpopular. Elliott *et al.* (1988) have shown that monthly group meetings with a health visitor or psychologist during pregnancy halved rates of subsequent postnatal depression. However, many women were reluctant to participate: 35% of women identified as being at risk did not attend any of the meetings offered. In a similar study, only 31% of mothers attended the support groups and there was no effect on rates of subsequent postnatal depression (Stamp *et al.*, 1995).

Midwifery support

Another response to the difficulty in providing accessible care has been the development of specialist midwifery services for high-risk women (Kumar *et al.*, 1995b). The key feature of such services is continuity of midwifery care rather than specialized training, for example, counselling training, as a main aim is to deploy *existing* midwifery resources to good effect. Continuity of care is thought to have a preventative role by providing social support to mothers, enhancing the likelihood of detection of prodromal symptoms and improving take-up rates if referrals are made to other professionals (cf. Briscoe, 1986). There is evidence, too, that continuity of midwifery care may have direct beneficial effects. It has been shown to reduce postnatal 'blues' (Odent, 1984), labour times and obstetric complications in both mother and baby (Sosa *et al.*, 1980; Klaus *et al.*, 1986; Kennell *et al.*, 1991) and it is thought that it may also contribute to enhanced maternal postnatal mood. Indications are that this form of support is very popular with high-risk women. The impact on maternal psychopathology after delivery is currently being assessed.

Bipolar depression in the postnatal period

Bipolar affective illness in the postnatal period raises issues which are different from bipolar illness elsewhere in the life cycle and unipolar illness following childbirth. First, the month after delivery is the time of the highest risk for manic illness (Kendell *et al.*, 1987) and for women with histories of bipolar affective disorder, the risk of a further episode of illness after subsequent deliveries is 40–50% (Reich & Winokur, 1970; Schopf *et al.*, 1984; Marks *et al.*, 1992a). The risk of recurrence is further influenced by the time which has elapsed since the last episode of illness and women who have been admitted in the 2 years preceding delivery are particularly at risk (Marks *et al.*, 1992a). For women with histories of bipolar disorder, the risk of a purely depressive episode postpartum is similar to that of women with histories of unipolar disorder (Marks *et al.*, 1991). However, many puerperal manic episodes are followed by depressions which are sometimes very severe.

Phenomenology of postpartum bipolar relapse

It is estimated that 80–90% of manic episodes begin within 2 weeks postpartum (Brockington & Cox-Roper, 1988; Klompenhouwer & van Hulst, 1991; Kumar *et al.*, 1995a). Thereafter the rate of relapse falls exponentially. None the less, it remains elevated until at least 2 years postpartum (Kendell *et al.*, 1987). Bipolar illnesses occurring in the puerperium have onsets which are more acute. Otherwise the phenomenology appears to be similar to those occurring outside the postnatal period (Schopf & Rust, 1994).

Aetiology of postpartum bipolar relapse

While the mechanisms responsible for the vulnerability of bipolar patients to the puerperium are not yet known, it is thought that the physiological concomitants of pregnancy and parturition are probably implicated. One hypothesis is that there is an enhanced sensitivity of dopamine function to oestrogen and progesterone withdrawal. Neuroendocrine evidence in support of this hypothesis has been published (Wieck *et al.* 1991, 1997). However, the critical test of the hypothesis will be whether or not puerperal relapse can be reduced by lowering the rate of fall of brain concentrations of oestrogen and progesterone, and this is currently being investigated.

There is some evidence to suggest that psychosocial factors, for example, life events, are implicated in bipolar depressive episodes after childbirth, as with unipolar puerperal depression, but that they are less important in manic episodes (Marks *et al.*, 1991). The quality of the marital relationship, however, may have an impact on manic breakdown (Marks *et al.*, 1992a,b).

Impact of maternal bipolar disorder on the infant

There are very few studies of the impact of early exposure to maternal bipolar illness on the infant and the findings are inconsistent. One study found that children whose mothers were currently depressed but had had a previous manic illness were more likely to have insecure attachment patterns and to have more disturbed peer relationships and more behavioural disturbance than children of mothers who had suffered unipolar depressions (De Mulder & Radke-Yarrow, 1991). This contrasts with other studies which suggest that children of mothers with bipolar disorder may be at decreased risk compared to those of unipolar mothers, in terms of social competence and disturbed behaviour (Connors *et al.*, 1979; Winters *et al.*, 1981), security of attachment and persistence in play tasks (Hipwell *et al.*, 1997), and that there is no long-term impact on the infant's cognitive and social development (Davies *et al.*, 1996). It may be that in contrast to mothers who are depressed, when a mother becomes manic she is more obviously not safe with her infant, and that the care of the infant is therefore more likely to be supervised and taken over by others when necessary, thereby protecting the child from the full impact of maternal illness. However, the handful of studies completed to date have consisted of very small and unrepresentative samples. Future research, using methodology designed to test more precise hypotheses about bipolar mothers' relationships with their infants, may yet demonstrate a specific impact of maternal bipolar illness on the infant.

Management of postpartum bipolar illness

In general, women who become manic after delivery will require psychiatric admission and usually mother and infant are admitted together, either to a general psychiatric ward or to a specialized psychiatric mother and baby unit. Initially all contact between mother and baby needs to be supervised by nursing staff, and as the mother's condition improves contact with her baby to be increased accordingly. Physical treatment is dictated by the clinical picture, as with bipolar illnesses occurring at other times, and neuroleptics, antidepressants, mood stabilizers and electroconvulsive therapy are all used.

Prevention of postpartum bipolar relapse

The use of lithium as a prophylaxis has been tested in two open clinical trials which showed some reduction in relapse rates (Stewart *et al.*, 1991; Austin, 1992). Transdermal oestrogen administered after delivery and continued for the first two postpartum weeks has had no impact on relapse (Kumar *et al.*, in prep.). For both these treatments, breastfeeding is contraindicated and therefore unwelcome to women who are currently well and wish to breastfeed.

Conclusions

Most postnatal depressions are mild and short lived, and can be cared for in the community with minimal intervention. It is important, however, that carers are alert to the possibility that sometimes the condition can become severe and intransigent, and that it may have a long-term, possibly fatal impact on the infant. At present, treatment strategies are similar to those used for depressions occurring at other times although different modes of delivery of care, particularly those involving health visitors and midwives are currently evolving. Research into the efficacy of different types of pharmacological treatment for this condition has yet to be done as have investigations into women whose depressions occur only after childbirth.

References

Ainsworth, M.D.S., Blehar, M.C. & Wall, S. (1978) *Patterns of Attachment*. Erlbaum, Hillsdale, NJ.

American Psychiatric Association (1987) *Diagnostic and Statistical Manual of Mental Disorders*, revised 3rd edn. American Psychiatric Association, Washington, DC.

Appleby, L. (1991) Suicide during pregnancy and in the first postnatal year. *British Medical Journal*, **302**, 137–140.

Appleby, L. (1996) Suicide behaviour in childbearing women. *International Review of Psychiatry*, **8**, 107–115.

Appleby, L., Fox, H., Shaw, M. & Kumar, R. (1989) The psychiatrist in the obstetric unit. Establishing a liaison service. *British Journal of Psychiatry*, **154**, 510–515.

Appleby, L., Gregoire, A., Platz, C. & Kumar, R. (1994) Screening women for high risk of postnatal depression. *Journal of Psychosomatic Research*, **38**, 539–545.

Appleby, L., Warner, R., Whitton, A. & Faragher, B. (1997) A controlled study of fluoxetine and cognitive-behavioural counselling in the treatment of postnatal depression. *British Medical Journal*, **314**, 932–936.

Austin, M.P. (1992) Puerperal affective psychosis: is there a case for lithium prophylaxis? *British Journal of Psychiatry* **161**, 692–694.

Ballard, C. & Davies, R. (1996) Postnatal depression in fathers. *International Review of Psychiatry*, **8**, 65–71.

Ballard, C.G., Davies, R., Cullen, R.N., Mohan, R.N. & Dean, C. (1994) Prevalence of postnatal psychiatric morbidity in mothers and fathers. *British Journal of Psychiatry*, **164**, 782–788.

Bebbington, P.E., Dean, C., Der, G., Hurry, J. & Tennant, C. (1991) Gender, parity, and the prevalence of minor affective disorder. *British Journal of Psychiatry*, **158**, 40–45.

Bowlby, J. (1980) *Attachment and Loss*, Vol. 3: *Loss*. Basic Books, New York.

Boyce, P., Hickie, I. & Parker, G. (1991) Parents, partners or personality? Risk factors for postnatal depression. *Journal of Affective Disorders*, **21**, 245–255.

Briscoe, M. (1986) Identification of emotional problems in postpartum women by health visitors. *British Medical Journal*, **292**, 1245–1247.

Brockington, I. & Cox-Roper, A. (1988) The nosology of puerperal mental illness. In: *Motherhood and Mental Illness*, Vol. 2: *Causes and Consequences* (eds R. Kumar and I. F. Brockington), pp. 1–16. Wright, London.

Brown, G.W., Bifulco, A., Veiel, H.O.F. & Andrews, B. (1990a) Self esteem and depression. II: Social correlates of self esteem. *Social Psychiatry and Psychiatric Epidemiology*, **25**, 225–234.

Brown, G.W., Bifulco, A. & Andrews, B. (1990b) Self-esteem and depression. III: Aetiological issues. *Social Psychiatry and Psychiatric Epidemiology*, **25**, 235–243.

Buist, A., Norman, T.R. & Dennerstein, L. (1990) Breastfeeding and the use of psychotropic medication: a review. *Journal of Affective Disorders*, **19**, 197–206.

Carothers, A.D. & Murray, L. (1990) Estimating psychiatric morbidity by logistic regression. *Psychological Medicine*, **20**, 695–702.

Cogill, S.R., Caplan, H.L., Alexandra, H., Robson, K.M. & Kumar, R. (1986) Impact of maternal postnatal depression on cognitive development in young children. *British Medical Journal,* **292,** 1165–1167.

Conners, C., Himmelhock, J., Goyette, C., Ulrich, R. & Neil, J. (1979) Children of parents with affective disorders. *Journal of Academy of Child Psychology,* **18,** 600–607.

Cooper, P.J., Campbell, E., Day, A., Kennerley, H. & Bond, A. (1988) Non-psychotic disorder after childbirth: a prospective study of prevalence, incidence, course and nature. *British Journal of Psychiatry,* **152,** 799–806.

Cooper, P.J. & Murray, L. (1995) Course and recurrence of postnatal depression: evidence for the specificity of the diagnostic concept. *British Journal of Psychiatry,* **166,** 191–195.

Cooper, P.J. & Murray, L. (1997) The impact of psychological treatments of postnatal depression on maternal mood and infant development. In: *Postpartum Depression and Child Development* (eds L. Murray & P. J. Cooper), pp. 201–220. Guilford, New York.

Cox, J.L., Connor, Y. & Kendell, R.E. (1982) Prospective study of the psychiatric disorders of childbirth. *British Journal of Psychiatry,* **140,** 111–117.

Cox, J.L., Murray, D. & Chapman, G. (1993a) A controlled study of the onset, duration and prevalence of postnatal depression. *British Journal of Psychiatry,* **163,** 27–31.

Cox, J.L., Gerrard, J., Cookson, D. & Jones, J.M. (1993b) Development and audit of Charles Street Parent and Baby Day Unit, Stoke-on-Trent. *Psychiatric Bulletin,* **17,** 711–713.

Cutrona, C.E. (1984) Social support and stress in the transition to parenthood. *Journal of Abnormal Psychology,* **92,** 161–172.

Dalton, K. (1980) *Depresssion after Childbirth.* Oxford University Press, Oxford.

Davies, L., Hipwell, A. & Kumar, R. (1994) Severe postnatal mental illness and the psychological development of the 4 year old: a controlled follow-up study. *Infant Behaviour and Development,* **17,** 594.

De Mulder, E. & Radke-Yarrow, M. (1991) Attachment with affectively ill and well mothers: concurrent behavioural correlates. *Development and Psychopathology,* **3,** 227–242.

Ditkoff, E.C., Crary, W.G., Cristo, M. & Lobo, R.A. (1991) Oestrogen improves psychological function in asymptomatic post-menopausal women. *Obstetrics and Gynaecology,* **78,** 991–995.

Dowlatshahi, D. & Paykel, E.S. (1990) Life events and social stress in puerperal psychoses: absence of effect. *Psychological Medicine,* **20,** 655–662.

Edwards, D.R.L., Porter, S.A.M. & Stein, G.S. (1994)

A pilot study of postnatal depression following caesarian section using two retrospective self-rating instruments. *Journal of Psychosomatic Research,* **38,** 111–117.

Elliott, S.A., Sanjak, M. & Leverton, T. (1988) Parent groups in pregnancy: a preventative intervention for postnatal depression? In: *Marshalling Social Support: Formats, Processes and Effects* (ed. B. H. Gottlieb), pp. 87–110. Sage, Beverly Hills, CA.

Field, T.M., Healy, B., Goldstein, S. *et al.* (1988) Infants of depressed mothers show 'depressed' behaviour even with nondepressed adults. *Child Development,* **59,** 1569–1579.

Gater, R.A., Dean, C. & Morris, J. (1989) The contribution of childbearing to the sex difference in first admission rates for affective psychosis. *Psychological Medicine,* **19,** 719–724.

Gotlib, I.H., Whiffen, V.E., Wallace, P.M. & Mount, J.H. (1991) Prospective investigation of postpartum depression: factors involved in onset and recovery. *Journal of Abnormal Psychology,* **100,** 122–132.

Gregoire, A.J.P., Kumar, R., Everitt, B., Henderson, A.F. & Studd, J.W.W. (1996) Transdermal oestrogen for severe postnatal depression. *Lancet,* **347,** 930–933.

Harris, B. (1996) Hormonal aspects of postnatal depression. *International Review of Psychiatry,* **8,** 27–36.

Harvey, I. & McGrath, G. (1988) Psychiatric morbidity in spouses of women admitted to a mother and baby unit. *British Journal of Psychiatry,* **152,** 506–510.

Hipwell, A.E., Goosens, F.A., Melhuish, E.C. & Kumar, R. (1997) Severe maternal psychopathology, joint hospitalisation and infant–mother attachment. *Development and Psychopathology.* (In press.)

Holden, J. (1996) The role of health visitors in postnatal depression. *International Review of Psychiatry,* **8,** 79–86.

Holden, J.M., Sagovski, R. & Cox, J.L. (1989) Counselling in a general practice setting: controlled study of health visitor intervention in treatment of postnatal depression. *British Medical Journal,* **298,** 223–226.

Kendell, R.E., Wainwright, S., Hailey, A. & Shannon, B. (1976) The influence of childbirth on psychiatric morbidity. *Psychological Medicine,* **6,** 297–302.

Kendell, R.C., Chalmers, J.C. & Platz, C. (1987) Epidemiology of puerperal psychoses. *British Journal of Psychiatry,* **150,** 662–673.

Kennell, J., Klaus, M. & McGrath, S. *et al.* (1991) Continuous emotional support during labour in a US hospital: a randomised controlled trial. *Journal of the American Medical Association,* **265**, 2197–2201.

Klaus, M.H., Kennell, J.H., Roberson, S.S. & Sosa, R. (1986) Effects of social support during parturition on maternal and infant morbidity. *British Medical Journal,* **6**, 585–587.

Klompenhouwer, J.L. & van Hulst, A.M. (1991) Classification of postpartum psychosis: a study of 250 mother and baby admissions in the Netherlands. *Acta Psychiatrica Scandinavica,* **84**, 255–261.

Kumar, R. (1997) Anybody's child: 44 mothers with post-partum onset of disturbances of maternal affection and of the mother–infant relationship. *British Journal of Psychiatry.* (In press.)

Kumar, R. & Robson, K. (1984) A prospective study of emotional disorders in childbearing women. *British Journal of Psychiatry,* **144**, 35–47.

Kumar, R., Marks, M.N., Platz, C. & Yoshida, K. (1995a) Clinical survey of a psychiatric mother and baby unit: characteristics of 100 consecutive admissions. *Journal of Affective Disorders,* **33**, 11–22.

Kumar, R., Marks, M.N. & Jackson, K. (1995b) Prevention and treatment of postnatal psychiatric disorders: the role of the midwife. *British Journal of Midwifery,* **3**, 314–317.

Kumar, R., Marks, M.N., Campbell, I.C. & Checkley, S.A. Transdermal oestrogen and postpartum biploar relapse. (In preparation.)

Lovestone, S. & Kumar, R. (1993) Postnatal psychiatric illness: the impact on spouses. *British Journal of Psychiatry,* **68**, 157–168.

McIntosh, J. (1993) Postpartum depression: women's help-seeking behaviour and perceptions of cause. *Journal of Advanced Nursing,* **18**, 178–184.

McIvor, R.J., Davies, A., Wieck, A. *et al.* (1996) The growth hormone response to apomorphine at 4 days postpartum in women with histories of major depression. *Journal of Affective Disorders,* **40**, 131–136.

Magos, A.L., Brewster, E. & Sing, H. *et al.* (1986) The effects of norethisterone in post-menopausal women on oestrogen replacement therapy: a model for the pre-menstrual syndrome. *British Journal of Obstetrics and Gynaecology,* **93**, 1290–1296.

Margison, F. (1982) The pathology of the mother–infant relationship. In: *Motherhood and Mental Illness* (eds I.F. Brockington & R. Kumar), pp. 191–222. Wright, London.

Marks, M.N. & Lovestone, S. (1995) The role of the father in parental postnatal mental health. *British Journal of Medical Psychology,* **68**, 157–168.

Marks, M.N., Wieck, A., Checkley, S.A. & Kumar, R. (1991) Life stress and postpartum psychosis: a preliminary report. *British Journal of Psychiatry,* **158** (Suppl. 10), 45–49.

Marks, M.N., Wieck, A., Checkley, S.A. & Kumar, R. (1992a) Contribution of psychological and social factors to psychotic and non-psychotic relapse after childbirth in women with histories of affective disorder. *Journal of Affective Disorders,* **29**, 253–264.

Marks, M.N., Wieck, A., Seymour, A., Checkley, S.A. & Kumar, R. (1992b) Women whose mental illnesses recur after childbirth and partners levels of expressed emotion during late pregnancy. *British Journal of Psychiatry,* **161**, 211–216.

Marks, M.N., Wieck, A., Checkley, S.A. & Kumar, R. (1996) How does marriage protect women with histories of affective disorder from postpartum relapse? *British Journal of Medical Psychology,* **69**, 329–342.

Martin, C.J., Brown, G.W., Goldberg, D.P. & Brockington, I.F. (1989) Psychosocial stress and puerperal depression. *Journal of Affective Disorders,* **16**, 283–293.

Mitchell, E.A., Thompson, J.M.D., Stewart, A.W. *et al.* (1992) Postnatal depression and SIDS: a prospective study. *Journal of Paediatric Child Health,* **28** (Suppl. 1), S13–16.

Murray, L. (1992) The impact of postnatal depression on infant development. *Journal of Child Psychology and Psychiatry,* **33**, 543–561.

Murray, L., Kempton, C., Woolgar, M. & Hooper, R. (1993) Depressed mothers' speech to their infants and its relation to infant gender and cognitive development. *Journal of Psychology and Psychiatry,* **34**, 1083–1102.

Murray, L., Stanley, C., Hooper, R., King, F. & Fiori-Cowly, A. (1996) The role of infant factors in postnatal depression and mother infant interactions. *Developmental Medicine and Child Neurology* **38**, 109–119.

Oates, M. (1988) The development of an integrated community oriented service for severe postnatal mental illness. In: *Motherhood and Mental Illness* (eds R. Kumar & I. F. Brockington), pp. 133–158. Wright, London.

Oates, M. (1989) Management of major mental illness in pregnancy and the puerperium. In: *Psychological Aspects of Obstetrics and Gynaecology.* (ed M Oates), pp. 905–920. *Ballière's Clinical Obstetrics and Gynaecology,* 3.

Odent, M. (1984) *Birth Reborn.* Souvenir Press, London.

O'Hara, M.W. (1986) Social support, life events and depression during pregnancy and the puerperium. *Archives of General Psychiatry,* **43**, 569–573.

O'Hara, M.W. & Swain, A.M. (1996) Rates and risk

of postpartum depression—a meta-analysis. *International Review of Psychiatry*, **8**, 37–54.

O'Hara, M.W. & Zekoski, E. (1988) Post-partum depression: a comprehensive review. In: *Motherhood and Mental Illness* (eds R. Kumar & I.F. Brockington), pp. 17–63. Wright, London.

O'Hara, M.W., Neunaber, D.J. & Zekoski, E.M. (1984) Prospective study of postpartum depression: prevalence, course and predictive factors. *Journal of Abnormal Psychology*, **93**, 158–171.

O'Hara, M.W., Zekoski, E.M., Phillips, L.H. & Wright, E.J. (1990) Controlled prospective study of postpartum mood disorders: comparison of childbearing and non-childbearing women. *Journal of Abnormal Psycholgy*, **99**, 3–15.

Paffenbarger, R.S., Jr (1964) Epidemiological aspects of postpartum mental illness. *British Journal of Preventative and Social Medicine*, **18**, 189–195.

Paykel, E.S., Emms, E.M., Fletcher, J. & Rassaby, E.S. (1980) Life events and social support in puerperal depression. *British Journal of Psychiatry*, **136**, 339–346.

Pitt, B. (1968) Atypical depression following childbirth. *British Journal of Psychiatry* **114**, 1325–1335.

Pitts F. (1995) Comrades in adversity: the group approach. *Health Visitor*, **68**, 144–145.

Pugh, T.F., Jerath, B.K., Schmidt, W.M. & Reed, R.B. (1963) Rates of mental disease relating to childbearing. *New England Journal of Medicine*, **268**, 1224–1228.

Reich, T. & Winokur, G. (1970) Postpartum psychoses in patients with manic depressive disease. *Journal of Nervous Mental Disorders*, **151**, 60–68.

Romaine, S., Jones, A. & Watts, T. (1995) Postnatal depression: facilitating peer group support. *Health Visitor*, **68**, 153.

Ruble, D.N., Brooks-Gunn, J., Fleming, A.S., Fitzmaurice, G., Stangor, C. & Deutsch, F. (1990) Transitions to motherhood and the self: measurement, stability and change. *Journal of Personal and Social Psychology*, **58**, 450–463.

Sanderson, C.A., Cowden, B. & Hall, D.M.B. (1996) *Is postnatal depression a risk factor for 'cot death'?* Paper presented to the biennial meeting of the Marce Society, September 4–7, 1996.

Schopf, J. & Rust, B. (1994) Follow-up and family study of postpartum psychoses. Part I: Overview. *European Archives Psychiatry Clinical Neuroscience*, **244**, 101–111.

Schopf, J., Bryois, C., Jonquiere, M. & Le, P.K. (1984) On the nosology of severe psychiatric postpartum disorders. *European Archives of Psychiatry, and Neurological Sciences*, **234**, 54–63.

Sharp, D., Hay, D., Pawlby, S., Schmucker, G.,

Allen, H. & Kumar, R. (1995) The impact of postnatal depression on boys' intellectual development. *Journal of Child Psychology and Psychiatry*, **36**, 1315–1336.

Sherwin, B.B. (1991) The impact of different doses of oestrogen and progestin on mood and sexual behaviour in post-menopausal women. *Journal of Clinical Endocrinology and Metabolism*, **72**, 336–343.

Sherwin, B.B. & Gelfand, M.M. (1985) Sex steroids and affect in the surgical menopause: a double-blind cross-over study. *Psychoneuroendocrinology*, **10**, 325–335.

Singer, J.M. & Fagan, J.W. (1992) Negative affect, emotional expression and forgetting in young infants. *Developmental Psychology*, **28**, 48–57.

Sosa, R., Kennell, J.H., Klaus, M.H. & Urruttia, J. (1980) The effect of a supportive companion on perinatal problems, length of labour and mother–infant interaction. *New England Journal of Medicine*, **303**, 597–600.

Spitzer, R.L., Endicott, J. & Robbins, E. (1978) Research diagnostic criteria: rationale and reliability. *Archives of General Psychiatry*, **35**, 773–782.

Stamp, G.E., Williams, A.S. & Crowther, C.A. (1995) Evaluation of antenatal and postnatal support to overcome postnatal depression: a randomized, controlled trial. *Birth*, **22** (3), 138–143.

Stewart, D.E., Klompenhouwer, J.L., Kendell, R.E. & van Hulst, A.M. (1991) Prophylactic lithium in puerperal psychosis: the experience of three centres. *British Journal of Psychiatry* **158**, 393–397.

Watson, J.P., Elliott, S.A., Rugg, A.J. & Brough, D.I. (1984) Psychiatric disorder in pregnancy and the first postnatal year. *British Journal of Psychiatry*, **144**, 453–462.

Wieck, A. (1989) Endocrine aspects of postnatal mental disorders. In: *Psychological Aspects of Obstetrics and Gynaecology* (ed. M. Oates), pp. 857–877. Balliere Tyndall, London.

Wieck, A. (1996) Ovarian hormones, mood and neurotransmitters. *International Review of Psychiatry*, **8**, 17–25.

Wieck, A., Kumar, R., Hirst, A.D., Marks, M.N., Campbell, I.C. & Checkley, S.A. (1991) Increased sensitivity to dopaminergic stimulation precedes recurrence of affective psychosis after childbirth. *British Medical Journal*, **303**, 613–616.

Wieck, A., Davies, R.A. & Kumar, R. *et al.* (1997) Increased D2 hypothalamic receptor sensitivity: a trait marker for puerperal manic-depressive illness? (Submitted for publication.)

Whiffen, E.V. & Gotlib, I.A. (1993) Comparison of postpartum and nonpostpartum depression: clinical presentation, psychiatric history and psychosocial functioning. *Journal of Consulting* and *Clinical Psychology*, **61**, 485–494.

Winters, K.C., Stone, A.A., Weintraub, S. & Neale, J.M. (1981) Cognitive and attentional deficits in children vulnerable to psychopathology. *Journal of Abnormal Child Psychology*, **9**, 435–453.

Wisner, K.L. & Wheeler, S.B. (1994) Prevention of recurrent postpartum major depression. *Hospital and Community Psychiatry* **45**, 1191–1196.

Yoshida, K. & Kumar, R. (1996) Breastfeeding and psychotropic drugs. *International Review of Psychiatry*, **8**, 117–124.

Yoshida, K., Marks, M.N., Kibe, N., Kumar, R., Nakahano, H. & Tashiro, N. (1997) Postnatal depression in Japanese women who have given birth in England. *Journal of Affective Disorders*, **43**, 69–77.

18 The management of depression in the elderly

LUCY C. AITKEN AND
ROBERT C. BALDWIN

The object of this chapter is to review those aspects of the treatment of depression in old age which are different from the treatment of depression in younger people. The main differences concern diagnosis, which can be more uncertain in the elderly, the assessment of memory loss, the presence of physical illness and social isolation, and the implications of these both for physical and psychosocial management.

Diagnostic difficulties

There are factors which may modify the expression of depressive illness in elderly people. Some are due to generational differences in the perception of psychological and physical health, others occur because of the frequent overlap of depressive symptoms and physical illness. Sometimes these factors may accentuate certain aspects of the clinical picture whilst others may obscure the diagnosis. Factors which may alter the presentation of depression in older people are summarized in Table 18.1.

Table 18.1 Factors which modify the presentation of depression in old age.

Overlap of medical and psychiatric symptoms
Minimal expression of sadness
Somatization or disproportionate complaints associated with physical disorder
Neurotic symptoms of recent onset
Deliberate self-harm (especially medically 'trivial')
'Pseudodementia'
Depression superimposed upon dementia
Conduct disorder
Accentuation of abnormal personality traits
Late onset alcohol dependency syndrome

Associated physical ill-health may lead to an overlap of symptoms. DSM-IV criteria (American Psychiatric Association, 1994) require that symptoms due to associated physical illness should be discounted when diagnosing depression. In practice this is not always easy. An older individual with chronic obstructive airways disease may experience insomnia, fatigue and poor appetite equally from the chest disease or from an associated depression. If attention is paid to the following points, difficulties can often be resolved. First, the history may indicate on closer enquiry that some symptoms are new: for example, early morning wakening may emerge from a background of more generalized sleep disturbance due to dyspnoea. Second, for those with limited mobility or exercise tolerance, questions about energy and activity must be appropriate: 'Do you feel tired even when resting?', not 'Have you no energy?'. Third, patients who dismiss depression as purely 'understandable' because of ill-health can easily wrong-foot an inexperienced clinician. A history not only from the patient but also from an informant is thus essential. It may demonstrate, for example, a recent decline in interests at a time of static physical health. Cohen-Cole and Stoudemire (1987) provide a useful overview of the problems of diagnosing depression in the presence of major physical illness. Essentially the clinician can opt to be restrictive, that is to allow only those symptoms which are unequivocally due to depression rather than physical ill-health; or over-inclusive, in which case symptoms which might be due either to depression or physical ill-health are counted as depressive in origin. Many would agree with Cohen-Cole and Stoudemire that whereas strict criteria are necessary for research, clinicians may wish to take the less restrictive option in order to avoid overlooking depression in complex cases.

Another difficulty arises because of the well-recognized tendency of elderly people to minimize feelings of sadness (Georgotas *et al.*, 1983), presumably reflecting a cohort of people brought up not to bother their doctors with emotional difficulties. It is essential to ask about two areas: *anhedonia*, the inability to experience pleasure, and *depressive thoughts*, especially reduced self-esteem, guilt, worthlessness and suicidal ideation. Even if depression is denied or somatized, as it often is in older people, some of these symptoms will be present if the patient has a depressive illness.

An obscure pain may occasionally have its origin in undiagnosed depression which an accurate history will usually uncover. Similar to this is Post's observation that occasional cases of severe tinnitus are relieved when an underlying depression is treated (Post, 1982). More common though is the presentation of an unreassurable elderly person with physical complaints disproportionate to known pathology. Again the key is a good history, especially noting recent changes in pain threshold, plus a careful physical review.

A serious error is that of taking at face value neurotic symptoms of recent onset. The sudden emergence of severe anxiety, obsessional compulsive phenomena, hysteria or hypochondriasis in an elderly person not previously prone to such disorders should lead to a careful search for depressive illness, which is the usual cause (Baldwin, 1988a). Likewise, at all levels of severity of depression, anxiety is a common accompanying symptom (Post, 1972). If it dominates the clinical picture the unwary may miss the underlying depression.

Another trap is to dismiss an act of deliberate self-harm in an older person because the medical consequences appear to be trivial. There is no reliable correlation between the medical severity of deliberate self-harm and any associated psychiatric illness; nor is it necessarily the most severely depressed patients who kill themselves (Barraclough, 1971). Elderly people rarely take 'manipulative' overdoses. Most have depressive illness (Post & Shulman, 1985) and *all* require psychiatric referral.

'Pseudodementia' is defined by Lishman (1987) as 'a number of conditions [in which] a clinical picture resembling dementia presents for attention yet physical disease proves to be little if at all responsible'. In the setting of depression it is sometimes referred to as 'dementia of depression' (Pearlson *et al.*, 1989) or 'depressive pseudodementia' and is thought to be more common in the elderly. These terms are used in several different ways.

The first and least helpful way is when an elderly person, usually clearly depressed, fails a routine 'bedside' screening test for dementia. Since dementia is defined clinically and not on the basis of single test results, this usage is not acceptable. A second and more common application of the term 'pseudodementia' is to a characteristic and somewhat dramatic clinical presentation of severe depressive illness in an older person. Post (1982) has summarized the clinical picture. Informants are always aware of memory impairment and can usually date the onset accurately, unlike the onset of dementia which is much more insidious. The patients often complain vociferously about their memory, and occasionally other cognitive difficulties, again unlike most dementia sufferers. Questions about cognitive function often lead to 'don't know' responses, sometimes accompanied by marked irritation, in contrast to those with dementia who try their best but are inaccurate. Patients with pseudodementia convey a great deal of despair, often non-verbally, during the interview. The history is often short and sometimes a previous personal or family history of depression is uncovered. Nursing observation may reveal insomnia, diurnal mood change and the chance comment to suggest depressive ideation, for example, 'I've nowhere to live'; 'I'm ruined'. These patients are often perplexed and inaccessible. Post argues that depressive pseudodementia should only be diagnosed in patients who *can* be tested, rather than those who appear confused but are inaccessible and hence not really testable.

Third, the term 'pseudodementia' is sometimes applied to a clearly depressed patient who is found to have subtle but measurable cognitive impairment. Sometimes this may be global impairment although more usually it is specific, for example an amnesia. Reynolds *et al.* (1989) have reviewed the literature and found that cognitive impairment was reported in 10–20% of depressed elderly patients. However, deficits in higher cortical function (aphasia, agraphia, etc.) are rarely present. Yet if 'pseudodementia' were to be defined purely on the basis of *any* degree of cognitive dysfunction occurring in a depressed patient, then most elderly depressives could be deemed to be cases of 'pseudodementia', since most have subtle deficits (Abas *et al.*, 1990). The term then becomes redundant.

Post (1982) argues that depressive 'pseudodementia' is a term with limited clinical utility: for severe depressive symptoms in a patient require treatment, whether or not it is thought that dementia is present. Perhaps then the term serves its purpose best by acting as a reminder that sometimes apparently demented patients may be suffering from severe depression. 'Depression on dementia', in contrast, refers to the superimposition of depression on an established dementing disorder.

Elderly people sometimes present their depression as a disorder of behaviour. Pitt (1982) points to certain patterns. These include presentations with food refusal, 'incontinence' (for example, a perverse ability to eliminate in almost any place other than the toilet, unlike the incontinence of dementia), screaming and outwardly aggressive behaviour. Often the location is a residential or nursing home facility and the context a resentful dependency. A good history is crucial. This is best given either by the resident's key nurse or a care assistant who knows the resident well. A family member and/or close friend can amplify this and give details of any previous psychiatric history, information which is often not known to those caring for the individual. Besides the usual neurovegetative symptoms of depression, a history of a relatively recent *change* in behaviour can be very illuminating. This may take the form of social withdrawal and loss of interest in self and the environment, as well as the more obviously disruptive behaviours described by Pitt.

Depressive illness may also lead to an accentuation of premorbid personality traits. The advent of depressive illness may lead to dramatic theatricality and ceaseless importuning to several agencies simultaneously—for example, social services and primary care. The key is an accurate appreciation of change in the light of known premorbid personality traits. Also within the area of behaviour disturbance it is worth recalling that sometimes a conduct disorder, such as shoplifting, may be a behavioural correlate of depressive illness in an older person, as is an alcohol dependence syndrome acquired for the first time. Finally, a complaint of loneliness from an individ-

Table 18.2 Causes of organic depressions.

Occult carcinoma	*Infections*
Lung	Post-viral infections
Pancreas	Myalgic encephalomyelitis
	Brucellosis
Metabolic/endocrine	Neurosyphilis
Hypothyroidism	
Hypercalcaemia	*Organic brain disease*
Cushing's disease	Space-occupying lesion
B_{12} deficiency	Dementia
Drugs	
Steroids	
Beta-blockers	
Methyldopa	
Clonidine	
Nifedipine	
Digoxin	
L-dopa	
Tetrabenazine	

ual who has hitherto coped quite well alone, usually accompanied by a request to be re-housed, should lead to a search for depressive illness.

Laboratory investigation

The laboratory investigation of depression is particularly important in the elderly in view of the associated medical causes of depression. These are listed in Table 18.2.

Investigation should include haemoglobin and red blood cell indices which may point to possible B_{12} deficiency or alcohol excess. B_{12} estimation should be undertaken in a first episode. Where depression has been present for many weeks folate levels should be checked, as subclinical nutritional deficits may have developed. For similar reasons urea and electrolyte estimations are important. A low serum potassium will lead to electroconvulsive therapy (ECT) being delayed and an elevated calcium is occasionally associated with depression, as in primary hyperparathyroidism (Peterson, 1968) and metastatic cancer.

One principle to guide investigation is an awareness that elderly people have less physiological reserve. Severe depression in a 75-year-old may lead to quite serious metabolic derangement which would be unlikely in a fit 40-year-old. Thyroid function testing should be performed because of the well-known association of depression with hypothyroidism, which may be overlooked in the elderly, and because 'apathetic hyperthyroidism' can be mistaken for depression. Table 18.3 summarizes investigations appropriate

Table 18.3 Investigations for depression in later life.

Investigation	First episode	Recurrence
Full blood count	Yes	Yes
Urea and electrolytes	Yes	Yes
Calcium	Yes	If indicated
Thyroid function	Yes	If indicated, or more than 12 months previously
B_{12}	Yes	If indicated, or more than 2 years
Folate	Yes	If indicated by nutritional state
Liver function	Yes	If indicated (e.g. alcohol abuse)
Syphilitic serology	Yes	Only if not already done
CT (brain)	If clinically indicated	Only if neurologically indicated
EEG	If clinically indicated	Only if neurologically indicated

for a first episode of depression and a recurrence. Regarding the electro-encephalogram (EEG), there are no diagnostic changes specific to depression on the standard 12-lead EEG. The main clinical benefit of an EEG is to help differentiate depression from an organic brain syndrome.

Another approach to diagnosis is the use of screening questionnaires. The most widely used rating instruments in depression are the Zung Depression Rating Scale, which may require adjustment of its cut-off for 'caseness' in older people (Zung, 1967), and the Beck Depression Inventory (Beck *et al.*, 1961). Neither of these was designed specifically for use with elderly people and both use a multiple choice format which some elderly people find confusing. For this reason the Geriatric Depression Scale (GDS) has been introduced (Yesavage *et al.*, 1983). It focuses almost entirely on the cognitive aspects of depressive illness, rather than physical depressive symptomatology, and has a simple 'yes/no' format. Even so, the full version has 30 questions (Table 18.4) and the original validation was carried out on a physically fit group of depressives which contained individuals as young as 55 years. A cut-off score of 11 or above indicates probable depression. The same cut-off was found to give satisfactory sensitivity and specificity in hospitalized elderly patients with concurrent medical illness (Koenig *et al.*, 1988; Jackson & Baldwin, 1993). A shorter version is available (Yesavage, 1988); the relevant items, for which a score of 5 and above indicate probable depression, are highlighted in bold. Whether the GDS is a useful means of detecting depressive illness in the presence of *dementia* is less clear. In one study of patients referred to a geriatric medical service it was poor at detecting depression associated with Alzheimer's disease (Burke *et al.*, 1989) whilst in another it fared reasonably well (O'Riordan *et al.*, 1990), at least for patients with mild dementia. New scales—for example, the Cornell Scale for Depression in Dementia (Alexopoulos *et al.*, 1988)—have been introduced to address this difficult area. The latter incorporates information from a carer.

Table 18.4 The Geriatric Depression Scale.

Instructions: Choose the best answer for how you have felt over the past *week*.	
1 Are you basically satisfied with your life?	No
2 Have you dropped many of your activities and interests?	Yes
3 Do you feel your life is empty?	Yes
4 Do you often get bored?	Yes
5 Are you hopeful about the future?	No
6 Are you bothered by thoughts you can't get out of your head?	Yes
7 Are you in good spirits most of the time?	No
8 Are you afraid something bad is going to happen to you?	Yes
9 Do you feel happy most of the time?	No
10 Do you often feel helpless?	Yes
11 Do you often get restless and fidgety?	Yes
12 Do you prefer to stay at home, rather than going out and doing new things?	Yes
13 Do you frequently worry about the future?	Yes
14 Do you feel you have more problems with your memory than most?	Yes
15 Do you think it is wonderful to be alive now?	No
16 Do you often feel down-hearted and blue (sad)?	Yes
17 Do you feel pretty worthless the way you are?	Yes
18 Do you worry a lot about the past?	Yes
19 Do you find life very exciting?	No
20 Is it hard for you to start on new projects (plans)?	Yes
21 Do you feel full of energy?	No
22 Do you feel that your situation is hopeless?	Yes
23 Do you think most people are better off (in their lives) than you are?	Yes
24 Do you frequently get upset over little things?	Yes
25 Do you frequently feel like crying?	Yes
26 Do you have trouble concentrating?	Yes
27 Do you enjoy getting up in the morning?	No
28 Do you prefer to avoid social gatherings (get-togethers)?	Yes
29 Is it easy for you to make decisions?	No
30 Is your mind as clear as it used to be?	No

'Yes' or 'no' responses are those which score '1'.
Phrases in parentheses refer to alternative ways of expressing the questions to a UK population, as used by the authors.

It is important to place questionnaires in their proper context. They do not 'make' a diagnosis. In fact, their use requires careful thought. False positives are bound to occur and could lead to increased referrals to secondary agencies. With these provisos, instruments such as the GDS may have a useful role in settings such as geriatric wards where the prevalence of depressive illness is high (25% in the study of Jackson & Baldwin, 1993), and where non-psychiatrically trained staff wish to improve their ability to detect it.

Aspects of physical treatment relevant to elderly depressed patients

Although drug treatment is covered elsewhere, some aspects relevant to elderly depressed patients need to be emphasized. Failure to meet fully the diagnostic criteria outlined earlier for major depression is not necessarily a reason to withhold antidepressant treatment. Patients with fewer symptoms than are specified within diagnostic criteria such as ICD-10 (World Health Organization, 1992) and DSM-IV may nevertheless benefit from treatment. ICD-10 partly recognizes this by introducing categories such as 'mild' depressive episode. Factors to consider are: subjective distress, degree of social and functional impairment, and extent of loss of interests. If one is unsure about whether to prescribe an antidepressant, and there often is more uncertainty when assessing older people, it is often helpful to see the patient two or even three times over a few weeks and to reassess. A proportion of depressive syndromes resolve spontaneously. An alternative to this 'wait and see' approach is to conduct a therapeutic trial of an antidepressant. Involving a community psychiatric nurse (CPN) to monitor symptoms and response can be helpful. The patient's mood should be reassessed 3–4 weeks after being on a therapeutic dose of an antidepressant. At that point, if there has been some response, the antidepressant should be continued. If the patient remains unchanged, then a re-evaluation will be required, with special attention to dosage of the antidepressant, compliance and possible maintaining psychosocial factors. For example, an elderly lady who lived alone developed low mood, insomnia, pervasive anxiety and poor concentration following a burglary. Her sleep pattern improved after a trial of an antidepressant, but her mood remained low. However, with support from a CPN, she moved to sheltered housing and this resulted in rapid improvement in her mood.

Acute treatment

Building a partnership with the patient is therefore crucial. This begins with an *explanation* that depression which warrants treatment with tablets is an illness, and that it is common, treatable and not a sign of moral weakness. Many patients need *reassurance* that the tablets they will be asked to take are not addictive, and that depression is neither 'senility' nor a harbinger of dementia. They should be *involved* in the treatment. They need to be told, in lay terms, why they should not expect immediate results. They and the clinician should agree on a plan of treatment. For example, a patient should be informed that antidepressants will relieve their depressive symptoms, but that further help to manage anxiety or address a bereavement, for example, is also indicated. Nowadays, almost all psychiatrists specializing in the care of older people work as part of a multidisciplinary team. A 'key worker' from this team should be appointed who can coordinate the care delivered and act as a point of contact for the patient and family.

Pharmacological aspects

This requires an understanding of the age-associated changes in the distribution, metabolism and excretion of therapeutic drugs. The following points are important. First, in elderly people levels of circulating serum albumin are lower, reducing the capacity for protein binding and resulting in elevated unbound drug concentrations. The rates of both hepatic metabolism of the drugs and renal excretion of the metabolites will be lower than among younger patients. Any resultant accumulation can lead to exaggerated side-effects. Second, as a result of normal physiological changes, the pharmacokinetics of tricyclic antidepressants differ in the elderly from those in younger adults. Consequently, considerably higher steady-state plasma levels may develop in older patients. Third, an increase in inter-individual variability is found in the elderly, making prediction of the therapeutic dose of tricyclics particularly difficult. Some require dosages one-third or half of those recommended for younger adults, others the full dose. Time can thus be lost 'titrating' tricyclics in this way. Fourth, some of the selective serotonin re-uptake inhibitors (SSRIs) (fluoxetine, fluvoxamine and paroxetine) have proved to be inhibitors of hepatic enzymic oxidation (cytochrome P450 2D6—debrisoquine hydrochloride (Crewe *et al.*, 1992)). These drugs can alter the pharmacokinetics of other, hepatically oxidized drugs, leading to drug interactions. Drugs metabolized by this enzyme, and hence likely to be affected by these new antidepressants are: tricyclic antidepressants and trazodone; neuroleptics; lipophilic beta-blockers (e.g. metoprolol); some antiarrhythmics, and triazolobenzodiazepines, such as alprazolam. Lastly, because depression and physical illness are closely linked in old age, and because the burden of physical morbidity is invariably the greatest in older people, there are considerable risks of adverse interactions with drugs for medical disorders. Particular problems may arise with coadministration of diuretics, antiarrhythmics, calcium-channel blockers, some ulcer-healing drugs, hypnotics and other sedative drugs and, of course, alcohol, the abuse of which is frequently unsuspected in an older person.

Response times to recovery are longer than younger patients (Schneider *et al.*, 1994). Whilst most patients respond within 6 weeks, a sizeable minority may take up to 9 weeks (Georgotas & McCue, 1989).

Delusional (psychotic) depression

This rarely remits with an antidepressant alone. As with other age groups, either a combination of an antidepressant plus an antipsychotic will be required, or electroconvulsive therapy (ECT) (Baldwin, 1988b).

Choosing an antidepressant

Knowledge of class-specific contraindications to, and side-effects of, particular antidepressants is crucial. This is covered elsewhere and only those points relevant to older patients will be stressed.

Postural hypotension is a common and dangerous problem and occurs most in frail patients and those with reduced left ventricular output, and/or those on diuretics. To reinforce this, a case-control study in America (Ray *et al.*, 1987) highlighted a significant increase in hip fracture in elderly people taking tricyclic antidepressants. This is clearly an avoidable tragedy and is arguably one of the most potent arguments against the use of the older tricyclics in frail older people. Delirium is also a problem with the older tricyclics, and occurs most often in patients who are medically ill; amitriptyline is the worst offender. Cardiotoxicity is a risk in the face of a cardiac rhythm disturbance or a clinically relevant conduction disorder. These effects are much more likely if plasma levels are allowed to rise above therapeutic levels. In general, though, the cardiotoxicity of tricyclic drugs has been overstated. Weight gain, however, is understated and, at a time when it is argued that many elderly patients with major depression should be given long-term maintenance therapy (Old Age Depression Interest Group, 1993), this can be a real problem in an older patient: aggravating arthritis, chronic bronchitis and lowering self-esteem. All these problems are encountered less with lofepramine, which is why it is a popular choice in the elderly. Postural hypotension and anticholinergic effects are worse with tertiary amine tricyclics (amitriptyline and imipramine).

SSRIs, in contrast, have hardly any action on cholinergic or histaminergic pathways and little effect on alpha$_1$ adrenoreceptors. The main unwanted effects are: nausea (around 15%); diarrhoea (around 10%), insomnia (5–15%), anxiety and agitation (2–15%), headache and weight loss. Many of these effects are mild and transient. Nausea is the most frequent. Side-effects do not differ between younger and older patients.

Postural hypotension also limits the use of the traditional monoamine oxidase inhibitors. For moclobemide, a reversible inhibitor of monoamine oxidase A, the side-effect profile seems relatively benign, although nausea, dizziness, headache, agitation and insomnia may occur. The latter may require coprescription of a benzodiazepine for the first 2 weeks of treatment. Because it lacks significant anticholinergic effects and is non-cardiotoxic, mianserin is still occasionally prescribed to older patients. However, the risk of aplastic anaemia, with a requirement for regular blood tests, limits its use.

Trazodone is moderately sedative and lacks adverse cardiovascular effects. Experience to date with venlafaxine and nefazadone is too limited with regard to age-associated side-effects to make any comment.

Behavioural toxicity (affecting vigilance, reaction times, etc.) has been largely ignored among elderly people. With increasing numbers of them driving and pursuing other activities demanding high levels of vigilance, this must be taken more seriously. Sherwood and Hindmarch (1993) found that among five commonly prescribed antidepressants, lofepramine, fluoxetine and paroxetine had more favourable profiles with respect to measures of skilled performance thought to reflect everyday activities, than amitriptyline and dothiepin.

Efficacy in special patient groups

Elderly patients with dementia

Reifler *et al.* (1989) reported improvement in depression in 28 elderly patients with underlying Alzheimer's disease in a trial of imipramine lasting 8 weeks, but comparable improvement was also noted in a placebo group! The average dose was 80 mg. Of the newer drugs, Hebenstreit *et al.* (1991) demonstrated highly significant therapeutic efficacy of moclobemide (400 mg) over placebo in 726 elderly patients with unspecified dementia who were also depressed. Postma and Vranesic (1985) describe 10 demented depressives who responded well to moclobemide at a much lower dose (maximum 225 mg).

In a recent study (Roth *et al.*, 1996) moclobemide was also found to be effective in elderly depressed patients with cognitive impairment. Improvement was noted in both those with depression and comorbid dementia ($n = 511$) and those with depression and subtle cognitive impairment but without dementia ($n = 183$). Those treated with moclobemide also had measurable improvement in cognitive function, although this was only significant for the group without dementia.

Depression associated with general systemic disease

Intolerance to antidepressants occurs in about one-third of patients with depression and comorbid medical problems (Lipsey *et al.*, 1984; Katz *et al.*, 1990) and Koenig *et al.* (1989) had to abandon a proposed drug trial using nortriptyline in physically ill older patients because virtually all had contraindications or were intolerant of the drug. Physically ill depressives have been treated in an open trial for up to 1 year with fluoxetine 20 mg daily (Evans, 1993). The drug was tolerated well in a range of serious medical disorders, many grave. More recently, Roose *et al.* (1994) found that 22 depressed patients with heart disease with a mean age of 73 years responded less well to fluoxetine than 42 comparable patients treated with nortriptyline (mean age, 70). Indeed, only five of the 22 fluoxetine-treated patients responded; those with melancholic subtype of major depression (the majority) did especially poorly. The number of dropouts in each group was similar.

So, although the newer antidepressants appear to have a niche here, the evidence that they are more appropriate than established antidepressants is not totally convincing and it is surprising how little evaluation of them there has been in this context.

Electroconvulsive therapy

ECT is well tolerated in elderly patients (Benbow, 1989). All contraindications are relative if it is given as a life-saving procedure. It is best avoided within 3 months of a stroke or myocardial infarct, or if pulmonary function is poor. Since most complications of ECT in older people are cardiovascular (Benbow, 1989), with a higher risk of asystole (Abrams, 1991), this system should be examined carefully, and a past history of an arrythmia accurately determined, plus a cardiac opinion if there is any concern or doubt. Unilateral electrode placement is often the choice in elderly patients to minimize memory disturbance. However, whilst this is measurably worse with bilateral ECT, it may not be of any practical significance, and some argue that bilateral placement is more effective in older depressed patients (Benbow, 1989). A pacemaker is not a contraindication provided the patient's bed is insulated from the ground, the patient is not touched and the monitoring equipment properly earthed. Symptoms which predict a good response are similar at all ages, but one area of difference is that older patients with marked anxiety, often regarded as poor prognosis in younger adults, do just as well (Benbow, 1989).

Treatment resistance

There have been four prospective studies of lithium augmentation in elderly patients to date. Zimmer *et al.* (1988) and Flint and Rifat (1994) found response rates of 20% and 23%, respectively, much lower than open studies of younger adults. Parker *et al.* (1994) compared a group treated with a single antidepressant (*n* = 23) with a lithium augmented group (*n* = 21) in a prospective study. The latter group were found to have significantly lower depression severity scores on the Montgomery–Asberg Depression Scale at follow-up and a trend for lower scores on the Geriatric Depression Scale. Although all but one patient in the lithium augmentation (LA) group experienced side-effects, the total burden of side-effects was greater in the antidepressant alone group. The results can only be viewed as encouraging but preliminary. In elderly patients, LA is associated with a higher rate of lithium side-effects than in younger patients. Therefore the necessary dose level is usually one-third to one-half that of younger patients.

Georgotas *et al.* (1983) gave phenelzine to 20 elderly refractory patients with a 65% recovery rate. However, many older patients are intolerant of the older monoamine oxidase inhibitors. A fashionable strategy, that of combining a tricyclic with a serotonin re-uptake inhibitor, is reportedly beneficial to older patients with resistant depression (Seth *et al.*, 1992), but it has not been properly evaluated.

Practice points

There is no agreed strategy for the drug management of an older patient with depressive illness. The following points should be considered. First, a trial of an antidepressant, chosen by tailoring the drug to the patient, should be given for a minimum of 6 weeks provided, of course, it is safe and humane to do so. Second, if this fails, then assuming compliance and adequate dosaging, and after a review of psychosocial maintaining factors (see below), then two options appear possible. One is to change to an antidepressant from another class for a further 6 weeks. This strategy is popular in general adult psychiatry but there has been no evaluation of it among older patients. Third, if these strategies fail or the patient's condition is deteriorating, then either ECT or lithium augmentation can be given. These are the only strategies with evidence for efficacy in resistant depression in older patients. In older patients continuation therapy should be for a minimum of 12 months (Flint, 1992) or longer for younger patients.

Social factors in the management of old-age depression

Services for older people with mental illness arose as a response to the growing challenge of dementia, and social management has always been a major component in old-age psychiatry. Depression no less than dementia requires a multidisciplinary approach, able to address social and psychological as well as medical needs. Ideally, a team serving the needs of older people with depression will include a specialist psychiatrist, CPNs, an occupational therapist, a social worker and a psychologist. Most parts of the UK now have such services, although not all have a full compliment of disciplines. In fact there is little research evidence that manipulation of social factors is of benefit in managing old-age depression, but clinical experience is compelling enough to encourage services to address these factors wherever possible. Here, social factors are discussed under the headings: predisposing, precipitating, and maintaining factors, albeit with some overlap between these categories. Although the first two seem more relevant to aetiology than management, an appreciation of them is important in planning social care. Accordingly, they will be briefly discussed first.

Predisposing factors

Age

There is an increased prevalence of depressive symptoms in the elderly compared with the younger population, although not an increased prevalence of
depressive disorder as defined by standard diagnostic criteria. Within elderly
populations some suggest that there is a slightly increased risk of depression
in the very old (Blazer *et al.*, 1987; Warheit *et al.*, 1975).

Gender

In younger people, females are at greater risk of depression than males, but in
extreme old age this sex difference is less obvious (Krause, 1986c; George,
1988, 1992).

Race

In the elderly, any differences are very small, although some suggest non-
whites are at slightly greater risk of depression (Warheit *et al.*, 1975; Myers *et
al.*, 1984; Blazer *et al.*, 1985; George, 1992).

Urban vs. rural residence

Crowell *et al.* (1986) and George (1992) found minimal differences in rates of
depression in the old in contrast to some studies of younger people which
have suggested depression is more prevalent in urban residents.

Socioeconomic status

Indicators of low socioeconomic status such as low income or occupational
status are risk factors for depression in mixed age samples. George (1992)
suggests that in the elderly these risk factors may be less significant.

Marital status

The never-married and even more so the divorced or separated are at greater
risk of depression than those who are married, and marriage may be a stronger
protective factor in the old than in the young (George, 1992).

Early life experience

Parental loss, childhood poverty and sexual assault have been shown to predispose to depression in the elderly (Kaminsky, 1978; McMordie & Blom, 1979) as well as younger people.

Education

Lower levels of education have been shown to be related to greater risk of depression in later life in age heterogenous samples. However, a study by George (1992) suggests this relationship may be weaker in the old.

Social support

Brown and Harris (1978) proposed that lack of social support is one of a number of vulnerability factors which may increase the risk of depression in the presence of a provoking agent. Older people generally have fewer social contacts and sources of support. Murphy (1982) suggests that among the elderly a confidant may act as a buffer against social losses and therefore against depression. Older people with a life-long inability to form intimate relationships are more susceptible to depression given an adverse life event. Emmerson *et al.* (1989) found the absence of a confidant to be a striking risk factor for depression, particularly in men. Pahkala (1990) did not find such an association for men, but did for women. Lastly, Henderson *et al.* (1986) found depressed elderly patients at home did not report a lack of confiding relationships, but did report a lack of more diffuse relationships. Studies of older people suggest that those with greater social support have lower rates of depression (Dimond *et al.*, 1987; Holahan & Holahan, 1987; Krause, 1987a; Norris & Murrell, 1984). There is a suggestion that tangible support as well as perception of support is important in the elderly (Krause, 1986a, 1987c; George, 1992). A few studies have found that participation in formal aspects of social structure, for example religious or voluntary organizations, protects against psychiatric disorder in the elderly (Idler, 1987; Koenig *et al.*, 1989).

Implications for management

Theoretically, at least, addressing one of these predisposing factors, social support, may reduce the risk of depression developing in an older person.

A social worker can assess the financial circumstances of the patient, ensuring that the correct benefits are received. Social support may be improved by introducing the patient to a day centre or luncheon club, or voluntary organizations such as Help the Aged or Age Concern. There may be opportunities for promoting new social roles and increasing self-esteem through these organizations. They may offer an opportunity for confiding relationships to develop. Similarly, aftercare visits by community psychiatric nurses or social workers attached to the old-age psychiatry team may serve to increase perceived social support and allow the development of a supportive relationship. In contrast to younger depressed patients, this will often be a long-term commitment, given the high rate of recurrence of depression in older patients.

Lastly, in theory at least, improved public awareness of the potential benefits of social supports in ameliorating or even preventing depression could lead to improved social networks within the community. The Royal College of Psychiatrist's 'Defeat Depression' campaign has resulted in leaflets aimed at the general public; one of these offers advice specifically for older depressed people and their carers.

Although many of these interventions are most likely to act as a buffer against relapse and/or recurrence they may also help with management of the acute episode. Waterreus *et al.* (1994) describe the positive impact of interventions by a CPN to elderly patients with depression in an inner London study. The group with CPN involvement ($n = 47$) had significantly lower depression scores at the end of the study than those who were followed up by primary care services ($n = 49$). The interventions described in this study are informative and included: personal supportive therapy, behaviour therapy and teaching relaxation, encouragement to seek medical advice regarding physical health problems, family and marital work and bereavement counselling. However, the biggest impact in this study appears to have been via improved medication education.

Precipitating factors

Life events

Usually in the form of sudden, undesirable, losses these have been shown to have a significant temporal relationship to the onset of depression. In most studies, depressed patients report an excess of life events in the months preceding the onset of depression (Holmes & Rahe 1967; Paykel *et al.*, 1969; Brown & Harris, 1978; George, 1992). This has also been found in studies of older people (Holahan *et al.*, 1984; Norris & Murrell, 1984; Krause, 1986a). Certain types of loss event are common in old age, for example, loss of significant others through bereavement, loss of health, loss of independence, loss of role, loss of status and loss of income. These events are particularly likely to provoke depression (Paykel *et al.*, 1969). Murphy (1982) found that almost half of a sample of elderly depressed patients had experienced at least one severe adverse life event in the preceding year. However, many older people experience such events without becoming depressed. Interestingly in an Australian study by Emmerson and colleagues (1989), a depressed community sample reported serious life events no more than a healthy control group.

Brown and Harris (1978) and Brown *et al.* (1986) proposed that long-term major difficulties (or chronic stressors) such as marital and family conflict, physical ill health, housing and financial difficulties may also act as precipitating factors for depression in the same way as adverse life events. Similar findings have come from studies of older people (Aneshensel *et al.*, 1984; Ross & Huber, 1985; Krause, 1987b; George *et al.*, 1989). As chronic physical illness is more likely in old age, income is generally low, housing often inadequate and family conflict no less likely, this research is of particular concern.

Implications for management

Management of depression in an older person should aim to reduce the impact of adverse life events wherever possible. These in the main involve loss and it is essential to address such triggers as soon as practically possible, that is after depressive symptoms have remitted sufficiently. Specific areas to address are bereavement (see next section) and help to adjust to altered (lost) physical health. The strategies employed are no different from those adopted with younger patients.

Change in physical health should be thoroughly assessed and treatment optimized. Referral to other medical specialists should not be ignored because of age. Many old-age psychiatric services have specific types of liaison with colleagues in geriatric medicine. For example, our own practice in Manchester consists of a weekly joint clinic attended by both a senior psychiatrist and a geriatrician. It may be possible to increase physical independence with aids for activities of daily living and a full assessment of functional abilities and disabilities by an occupational therapist from within the team is helpful.

Chronic housing or financial difficulties may be eased following social assessment by a social worker. Services required may range from financial help with heating or cleaning, to help in finding suitable alternative accommodation. However, although many older depressed people request a housing move, often this preoccupation diminishes with successful treatment of the underlying depressive illness. Anecdotally, it is not infrequent to find a well-meaning relative who has found alternative accommodation for a depressed older person, who then later regrets the move.

It is important to try and understand the dynamics of family and marital conflict where this may have served to precipitate depression. This requires interviews with family members as well as the patient, both separately and together, and is discussed in the next section.

Most patients can be managed in the community. For some an in-patient admission may be required, for others a period of increased support and supervision may be best delivered through a psychiatric day hospital. Once again, whatever the setting, the key to managing psychosocial factors in late-life depression is multidisciplinary teamwork.

Maintaining factors

These are factors which are implicated in delaying recovery from an episode of depression or in precipitating a relapse of symptoms during the course of recovery. There is a need for much more research on the maintaining factors of old-age depression.

Age

There are few longitudinal studies exploring the relationship between age and recovery from depression, but the prognosis seems poorer for older people (Post, 1972; Mann *et al.*, 1981; Cole, 1983; Murphy, 1983; Keller *et al.*, 1986).

Sex

Women seem more likely to recover than men (George *et al.*, 1989).

Marital status

George (1989) found that among the old, married people were less likely to recover from depression than unmarried. Although counter intuitive, the explanation probably lies in the quality of the marital relationship, which may not, in some cases, withstand severe depression.

Expressed emotion

It has been shown that living with a hostile or critical relative and therefore with a high level of expressed emotion increases the risk of relapse in depression (Vaughn & Leff, 1976; Hooley *et al.*, 1986). Clinical experience suggests this is also true for the elderly depressed.

Social support

Adequate social support has been found to predict recovery from depression in the old (George, 1989; Henderson & Moran, 1983). In the study by George, social factors were more strongly related to recovery than a number of clinical factors. Murphy (1983), however, did not find that one form of social support, a confiding relationship, protected against relapse.

Life events

Recovery from depression in old age may be influenced adversely by continuing stressful life events, as found by Murphy (1983), although these findings were not confirmed by George (1989).

Chronic stressors

These may also play a part in maintaining depression. In the case of chronic physical ill health, several studies have found this factor reduces the likelihood of recovery from depression in the elderly (Mann *et al.*, 1981; Murphy, 1983; Baldwin & Jolley, 1986; Schulberg *et al.*, 1987; Wells *et al.*, 1989; Keitner *et al.*, 1991).

Carer stress

Another source of chronic stress which is particularly relevant to the elderly population is the role of a carer which many people (particularly women) have to take on. The dependent relative is usually a parent or spouse, often with physical and/or cognitive problems. Studies have shown high rates of depression in carers (Coppel *et al.*, 1985; Cohen & Eisdorfer, 1988; Gallagher *et al.*, 1989; Schulz *et al.*, 1990), so that interventions aimed at relieving their stress are commonly taken on by the old-age psychiatric team. Hinrichsen and Hernandez (1993) have shown that three factors, psychiatric symptoms in the carer, reported difficulties and poorer carer health, were all associated with poorer outcome at one year from major depression in a cohort of patients with a mean age of just over 70 years. Attention to carers may thus enhance the prognosis of the designated patient.

Implications for management

Many of the psychosocial factors implicated in increasing the risk and precipitating the onset of depression in the elderly also seem to be associated with maintaining it. Continued attendance at a day hospital to reduce the time spent with a hostile or critical relative, to encourage involvement in activities, or to increase social support or the opportunity for confiding relationships may be required. In many circumstances attendance at a day centre or involvement in voluntary activities can provide similar benefits. Regular visits by community psychiatric nurses or social workers to monitor the patient's progress may also be perceived as increased social support and foster confiding relationships, as already discussed. Such visits are particularly important at critical times for relapse of depression such as the anniversary of a bereavement. The burden of care on families looking after a chronically depressed elderly person can be considerable and regular visits may help by educating families about how to manage particular behaviours, or how their own behaviour may be altered to reduce the patient's symptoms. Very occasionally a patient may require regular admissions to respite care in a residential facility to reduce the level of expressed emotion at home and may eventually decide on a permanent move.

Psychological interventions in old-age depression

Paucity of research in this area is disappointing, particularly in view of the problems associated with drug treatment in the elderly, such as increased sensitivity to side-effects and drug interactions, more medical contraindications and frequent voluntary non-compliance. Proven effective alternatives to drug treatment would be very welcome. Some psychological therapies will be briefly reviewed.

Counselling

Since bereavement is such a common precipitant of depression, it is useful to ensure that at least one member of an old-age psychiatric team is skilled in bereavement counselling.

Anxiety management

It is not uncommon for patients recovering from late-life depression to suffer from residual anxiety symptoms. They can usefully be addressed by relatively low key interventions, such as teaching relaxation techniques either individually or in a group.

After a prolonged episode of depression, and older patients do take longer to recover (Schneider *et al.*, 1994), an avoidance fuelled by anxiety may develop to everyday activities. Simple graded tasks carried out with a suitably trained member of the team, or a 'graded discharge' (that is increasing the amount of time at home gradually) if in hospital, can be extremely effective.

Cognitive-behavioural therapy

In elderly patients, this is the most extensively researched psychological treatment. The theoretical model underlying it proposes that cognitive and behaviour disturbances of a particular kind precipitate and maintain depression. Cognitive-behavioural therapy (CBT) has been shown to be more effective than no treatment and comparable to pharmacotherapy in treating depression in younger adults (Kovacs *et al.*, 1981; Teri & Lewinsohn, 1986) (see Chapter 11). Clinical reports suggest CBT is also effective in treating older depressed patients (for example, Yost *et al.*, 1986; Teri & Umoto, 1991). Research with older patients is, however, limited and what exists has methodological flaws. Gallagher and Thompson (1982; 1983), for example, who have made the most substantial contribution to date, used data from a group of self-selected middle-class elderly depressed, who are not representative of the general population of elderly depressed. Therefore results should be viewed with caution, but generally they point to findings comparable with research in younger depressed people.

Comparing groups treated with short-term cognitive therapy, behaviour therapy and insight/relational therapy, Gallagher and Thompson found a decrease in depression in all three groups, but only the cognitive and behaviour therapy groups had maintained treatment gains at 1-year follow-up (Gallagher & Thompson, 1982). In another study comparing three similar treatment groups (cognitive, behaviour and brief dynamic therapy), but with an additional delayed treatment control group, an initial significant decrease in depressive symptoms in all four groups was noted (Thompson & Gallagher, 1984). At 1-year follow-up, 27% met diagnostic criteria for major depression but there was no significant difference between the groups. Similar findings were found at 2-year follow-up (Thompson *et al.*, 1987, 1988; Gaston *et al.*, 1988, 1989; Marmar *et al.*, 1989; Gallagher *et al.*, 1990).

Thompson and colleagues. (1991) compared drug therapy (desipramine) with CBT, and combined drug and CBT. The combined therapy group improved more than the drug-only group, but not more than the CBT-only group, using two measures of outcome (Beck Depression Inventory and Hamilton scale). No significant differences were found between the combined therapy and drug therapy-only groups at post-treatment follow-up. However, on a third outcome measure (Research Diagnostic Criteria) there were no significant differences between the three groups from pre- to post-treatment.

Jarvik *et al.* (1982) also compared drug treatment to CBT and found 45% recovered in the drug treatment group (imipramine or doxepin) compared to 12% in the CBT group. However, the patients were not randomly assigned to treatment.

A few studies have examined the application of CBT to subgroups of depressed patients. Evans *et al.* (1982) found problem-solving to be more effective than no treatment in a group of elderly depressed blind patients. Steuer *et al.* (1984) found that CBT and psychodynamic therapy were equally as effective in reducing depressive symptoms in patients with chronic physical illness. Lovett and Gallagher (1988) reported that depression in caregivers was significantly reduced by CBT or behaviour therapy, and both were significantly more effective than being placed on a treatment waiting list.

Results of other studies suggest factors which may influence the outcome of treatment with CBT. Those with more endogenous depressions respond less well (Gallagher & Thompson, 1983), as do patients with personality disorders (Thompson *et al.*, 1988), or with severe symptoms at the onset of treatment (Beckham, 1989). Also important are patients' expectancies of change and the role they play in the development of a therapeutic alliance (Gaston *et al.*, 1988, 1989; Marmar *et al.*, 1989).

Psychodynamic therapy

Studies by Gallagher and Thompson mentioned in the previous section on CBT suggest that psychodynamic therapy is more effective than no treatment for elderly depressed patients and is as effective as CBT, particularly in the acute phase of treatment. One study has found interpersonal therapy (IPT) to be equally as effective as nortriptyline in the treatment of the elderly depressed (Sloane *et al.*, 1985). Klerman *et al.* (1984) suggests IPT treatment adapted for elderly people is useful in combination with drug treatment. A specific adaptation of IPT for elderly patients exists (Frank *et al.*, 1993). IPT focuses on interpersonal factors that are highly relevant to the elderly. They include role transitions, interpersonal role disputes, interpersonal deficits and grief. Reynolds *et al.* (1992) reports evidence for greater efficacy in the treatment of depression by combining IPT and nortriptyline.

Family therapy

Most old people are part of a family network, and for many elderly mentally ill people the family is the main source of support. Families continue to develop and relationships change as the members age. Family relationships can, of course, have negative as well as positive aspects, and there is evidence that family relationships can affect the course of mental illness.

Ratna and Davis (1984) found 60% of referrals to a community psychogeriatric service were precipitated by events which might be seen to represent a change of some sort in a significant relationship, such as retirement, illness in a carer or a bereavement. Clinical practice suggests that conflict in relationships often plays a significant part in the course of mental illness in the elderly, although research in this area is scarce.

Further progress has been made in this field in recent years. Benbow (1988) describes the development of a family therapy clinic in the old-age psychiatry department in Manchester. Two members of a multidisciplinary team interviewed the family while the rest of the team observed from behind a two-way screen. Following the assessment or therapy session of about 45 min, the team met to discuss the case and the session was then reconvened to feed-back to the family. Although depression was not the problem in all the families described by Benbow and colleagues, the perceived uses of the clinic, for example promoting understanding of a problem within the family context and coordinating support between different family members and between family members and services, suggests that, in the management of depression in the elderly, family therapy could be useful in certain cases. However, there has been no systematic evaluation of family therapy in older depressed patients.

References

Abas, M.A., Sahakian, B.J. & Levy, R. (1990) Neuropsychological deficits and CT scan changes in elderly depressives. *Psychological Medicine*, **20**, 507–520.

Abrams, R. (1991) Electroconvulsive therapy in the medically compromised patient. *Psychiatric Clinics of North America*, **14**, 871–885.

Alexopoulos, G.S., Abrams, R.C., Young, R.C. & Shamoian, C.A. (1988) Cornell Scale for depression in dementia. *Biological Psychiatry*, **23**, 271–284.

American Psychiatric Association (1994) *Diagnostic and Statistical Manual of Mental Disorders*, 4th edn. American Psychiatric Association, Washington, DC.

Aneshensel, C.S., Frerichs, R.R. & Huba, G.J. (1984) Depression and physical illness: a multiwave, non-recursive model. *Journal of Health and Social Behaviour*, **25**, 350–371.

Baldwin, R.C. & Jolley, D.J. (1986) The prognosis of depression in old age. *British Journal of Psychiatry*, **149**, 574–583.

Baldwin, R. (1988a) Late life depression—undertreated? *British Medical Journal*, **296**, 519.

Baldwin, R. (1988b) Delusional and non-delusional depression in late life: evidence for distinct subtypes. *British Journal of Psychiatry*, **152**, 39–44.

Barraclough, B.M. (1971) Suicide in the elderly. In: *Recent Developments in Psychogeriatrics* (eds D.W.K. Kay & A. Walk). Headley Bros., Kent.

Beck, A.T., Ward, C.H., Mendelson, M., Mock, J.E. & Erbaugh, J. (1961) An inventory for measuring depression. *Archives of General Psychiatry*, **4**, 561–571.

Beckham, E.E. (1989) Improvement after evaluation in psychotherapy of depression: evidence of a placebo effect? *Journal of Clinical Psychology*, **45**, 945–950.

Benbow, S.B. (1989) The role of electroconvulsive therapy in the treatment of depressive illness in old age. *British Journal of Psychiatry*, **155**, 147–152.

Benbow, S.M. (1988) Family therapy in the elderly. In: *Current Approaches in Affective Disorders in the Elderly* (eds E. Murphy & S. W. Parker) pp. 44–48. Duphar Laboratories Ltd, Southamptom.

Blazer, D. (1989) Affective disorders in late life. In: *Geriatric Psychiatry* (eds E. Busse & D. Blazer), pp. 369–401. Cambridge University Press, Cambridge.

Blazer, D., George, L.K. & Landerman, R. *et al.* (1985) Psychiatric disorders: a rural/urban comparison. *Archives of General Psychiatry*, **42**, 651–656.

Blazer, D., Hughes, D.C. & George, L.K. (1987) The epidemiology of depression in an elderly community population. *American Journal of Epidemiology*, **11**, 521–37.

Brown, G.W. & Harris, T.O. (1978) *Social Origins of Depression: A Study of Psychiatric Disorder in Women*. Tavistock, London.

Brown, G.W., Bifulco, A. & Harris, T. *et al.* (1986) Life stress, chronic subclinical symptoms and vulnerability to clinical depression. *Journal of Affective Disorders*, **11**, 1–9.

Burke, W.J., Houston, M.J., Boust, S.J. & Roccaforte, W.H. (1989) Use of the Geriatric Depression Scale in dementia of Alzheimer type. *Journal of American Geriatric Society*, **37**, 856–860.

Cohen, D. & Eisdorfer, C. (1988) Depression in family members: caring for a relative with Alzheimer's Disease. *Journal of the American Geriatric Society*, **36**, 885–889.

Cohen-Cole, S.A. & Stoudemire, A. (1987) Major depression and physical illness: special considerations in diagnosis and biologic treatment. *Psychiatric Clinics of North America*, **10**, 1–17.

Cole, M.G. (1983) Age, age of onset and course of primary depressive illness in the elderly. *Canadian Journal of Psychiatry*, **28**, 102–104.

Coppel, D.B., Burton, C., Becker, J. *et al.* (1985) The relationships of cognitions associated with coping reactions to depression in spousal caregivers of Alzheimer's Disease patients. *Cognitive Therapy and Research*, **9**, 253–266.

Crewe, H.K., Lennard, M.S., Tucker, G.T., Woods, F.R. & Haddock, R.E. (1992) The effect of selective serotonin re-uptake inhibitors on cytochrome P4502D6 (CYP2D6) activity in human liver microsomes. *British Journal of Clinical Pharmacology*, **34**, 262–265.

Crowell, B.A., Jr, George, L.K. & Blazer, D. *et al.* (1986) Psychosocial risk factors and urban/rural differences in the prevalence of major depression. *British Journal of Psychiatry*, **149**, 307–314.

Dimond, M., Lund, D.A. & Caserta, M.S. (1987) The role of social support in the first two years of bereavement in an elderly sample. *Gerontologist*, **27**, 599–604.

Emmerson, J.P., Burvill, P.W., Finlay-Jones, R. & Hall, W. (1989) Life events, life difficulties and confiding relationships in the depressed elderly. *British Journal of Psychiatry*, **155**, 787–792.

Evans, R.L., Werkhoven, W. & Fox, H.R. (1982) Treatment of social isolation and loneliness in a sample of visually impaired elderly persons. *Psychology Report*, **51**, 103–108.

Evans, M.E. (1993) Depression in elderly physically ill inpatients: a 12-month prospective study. *International Journal of Geriatric Psychiatry*, **8**, 587–592.

Flint, A.J. (1992) The optimum duration of antidepressant treatment in the elderly. *International Journal of Geriatric Psychiatry*, **7**, 617–619.

Flint, A.J. & Rifat, S.L. (1994) A prospective study of lithium augmentation in antidepressant-resistant geriatric depression. *Journal of Clinical Psychopharmacology*, **14**, 353–356.

Frank, E., Frank, N., Cornes, C. *et al.* (1993) Interpersonal psychotherapy in the treatment of late-life depression. In: *New Applications of Interpersonal Psychotherapy* (eds G.L. Klerman & M.M. Weissman), pp. 167–198. American Psychiatric Association, Washington, DC.

Gallagher, D. & Thompson, L.W. (1982) Differential effectiveness of psychotherapies for the treatment of major depressive disorder in older adult populations. *Psychotherapy: Theory, Research and Practice*, **19**, 482–490.

Gallagher, D. & Thompson, L.W. (1983) Effectiveness of psychotherapy for both endogenous and nonendogenous depression in older adult outpatients. *Journal of Gerontology*, **38**, 707–712.

Gallagher, D., Rose, J. & Rivera, P. *et al.* (1989) Prevalence of depression in family care-givers. *Gerontologist*, **29**, 449–456.

Gallagher, D., Hanley-Peterson, P. & Thompson, L.W. (1990) Maintenance of gains vs. relapse following brief psychotherapy for depression. *Journal of Consulting and Clinical Psychology*, **58**, 371–374.

Gaston, L., Marmar, C.R. & Thompson, L.W. *et al.* (1988) Relation of patient pretreatment characteristics to the therapeutic alliance in diverse psychotherapies. *Journal of Consulting and Clinical Psychology*, **56**, 483–489.

Gaston, L., Marmar, C.R. & Gallagher, D. *et al.* (1989) Impact of confirming patient expectations of change processes in behavioral, cognitive, and brief dynamic psychotherapy. *Psychotherapy*, **26**, 296–302.

George, L.K. (1988) Social participation in later life: black/white differences. In: *The Black American Elderly: Research on Physical and Psychosocial Health*, (ed J.S. Jackson), pp. 99–126. Springer, New York.

George, L.K. (1989) Social-economic factors in geriatric psychiatry. In: *Geriatric Psychiatry* (eds J. Brody & G.L. Maddox), pp. 203–234. American Psychiatric Press, Washington, DC.

George, L.K. (1992) Social factors and the onset and outcome of depression. In: *Aging, Health Behaviours and Health Outcomes* (eds J.W. Schaie, J.S. House & D.G. Blazer), pp. 137–160. Lawrence Erlbaum, Hillsdale, NJ.

George, L.K., Blazer, D.G., Hughes, D.C. *et al.* (1989) Social support and the outcome of major depression. *British Journal of Psychiatry*, **154**, 478–485.

Georgotas, A. & McCue, R. (1989) The additional benefit of extending an antidepressant trial past seven weeks in the depressed elderly. *International Journal of Geriatric Psychiatry*, **4**, 191–195.

Georgotas, A., Friedman, E., McCarthy, M. *et al.*, (1983) Resistant geriatric depressions and therapeutic response to monoamine oxidase inhibitors. *Biological Psychiatry*, **18**, 195–205.

Hebenstreit, G.F., Baumhackl, U., Chan-Palay, V. *et al.* (1991) *Proceedings of the Fifth Congress of the*

International Psychogeriatric Association, p.31, July 1991, Rome.

Henderson, A.S. & Moran, P.A.P. (1983) Social relationships during the onset and remission of neurotic symptoms: a prospective community study. *British Journal of Psychiatry,* **143,** 467–472.

Henderson, A.S., Grayson, D.A., Scott, R. *et al.* (1986) Social support, dementia and depression among the elderly living in the Hobart Community. *Psychological Medicine,* **16,** 379–390.

Hinrichsen, G.A. & Hernandez, N.A. (1993) Factors associated with recovery from and relapse into major depressive disorder in the elderly. *American Journal of Psychiatry,* **150,** 1820–1825.

Holahan, C.K., Holahan, C.J. & Belk, S.S. (1984) Adjustment in aging: the role of life stress, hassles, and self efficacy. *Health Psychology,* **3,** 315–328.

Holahan, C.K. & Holahan, C.J. (1987) Self efficacy, social support and depression in aging: a longitudinal analysis. *Journal of Gerontology,* **42,** 65–68.

Holmes, T.H. & Rahe, R.H. (1967) The Social Readjustment Rating Scale. *Journal of Psychosomatic Research,* **11,** 213–218.

Hooley, J.M., Orley, J. & Teasdale, J.D. (1986) Levels of expressed emotion and relapse in depressed patients. *British Journal of Psychiatry,* **148,** 642–647.

Idler, E.L. (1987) Religious involvement and the health of the elderly: some hypotheses and an initial test. *Social Forces,* **66,** 226–238.

Jackson, R. & Baldwin, B. (1993) Detecting depression in elderly medically ill patients: the use of the Geriatric Depression Scale compared with medical and nursing observations. *Age and Ageing,* **22,** 349–353.

Jarvik, L.F., Mintz, J.M. & Steuer, J. *et al.* (1982) Treating geriatric depression: a 26-week interim analysis. *Journal of the American Geriatric Society,* **30,** 713–717.

Kaminsky, M. (1978) Pictures from the past: the uses of reminiscence in case work with the elderly. *Journal of Gerontological Social Work,* **1,** 19–31.

Kastenbaum, R. (1987) Prevention of age related problems. In: *Handbook of Clinical Gerontology* (eds L.L. Carstensen & B.A. Edelstein), pp. 322–353. Pergamon, New York.

Katz, I.R., Simpson, G.M., Curlik, S.M., Parmelee, P.A. & Muhly, C. (1990) Pharmacologic treatment of major depression for elderly patients in residential settings *Journal of Clinical Psychiatry,* **51** (Suppl. 4); 41–47.

Keitner, G.I., Ryan, C.E. & Miller, J.W. *et al.* (1991) Twelve-month outcome of patients with major depression and co-morbid psychiatric or medical illness (compound depression). *American Journal of Psychiatry,* **148,** 345–350.

Keller, M.B., Lavori, P.W. & Rice, J. *et al.* (1986) The persistant risk of chronicity in recurrent episodes of nonbipolar major depressive disorder: a prospective follow-up. *American Journal of Psychiatry,* **143,** 24–28.

Klerman, G.L., Weissman, M.M. & Rounsaville, B.J. *et al.* (1984) *Interpersonal Psychotherapy of Depression.* Basic Books, New York.

Koenig, H.G., Meador, K.G., Cohen, H.J. & Blazer, D. (1988) Depression in elderly hospitalised patients with medical illness. *Archives of Internal Medicine,* **148,** 929–936.

Koenig, H.G., Goli, V., Shelp, F. *et al.* (1989) Antidepressant use in elderly medical patients: lessons from an attempted clinical trial. *Journal of General Internal Medicine,* **4,** 498–505.

Koenig, H.G., Siegler, I.C. & George, L.K. (1989) Religious and non religious coping: impact on adaptation in later life. *Journal of Religion and Aging,* **5,** 73–94.

Kovacs, M., Rush, A.J., Beck, A.T. *et al.* (1981) Depressed outpatients treated with cognitive therapy or pharmacotherapy. *Archives of General Psychiatry,* **38,** 33–39.

Krause, N. (1986a) Social support, stress and well being among older adults. *Journal of Gerontology,* **41,** 512–519.

Krause, N. (1986b) Stress and coping: reconceptualizing the role of locus of control beliefs. *Journal of Gerontology,* **41,** 617–622.

Krause, N. (1986c) Stress and sex differences in depressive symptoms among older adults. *Journal of Gerontology,* **41,** 727–731.

Krause, N. (1987a) Chronic financial strain, social support and depressive symptoms among older adults. *Psychology of Aging,* **2,** 185–192.

Krause, N. (1987b) Chronic strain, locus of control, and distress in older adults. *Psychology of Aging,* **2,** 375–382.

Krause, N. (1987c) Life stress, social support and self-esteem in the elderly population. *Psychology of Aging,* **2,** 349–356.

Lipsey, J.R., Robinson, R.G., Pearlson, G.D., Rao, K. & Price, T.R. (1984) Nortriptyline treatment of post-stroke depression: a double-blind study. *Lancet,* **333,** 297–300.

Lishman, W.A. (1998) *Organic Psychiatry,* 3rd edn. Blackwell Science, Oxford.

Lovett, S. & Gallagher, D. (1988) Psychoeducational interventions for family caregivers: preliminary efficacy data. *Behavior Therapy,* **19,** 321–330.

Mann, A.H., Jenkins, R. & Besley, E. (1981) The

twelve month outcome of patients with neurotic illness in general practice. *Psychological Medicine*, **11**, 535–550.

Marmar, C.R., Gaston, L., Gallagher, D. *et al.* (1989) Alliance and outcome in late life depression. *Journal of Nervous and Mental Disorders*, **177**, 464–472.

McMordie, W.R. & Blom, S. (1979) Life review therapy: psychotherapy for the elderly. *Perspectives in Psychiatric Care*, **4**, 162–166.

Murphy, E. (1982) Social origins of depression in old age. *British Journal of Psychiatry*, **141**, 135–142.

Murphy, E. (1983) The prognosis of depression in old age. *British Journal of Psychiatry*, **142**, 111–119.

Myers, J.K., Weissman, M.M. & Tischler, G.L. *et al.* (1984) Six-month prevalence of psychiatric disorders in three communities. *Archives of General Psychiatry*, **41**, 959–970.

Norris, F.H. & Murrell, S.A. (1984) Protective function of resources related to life events, global stress and depression in older adults. *Journal of Health and Social Behaviour*, **25**, 424–437.

O'Riordan, T.G., Hayes, J.P., O'Neill, D., Shelley, R., Walsh, J.B. & Coakley, D. (1990) The effect of mild to moderate dementia on the Geriatric Depression Scale and on the General Health Questionnaire. *Age and Ageing*, **19**, 57–61.

Old Age Depression Interest Group (1993) How long should the elderly take antidepressants? A double blind placebo-controlled study of continuation/prophylaxis therapy with dothiepin. *British Journal of Psychiatry*, **162**, 175–182.

Pahkala, K. (1990) Social and enviromental factors and depression in old age. *International Journal of Geriatric Psychiatry*, **2**, 119–123.

Parker, K.L., Mittmann, N. & Shear, N. H. (1994) Lithium augmentation in geriatric depressed outpatients: A clinical report. *International Journal of Geniatric Psychiatry*, **9**, 995–1002.

Paykel, E.S., Myers, J.K. & Dienelt, M.N. *et al.* (1969) Life events and depression: a controlled study. *Archives of General Psychiatry*, **21**, 753–761.

Pearlson, G.D., Rabins, P.V., Kim, W.S. *et al.* (1989) Structural brain CT changes and cognitive deficits with and without reversible dementia ('pseudodementia'). *Psychological Medicine*, **19**, 573–584.

Peterson, P. (1968) Psychiatric disorders in primary hyperparathyroidism. *Journal of Clinical Endocrinology and Metabolism*, **28**, 1491–1495.

Pitt, B. (1982) *Psychogeriatrics*, 2nd edn. Churchill Livingstone, Edinburgh.

Post, F. (1972) The management and nature of depressive illnesses in late life: a follow-through study. *British Journal of Psychiatry*, **121**, 393–404.

Post, F. (1982) Functional disorders. In: *The Psychiatry of Late Life* (eds R. Levy & F. Post), pp. 176–196. Blackwell Scientific Publications, Oxford.

Post, F. & Shulman, K. (1985) New views on old age affective disorders. In: *Recent Advances in Psychogeriatrics*, Vol. 1 (ed. T. Arie), pp. 119–140. Churchill Livingstone, Edinburgh.

Postma, J.U. & Vranesic, D. (1985) Moclobemide in the treatment of depression in demented geriatric patients. *Acta Therapeutica*, **11**, 1–4.

Ratna, L. & Davis, J. (1984) Family therapy with the elderly mentally ill: some strategies and techniques. *British Journal of Psychiatry*, **145**, 311–315.

Ray, W.A., Friffin, M.R., Schaffner, W., Baugh, U.K. & Melton, L.J. (1987) Psychotropic drug use and the risk of hip fracture. *New England Journal of Medicine*, **316**, 363–369.

Reynolds, C.F., Perel, J.M., Cornes, C. & Kupfer, D.J. (1989) Open-trial maintenance pharmacotherapy in late-life depression: survival analysis. *Psychiatric Research*, **27**, 225–231.

Reynolds, C.F., Frank, E. & Perel, J.M. *et al.* (1992) Combined pharmacotherapy and psychotherapy in the acute and continuation treatment of elderly patients with recurrent depression: a preliminary report. *American Journal of Psychiatry*, **149**, 1687–1692.

Reifler, B.V., Teri, L. & Raskind, M. *et al.* (1989) Double-blind trial of imipramine in Alzheimer's disease patients with and without depression. *American Journal of Psychiatry*, **146**, 45–49.

Roose, S.P., Glassman, A.H., Attia, E. & Woodring, S. (1994) Comparative efficacy of selective serotonin reuptake inhibitors and tricyclics in the treatment of melancholia. *American Journal of Psychiatry*, **151**, 1735–1739.

Ross, C.E. & Huber, J. (1985) Hardship and depression. *Journal of Health and Social Behaviour*, **26**, 312–327.

Roth, M., Mountjoy, C.Q. & Amrein, R. (1996) Moclobemide in elderly patients with cognitive decline and depression: an international double-blind placebo-controlled trial. *British Journal of Psychiatry*, **168**, 149–157.

Schneider, L.S., Reynolds, C.F., Lebowitz, B.D. & Friedhoff, A.J. (1994) *Diagnosis and Treatment of Depression in Late Life*. American Psychiatric Press, Washington, DC.

Schulberg, H.C., McClelland, M. & Burns, B.J. (1987) Depression and physical illness: the prevalence, causation and diagnosis of co-morbidity. *Clinical Psychology Review*, **7**, 145–167.

Schulz, R., Visintainer, P. & Williamson, G.M. (1990) Psychiatric and physical morbidity: effects on caregiving. *Journal of Gerontological and Psychological Science*, **45**, 181–191.

Seth, R., Jennings, A.L., Bindman, J., Phillips, J. & Bergmann, K. (1992) Combination treatment with noradrenalin and serotonin reuptake inhibitors in resistant depression. *British Journal of Psychiatry*, **161**, 562–565.

Sherwood, N. & Hindmarch, I. (1993) A comparison of five commonly prescribed antidepressants with particular reference to behavioural toxicity. *Human Psychopharmacology*, **8**, 417–422.

Sloane, R.B., Staples, F.R. & Schneider, L.S. (1985) Interpersonal therapy vs. nortriptyline for depression in the elderly. In: *Clinical and Pharmacological Studies in Psychiatric Disorders* (eds G.D. Burrows, T.R. Norman & L. Dennerstein), pp. 344–346. John Libbey, London.

Steuer, J.L., Mintz, J. & Hammen, C.L. *et al.* (1984) Cognitive-behavioral and psychodynamic group psychotherapy in treatment of geriatric depression. *Journal of Consulting and Clinical Psychology*, **52**, 180–189.

Teri, L. & Lewinsohn, P.M. (1986) Individual and group treatment of unipolar depression: comparison of treatment outcome and identification of predictors of successful treatment outcome. *Behaviour Therapy*, **17**, 215–228.

Teri, L. & Umoto, J. (1991) Reducing excess disability in dementia patients: training caregivers to manage patient depression. *Clinical Gerontologist*, **10**, 49–63.

Thompson, L.W. & Gallagher, D. (1984) Efficacy of psychotherapy in the treatment of late life depression. *Advances in Behavioral Research and Therapy*, **6**, 127–139.

Thompson, L.W., Gallagher, D. & Beckenridge, J.S. (1987) Comparative effectiveness of psychotherapies for depressed elders. *Journal of Consulting and Clinical Psychology*, **55**, 385–390.

Thompson, L.W., Gallagher, D. & Czirr, R. (1988) Personality disorder and outcome in the treatment of late life depression. *Journal of Geriatric Psychiatry and Neurology*, **21**, 133–146.

Thompson, L.W., Gallagher, D., Thompson, D. *et al.* (1991) Treatment of late life depression with cognitive/behavioural therapy or desipramine.

Proceedings of the 99th meeting of the American Psychological Association, San Francisco, Calif., August.

Vaughn, C.E. & Leff, J.P. (1976) Influence of family and social factors on the course of psychiatric illness. *British Journal of Psychiatry*, **129**, 125–137.

Warheit, G.L., Holzer, C.E. & Arey, S.A. (1975) Race and mental illness: an epidemiologic update. *Journal of Health and Social Behaviour*, **16**, 243–256.

Waterreus, A., Blanchard, M. & Mann, A. (1994) Community psychiatric nurses for the elderly: few side-effects and effective in the treatment of depression. *Journal of Clinical Nursing*, **3**, 299–306.

Wells, K.B., Stewart, A. & Hays, R.D. *et al.* (1989) The functioning and well-being of depressed patients: results from the Medical Outcomes Study. *Journal of the American Medical Association*, **262**, 914–919.

World Health Organization (1992) *Tenth Revision of the International Classification of Diseases*. World Health Organization, Geneva.

World Health Organization (1993) *The ICD-10 Classification of Mental and Behavioural Disorders: Research Criteria*. World Health Organization, Geneva.

Yesavage, J.A. (1988) Geriatric Depression Scale. *Psychopharmacology Bulletin*, **24**, 709–710.

Yesavage, J.A., Brink, T.L., Rose, T.L. & Lum, O. (1983) Development and validation of a geriatric depression screening scale: a preliminary report. *Journal of Psychiatric Research*, **17**, 37–49.

Yost, E., Beutler, L., Corbishley, M.A. *et al.* (1986) *Group Cognitive Therapy: A Treatment Approach for Depressed Older Adults*. Pergamon, New York.

Zung, W.W.K. (1967) Depression in the normal aged. *Psychosomatics*, **8**, 287–292.

Zimmer, B., Rosen, J., Thornton, J.E., Peral, J.M. & Reynolds, C.F. (1988) Adjunctive low dose lithium carbonate in treatment resistant depression: a placebo-controlled study. *Journal of Clinical Psychopharmacology*, **8(2)**, 120–124.

19 The management of depression in physical illness

MATTHEW HOTOPF AND
SIMON WESSELY

Depression in patients with physical illness is common, frequently unrecognized and leads to dilemmas in diagnosis and treatment. Depression may worsen disability caused by the physical illness, accentuate pain, affect prognosis and reduce compliance with physical treatments. Physical illness may restrict treatment options for, and worsen the prognosis of, depression. In this chapter we shall give an overview of the literature on prevalence and predictors of depression in the physically ill and some of the diagnostic difficulties implicit in the relationship. We shall then review the literature on physical, social and psychological treatments and their efficacy in the management of depression in the physically ill. This review is based on a MEDLINE search of depression in the context of specific diseases and physical illness in general, plus extensive use of cross-referencing from previous reviews.

Epidemiology of depression in physical illness

There is an extensive literature on the prevalence of depression in physical illness, reviewed in more detail elsewhere (Mayou & Hawton, 1986; Lishman, 1987; Fann & Tucker, 1995). The following is a brief resumé. Prevalence studies have used two broad designs, single disease studies and studies of mixed clinical populations. One of the most studied diseases is cancer, reviewed by McDaniel et al. (1995). Rates of depression ranged from 1.5–50% over 20 studies, with a median value of 22%. Most of these estimates were based on interviews and relatively stringent definitions of depression. Similarly, Cummings (1992) has reviewed the relationship between depression and Parkinson's disease and estimated prevalence from 4 to 70%. There are similar reviews for depression and heart disease (Dalack & Roose, 1990) and stroke (Robinson et al., 1990).

Studies of single diseases and depression allow links between disease process and depression to be explored, and may cast light on our understanding of 'primary' depression. For example, the finding of very high rates of depression in Cushing's Syndrome was an early piece of evidence for the role of corticosteroids in the pathophysiology of depression (Jeffcoate et al., 1979).

Likewise, stroke is strongly associated with depression and there is some evidence to suggest left hemisphere stroke is more strongly associated with depression than right hemisphere stroke (Robinson & Price, 1982), although this has not been replicated (Sharpe *et al.*, 1990; Schwartz *et al.*, 1993). These examples might suggest specific mechanisms in the aetiology of depression, but say less about the overall burden of depression in the physically ill. We know of no physical illness which is *not* associated with depression! This indicates that whilst specific biomedical mechanisms may play a role, the effect of illness and its resulting disability are likely to be important non-specific stressors.

The second approach to measuring prevalence of depression is to use a heterogeneous sample of physically-ill patients among clinical populations. These studies are often motivated more for public health ends than a specific interest in aetiological research, and aim to inform planners and policy makers of prevalence as well as consider issues such as recognition and management. Again, high rates of depression among clinical populations have been found. In broad terms there is a tendency for rates to increase from primary care, to secondary-care (Katon & Sullivan, 1990). From Mayou and Hawton's (1986) review, rates range from 13–61% in medical in-patients and 14–52% in medical out-patients. These estimates depend on the case definition used, the higher estimates being based simply on scoring above threshold on the General Health Questionnaire (GHQ) (Goldberg, 1972). When studies are restricted to those which used the Clinical Interview Schedule (CIS) (Lewis *et al.*, 1992) or Present State Examination (PSE) (Wing *et al.*, 1974) prevalence falls to 13–39% for medical in-patients and 20–45% for out-patients, indicating higher rates than seen in community samples. The prevalence of studies on which these estimates are based use mixed populations of patients, and it is often unclear what proportion have a defined physical disease. Physical illness is not always distinguished from somatization, which is also associated with high rates of depression and follows a similar pattern of increasing prevalence in different clinical settings. Van Hemert *et al.* (1993) addressed this issue in a survey of newly referred medical out-patients. Just under one half of the patients seen had a clear medical explanation for their symptoms and their prevalence of psychiatric disorder was 15%. The remainder with doubtful or no medical diagnosis had rates of 40%. High rates might also be a result of different referral patterns among depressed and non-depressed physically ill individuals. Depression may modify illness behaviour in individuals with physical disease and increase their chance of consulting. In other words, there may be an interaction between physical illness and depression leading to increased consultation.

One recent prevalence survey got around some of these problems using DSM-IV (American Psychiatric Association, 1994) criteria to diagnose psychiatric disorder in 313 acute medical in-patients (Silverstone, 1996). Psychiatric disorder was diagnosed in 27.2% and only 5.1% had major depression. This relatively modest figure (which is still higher than community studies) is probably due to the inclusion of acute patients admitted only, who were then interviewed 7 days following admission, and the use of a stringent modified criteria for depression (Endicott, 1984).

Which patients with physical illness become depressed?

Severity of physical illness is associated with degree of psychiatric disorder, but not as strongly as some might think. In predicting depression in the context of physical illness there is a need to take note of premorbid factors such as personality and past psychiatric history; aspects of the illness, including its prognosis and chronicity; particular symptoms such as pain; treatments, especially those which are painful or mutilating; and social factors such as social support or the effects of the illness on employment prospects.

Mayou and Hawton (1986) identified a few general themes regarding those at increased risk. They suggest that younger patients, women and those with previous psychiatric illness have higher risk. Social problems such as housing, social isolation and unemployment also appear important. These risk factors are similar to those seen in community studies of depression. In a review of risk factors for depression in cancer patients, Harrison and Maguire (1994) identified similar demographic factors, premorbid psychiatric illness or neuroticism, and lack of social support as factors which appear to predict depression independent of disease severity. There is a risk of circularity in determining who is at greatest risk. For example, Godding *et al.* (1995) in a cross sectional study found poor quality of life was a predictor of depression in patients with cancer. Since quality of life is assessed using highly mood dependent ratings, it is not clear whether this is a causal relationship.

Detection of depression

There is an extensive literature on the detection of psychiatric disorder in primary care. There has been less extensive research in hospital samples, but there are grounds to suspect that even fewer patients are detected. Maguire *et al.* (1974) screened medical in-patients with a clinical interview and used case-note evidence to determine whether the clinical team were aware of cases of psychiatric disorder. They found approximately half the cases had been recognized. Factors which increased the likelihood of recognition were uncooperative noisy patients and those with a past psychiatric history. Wilkinson *et al.* (1987) applied a two-stage screening method to detect psychiatric 'cases' on the Clinical Interview Schedule (CIS) among diabetic patients and compared this to physician's ratings. Using these criteria they found that approximately two-thirds of cases would have been undetected. Similar findings have been reported by Bridges and Goldberg (1984) who found 72% of depressed neurological patients were not diagnosed and Pérez-Stable *et al.* (1990) who found that among medical out-patients only 37% of cases on the Diagnostic Interview Schedule (Robin *et al.* 1981) were recognized by their physicians. This study also demonstrated quite frequent misdiagnosis by physicians. Finally, Silverstone (1996) demonstrated that DSM-IV cases were more likely to be recognized by nurses (61%) than doctors (41%). In our clinical experience there is considerable variation between medical specialities in their ability to detect depression. Traditionally, oncologists and palliative care physicians, and more recently HIV physicians, have been unable to ignore the devastating psychological impact of the illnesses they treat. This interest is demonstrated by the predominance of these illnesses in the psychotherapy literature.

Diagnostic dilemmas

One reason for the low detection rates of depression may be that it is seen as an understandable consequence of physical illness. The psychological aspects of depression are 'understandable' in the context of what may be a devastating physical illness. Thus it could be argued that we are not detecting high rates of depression as an illness, but high rates of distress as a normal part of the process of adjustment to disability, handicap or impending death. Furthermore, symptoms of depression and physical illness overlap. Fatigue, sleep disturbance, pain, loss of appetite and loss of weight are features of many physical illnesses as well as being symptoms of depression (Mathew *et al.*, 1981). The overlap in these symptoms could lead to artefactual finding of high rates of depression in the physically ill.

House (1988) has argued that the diagnosis of depression, based on subjective symptoms, is a phenomenological one. Depression is a syndrome, not a disease entity which can be reliably diagnosed on the basis of objective investigations. Psychiatric epidemiologists and liaison psychiatrists require criteria to base the diagnosis on, and if there is overlap between the symptoms of physical illness and depression this does not alter the fact that the individual still meets criteria for depression. Thus studies which have used a standardized assessment such as the General Health Questionnaire (GHQ), Beck Depression Inventory (BDI) or CIS, are valid, because the diagnosis is reached in a consistent manner. If we ignore the problem of possible misclassification from cross sectional studies in physically-ill populations, the main question for clinicians and researchers becomes: 'Does the presence of depression matter in patients with physical illness?' The next section will attempt to address this question.

The implication of depression in physical illness

Depression worsens the prognosis of physical illness

It has long been known that patients with depression have a shorter life expectancy than the general population and that this is not due simply to higher suicide rates (Malzberg, 1937). There is an extensive literature on coping styles in cancer and survival (Greer, 1991). These studies indicate that either a 'fighting spirit' or denial are protective and more depressive coping styles are associated with a poorer outcome. Furthermore, there has been growing interest in depression itself as a risk factor for poor prognosis of physical illness. For example, Silverstone (1990) demonstrated that acutely ill patients admitted to hospital with myocardial infarction, pulmonary embolus, gastro-intestinal haemorrhage or stroke, were more likely to die if they reported symptoms of depression. This finding did not take into account possible confounders; however, the results were striking. We calculated the risk ratio of death in those with depression to be 5.8 (95% Confidence Interval: 4.4–7.6). Subsequently, Frasure-Smith *et al.* (1993) have shown that major depression at the time of a myocardial infarction is an independent risk factor for death at 6 months (Hazard Ratio 4.3; 95% CI 3.1–5.4). Given the high prevalence of depression in this study (15.7%), this result implies that depression could be an important and theoretically preventable cause of death in patients suffering myocardial infarctions.

It is unclear whether these results generalize to other physical illnesses. Similar findings have been reported for patients with stroke (Morris *et al.*, 1993). Our research into chronic fatigue syndrome indicates the importance of a past history of depression as an independent risk factor for poor prognosis (i.e. prolonged fatigue) following trivial (Wessely *et al.*, 1995) and serious (Hotopf *et al.*, 1996b) viral infections. It has been shown that there is a modest correlation between depressive symptoms and hospital length of stay for stroke patients and amputees (Schubert *et al.*, 1992), but we are not aware of stringently designed studies which have found an increase in mortality among those diagnosed with depression in other illnesses.

There are many possible reasons why depression might be a poor prognostic indicator in physical disease. Social class could confound the relationship since individuals from lower socioeconomic groups are likely to have both a worse prognosis of physical disease and a higher prevalence of depression. Depression may lead to poor compliance and motivation to change lifestyle. This is supported by Ladwig and colleagues (1994) finding that patients with depression were less likely to stop smoking following a myocardial infarction, and the finding that depression reduces participation in cardiac rehabilitation programmes (Ades *et al.*, 1992). Similarly, there are reports that compliance is poor in depressed renal dialysis patients (Rodin *et al.*, 1981). It seems probable that a web of other psychosocial risk factors are responsible, for example low social support appears to be a risk factor for dying following a heart attack (Case *et al.*, 1992). Alternatively, specific organic processes may account for the relationship. It is well documented that depression is associated with a wide variety of changes involving catecholamines, corticosteroids and the immune system. These changes could modify the disease process in physical illness. Nevertheless, fashionable though such theories are at present, we are unaware of any compelling evidence to support them.

If the relation between depression and poor outcome for some physical illnesses were genuine, what would this imply for management? In the absence of clear understanding of the causal pathway, it is difficult to be sure whether more aggressive treatment and rehabilitation of depressed patients with physical illness would improve their outcome. Although there are some studies examining the efficacy of identifying depressed physically-ill patients in hospital settings and using proximal outcomes such as duration of hospital stay to assess the efficacy of any intervention chosen by the psychiatrist, unfortunately these studies have not given encouraging results (Levenson *et al.*, 1992). This may be because the psychiatric intervention has been minimal and the outcome determined by powerful additional factors related to physical disease. It remains to be seen whether aggressive identification and treatment of depression in physically ill people affects their prognosis. A more proximal and probably more realistic aim should be to improve quality of life among those suffering from physical disease. For example, it is possible to have cancer and a good quality of life. It is barely possible to have cancer, depression and a good quality of life.

The implication of physical illness in depression

Coexistent physical illness has been linked with a worse prognosis of depression especially in elderly patients (Lyness *et al.*, 1993; Caine *et al.*, 1993). If the onset of the physical illness was responsible for the depression, it is probable that a chronic illness will act as a chronic stressor, so the relationship between physical illness and poor prognosis of depression is perhaps unsurprising. This viewpoint may be overly pessimistic: depression in these patients often may go unrecognized and untreated.

Assessment

Whilst we agree with House's comments on the need to maintain a phenomenological approach in research, in clinical practice it is sensible to give more weight to the symptoms of depression which are not likely to be a direct result of the physical disease. As we shall see, there is relatively little information on efficacy of treatments in this group, so much of the advice on assessment and treatment is little different than that for depression in other settings.

1 *The referral.* Liaison psychiatrists often emphasize the importance of sensitive handling of the referral, usually in the context of patients with medically unexplained symptoms. Even in physically ill patients, referral to a psychiatrist may be interpreted as a sign that the physician is trivialising the physical illness. It is useful to acknowledge the unpleasant nature of the physical illness and then go on to mention how this could be stressful or depressing. Good liaison between the physician and psychiatrists is important, ideally with the psychiatrists based within the general hospital and attached to specific clinical teams to aid prompt referral.

2 *Starting the assessment.* It is often best to start the assessment by reviewing the history of the physical illness. This serves two purposes: reassuring the patient that the physical complaints are being taken seriously and understanding the impact of the illness. If loss is central to the psychology of depression, there are plenty of opportunities for patients with physical illness to experience it. These may include loss of ability to work; financial loss; loss of their role in the family; sexual dysfunction and loss of ability to have children, as well as the more obvious threat of loss of life. The psychiatric history should seek to draw an understanding of these life changes.

It is also useful to gain an understanding of the impact of the physical illness on day-to-day activities. Asking how the patient spends a 'typical day' may be helpful to assess this, and gives an idea of the amount of social support available, and the limits illness may put on them. It is often surprising how little a patient with a serious physical illness may know of its prognosis, or even why they are in hospital. Sensitive questioning about their understanding of the implications of illness may reveal bewilderment and profound ignorance or denial. Patients may have fantasies based on misunderstandings of diagnosis or prognosis, or may not have had the opportunity to discuss aspects of diagnosis with physicians. If this is the case, it is useful to feed this back to the medical team. Finally, there may be aspects of the physical illness which contribute to depression directly, for example the use of depressogenic drugs such as corticosteroids.

3 *Diagnosis of depression.* Since physical illness may cause many biological symptoms of depression, there are specific cognitive features of the mental state examination which should be given special weight. It is for this reason that the Hospital Anxiety and Depression Scale (HADS) was developed (Zigmond & Snaith, 1983). Features of the mental state which should be given more weight include anhedonia, failure of the mood to react to positive events, hopelessness, worthlessness and guilt. The view that such emotions are

understandable and therefore cannot be treated is unhelpful. Physical illness is a risk factor for suicide, so it is important to assess suicidal risk carefully in the normal way, and also to be aware of additional means to this, such as access to lethal drugs.

4 *Aspects of the physical illness which alter treatment of depression.* Physical illnesses may limit or contraindicate the use of antidepressants and electroconvulsive therapy (ECT), as discussed later in this chapter. The patient may be on medication with the potential to interact with antidepressants.

5 *Cognitive assessment.* Dementia is an important differential diagnosis of depression in this setting, especially in neurological diseases such as stroke, motor neurone disease, or multiple sclerosis. Alzheimer's disease is not infrequent in many of the older patients with physical illness and depression may be an early sign.

6 *Effects of the illness on family members.* Close family members are often intimately involved in the care of patients especially if they are severely disabled. The illness may profoundly change relationships, with the patient suddenly becoming dependent. This may lead to resentments and tensions developing in the relationship and spouses are at increased risk of emotional disorder. It is, therefore, useful to see the spouse or other close family members or carers.

Treatment

General comments on treatment

The approach to treatment of depression in the physically ill need not differ dramatically from treating depression in other settings. The complications of suffering at least two illnesses increases the need to take an interdisciplinary approach and good liaison between psychiatrists, physicians, general practitioners (GPs), nurses (both in hospital and the community), occupational therapists, psychologists and social workers is desirable, but probably rare. We shall concentrate on treatments which have been systematically evaluated, but before doing so a few general comments on the evaluations published are necessary.

Randomized controlled trials (RCTs) of intervention for depression in physical illness suffer from several common faults: they are all small, some with as few as 10 patients in each group. This lack of statistical power is compounded by their tendency to compare several treatments simultaneously. Another problem for researchers is the temptation to examine multiple outcomes, such as measures of depression, quality of life, specific outcomes of relevance to the physical disease (such as physiological measure and inventories of specific symptoms), behavioural changes (such as smoking habits) and so on. Multiple endpoints, whilst desirable from the clinician's point of view, lead to serious statistical problems and raise the likelihood of type I error, whereby the null hypothesis is rejected incorrectly. As if this was not bad enough many of the trials (both antidepressant and psychotherapy) compared several treatments simultaneously. This combination means there are often more endpoints compared between treatments than patients randomized into the trial! Future trials would benefit by specifying *a priori* outcomes such as quality of life.

Physical treatments

Antidepressants and physical illness

The trials we identified of antidepressants in physical illness are summarized in Table 19.1. Placebo-controlled trials of antidepressants in this group indicate in the main that active medication is superior to placebo in terms of recovery from depression. The majority of placebo-controlled RCTs have used tricyclic antidepressants, and found that most patients could tolerate side-effects. Some studies have attempted to demonstrate improvements in physical disease with active medication. Where subjective measures of disease activity are reported there is a relationship between remission from depression and improvement in physical symptoms. However, these changes are not usually paralleled by improvements in objective measures of disease status.

We were unable to find any placebo-controlled trials of newer antidepressants in treating this patient group, although descriptions of non-randomized case series exist for SSRIs (Huyse *et al.*, 1994) and methylphenidate (Katon & Raskind, 1980). There have been few direct comparisons between different antidepressants. The well-documented side-effects of the tricyclics potentially restricts their use in patients with a wide range of physical illnesses. There has been one trial of a tricyclic vs. a SSRI in patients with heart disease which, perhaps surprisingly, found both drugs were equally well tolerated but the tricyclic (nortriptyline) was more efficacious (Roose *et al.*, 1994).

If antidepressants work in RCTs how easy are they to give in clinical practice? In a retrospective study, Popkin *et al.* (1985) reviewed 1649 psychiatric consultations in a general hospital setting. Seventy-eight cases, were selected, as they met the criteria of being consultations for depression in which antidepressants were prescribed and a primary medical illness had been diagnosed. Outcome was assessed using case-note information on the success of treatment. In all, they found only 40% had a good response (i.e. a clinical recovery was noted), 28% had no response and 32% had to be withdrawn from antidepressant treatment due to side-effects. Half of the withdrawals due to side-effects were for delirium. The authors concluded this disappointing result was at odds with patterns of efficacy observed for primary affective disorder.

This study illustrates some of the problems of inferring from the results of observational data. Without a comparison group it is unclear how many of the side-effects were directly attributable to antidepressant therapy, although the overall level of treatment withdrawals is remarkably similar to that observed in RCTs (Hotopf *et al.*, 1997). Nor is it possible to determine the number of remissions which would have taken place spontaneously. None the less this study points to the importance of proper supervision of antidepressants.

Choice of antidepressants

SSRIs have the advantage of greater safety in overdose and being marginally better tolerated than tricyclics. It may, therefore, be tempting to conclude that these should be first-line treatment for this group of patients. The SSRIs are considerably more expensive, however, and the disadvantages of the tricyclics may have been overstated (Hotopf *et al.* 1996a). Tricyclics also have analgesic properties which may be useful in many settings where pain is hard to control, for example diabetic neuropathy (Max *et al.*, 1992). We would recommend that tricyclics are used first line, except where there is a clear medical contraindication, high perceived suicide risk or they were not tolerated in a previous episode. We would not recommend the use of monoamine-oxidase inhibitors in the setting of medical illness due to their interactions with other drugs. Lithium is contraindicated or should be used with caution in many illnesses (see Table 19.2). The usual indications for lithium apply.

The specific conditions in which antidepressants must be used with caution have been reviewed extensively (Cunningham, 1994; Series, 1991; Cavanaugh, 1991; Fava & Sonino, 1996) and are shown in Table 19.2. In general terms the metabolism of antidepressants in the physically ill may be altered by poor renal or hepatic function, low plasma protein and pharmacokinetic drug interactions. Whilst some patients require full doses of antidepressants it is prudent to use a lower starting dose and build it up more gradually. Cavanaugh (1991) recommends taking tricyclic levels 5 days after the patient has been maintained on the lower therapeutic dose.

Electroconvulsive therapy (ECT)

The traditional importance of ECT in the management of depression in the physically ill may have diminished, as the advent of the SSRIs has allowed safe treatment of depression in patients with heart disease. ECT is useful in certain situations where there is urgency to treat the depression quickly, or in

Table 19.1 Randomized controlled trials of antidepressants in the treatment of physical illness.

Author	Design (duration in weeks)	Treatments	Physical illness	n^*	Main outcome	Comments
Veith et al. (1982)	RCT (4)	Placebo, imipramine, doxepin	Male heart disease	24	HRSD: significant improvement on both active drugs, superior to placebo	Extensive cardiac testing
Robertson and Trimble (1985)	RCT (6)	Placebo, amitriptyline, nomifensine	Epilepsy	49	HRSD: no difference between drugs and placebo at 6 weeks	Additional 12-week comparison of high dose
Costa et al. (1985)	RCT (4)	Mianserin, placebo	Female cancer patients	73	HRSD and Zung: mianserin > placebo	
Anderson et al. (1980)	Cross-over (8/8)	Nortriptyline, placebo	L-DOPA treated Parkinson's patients	22	Andersen ratings nortriptyline > placebo	Assessed neurological outcome
Schiffer and Wineman (1990)	RCT (5)	Desipramine, placebo	Multiple sclerosis	28	HRSD: desipramine > placebo; BDI: no significant difference	
Rifkin et al. (1985)	RCT (6)	Trimpramine, placebo	Out-patients with mixed physical illnesses	59	HRSD: non-significant difference	Sample included functional somatic symptoms
Tan et al. (1994)	RCT (4)	Low dose lofepramine, placebo	Elderly mixed medically ill in-patients	63	GDS: no overall advantage on lofepramine	Subgroup analyses suggested advantage of lofepramine in more severely depressed

Study	Design	Drugs	Condition	N*	Results	Comments
Schifano et al. (1990)	RCT (4)	Mianserin, maprotiline	Elderly mixed diagnosis in-patients	48	GDS: no difference HSCL-D: mianserin > maprotiline	
Roose et al. (1987)	Cross-over (3/3)	Imipramine, bupropion	Elderly congestive cardiac failure	10	Discontinuation for side effects: 50% on imipramine had severe orthostatic hypotension	
Reding et al. (1986)	RCT	Trazodone, placebo	Stroke	27	Barthel activities of daily living improved more on trazodone if depressed at outset	
Rabkin et al. (1994)	RCT (6)	Imipramine, placebo	HIV	97	Response rate on HRSD 74% for imipramine, 26% on placebo	Immune measure examined, no difference
Lipsey et al. (1984)	RCT (6)	Nortriptyline, placebo	Post-stroke	34	HRSD: nortriptyline > placebo	
Roose et al. (1994)	RCT (7)	Nortriptyline, fluoxetine	Heart disease	64	HRSD: nortriptyline > fluoxetine	Equally well tolerated
Lakshmanan et al. (1986)	RCT (3)	Doxepin, placebo	Mixed elderly rehabilitation patients	45	HRSD: doxepin > placebo	
Borson et al. (1992)	RCT	Nortriptyline, placebo	Chronic obstructive pulmonary disease	30	Nortriptyline > placebo	Subjective improvement in pulmonary symptoms

* Number randomized altogether.

RCT, randomized controlled trial; GDS, Geriatric Depression Scale; BDI, Beck Depression Inventory; HRSD, Hamilton Rating Scale for Depression; HIV, Human Immunodeficiency Virus.

Table 19.2 Physical illness and physical treatment of depression.

Disease	Treatment
Cardiovascular disease:	
Recent myocardial infarction	Tricyclics contraindicated
Heart block	Tricyclics contraindicated
Congestive cardiac failure	MAOIs contraindicated
	Tricyclics: risk postural hypotension—avoid
	Lithium excretion lowered by ACE inhibitors and diuretics
Aortic or cerebral aneurysm	ECT contraindicated
Hypertension	Lithium excretion reduced by diuretics
	Neurotoxicity of lithium with methyldopa
	MAOIs enhance antihypertensives
Eye disease: Glaucoma	Tricyclics contraindicated
Genito-urinary diseases	
Prostatic hypertrophy	Tricyclics worsen symptoms—risk of retention of urine
Renal failure	Risk of toxicity from tricyclics and lithium
Neurological disease	
Epilepsy	All antidepressants lower seizure threshold
	Maprotiline contraindicated
	Interactions between SSRIs and anticonvulsants (raised levels of phenytoin, carbamazepine)
	Avoid carbamazepine with MAOIs
Intracranial space occupying lesion	ECT contraindicated
Raised intracranial pressure	ECT contraindicated
Cerebrovascular accident	ECT potentially dangerous
	MAOIs contraindicated
Parkinson's disease	Interaction between fluoxetine and selegiline (confusional state)
Migraine	Interaction between lithium and sumatriptine (CNS toxicity)
Liver failure	Decrease dose of all antidepressants
	If severe, tricyclics contraindicated
Gastro-intestinal disease	
Upper GI tract disease	SSRIs may worsen nausea
Lower GI tract disease	Tricyclic levels raised by cimetidine
Severe diarrhoea	Tricyclics may worsen constipation
	Lithium contraindicated
Endocrine disease	
Addison's syndrome	Lithium contraindicated
Hypothyroidism	Lithium contraindicated
Phaeochromocytoma	MAOIs and moclobemide contraindicated
Hyperthyroidism	Tranylcypromine and moclobemide contraindicated
Blood disorders	
Agranulocytosis	Tricyclics and mianserin contraindicated
Sickle cell disease	Caution with ECT, anaesthetic risk
Others: Porphyria	Avoid tricyclics

resistant depression. ECT is contraindicated in patients with a recent cerebral bleed, raised intracranial pressure, brain tumour or recent ventricular dysrhythmia. There is some evidence to suggest that ECT is safe and effective even in poststroke depression (Murray *et al.*, 1986), which had previously been considered a contraindication for ECT. Unfortunately this report involved small numbers and one would be reluctant to make generalizations of the safety of ECT in this setting. A thorough anaesthetic assessment is essential before ECT is given to patients with physical illness.

Psychological interventions

Psychological interventions have been widely and successfully used in liaison psychiatry for the treatment of functional syndromes such as chronic fatigue syndrome and irritable bowel syndrome (Guthrie *et al.*, 1993; Sharpe *et al.*, 1996; Deale *et al.*, 1997). However, the literature is less clear for those with a defined physical illness. The majority of psychotherapeutic treatments which have been evaluated in patients with physical illness have aimed to improve adjustment to the illness and thereby improve quality of life. These studies have focused on outcomes such as behaviours, compliance and psychological adjustment, and might be considered as preventive trials in that most of the subjects did not suffer depression at the outset.

Guthrie (1996) has reviewed the literature on psychotherapy in chronic illness and comments that relatively brief, focused interventions have been shown to have long-lasting efficacy in serious illnesses if they are given early. Thus Thompson and Meddis (1990) showed reduced anxiety and better adjustment when men were given a brief package of counselling following heart attacks. This study used coronary care nurses, which implies that the intervention could be widely available. Other studies in cancer (Burton *et al.*, 1991; Greer *et al.*, 1992; Forester *et al.*, 1993) have shown similar benefits again with relatively brief focused psychotherapies; further studies in cancer are reviewed elsewhere (Fawzy *et al.*, 1995).

Psychotherapy for depression

A range of different psychotherapies, discussed in greater detail elsewhere in this book, may be useful in patients with physical illness and depression. As we have emphasized elsewhere in this chapter, it is important not to dismiss the symptoms of depression in this context as simply 'understandable' (especially in the elderly) and therefore not worthy of treatment. Many of the preventive trials emphasize the importance of relatively simple interventions. Psychoeducation is especially important, given the bewilderment many patients feel for their illnesses. It is worthwhile explaining to patients how symptoms occur and, where appropriate, to describe strategies to overcome symptoms. These might involve giving them a rational approach to self-medication or using simple behavioural techniques, such as relaxation or distraction to deal with pain.

Problem-solving has been assessed in primary care (Mynors-Wallis *et al.*, 1995) and is a brief therapy which may be given by general practitioners or general nurses, so has the advantage of potentially being more widely available than other therapies. Much of the emphasis of problem-solving is on dealing with social isolation and boredom, which are common consequences of physical illness. Cognitive-behavioural therapy has been assessed in two randomized controlled trials (RCTs), described below. As in other cases of depression the emphasis is on understanding mood in terms of involuntary thought patterns. In this setting the therapist would focus particularly on automatic negative thoughts related to the physical illness. For example, following a heart attack many individuals imagine their heart to be a battery which is low in power and have automatic negative thoughts such as: 'if I do too much I will have another heart attack'. Such thoughts are likely to have profound behavioural consequences, and lead to avoidance of activities and adoption of a maladaptive sick role. Cognitive therapy would aim to challenge them and replace them with more adaptive thoughts related to their illness. Psychodynamic interventions have not been assessed in this setting. They are likely to be of most use in patients where feelings of loss are prominent, and adjustment to the physical illness involves demanding changes in role.

Only a handful of studies of psychotherapy in the specific context of depression and physical illness have been identified, and these are reviewed below.

Evans and Connis (1995) examined two group therapies for the treatment of depression in cancer patients undergoing radiotherapy. They randomized 78 patients to receive either social support, cognitive therapy, or a no-treatment comparison. The therapies were given over 8 weeks. All patients were depressed at the start of the trial. Six had died at 6 months when the final evaluation was performed. The main finding was that both active treatments were associated with less depression measured on the Symptom Checklist 90 (Derogatis, 1975) at 8 weeks, but only in the social support group was this improvement maintained at 6 months.

Kelly *et al.* (1993) randomized 68 depressed men with HIV infection to receive either a cognitive therapy group, a social support group or a no-treatment condition. Both therapies were brief (8 weeks) and took place in small groups. They found only modest non-significant improvement for the active treatment groups compared with no treatment. There was some evidence that treatment was associated with some improvement in dangerous behaviours such as unprotected anal intercourse or illicit drug use.

Larcombe and Wilson (1984) compared group cognitive-behavioural therapy with waiting list controls for depressed patients with multiple sclerosis. Subjects were all moderately to severely depressed on the Beck Depression Inventory (BDI). The treatment consisted of 90 min, small group sessions for 6 weeks. The therapy aimed to increase social interactions and give patients a cognitive model of depression. Despite small numbers (only 20 randomized) they were able to demonstrate impressive benefits of treatment expressed as change in the BDI score, which appeared to be maintained at 6-month follow-up.

Interpersonal therapy for depression in human immunodeficiency virus (HIV) positive individuals has been assessed in an uncontrolled pilot study by Markowitz *et al.* (1992). The therapy took place over 16 weekly sessions and used a mixture of psychoeducation and behavioural strategies plus more in-depth discussion of emotions related to grief and interpersonal situations. Within the limits of the design this intervention appears to have been successful with resolution of depression in 20 of the 23 patients.

With so few studies it is difficult to have a clear idea of the role of psychotherapy in the treatment of depression in the setting of chronic physical illness. The results of some of this research are none the less encouraging. If relatively brief, focused therapies could make a clinically meaningful difference to depression and quality of life in physically-ill patients, they might be the treatment of choice as they would avoid possible harmful side-effects or interactions and have the theoretical advantage of bringing about long-term change. Without more complete assessment of these therapies it would be difficult to justify their widespread provision.

Social measures

One of the key parts of the psychological interventions described above is to deal with the social consequences of physical illness and depression. Many losses patients are faced with are social ones, which social measures may ameliorate. A detailed social history and referral to a social worker or occupational therapist is important in any chronic medical illness, especially if it involves substantial physical disability. These measures have not been evaluated specifically in this setting.

Conclusions

In summary, depression in patients with physical illness is common, though by no means inevitable. None the less it is frequently not detected and the consequences of this are likely to be grave in terms of reducing quality of life and worsening prognosis for both illnesses. There is some evidence that antidepressants are useful in a wide variety of physical illnesses. There is rather less evidence for psychological interventions, however, from the evidence available, we suspect that focused treatments which rely on a mixture of supportive, behavioural, educational and cognitive elements are likely to be helpful. Future research should concentrate on the role of simple psychotherapeutic interventions in the patients with physical illness and depression and should concentrate on long-term outcomes such as survival and quality of life.

Table 19.3 Key points.

Depression is common in all physical illnesses.

Depression frequently goes undiagnosed among patients with physical illness, especially in hospital settings.

Depression worsens quality of life and possibly survival for some physical illnesses.

Special emphasis should be placed on symptoms such as guilt, low self-esteem and worthlessness in the diagnosis of depression in patients with physical illness.

Antidepressants are more effective than placebo, although there is no clear evidence that any one class of antidepressants is superior. Choice of antidepressants depends on specific contraindications of the physical illness.

Psychotherapies have not been extensively evaluated in this setting, but there is some evidence to suggest brief structured psychotherapies are effective.

References

Ades, P.A., Waldmann, M.L., McCann, W.J. & Weaver, S.O. (1992) Predictors of cardiac rehabilitation participation in older coronary patients. *Archives of Internal Medicine*, **152**, 1033–1035.

American Psychiatric Association (1994) *Diagnostic and Statistical Manual of Mental Disorders: DSM IV*, IV edn. APA, Washington DC.

Anderson, J., Aabro, E., Gulmann, N., Hjelmsted, A. & Pederson, H.E. (1980) Anti-depressive treatment in Parkinson's disease. *Acta Psychiatrica Scandinavica*, **62**, 210–219.

Borson, S., McDonald, G.J., Gayle, T., Deffebach, M., Lakshiminarayan, S. & VanTuinen, C. (1992) Improvement in mood, physical symptoms, and function with nortriptyline in patients with chronic obstructive airways disease. *Psychosomatics*, **33**, 190–201.

Bridges, K.W. & Goldberg, D.P. (1984) Psychiatric illness in inpatients with neurological disorders: patients' views on discussion of emotional problems with neurologists. *British Medical Journal*, **289**, 654–658.

Burton, M.V., Parker, R.W. & Wollner, J.M. (1991) The psychotherapeutic value of a 'chat': a verbal response modes study of a placebo attention control with breast cancer patients. *Psychotherapy Research*, **1**, 39–61.

Caine, E.D., Lyness, J.M. & King, D.A. (1993) Reconsidering depression in the elderly. *American Journal of Geriatric Psychiatry*, **1**, 4–20.

Case, R.B., Moss, A.J., Case, N., McDermott, M. & Eberly, S. (1992) Living alone after myocardial infarction: impact on prognosis. *Journal of the American Medical Association*, **267**, 515–519.

Cavanaugh, S.v.A. (1991) Depression in the medically ill. In: *Handbook of Studies on General Hospital Psychiatry* (eds. Judd, Burrows and Lipsitt), pp. 281–303. B.V. Elsevier, Amsterdam.

Costa, D., Mogos, I. & Toma, T. (1985) Efficacy and safety of mianserin in the treatment of depression of women with cancer. *Acta Psychiatrica Scandinavica*, **72** (Suppl. 320), 85–92.

Cummings, J.L. (1992) Depression and Parkinson's Disease: a review. *American Journal of Psychiatry*, **149**, 443–454.

Cunningham, L.A. (1994) Depression in the medically ill: choosing an antidepressant. *Journal of Clinical Psychiatry*, **55**, 90–97.

Dalack, G.W. & Roose, S.P. (1990) Perspectives on the relationship between cardiovascular disease and affective disorder. *Journal of Clinical Psychiatry*, **51** (Suppl. 7), 4–9.

Deale, A., Chalder, T., Marks, I. & Wessely, S. (1997) A randomised controlled trial of cognitive behavior therapy for chronic fatigue syndrome. *American Journal of Psychiatry*, **154**, 408–414.

Derogatis, L.R. (1975) *The SCL-90*. Johns Hopkins University, Baltimore.

Endicott, J. (1984) Measurement of depression in patients with cancer. *Cancer*, **53** (Suppl.), 2243–2248.

Evans, R.L. & Connis, R.T. (1995) Comparison of brief group therapies for depressed cancer patients receiving radiation treatment. *Public Health Reports*, **11**, 306–311.

Fann, J.R. & Tucker, G.J. (1995) Mood disorders with general medical conditions. *Current Opinion in Psychiatry*, **8**, 13–18.

Fava, G.A. & Sonino, N. (1996) Depression associated with medical illness. *Drug Therapy*, **5**, 175–189.

Fawzy, F.I., Fawzy, N.W., Arndt, L.A. & Pasnau, R.O. (1995) Critical review of psychosocial interventions in cancer care. *Archives of General Psychiatry*, **52**, 100–113.

Forester, B., Kornfeld, D.S., Fleiss, J.L. & Thompson, S. (1993) Group psychotherapy during radiotherapy: effects on emotional and physical distress. *American Journal of Psychiatry*, **150**, 1700–1706.

Frasure-Smith, N., Lesperance, F. & Talajic, M. (1993) Depression following myocardial infarction: impact on 6-month survival. *Journal of the American Medical Association*, **270**, 1819–1825.

Godding, P.R., McAnulty, R.D., Wittrock, D.A., Britt, D.M. & Khansur, T. (1995) Predictors of depression among male cancer patients. *Journal of Nervous Mental Disorders*, **183**, 95–98.

Goldberg, D. (1972) *The Detection of Psychiatric Illness by Questionnaire*. Oxford University Press, London.

Greer, S. (1991) Psychological response to cancer and survival. *Psychological Medicine*, **21**, 43–49.

Greer, S., Moorey, S., Baruch, J.D.R. *et al.* (1992) Adjuvant psychological therapy for patients with cancer: a prospective randomised trial. *British Medical Journal*, **304**, 675–680.

Guthrie, E. (1996) Emotional disorder in chronic illness: psychotherapeutic interventions. *British Journal of Psychiatry*, **168**, 265–273.

Guthrie, E., Creed, F., Dawson, D. & Tomenson, B. (1993) A randomised controlled trial of psychotherapy in patients with refractory irritable bowel syndrome. *British Journal of Psychiatry*, **163**, 315–321.

Harrison, J. & Maguire, P. (1994) Predictors of psychiatric morbidity in cancer patients. *British Journal of Psychiatry*, **165** (5), 593–598.

Hotopf, M., Hardy, R. & Lewis, G. (submitted) Discontinuation rates of SSRIs and tricyclic anti-depressants: a meta-analysis and investigation of heterogeneity. *British Journal of Psychiatry*, **170**, 120–127.

Hotopf, M.H., Lewis, G. & Normand, C. (1996a) Are SSRIs a cost effective alternative to tricyclics? *British Journal of Psychiatry*, **168**, 404–409.

Hotopf, M.H., Noah, N. & Wessely, S. (1996b) Chronic fatigue and psychiatric morbidity following viral meningitis: a controlled study. *Journal of Neurology, Neurosurgery and Psychiatry*, **6**, 504–509.

House, A. (1988) Mood disorders in the physically ill—problems of definition and measurement. *Journal of Psychosomatic Research*, **32**, 345–353.

Huyse, F.J., Zwaan, W.A. & Kupka, R. (1994) The applicability of antidepressant in the depressed medically ill: an open clinical trial with fluoxetine. *Journal of Psychosomatic Research*, **38**, 695–702.

Jeffcoate, W.J., Silverstone, J.T., Edwards, C.R.W. & Besser, G.M. (1979) Psychiatric manifestations of Cushing's Syndrome: response to lowering of plasma cortisol. *Quarterly Journal of Medicine*, **191**, 465–472.

Katon, W. & Raskind, M. (1980) Treatment of depression in the medically ill elderly with methylphenidate. *American Journal of Psychiatry*, **137**, 963–965.

Katon, W. & Sullivan, M.D. (1990) Depression and chronic medical illness. *Journal of Clinical Psychiatry*, **51**, 3–11.

Kelly, J.A., Murphy, D.A., Bahr, G.R. *et al.* (1993) Outcome of cognitive-behavioural and support group brief therapies for depressed, HIV infected persons. *American Journal of Psychiatry*, **150**, 1679–1686.

Ladwig, K.H., Roll, G., Breithardt, G., Budde, T. & Borggrefe, M. (1994) Post-infarction depression and incomplete recovery 6 months after acute myocardial infarction. *Lancet*, **343**, 20–23.

Lakshmanan, M., Mion, L.C. & Frengly, J.D. (1986) Effective low dose tricyclic antidepressant treatment for depressed geriatric rehabilitation patients: a double-blind study. *Journal of the American Geriatric Association*, **34**, 421–426.

Larcombe, N.A. & Wilson, P.H. (1984) An evaluation of cognitive-behaviour therapy for depression in patients with multiple sclerosis. *British Journal of Psychiatry*, **145**, 366–371.

Levenson, J.L., Hamer, R.M. & Rossiter, L.F. (1992) A randomized controlled study of psychiatric consultations by screening general medical inpatients. *American Journal of Psychiatry*, **149**, 631–637.

Lewis, G., Pelosi, A.J., Araya, R. & Dunn, G. (1992) Measuring psychiatric disorder in the community: a standardised assessment for lay interviewers. *Psychological Medicine*, **22**, 465–486.

Lipsey, J.R., Robinson, R.G., Pearlson, G.D., Rao, K. & Price, T.R. (1984) Nortriptyline treatment of post-stroke depression: a double blind study. *Lancet*, **1**, 297–300.

Lishman, W.A. (1998) *Organic Psychiatry*, 3rd edn. Blackwell Science, Oxford.

Lyness, J.M., Caine, E.D., Conwell, Y., King, D.A. & Cox, C. (1993) Depressive symptoms, medical illness, and functional status in depressed psychiatric inpatients. *American Journal of Psychiatry*, **15**, 910–915.

Maguire, G.P., Julier, D.L., Hawton, K.E. & Bancroft, J.H.J. (1974) Psychiatric morbidity and referral on two general medical wards. *British Medical Journal*, **1**, 268–270.

Malzberg, B. (1937) Mortality among patients with involution melancholia. *American Journal of Psychiatry*, **93**, 1231–1238.

Markowitz, J.C., Klerman, G.L. & Perry, S.W. (1992) Interpersonal psychotherapy of depressed HIV positive outpatients. *Hospital Community Psychiatry*, **43**, 885–890.

Mathew, R.J., Weinman, M.L. & Mirabi, M. (1981) Physical symptoms of depression. *British Journal of Psychiatry*, **139**, 293–296.

Mayou, R. & Hawton, K. (1986) Psychiatric disorder in the general hospital. *British Journal of Psychiatry*, **149**, 172–190.

Max, M.B., Lynch, S.A., Muir, J., Shoaf, S.E., Smoller, B. & Dubner, R. (1992) Effects of desipramine, amitriptyline, and fluoxetine on pain in diabetic neuropathy. *New England Journal of Medicine*, **326**, 1250–1256.

McDaniel, J.S., Musselman, D.L., Porter, M.R., Reed, D.A. & Nemeroff, C.B. (1995) Depression in patients with cancer: diagnosis, biology and treatment. *Archives of General Psychiatry*, **52**, 89–99.

Morris, P.L.P., Robinson, R.G. & Samuels, J. (1993) Depression, introversion and mortality following stroke. *Australian and New Zealand Journal of Psychiatry*, **27**, 443–449.

Murray, G.B., Shea, V. & Conn, D.K. (1986) Electroconvulsive therapy for poststroke depression. *Journal of Clinical Psychiatry*, **47**, 258–260.

Mynors-Wallis, L.M., Gath, G.H., Lloyd-Thomas, A.R. & Tomlinson, D. (1995) Randomised controlled trial comparing problem solving treatment with amitriptyline and placebo for major depression in primary care. *British Medical Journal*, **310**, 441–445.

Pérez-Stable, E.J., Miranda, J., Munoz, R.F. & Ying, Y.W. (1990) Depression in medical outpatients: underrecognition and misdiagnosis. *Archives of Internal Medicine*, **150**, 1083–1088.

Popkin, M.K., Callies, A.L. & Mackenzie, T.B. (1985) The outcome of antidepressant use in the medically ill. *Archives of General Psychiatry*, **42**, 1160–1163.

Rabkin, J.G., Rabkin, R., Harrison, W. & Wagner, G. (1994) Effect of imipramine on mood and enumerative measures of immune status in depressed patients with HIV disease. *American Journal of Psychiatry*, **151**, 516–523.

Reding, M.J., Orto, L.A., Winter, S.W., Fortuna, I.M., Di Ponte, P. & McDowell, F.H. (1986) Antidepressant therapy after stroke. *Archives of Neurology*, **43**, 763–765.

Rifkin, A., Reardon, G., Siris, S. *et al.* (1985) Trimipramine in physical illness with depression. *Journal of Clinical Psychiatry*, **46**, 4–8.

Robertson, M.M. & Trimble, M.R. (1985) The treatment of depression in patients with epilepsy: a double blind trial. *Journal of Affective Disorders*, **9**, 127–136.

Robin, L.N., Helzer, J.E., Croughan, J. & Ratcliff, K.S. (1981) National Institute of Mental Health Diagnostic Interview Schedule; its history, characteristics and validity. *Archives of General Psychiatry*, **38**, 381–389.

Robinson, R.G., Morris, P.L.P. & Federoff, J.P. (1990) Depression and cerebrovascular disease. *Journal of Clinical Psychiatry*, **51** (Suppl. 7), 26–31.

Robinson, R.G. & Price, T.R. (1982) Post-stroke depressive disorder: a follow-up study of 103 patients. *Stroke*, **13**, 635–641.

Rodin, G.M., Chmara, J. & Ennis, J. (1981) Stopping life-sustaining medical treatment: psychiatric considerations in the termination of renal dialysis. *Canadian Journal of Psychiatry*, **26**, 540–544.

Roose, S.P., Glassman, A.H., Giardina, E.G.V., Johnson, L.L., Walsh, B.T. & Bigger, J.T. (1987) Cardiovascular effects of imipramine and bupropion in depressed patients with congestive cardiac failure. *Journal of Clinical Psychopharmacology*, **7**, 247–251.

Roose, S.P., Glassman, A.H., Attia, E. & Woodring, S. (1994) Comparative efficacy of selective serotonin reuptake inhibitors and tricyclics in the treatment of melancholia. *American Journal of Psychiatry*, **151**, 1735–1739.

Schifano, F., Garbin, A., Renesto, V. *et al.* (1990) A double-blind comparison of mianserin and maprotiline in depressed medically ill elderly people. *Acta Psychiatrica Scandinavica*, **81**, 289–294.

Schiffer, R.B. & Wineman, N.M. (1990) Antidepressant pharmacotherapy of depression associated with multiple sclerosis. *American Journal of Psychiatry*, **147**, 1493–1497.

Schubert, D.S.P., Burns, R., Paras, W. & Sioson, E. (1992) Increase of medical hospital length of stay by depression in stroke and amputation patients: a pilot study. *Psychotherapy and Psychosomatics* **57**, 61–66.

Schwartz, J.A., Speed, N.M., Brunberg, J.A., Brewer, T.L., Brown, M. & Greden, J.F. (1993) Depression in stroke rehabilitation. *Biological Psychiatry*, **33**, 694–699.

Series, H.G. (1991) Drug treatments of depression in medically ill patients. *Journal of Psychosomatic Research*, **36**, 1–16.

Sharpe, M., Hawton, K., House, A. *et al.* (1990) Mood disorders in long-term survivors of stroke: associations with brain lesion location and volume. *Psychological Medicine*, **2**, 815–828.

Sharpe, M., Hawton, K., Simkin, S. *et al.* (1996) Cognitive therapy for chronic fatigue syndrome: a randomized controlled trial. *British Medical Journal*, **312**, 22–26.

Silverstone, P.H. (1990) Depression increases mortality and morbidity in acute life-threatening medical illness. *Journal of Psychosomatic Research*, **34**, 651–657.

Silverstone, P.H. (1996) Prevalence of psychiatric disorders in medical inpatients. *Journal of Nervous and Mental Disease*, **184**, 43–51.

Tan, R.S.H., Barlow, R.J., Abel, C. *et al.* (1994) The effect of low dose lofepramine in depressed elderly patients in general medical wards. *British Journal of Clinical Pharmacology*, **37**, 321–324.

Thompson, D.R. & Meddis, R. (1990) A prospective evaluation of in-patient counselling for first time myocardial infarction in men. *Journal of Psychosomatic Research*, **34**, 237–248.

Van Hemert, A.M., Hengeveld, M.W., Bolk, J.H., Rooijmans, H.G.M. & Vandenbroucke, J.P. (1993) Psychiatric disorder in relation to medical illness among patients of a general medical outpatient clinic. *Psychological Medicine*, **23**, 167–173.

Veith, R.C., Raskind, M.A., Caldwell, J.H., Barnes, R.F., Gumbretch, G. & Ritchie, J.L. (1982) Cardiovascular effects of tricyclic antidepressants in depressed patients with chronic heart disease. *New Engl and Journal of Medicine*, **306**, 954–959.

Wessely, S., Chalder, T., Hirsch, S., Pawlikowska, T., Wallace, P. & Wright, D.J.M. (1995) Postinfectious fatigue: prospective cohort study in primary care. *Lancet*, **345**, 1333–1338.

Wilkinson, G., Borsey, D.Q., Newton, R.W., Lind, C. & Ballinger, C.B. (1987) Psychiatric disorder in patients with insulin dependent diabetes mellitus attending a general hospital clinic: (i) two stage screening and (ii) detection by physicians. *Psychological Medicine*, **17**, 515–517.

Wing, J.K., Cooper, J.E. & Sartorius, N. (1974) *The measurement and classification of psychiatric symptoms*, Cambridge: Cambridge University Press.

Zigmond, A.S. & Snaith, R.P. (1983) The Hospital Anxiety and Depression Scale. *Acta Psychiatrica Scandinavica*, **67**, 361–370.

20 The management of resistant depression

STUART CHECKLEY

The aim of this final chapter is to make some practical suggestions for the assessment and management of patients with resistant depression. Preceding chapters have summarized what is known about the treatment of depression in the different settings and age groups in which it presents. Depressed patients who do not respond to the standard treatment as described in these chapters are frequently referred for a second opinion with a diagnosis of resistant depression.

Definition of resistant depression

The term resistant depression is used when a patient has made an inadequate clinical response to an adequate course of antidepressant treatment. The definition of what comprises an adequate course of treatment with, for example, electroconvulsive therapy (ECT), antidepressant medication or cognitive therapy is more difficult and will be discussed in this chapter. It will be seen that the assessment of the adequacy of prior treatment is one of the most important aspects of the assessment of patients with resistant depression. The assessment of the adequacy of the response to each treatment will also be discussed.

Although common usage refers to resistant depression as if it represented a distinct and exclusively biological variant of depression, there is no scientific basis for this view. The genetic studies which have been reviewed in Chapter 3 have demonstrated an environmental contribution to all forms of depression, and the environmental model of depression which has been described in Chapter 4 explains most of the variance in onset and much of the variance in rates of recovery in most forms of non-psychotic unipolar depression. This chapter will describe the assessment of the biological and psychosocial contributions to any case of resistant depression from which assessments follow the need for physical and psychosocial interventions.

The order to be followed in this chapter will be that followed in the assessment and treatment of a patient with resistant depression. The first assessment is of the diagnosis and time course of the depressive illness and of any associated (comorbid) mental or physical illness. The second assessment is of the respective contributions of biological and psychosocial factors to the onset and chronicity of the illness in question: discussion of psychological and psychosocial intervention in patients with resistant depression follows logically from discussion of the psychosocial causes. The third assessment is of the adequacy of prior physical treatments and the clinical response to them. The fourth section will describe the use of physical treatments in patients with resistant depression: most of this section will concern the physical treatment of resistant unipolar depression, but the special needs of patients with treatment resistant bipolar, winter, brief recurrent and psychotic depressions will also be discussed.

Assessment of the diagnosis and time course of depression and associated mental and physical illness

Although it is usually a simple matter to confirm a diagnosis of major depression in a patient referred with resistant depression, it is much more difficult to evaluate the time course of the illness which may extend back over several decades. The histories of such illness provide a wealth of information about the effects upon the illness of psychosocial stress on the one hand and physical and psychosocial treatments on the other. Help is needed from independant informants and past medical records if an accurate history is to be obtained. Often it is helpful to plot the course of the illness over time as illustrated in the chart in this chapter (Fig. 20.1)

Comorbidity

Although the diagnosis of depression is rarely altered in patients referred with a diagnosis of resistant depression, frequently a second (comorbid) diagnosis is made.

Dysthymia and depression ('double depression')

The distinction between major depression and dysthymia is important because in the case of depression higher expectations of the benefit of treatment can be raised than with dysthymia. The distinction between dysthymia and depression is not made by most patients, but with the aid of operational criteria such as DSM-IV (American Psychiatric Association (APA), 1994) it can be made with reasonable reliability (Holzer *et al.*, 1996). Both illnesses respond to antidepressant medication (Thase *et al.*, 1996) and so it is necessary to evaluate the effects of past treatment on the two disorders separately.

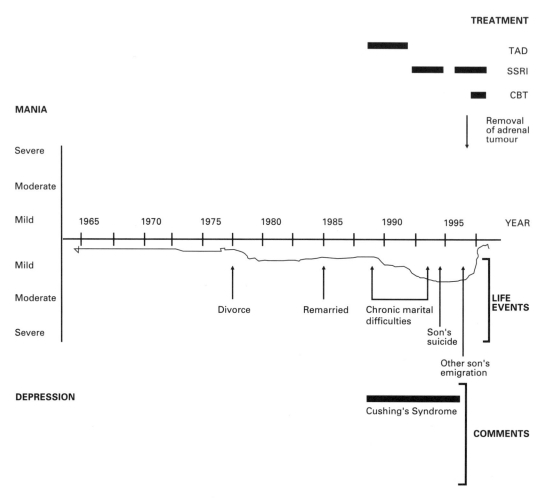

Fig. 20.1 A typical life chart of the course of a chronic depressive illness which shows the effects of treatment with tricyclic antidepressants (TADs), selective serotonin re-uptake inhibitors (SSRIs), cognitive behaviour therapy (CBT) and removal of an adrenal tumour. Also shown are the timing of a number of severe life events and chronic difficulties and the course of this patient's Cushing's Syndrome.

Depression with personality disorder

Confusion between personality disorder and depression should not arise if the episodes of depression are carefully charted and if the diagnosis of personality disorder is based on enduring personality characteristics as assessed in between episodes of depression. There is some evidence from controlled studies that the coexistence of personality disorder with depression results in poorer response to antidepressant medication (Sato *et al.*, 1993), to interpersonal psychotherapy (IPT) (Shea *et al.*, 1990, 1992) and to antidepressant medication with IPT (Frank & Kupfer, 1990). The presence of personality disorder may not effect the response of depression to cognitive behaviour therapy (CBT) (Shea *et al.*, 1990) and depressed patients with dysfunctional attitudes have a better response to pharmacotherapy combined with CBT than depressed patients without dysfunctional attitudes (Miller *et al.*, 1990; Whisman *et al.*, 1991). A particular CBT package has been developed for patients with borderline personality disorder (Linehan, 1993) and the use of cognitive techniques in the management of patients with personality disorder has been described by Thase and Rush (1995). The importance of measuring objectively depressive symptoms in patients with comorbid personality disorder is emphasized by the finding that although a second diagnosis of personality disorder predicted a poorer response to pharmacotherapy and IPT when social outcome was measured, very similar reductions in objective measures of depressive symptoms were found in depressed patients with and without personality disorder (Shea *et al.*, 1990).

Obsessive compulsive disorder with resistant depression

When a patient with resistant depression also has features of an obsessive compulsive disorder, then the time course of the two syndromes needs to be distinguished. The possibilities include:

1 depression secondary to obsessive compulsive disorder;
2 obsessive compulsive symptoms developing *de novo* in a depressed patient;
3 obsessive compulsive traits exacerbated by depression (and sometimes ameliorated by hypomania).

Once the two disorders have been separated it is then possible to target physical and psychological treatments towards each. It will be recalled from Chapter 10 that selective serotonin re-uptake inhibitors (SSRIs) have a particular role to play in the treatment of patients with depressive and obsessive compulsive symptoms (Goodman *et al.*, 1992).

Depression with anxiety disorder

As was the case with comorbid obsessive compulsive disorder, it is the same with comorbid anxiety disorder and panic disorder; and it is necessary to chart the time course of the different disorders. Cognitive therapy is particularly effective against panic attacks and both the SSRIs and the monoamine oxidase inhibitors (MAOIs) can be used to treat most forms of anxiety states. But before planning such treatments for comorbid disorders it is essential to have a good baseline assessment of the severity and the time course of the different disorders which require simultaneous treatment.

Depression with substance abuse

Substance abuse is associated with resistant depression (Rosenbaum *et al.*, 1995) and a systematic history of drug and alcohol intake will reveal undetected cases of substance abuse in some patients with resistant depression. Self-medication with alcohol and/ or benzodiazepines is not uncommon in resistant depression and both tolerance and dependence are seen. An important part of the assessment of such depressions is an attempt to withdraw the abused substances, if necessary with the patient as an in-patient, while trying to teach alternative coping strategies. When depression develops in the presence of substance abuse then the treatment of the substance abuse is the first part of the assessment: substance related mood disorders in DSM-IV are those which resolve spontaneously within 1 month of abstinence. Antidepressant medication has some therapeutic effect in recently abstinent alcoholics (Mason & Kocsis, 1991) in non-abstinent alcoholics (McGrath *et al.*, 1996) and in opiate addicts maintained on methadone (Nunes *et al.*, 1991).

Depression and undetected medical illness

Depression is associated with medical illnesses such as carcinoma, myxoedema and diabetes, therefore screening for these disorders is part of the evaluation of any patient with resistant depression. As with other comorbid disorders, the need is to distinguish between the time course of episodes of affective disorder and the time course of episodes of medical illness (Fig. 20.1). Any debilitating illness or one which imposes physical handicap is a risk factor for chronic depression (Prince *et al.*, 1992).

The effects on depression of treatment for comorbid medical illness

Depression is a well-known side-effect of hypotensive agents which act by inhibiting noradrenergic neurotransmission (Goodwin & Binney, 1971; Paykel *et al.*, 1982) but is also seen in patients treated with calcium channel blockers (Pascualy & Veith, 1989), steroid hormones (Lewis & Smith, 1986) and H_2 blockers (Billings *et al.*, 1981; Billings & Stein, 1986). When one of these drugs is prescribed for a patient with resistant depression then an alternative should be sought.

Depressive pseudodementia

Previously undetected cognitive decline is detected frequently when elderly patients with resistant depression are investigated. Cognitive decline by itself is not a cause of treatment resistance (Reynolds *et al.*, 1987; Reifler *et al.*, 1989; Stoudemire *et al.*, 1991). When cognitive decline is suspected in a case of resistant depression, memory testing is necessary to measure the baseline cognitive state which may deteriorate as a result of subsequent ECT. The differential diagnosis of pseudodementia is well described by Lishman (Lishman, 1987).

Re-assessment of the causes of the individual depression

The assessment of the causes of any depressive illness involves the separate but related assessment of possible *genetic*, biological, medical and psychosocial factors. The evidence for the genetic aetiology of depression has been reviewed earlier and varies considerably with depressive subtype. In the case of bipolar illness as much as 80% of the variance in lifetime risk is due to genetic factors (McGuffin & Katz, 1989), and in multiply affected families the genetic influence of lifetime risk is even greater. In the case of recurrent unipolar depression as seen in secondary and tertiary care, the genetic influence may explain 50% of lifetime risk (McGuffin & Katz, 1996) and in milder sporadic cases of depression, as typically seen in the community, the genetic contribution to lifetime risk is much less than 50% (Kendler *et al.*, 1992). Thus depressive subtype (bipolar and unipolar), course of illness (sporadic or recurrent) and family history are important evidence in the assessment of genetic aetiology.

As well as genetic evidence, other clinical evidence in favour of a *biological* (as opposed to exclusively psychosocial) aetiology of a given depression includes regular periodicity of the course of the illness, presence of the features of melancholia and severity of depression. Each of these indicate that neurobiological changes in sleep and neuroendocrine function are likely (Chapter 3) and that response to physical treatment is possible.

Important *medical* causes of depression include myxoedema (Cleare *et al.*, 1996), Cushing's Syndrome (Kelly *et al.*, 1983), hypercalcaemia, carcinoma and any debilitating or painful chronic disorder (Prince *et al.*, 1996). The careful screening of patients with resistant depression regularly identifies patients in which such medical conditions have been overlooked.

Whether or not the onset of any individual episode of depression is influenced by *psychosocial* factors is best determined by assessment of the psychosocial adversity and vulnerability as described in Chapter 4 of this

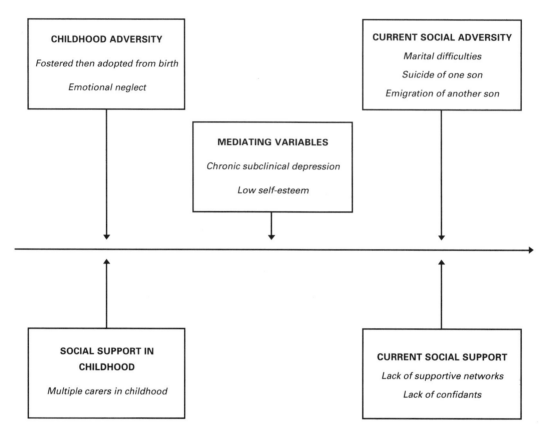

Fig. 20.2 A schematic summary of the psychosocial formulation of a depressed patient. The headings printed in bold type are assessed for all patients. The information in italics refers to the individual patient who is the same individual as in Figure 20.1.

volume. The author's depressed patients are routinely assessed as in Fig. 20.2, using the LEDS (Brown & Harris, 1978) for research purposes, with routine clinical enquiry for clinical assessment. There is evidence that psychosocial adversity and vulnerability explain most of the variance in onset of depression and much of the variance in rates of recovery (Brown & Moran, 1994; Brown *et al.*, 1994b). However, for recurrences of bipolar and psychotic/ melancholic episodes there is no such evidence (Brown *et al.*, 1994a). With the exception of recurrences (not inceptions) of bipolar and psychotic depression, it can be assumed that when psychosocial adversity (see Chapter 4), precedes an episode of depression then a causal relationship is likely. Furthermore, if such adversity continues while a patient remains chronically depressed, then it is likely that psychosocial factors are contributing to chronicity of illness.

Most of the psychosocial triggers for the onset of depression also serve to maintain a depressive illness (Chapter 4). These factors include persistent chronic difficulties (such as long-term marital discord) and additional life events involving loss. Childhood adversity and current lack of social support also predict chronicity (Brown & Moran, 1994; Brown *et al.*, 1994b). Conversely 'fresh start' events, like a new relationship or new job, which cancel out the effect of a depressogenic event or difficulty, predict good outcome (Brown *et al.*, 1992). There have been few detailed interview-based studies of the effects of these same psychosocial influences on response to medication (as measured in a placebo-controlled study), but in one such study social adversity (life events and chronic difficulties) had a greater effect on outcome than the administration of the antidepressant desipramine (Lam *et al.*, 1994). Whether ongoing social adversity and lack of social support interacts specifically in response to antidepressant medication (Lam *et al.*, 1994) or whether it has a direct effect on outcome (Brown *et al.*, 1994a) is a somewhat academic question: either way ongoing social adversity and lack of social support result in resistant depression. Since there are interventions which can influence the psychosocial forces bearing upon depression, it is necessary to identify social adversity when present and to formulate ways in which its effects can be minimized.

Psychosocial interventions

Social support is a critical variable in determining whether social adversity results in onset of depression: it also influences the chronicity of depression (Brugha *et al.*, 1987). The element of social support which has this protective effect is the presence of a confiding relationship, i.e. a close friendship within which it is possible to disclose personal difficulties and shortcomings (Brown *et al.*, 1986). For this reason it is helpful to see depressed patients with their spouses on one occasion to evaluate the communication that takes place between them. Sometimes the non-depressed spouse demonstrates a high level of expressed emotion (EE) and makes many critical remarks about the depressed patient who says little but communicates passively (Hooley, 1986). High levels of EE in the spouse predict depressive relapse in the patient (Vaughan & Leff, 1976; Hooley *et al.*, 1986): marital therapy can help such couples to communicate on a more satisfactory manner. The spouses of chronically depressed patients are themselves by definition exposed to a chronic difficulty and hence are vulnerable to depression. They suffer a restriction in social and leisure activities, a fall in family income and a strain on the marital relationship: 'negative' behaviour is particularly hard for them to bear (Fadden *et al.*, 1987). Family members often say that they need further information about the nature of the illness (Fadden *et al.*, 1987) and this can be provided, for example, in a single psychoeducational group meeting (Anderson *et al.*, 1986). Divorce and separation are seen in as many as 50% of the spouses of bipolar depressives and so this is another reason for offering marital assessment and/or therapy (Brodie & Leff, 1971). A behavioural approach to marital therapy has been shown to increase marital satisfaction even in the presence of significant depression (O'Leary & Beach, 1990). When a patient with resistant depression has little in the way of social support and in particular has no close confidant, then interventions to change this state of affairs are warranted. Patients with chronic depression and marital difficulties can be helped significantly by a combination of emotional and practical help given, for example, by a social worker (Corney, 1987). The effectiveness of a befriending scheme provided by trained lay volunteers has been described by Harris in Chapter 4. Finally, there are a number of excellent self-help and relative support groups which can provide information and contacts with others in similar situations. In the UK, the Manic Depression Fellowship and the Seasonal Affective Disorder Association are particularly recommended.

Psychological interventions

Psychological interventions such as cognitive-behavioural therapy (CBT) can interrupt the mechanisms whereby social adversity influences the course of depressive illness. Thus, low self-esteem (Negative Evaluation of the Self) which is a consequence of childhood adversity is also a vulnerability factor which increases the likelihood that social adversity will be followed by onset and chronicity of depression (Brown *et al.*, 1994a): conversely, high self-esteem (Positive Evaluation of the Self) predicts recovery from an established depression (Brown *et al.*, 1994b). Cognitive therapy addresses these negative cognitions and also the depressive schemata from which they arise (Teasdale & Barnard, 1993). The use of cognitive-behavioural therapy with pharmaco-therapy for depressed in-patients with resistant depression has been described by Scott (1988). Effective coping strategies have a protective effect against social adversity (see Chapter 4) and can be taught as part of a CBT package which includes problem-solving. They can also be taught to patients with bipolar illness who learn to recognize early signs of hypomania. The role of cognitive therapy in this situation is being evaluated at present (Chapter 5).

Assessment of the adequacy of previous physical treatments

Assessment of adequacy of compliance

Since compliance rates can be as low as 50% in depressed out-patients (Wilcox *et al.*, 1965) and even lower in elderly patients (Salzman, 1995) the first investigation to make in any patient with resistant depression is measurement of plasma drug concentrations, together with a pill count and an enquiry about compliance and side-effects. When investigation reveals total non-compliance it is necessary to find out the reasons. It may be that the patient has not received an adequate explanation of the wanted and unwanted effects of the drug, or there may have been troublesome side-effects prior to the onset of therapeutic response; on occasions non-compliance is an expression of the patient's negative cognitions concerning their future and their treatment. When compliance has been inadequate, it is important to ensure good compliance for a trial period of 6 weeks and to measure any symptom reduction using an observer rating scale. Frequent measurement of plasma drug concentrations is needed, and with in-patients medication can be given as syrup. Time spent on educating a patient in simple coping strategies (Cochran, 1984) can bring compliance rates up to 85% (Frank *et al.*, 1995).

Assessment of adequacy of dose and plasma drug concentration

In the absence of clear dose–response relationships for most antidepressant drugs (see Chapter 11) the recommended doses of tricyclic drugs are arbitrary. In the UK 150 mg daily is the recommended maximum (*British National Formulary*, 1996) whereas in the USA 250 mg daily would be considered an adequate dose of imipramine, amitriptyline and chlomipramine, whereas 200 mg daily is considered adequate for desipramine and trimipramine: higher doses are given when acceptable to patients (see Amsterdam & Hornig-Rohan, 1996 for further details). The relationship between dose and side-effects of SSRIs and other recently introduced antidepressants has been investigated more carefully and for these drugs similar ranges of dose and plasma drug concentrations are recommended in the USA, UK and the rest of Europe. In assessing the adequacy of dose of antidepressant it is sensible to ask first whether the locally recommended dose (and plasma drug level) has been followed and, second (in the case of tricyclic antidepressants), to ask whether the maximally tolerated dose of a tricyclic has been used with concurrent monitoring of plasma drug levels and electrocardiograph (ECG).

Assessment of adequacy of duration of antidepressant treatment

There is now much evidence that the time needed to evaluate the efficacy of an antidepressant drug is 6 weeks, most of the variance in outcome being seen during the first 4–6 weeks of treatment (AHCPR Depression Guideline Panel, 1993). One report suggests that much longer treatment periods (of 10–16 weeks) may be needed in patients with personality difficulties and social adversity (Frank & Kupfer, 1990); and in the case of fluoxetine there is some evidence that 8 weeks is needed for maximal antidepressant response (Schweizer *et al.*, 1990). A recent meta-analysis of published clinical trials has concluded that if there had been no symptom reduction after 4 weeks of treatment then future treatment with the same drug would not be of help, whereas if a small reduction in symptoms was seen after 4 weeks of treatment then further improvement over the next 2 weeks of treatment with the same drug was likely (Quitkin *et al.*, 1996). In general, an adequate duration of treatment can be considered to be one which has been continued at optimal dose for 6 weeks.

Assessment of adequacy of response to previous medication

The 'effect size' of any treatment can be defined as a change by one standard deviation in the baseline measure (see Chapter 11). The effect size of treatment with tricyclic antidepressant and placebo have been estimated to be 1.5 and 0.8, respectively (Quality Assurance Project, 1983) which means that compared with placebo treatment an antidepressant drug can be expected to reduce a depression rating by less than one standard deviation of the baseline measure. Fava and Davidson (1996) have reviewed a more recent cohort of clinical trials published between 1993 and 1995. They defined treatment resistance as a fall by less than 50% in the Hamilton Rating Scale after at least 6 weeks of treatment with an antidepressant given in the dose ranges recommended in the USA (see above): treatment resistance according to this definition was found in 29–30% of all studies sampled (Fava & Davidson, 1996). From this it follows that patients with resistant depression can at least be expected to have received only partial antidepressant benefit from prior antidepressant treatment: they may be too depressed and too negative in their thinking to be able to recall which of the many antidepressant drugs produced a small reduction in depressive symptoms. When different treatment regimes are given to patients with resistant depression it is essential to monitor treatment response using an objective measure of depression.

Assessment of adequacy prior to ECT treatment

Since guidelines vary between countries there is no absolute criterion for an adequate ECT stimulus. In the case of bilateral ECT a stimulus which is $2 \times$ threshold is certainly adequate (Sackeim *et al.*, 1990): a right unilateral $2.5 \times$ threshold stimulus is probably also adequate. The practice of titrating ECT stimulus against duration of seizure (Fink, 1992) cannot guarantee that an adequate stimulus has been given (Robin & De Tissera, 1982). This is particularly so in the case of unilateral ECT when a barely suprathreshold pulse can produce a seizure of 'adequate' duration but of no therapeutic value (Sackeim *et al.*, 1987). The titration of ECT stimulus against duration of seizure as recommended by the Royal College of Psychiatrists is, however, better than the use of arbitrary fixed low-dose stimulus which makes no allowance for variation in ECT threshold. The use of a fixed high-dose stimulus (Abrams *et al.*, 1991) is also an adequate therapeutic strategy, although one which may cause unnecessary memory loss.

There is even less empirical evidence to help the clinician evaluate whether previous courses of ECT have been given for a sufficient length of time. Different authorities have recommended that ECT be discontinued if no improvement has been seen after eight (Royal College of Psychiatrists, 1995), six to 10 (APA, 1990), 12 (Abrams, 1992) and even 15 (Devanand *et al.*, 1991) adequate seizures: the author's practice follows the most cautious of these recommendations.

Although there is doubt about the definition of an optimal course of ECT, there is sufficient consensus to be able to identify when a patient with resistant depression has received inadequate ECT treatment. A treatment in which none of the recommended methods for controlling the stimulus was used should be considered inadequate, as should a course which was abandoned on account of non-response before at least eight adequate seizures were produced. In view of the superior efficacy of bilateral ECT over unilateral ECT (see Chapter 12), an unsuccessful course of unilateral ECT should also be considered to be inadequate in a patient with resistant depression. Under all these circumstances a second course of ECT should be considered using bilateral placement of electrodes, stimulus dosing and recording of seizures, and measuring any symptomatic improvement with an observer rating scale after at least eight adequate seizures before concluding that ECT was ineffective.

Alternative treatment options in resistant depression

In the light of current evidence, the following treatment options can be considered in most patients with resistant depression.

Switching from TAD to an SSRI

Uncontrolled studies have shown that out-patients' resistant to tricyclic antidepressant(TAD) treatment have a 30–70% chance of responding to a change to an SSRI (Thase & Rush, 1995). Whether or not it is effective to adopt the converse strategy of changing from an SSRI to a TAD in cases of treatment resistance is not known.

441

Changing from a TAD or an SSRI to an MAOI

Response rates of over 50% have been reported in a number of controlled studies in which patients who had failed to respond to a tricyclic antidepressant were changed to an MAOI (Thase *et al.*, 1992; McGrath *et al.*, 1993). Patients with atypical depression are particularly likely to benefit (McGrath *et al.*, 1993). However, the usefulness of this intervention is limited by the need to have an adequate medication-free 'washout' period which should be 3 weeks for TCAs, 3 weeks for SSRIs (other than fluoxetine) and 6 weeks for fluoxetine. It is sometimes not possible to keep treatment resistant depressed patients drug-free in this way without causing a severe exacerbation of depression.

Augmenting a TAD, SSRI or MAOI with lithium

Similarly, response rates of around 50% have been reported in a number of controlled studies in which lithium treatment for at least 4 weeks has been added to a tricyclic or heterocyclic drug which had been given in adequate dose but with inadequate response (Thase & Rush, 1995). Lithium augmentation of SSRIs and MAOI's has been reported in a smaller number of studies, although features of the 5-HT syndrome have been seen with lithium-SSRI combinations (Fontaine *et al.*, 1991).

Augmentation of TAD with T_3

The evidence that T_3 augments the antidepressant effect of TADs is weaker than is the case for lithium augmentation, although some patients do benefit (Joffe *et al.*, 1993; Aronson *et al.*, 1996). T_3 can cause a moderate degree of weight loss and some anxiety but does have a place in the out-patient treatment of resistant depression.

A number of other treatments including ECT are worth considering in the out-patient treatment of resistant depression. In the author's experience when most of the above treatments have been given adequate trial on an out-patient basis and have not shown sufficient efficacy, then in-patient treatment with more detailed assessment and more vigorous physical and psychological treatment should be considered.

ECT

Resistant depression is a recognized indication for ECT and response rates of ≈50% are found in patients who have not responded to an adequate course of antidepressant drug (Prudic *et al.*, 1990, 1996). Although ECT is the most effective intervention it may be delayed in less depressed patients to allow for adequate trial of other treatments.

Relatively high dose TAD treatment

In the absence of an established therapeutic window for most antidepressant drugs, it is reasonable to conduct an empirical trial of the effectiveness of a maximally tolerated dose if there has been inadequate response to a recommended dose, provided that close supervision of unwanted drug effects is possible. This is particularly appropriate for TCAs providing that monitoring of ECG and plasma concentrations are possible (see Chapter 10 for adverse drug effects).

Precursor loading with tryptophan

The combination of tryptophan with an MAOI needs careful monitoring both on account of the 5-HT syndrome (Sternbach, 1991) and the possibility of the Eosinophilic Myalgic Syndrome (EMS) (see Chapter 10), but it is a treatment that has been shown to be effective in severely depressed patients who were resistant to MAOI treatment alone (Pare, 1963; Glassman & Platman, 1969).

Experimental treatments

For all of the treatments discussed so far there is either evidence from randomized controlled trials of efficacy in patients with resistant depression or, in the case of high dose antidepressant treatment, a clear rationale which is backed up by extensive experience. The mainstay of the physical treatment of resistant depression is the correct use of these treatments of proven efficacy (as discussed above) and most patients with resistant depression can be helped by these treatments, particularly when they are combined with optimal psychosocial interventions. A number of other biological treatments are currently being evaluated in specialist centres and, though they cannot be recommended for general use, several of these have been referred to elsewhere in this book. The combination of pindolol with an SSRI may result in accelerated or enhanced antidepressant response to an SSRI (Artigas *et al.*, 1994; Blier & Bergeron, 1995) as a consequence of blockade of the $5-HT_{1A}$ somatodendritic autoreceptors which normally inhibit 5-HT cell firing when 5-HT release is increased. Another strategy of theoretical interest is the inhibition of cortisol synthesis and/or the blockade of central corticosteroid receptors (Ghadirian *et al.*, 1985; O'Dwyer *et al.*, 1995).

Psychosurgery

As described in Chapter 3, the stereotactic operation of subcaudate tractotomy has been reported to be followed by response rates of 50% in severely depressed treatment resistant patients (Lovett *et al.*, 1989; Poynton *et al.*, 1995). Contraindications include personality disorder and drug and alcohol dependence, but in appropriately selected cases response rates of up to 50% have been reported in patients who have failed to respond to the main treatments for resistant depression. Epilepsy is seen in 1% of cases operated upon but other permanent unwanted effects of surgery are extremely rare. This treatment, which in the UK requires the approval of the Mental Health Act Commissioners, needs further evaluation and is only available at a few specialist centres.

In the case of all treatments for resistant depression it is necessary to monitor both the treatment (with plasma drug concentrations) and the response (using an observer rating scale). This chapter will conclude with a discussion of decision pathways between the above treatments, but before doing so the management of treatment resistant psychotic, bipolar, winter and brief recurrent depression will be considered.

Psychotic depression

ECT is the most effective treatment for psychotic depression and response rates of 50% (Sackeim *et al.*, 1990) and 88% (Spiker *et al.*, 1985) have been reported when ECT has been given to patients with psychotic depression who have not responded to combined treatment with neuroleptic medication and tricyclic antidepressants.

Although less effective than ECT (Parker *et al.*, 1992) the combination of a TAD with a neuroleptic drug achieves partial improvement in 70–80% of patients (Rothschild, 1996). When psychotic depression is resistant to treatment it is wise to use the maximally tolerated dose of TAD with a moderate dose of neuroleptic and to measure plasma tricyclic drug concentrations in view of the known ability of some neuroleptics to inhibit the metabolism of TADs. The combination of the SSRI fluoxetine with the neuroleptic perphenazine has been investigated in psychotic depression but resulted in extrapyramidal side-effects in half of the patients studied (Rothschild *et al.*, 1993). Several case reports of individual patients with treatment resistant psychotic depression who subsequently responded to treatment with clozapine (Wood & Rubinstein, 1990; Dassa *et al.*, 1993) are of interest and merit further investigation. Since most psychotic depressives relapse over a follow-up period of a year, long-term maintenance treatment with TAD is recommended. Neuroleptic drugs are usually withdrawn cautiously once patients have fully recovered in view of the risk of developing tardive dyskinesia: research on maintenance treatment with clozapine and risperid-one is needed since these atypical neuroleptics do not cause tardive dyskinesia.

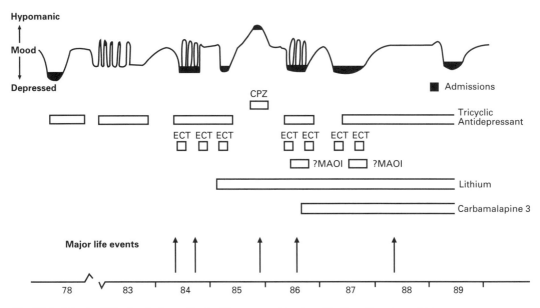

Fig. 20.3 A typical life chart of a patient with a severe bipolar affective disorder, which shows the effects of different treatments and life events. For discussion, see text.

The management of treatment resistant bipolar affective disorder

The physical treatments available for treatment resistant bipolar disorder have been reviewed earlier and will not be discussed further here. In this section of this chapter the general principles which have been developed for treatment resistant unipolar affective disorder will be applied to the treatment of resistant bipolar affective disorder.

1 The most important aspect of assessment is the charting of the illness over time with detailed attention to the number of admissions to hospital and the duration of illness on each trial of mood stabilizer (Fig. 20.3). The construction of such charts is time consuming and involves checking from records of plasma drug concentrations to determine whether prescribed mood stabilizers were in fact taken prior to relapses. Predictions can be made on the basis of the literature reviewed in Chapter 13, but the individual case-decisions about the use of mood stabilizers are made on empirical grounds. In the example cited in Fig. 20.3, charting of the illness revealed that neither lithium nor carbamazepine reduced the severity of illness, that both tricyclic antidepressants and ECT triggered hypomania, that rapid cycling only developed while tricyclic antidepressants were prescribed and that life events had no apparent effect on the course of the illness.

2 In general, the use of antidepressants is to be minimized in bipolar depression since hypomania or mania have been reported to develop in 31–70% of the series studied (Goodwin & Jamison, 1990). Antidepressants

may also trigger rapid cycling (Wehr & Goodwin, 1987) especially in patients in which antidepressants have induced hypomania (Altshuler *et al.*, 1995 and Fig. 20.3). In such patients lithium should be tried as an antidepressant using, if necessary, maximally tolerated plasma lithium concentration (i.e. up to 1.2 nM L^{-1}) (Sachs, 1996). Carbamazepine can also be used for the treatment of bipolar depression (Post *et al.*, 1983).

3 Lithium discontinuation is another hazard since it is followed by relapse in ≈50% of cases (Faedda *et al.*, 1993; Goodwin, 1994).

4 The puerperium is a time of greatly enhanced relapse with rates of up to 50% being reported (see Chapter 17). In view of its teratogenic effects, lithium should be withdrawn during the first trimester, if not for the whole of pregnancy. Fortunately, relapse is rare during pregnancy but in view of the very high risk of relapse during the puerperium, very close supervision is needed following childbirth.

5 The mood stabilizers, which are the mainstay of treatment, are those for which there is good evidence from controlled studies of long-term prophylactic efficacy. As has been described in Chapter 13, only lithium and carbamazepine and (possibly) valproate meet these criteria. It is therefore essential to ensure that adequate courses of each have been given and that the response to each is charted. When bipolar illness is truly resistant to adequate courses of treatment, both with lithium and carbamazepine, selection of future treatments is then made on theoretical rather than empirical grounds. Commonly adopted strategies in this situation are the combined use of lithium with carbamazepine and the addition of valproate and sometimes other anticonvulsants. The rationale for combining lithium and carbamazepine is that each is effective on its own but through different pharmacological mechanisms. The combination may therefore be expected to be more effective than the effectiveness of either drug given alone. The rationale for the use of anticonvulsants other than carbamazapine and valproate is that as carbamazepine and valproate are effective mood stabilizers, very careful charting of the effect of such experimental treatments is needed; but when a patient has frequent episodes then it is possible to determine on empirical grounds whether an experimental treatment such as valproate is of help in an individual case. Other preventative treatments for which there is less empirical evidence are reviewed in Chapter 13, including the use of other anticonvulsants.

6 Patients with good outcome often develop coping strategies such as avoiding sleep deprivation and the extremes of overwork. Some learn to recognize signs of incipent hypomania, such as insomnia, and have agreed with their psychiatrist medication changes to be made under such circumstances. The effect of cognitive, behavioural therapy in such patients is being evaluated at present (see Chapter 5).

7   Social adversity has little, if any, influence on the course of recurrent bipolar affective disorder and there is no reason to think that the course of such an illness can be changed by social management. However, depression is common and understandable in the spouses of such patients and rates of marital breakdown as high as 50% have been reported (Brodie & Leff, 1971). It is for this reason that time should be spent giving information and support to the families of patients with resistant bipolar affective disorder. Membership of self-help groups such as the Manic Depression Fellowship in the UK is recommended.

Light treatment for seasonal affective disorder

Although some patients with seasonal affective disorder (SAD) do not meet criteria for resistant depression, some do, and it is convenient to discuss SAD in the chapter devoted to resistant depression. SAD is, as its name suggests, an affective disorder which meets operational criteria for seasonality. The original criteria of seasonality were that major depression should be present in at least two consecutive previous years in which the depression developed during autumn or winter and remitted by the following spring or summer (Rosenthal *et al.*, 1984). The subsequent DSM-III-R (American Psychiatric Association, 1987) criteria were more specific and required that two-thirds of all onset occurred during the same 60-day window and that two-thirds of all offsets occurred during a second 60-day window. The DSM-IV criteria are less specific but remain controversial, and many SAD researchers still use Rosenthal's original criteria. SAD is characterized by the 'atypical' symptoms of increased sleeping, carbohydrate craving, and weight gain. Many, though not all, cases of SAD follow a bipolar I and a few a bipolar II course (Oren & Rosenthal, 1992).

The treatment of SAD is the same as for any other form of affective disorder with the exception that light treatment is used in the treatment of those SAD patients whose depressions are present only in winter. The best evaluated treatment regimes are those which involve 2500 lux of bright artificial daylight given in the morning from 7:00 to 10:00 and in the evening from 8:00 to 11:00. Treatment response is extremely rapid and most patients with SAD note a 50% reduction in symptoms after 4 days of treatment. Relapse occurs equally quickly after stopping light treatment; therefore if the treatment is effective it should be continued indefinitely throughout the winter months. More recently, to shorten the period of treatment, stronger light (10 000 lux) has been given for just half an hour early in the morning (Terman *et al.*, 1990) and two unpublished studies have found this to be more effective than a 'placebo' treatment which was provided by an ion generator. Despite this, doubts remain about the possibility of a placebo response to light treatment for a condition in which patients expect bright light to help them. As in all patients with resistant depression it is essential to use objective rating scales of the severity of depression—adapted for SAD—before and after the administration of light treatment and periodically thereafter (Terman *et al.*, 1992). When light treatment is effective it needs to be continued throughout the winter period. There is some evidence that light treatment given before the onset of depression can prevent relapses of SAD. In the UK, an excellent self-help group is available: the Seasonal Affective Disorder Association (SADA).

Brief recurrent depression

Brief recurrent depression is a variant of unipolar depression in which the full range and severity of depressive symptoms are present for episodes lasting no more than 2–14 days and recurring at least once a month for at least a year (Angst, 1994). Brief recurrent depression responds poorly to all antidepressant drugs (Montgomery, 1994).

Decision paths and the physical treatment of depression

The decisions which need to be made concerning the physical treatment of most patients with resistant depression can be summarized in four diagrams. Since each treatment decision takes 6 weeks to evaluate it is necessary to be economical in the selection of treatment options. The following selection is based on the critical evaluation of each of these options as described in Chapter 11. Inevitably the selection is a matter of judgement and alternative decision pathways have been described by others (e.g. Amsterdam & Horning-Rohan, 1996).

The first decision is whether the patient is best treated with a TAD, an SSRI or an MAOI. The factors which will influence this decision will include some evidence that TADs may be more effective than SSRIs and MAOIs in more severely depressed patients (Perry, 1996), some evidence that MAOIs may be more effective than other antidepressants in patients with atypical depression (Quitkin *et al.*, 1989), and the different profile of side-effects and drug interactions of the three classes of drugs (Chapter 9). Most important of all is the empirical evidence derived from the patient's history and, if necessary, confirmed by therapeutic trial of the differential effect of the three main classes of antidepressant upon the illness in question. The choice of the optimal class of antidepressants for each patient is therefore made partly on empirical grounds and partly with reference to the literature.

Despite the suggestion raised in Chapters 10 and 11 for several SSRIs and for venlafaxine it is not yet established that there are important within, class differences for the efficacy of individual drugs in resistant depression. The choice of the individual member of the class, therefore, can be made on the basis of the side-effect profiles as tabulated in Chapter 10. Once an individual drug has been selected it is essential to ensure that an adequate plasma drug concentration is obtained, that an adequate course of treatment as described above is given and that antidepressant response is measured using an observer-rated depression scale. The next decision is how to augment the probably modest antidepressant response to the first drug. A different decision tree applies to each of the three classes of antidepressant drug, although in each case the first option is lithium augmentation.

Enhancement of the antidepressant effect of a tricyclic antidepressant

Figure 20.4 lists the options to be considered in the augmentation of the antidepressant effect of a TAD. Lithium augmentation is considered first in view of the strength of the evidence from controlled trials that this is an effective intervention in treatment resistant depression (Chapter 10) and the acceptability by most patients of this treatment combination.

When lithium augmentation is contraindicated, for example by serious kidney disease, or when it has been tried adequately but without success, then the addition of T_3 can be considered. The evidence from controlled trials is positive (Aronson *et al.*, 1996) though not as strong as the case is with lithium augmentation (Joffe *et al.*, 1993). Care is needed since the T_3 may exacerbate anxiety and weight loss, and it may also cause cardiac arrhythmias.

Since lithium and T_3 are the only agents which have been shown in controlled studies to augment the antidepressant effect of TADs in resistant depression, the choice of treatment strategy if they have both failed is arbitrary. The use of high dose TAD treatment at this point is logical. Caution is needed

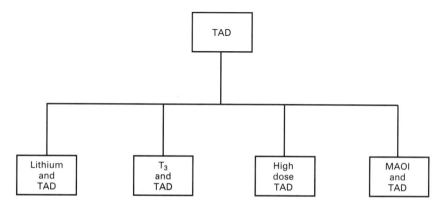

Fig. 20.4 Available options for trying to enhance the antidepressant action of a tricyclic antidepressant drug.

with the monitoring of all the usual side-effects of TADs and the monitoring of the ECG and plasma TAD concentrations is essential.

The final option to consider in the enhancement of the antidepressant effect of a TAD is the addition of an MAOI. Although the evidence for the effectiveness of TAD–MAOIs combinations in resistant depression is not strong (Chapter 11) the combination has been used for many years. The precautions that should be taken include strict adherence to a low tyramine diet, the avoidance of tranylcypramine and sympathomimetic agents, the avoidance of imipramine and chlomipramine (both of which cause features of the 5-HT syndrome in combination with MAOIs) and monitoring of pulse and blood pressure. A further reason for adding MAOIs is that if the combination is not effective then the TAD can be withdrawn and several options for enhancing the antidepressant effect of MAOIs (see below) can be explored. The same logic would also support the addition of an SSRI to a TAD, although again no evidence of efficacy from controlled trials is yet available for SSRI–TAD combinations in patients with resistant depression (Chapter 11).

Enhancement of the antidepressant effect of an SSRI

The first decision to consider in the attempted enhancement of an antidepressant action of an SSRI (Fig. 20.5) is whether or not to add lithium. Lithium augmentation is the only procedure which has been shown to enhance the antidepressant effect of SSRIs in controlled studies. Care is needed with the combination since both treatments increase the availability of 5-HT (Chapter 3) and features of the 5-HT syndrome have been reported with SSRI–lithium combination (Young & Cowen, 1994).

The addition of pindolol to an SSRI is worth considering. Pindolol is an antagonist at beta$_1$ and 5-HT$_{1A}$ receptors and through its action at 5-HT$_{1A}$ somatodendritic receptors has been shown to enhance the effect of SSRIs on

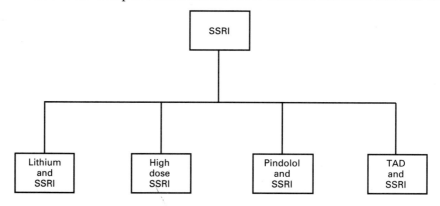

Fig. 20.5 Available options for trying to enhance the antidepressant effect of a selective serotonin re-uptake inhibitor.

5-HT neurotransmission by inhibiting negative feedback control of 5-HT cell firing by intrasynaptic 5-HT (Arborelius *et al.*, 1995). Pindolol might therefore be expected both to accelerate and to enhance the antidepressant effect of SSRIs as has recently been reported in two preliminary studies (Artigas *et al.*, 1994; Blier & Bergeron, 1995). Particular care is needed with pindolol–SSRI combination in view of the limited experience to date and the likely pharmacodynamic interactions between the two.

The fourth decision to make in the enhancement of the antidepressant effect of an SSRI is whether or not to add a TAD. However, the evidence that this combination is of value in the treatment of resistant depression comes only from uncontrolled studies (Weilburg *et al.*, 1989, 1991; Seth *et al.*, 1992).

Enhancement of the antidepressant effect of MAOIs

The safest and best established way to enhance the antidepressant effect of an MAOI is to add lithium (Fig. 20.6) (Johnson, 1991).

Combinations of tryptophan with MAOIs have been used for many years in the treatment of resistant depression and with encouraging results in severely depressed patients (Pare, 1963 and Glassman & Platman, 1969). The combination produces a powerful enhancement of 5-HT neurotransmissions in animals, and in man features of the 5-HT syndrome are seen which limit the dose of tryptophan to 2 g. More recently tryptophan has been withdrawn on account of the EMS. However, the EMS is thought to be caused by a contaminant in the preparation of tryptophan (Slutsher *et al.*, 1990). The tryptophan–MAOI combination should be considered seriously when and if tryptophan becomes readily available for clinical use.

The combined use of MAOI with TAD has already been discussed (above).

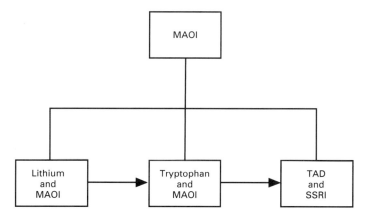

Fig. 20.6 Available options for trying to enhance the antidepressant action of a monoamine oxidase inhibitor.

When to give ECT

Perhaps the most important decision in the physical treatment of resistant depression concerns the timing of the use of ECT. No treatment has been shown to be more effective or more quickly effective in the treatment of resistant depression. Consequently, ECT is used either when there is a threat to the life of the patient (from suicide, starvation or dehydration), or when patient and doctor agree that the likely delays implicit in future drug treatments are not warranted. In the UK, though not always in the USA, it is normal practice for an antidepressant to be continued throughout the course of treatment. This is one reason why it is important to decide as soon as possible which class of antidepressant drug is most effective in an individual case.

Antidepressant 'cocktails'

The treatment combinations which have been discussed so far include the use of no more than two antidepressant drugs at any one time. Drug combinations involving three or more antidepressant drugs have been described (Hale *et al.*, 1987). The intention of such combinations is mostly to enhance 5-HT neurotransmission. Since features of the 5-HT syndrome are seen with several of the two drug combinations (e.g. lithium+SSRI and trypto-phan+MAOI) the theoretical case for a third or fourth drug is hard to justify. It is also more difficult to evaluate the effectiveness of the different components of such treatment combinations. To date, there is no evidence from randomized controlled trials that drug combinations which involve three or more psychotropic agents are more effective than those which employ two.

Conclusion

Most patients with resistant depression gain some benefit from the optimal use of the physical treatments for which there is good evidence from controlled studies of efficacy in resistant depression. The clinical challenge in these patients is to convert an improvement in physical symptoms into a reward-ing change in lifestyle using the behavioural and psychosocial strategies described elsewhere in this chapter. Meanwhile, research into new treatments for resistant depression continues.

References

Abrams, R. (1992) *Electroconvulsive Therapy*, 2nd edn. Oxford University Press, Oxford.

Abrams, R., Swartz, C.M. & Vedak, C. (1991) Anti-depressant effect of high-dose right unilateral electroconvulsive therapy. *Archives of General Psychiatry*, **48**, 746–748.

Altshuler, L.L., Post, R.M., Leverich, G.S. *et al.* (1995) Antidepressant-induced mania and cycle acceleration: a controversy revisited. *American Journal of Psychiatry*, **152**, 1130–1138.

American Psychiatric Association (1987) *Diagnostic and Statistical Manual of Mental Disorders*, revised 3rd edn. American Psychiatric Association, Washington, DC.

American Psychiatric Association (1990) *Clinical Guidelines for the Practice of ECT*. American Psychiatric Association, Washington, DC.

American Psychiatric Association (1994) *Diagnostic and Statistical Manual of Mental Disorders*, 4th edn. American Psychiatric Association, Washington, DC.

Amsterdam, J.D. & Hornig-Rohan, M. (1996) Treatment algorithms in treatment resistant depression. *Psychiatric Clinics of North America*, **19**, 371–386.

Anderson, C.M., Griffin, S., Rossi, A., Pagonis, I. *et al.* (1986) A comparative study of the impact of education vs. process groups for families of patients with affective disorders. *Family Process*, **25**, 185–205.

Angst, J. (1994) The history and concept of recurrent brief depression. *European Archives of Psychiatry and Clinical Neuroscience*, **244**, 171–173.

AHCPR (1993) Diagnosis and treatment of depression in late life: NIH Consensus Development Panel on depression in late life. *Journal of the American Medical Association*, **268**, 1018–1024.

Arborelius, A.Nomikos, G., Grillner, P., Hertel, P., Hook, B.B., Hacksell, U. & Svensson, T.H. (1995) 5-HT$_{1A}$ receptor antagonists increase the activity of serotonergic cells in the dorsal raphe nucleus in rats treated acutely or chronically with citalopram. *Naunyn Schmiedeberg's Archives of Pharmacology*, **352**, 157–165.

Aronson, R., Offman, H.J., Joffe, R.T. & Naylor, C.D. (1996) Triiodothyronine augmentation in the treatment of refractory depression. *Archives of General Psychiatry*, **53**, 842–848.

Artigas, F., Perez, V. & Alvarez, E. (1994) Pindolol induces a rapid improvement of depressed patients treated with serotonin reuptake inhibitors. *Archives of General Psychiatry*, **51**, 248–251.

Billings, R., Tang, S.W. & Rafkoff V.U. (1981) Depression associated with ranitidine. *American Journal of Psychiatry*, **743**, 915–916.

Blier, P. & Bergeron, R. (1995) Effectiveness of pindolol with selected antidepressant drugs in the treatment of major depression. *Journal of Clinical Psychopharmacology*, **15**, 217–222.

British National Formulary (1996) *British National Formulary*, 32 (Sept.). (ed C. F. George) British Medical Association and Royal Pharmaceutical Society of Great Britain, London.

Brodie, H.K.H. & Leff, M.J. (1971) Bipolar depres-

sion: a comparative study of patient characteristics. *America Journal of Psychiatry*, **127**, 1086–1090.

Brown, G.W. & Harris, T.O. (1978) *Social Origins of Depression: A Study of Psychiatric Disorder in Women*. Tavistock, London.

Brown, G.W. & Moran, P. (1994) Clinical and psychosocial origins of chronic depressive episodes. 1: A community survey. *British Journal of Psychiatry*, **165**, 447–456.

Brown, G.W., Andrews, B., Harris, T.O., Adler, Z. & Bridge, L. (1986) Social support, self-esteem and depression. *Psychological Medicine*, **16**, 813–831.

Brown, G.W., Lemyre, L. & Bifulco, A. (1992) Social factors and recovery from anxiety and depressive disorders: a test of the specificity. *British Journal of Psychiatry*, **161**, 44–54.

Brown, G.W., Harris, T.O. & Hepworth, C. (1994a) Life events and 'endogenous' depression: a puzzle re-examined. *Archives of General Psychiatry*, **51**, 525–534.

Brown, G.W., Harris, T.O., Hepworth, C. & Robinson, R. (1994b) Clinical and psychosocial origins of depression. 2: A patient enquiry. *British Journal of Psychiatry*, **165**, 457–465.

Cleare, A.J., MacGregor, A., & Chambers, S.M. *et al.* (1995) Thyroxine replacement increase central 5-hydroxytryptamine activity and reduces depressive symptoms in hypothyroidism. *Neuroendocrinology*, **64**, 65–69.

Cochran, S.D. (1984) Preventing medical non-compliance in the outpatient treatment of affective disorders. *Journal of Consulting and Clinical Psychology*, **52**, 54–60.

Corney, R. (1987) Marital problems and treatment outcome in depressed women: a clinical trial of social work intervention. *British Journal of Psychiatry*, **151**, 652–659.

Dassa, D., Kaladjian, A., Azorin, J.M. *et al.* (1993) Clozapine in the treatment of psychotic refractory depression. *British Journal of Psychiatry*, **163**, 822–824.

Depression Guideline Panel (1993) *Clinical Practice Guideline: Depression in Primary Care*. Vol. 2: *Treatment of Major Depression*. US Department of Health and Human Services, Washington DC.

Devanand, D.P., Sackeim, H.A. & Prudic, J. (1991) Electroconvulsive therapy in the treatment-resistant patient. *Psychiatric Clinics of North America*, **15**, 902–923.

Fadden, G., Bebbington, P. & Kuipers, L. (1987) Caring and its burdens: a study of the spouses of depressed patients. *British Journal of Psychiatry*, **151**, 660–667.

Faedda, G.L., Tondo, L., Baldessarinin, R.J.,

Suppes, T. & Tohen, M. (1993) Outcome after rapid vs. gradual discontinuation of lithium treatment in bipolar disorder. *Archives of General Psychiatry,* **50**, 448–455.

Fava, M. & Davidson, K.G. (1996) Definition and epidemiology of treatment-resistant depression. *Psychiatric Clinics of North America,* **19**, 179–200.

Fink, M. (1992) Electroconvulsive therapy. In: *Handbook of Affective Disorders* (ed. E. S. Paykel), pp. 359–368. Churchill Livingstone, Edinburgh.

Fontaine, R., Ontiveros, A. & Elie, R. *et al.* (1991) Lithium carbonate augmentation of desipramine and fluoxetine in refractory depression. *Biological Psychiatry,* **29**, 946–948.

Frank, E. & Kupfer, D.J. (1990) Axis II personality disorders and personality features in treatment-resistant and refractory depression. In: *Treatment Strategies for Refractory Depression* (eds S. P. Roose & A. H. Glassman), pp. 207–221. American Psychiatric Press, Washington DC.

Frank, E., Kupfer, D. & Siegel, L.R. (1995) Alliance not compliance: a philosophy of outpatient care. *Journal of Clinical Psychiatry,* **56** (Suppl. 1), 11–16.

Ghadirian, A.M., Engelsmann, F. & Dhar, V. *et al.* (1985) The psychotropic effects of inhibitors of steroid biosynthesis in depressed patients refractory to treatment. *Biological Psychiatry,* **37**, 368–375.

Glassman, A.H. & Platman, S.R. (1969) Potentiation of monoamine oxidase inhibitor by tryptophan. *Journal of Psychiatric Research* **7**, 83–88.

Goodman, W.K., McDougle, C.J. & Price, L.H. (1992) Pharmacotherapy of obsessive compulsive disorder. *Journal of Clinical Psychiatry,* **53** (Suppl 4) 29–37.

Goodwin, G.M. (1994) Recurrence of mania after lithium withdrawal: implications for the use of lithium in the treatment of bipolar affective disorder. *British Journal of Psychiatry,* **164**, 149–152.

Goodwin, F.K. & Bunney, W.E. (1971) Depression following reserpine: a re-evaluation. Seminars in Psychiatry, **3**, 435–448.

Goodwin, E.K. & Jamison, K.R. (1990) *Manic Depressive Illness.* Oxford University Press, New York.

Hale, A.S., Procter, A.W. & Bridges, P.K. (1987) Clomipramine, tryptophan and lithium in combination for resistant endogenous depression: 7 case studies. *British Journal of Psychiatry,* **151**, 213–217.

Holzer, C.E., Nguyen, H.T. & Hirschfield, R.M.A. (1996) Reliability of diagnosis in mood disorder. *Psychiatric Clinics of North America,* **19**, 73–84.

Hooley, J.M. (1986) Expressed emotion and depression: interactions between patients and high vs. low EE spouses. *Journal of Abnormal Psychology* **95**, 237–246.

Joffe, R.T., Singer, W., Levitt, A.J. *et al.* (1993) A placebo-controlled comparison of lithium and triiodothyrone augmentation of tricyclic antidepressants in unipolar refractory depression. *Archives of General Psychiatry,* **50**, 387–393.

Johnson, F.N. (1991) Lithium augmentation therapy for depression. *Reviews in Contemporary Pharmacotherapy,* **2**, 3–52.

Kelly, W.F., Checkley, S.A. & Bender, B.A. *et al.* (1983) Cushing's Syndrome and depression: a prospective study of 26 patients. *British Journal of Psychiatry,* **142**, 16–19.

Kendler, K.S., Neale, M.C., Kessler, R.C. *et al.* (1992) A population-based twin study of major depression in women: the impact of varying definitions of illness. *Archives of General Psychiatry,* **49**, 272–281.

Lackheim, H.A., Prudic, J. & Devanand, D.P. *et al.* (1993) Effects of stimulus intensity and electrode placement on the efficacy and cognitive effects of electroconvulsive therapy. *New England Journal of Medicine,* **328**, 839–846.

Lam DH, Green B and Power MJ *et al* (1994) The impact of social cognitive variables on the initial level of depression and recovery. *Journal of Affective Disorders,* **32**, 75–83.

Lewis, D.A. & Smith, R.E. (1983) Steroid induced psychiatric syndromes. *Journal of Affective Disorders,* **5**, 319–332.

Linehan, M.M. (1993) *Cognitive-behavioral Treatment of Borderline Personality Disorder.* Guilford Press, New York.

Lishman, W.A. (1987) *Organic Psychiatry: the Psychological Conquences of Cerebral Disorder,* 2nd edn. Blackwell Scientific Publications, Oxford.

Lovett, L.M., Crimmins, R. & Shaw, D.M. (1989). Outcome in unipolar affective disorder after stereotactic tractotomy. *British Journal of Psychiatry,* **155**, 547–550.

Mason, B.J. & Kocsis, J.H. (1991) Desipramine treatment of alcoholism. *Psychopharmacology Bulletin,* **27**, 155–161.

McGrath, P.J., Stewart, J.W., Nunes, E.V. *et al.* (1993) A double-blind crossover trial of imipramine and phenelzine for outpatients with treatment-refractory depression. *American Journal of Psychiatry,* **150**, 118–123.

McGrath, P.J., Nunes, E.V., Stewart, J.W. *et al.* (1996) Imipramine treatment of alcoholics with primary depression: a placebo controlled clinical trial. *Archives of General Psychiatry,* **53**, 232–240.

McGuffin, P. & Katz, R. (1989) The genetics of depression and manic depressive illness. *British Journal of Psychiatry,* **155**, 294–304.

McGuffin, P. & Katz, R. (1996) Nature, nurture and depression: a twin study. *Psychological Medicine,* **21,** 329–335.

Miller, I.W., Norman, W.H. & Keitner, G.I. (1990) Treatment response of high cognitive dysfunction depressed inpatients. *Comparative Psychiatry* **31,** 62–71.

Montgomery, D.B., Roberts, A., Green, M., Bullock, T., Baldwin, D. & Montgomery, S.A. (1994) Lack of efficacy of fluoxetine in recurrent brief depression and suicidal attempts. *European Archives of Clinical Psychiatry and Clinical Neuroscience,* **244,** 211–215.

Nunes, E., Quitkin, F.M., Brady, R. *et al.* (1991) Imipramine treatment of methadone maintenance patients with affective disorder and illicit drug use. *American Journal of Psychiatry,* **148,** 667–669.

O'Dwyer, A.M., Lightman, S.A. & Marks, M.N. *et al.* (1995) Treatment of major depression with metyrapone and hydrocortisone. *Journal of Affective Disorders,* **33,** 123–128.

O'Leary, K.D. & Beach, R.H. (1990) Marital therapy: a viable treatment for depression and marital discord. *American Journal of Psychiatry,* **147,** 229–235.

Oren, D.A. & Rosenthal, N.E. (1992) Seasonal affective disorder. In: *Handbook of Affective Disorders* (ed. E. S. Paykel), pp. 551–568. Churchill Livingstone, Edinburgh.

Pare, C.M.B. (1963) Potentiation of monoamine oxidase inhibitors by tryptophan. *Lancet,* **ii,** 527–528.

Parker, G., Roy, K., Hadzi-Pavovic, D. *et al.* (1992) Psychotic (delusional) depression: a meta-analysis of physical treatments. *Journal of Affective Disorders,* **24,** 17–24.

Pascualy, M. & Veith, R.C. (1989). Depression as an adverse drug reaction. In: *Aging and Clinical Practice* (eds R. G. Robinson & P.V. Rabin), pp. 132–151. Igaku Shoin, New York.

Paykel, E.S., Flemingero, R.F. & Watson, J.P. (1982). Psychiatric side effects of antihypertensives other than reserpine. *Journal of Clinical Psychopharmacology,* **2,** 14–39.

Perry, P.J. (1996) Pharmacotherapy for major depression with melancholic features: relative efficacy of tricyclic vs. selective serotonin reuptake inhibitor antidepressants. *Journal of Affective Disorders,* **39,** 1–6.

Post, R.M., Uhde, T.W., Ballenger, J.C. *et al.* (1983) Carbamazepine and its 10-, 11-epoxide metabolite in plasma and CSF: relationship to antidepressant response. *Archives of General Psychiatry,* **40,** 673–676.

Poynton, A.M., Kartsoukis, L.D. & Bridges, P.K.

(1995). A prospective clinical study of stereotactic subcaudate tractotomy. *Psychological Medicine,* **25,** 763–770.

Prince, M., Harwood, H., Blizard, R., Thomas, A. & Mann, A. (1997) Impairment, disability and handicap as risk factors for depression in old age. *Psychological Medicine,* **27,** 311–322.

Prudic, J., Sackeim, H.A. & Devanand, D.P. (1990) Medication resistance and clinical response to electroconvulsive therapy. *Psychiatry Research,* **31,** 287–296.

Prudic, J., Haskett, R.F., Mulsant, B. *et al.* (1996) Resistance to antidepressant medications and short-term clinical response to ECT. *American Journal of Psychiatry,* **153,** 985–992.

Quality Assurance Project (1983) A treatment outline for depressive disorders. *Australian and New Zealand Journal of Psychiatry,* **17,** 129–146.

Quitkin, F.M., McGrath, P.J. Stewart, J.W. *et al.* (1989). Phenelzine and imipramine in mood reactive depressives. *Archives of General Psychiatry,* **46,** 787–793.

Quitkin, F.M., McGrath, P.J., & Stewart, J.W. *et al.* (1996) Chronological milestones to guide drug change. *Archives of General Psychiatry,* **53,** 787–792.

Reifler, B.V., Teri, L., Raskind, M. *et al.* (1989) Double-blind trial of imipramine in Alzheimer's disease patients with and without depression. *American Journal of Psychiatry,* **146,** 45–49.

Reynolds, C.F., Perel, J.M., Kupfer, D.J. *et al.* (1987) Open trial response to antidepressant treatment in elderly patients with mixed depression and cognitive impairment. *Psychiatry Research,* **21,** 111–122.

Robin, A. & De Tissera, S. (1982) A double blind controlled comparison of the therapeutic effects of low and high energy electroconvulsive therapy. *British Journal of Psychiatry,* **141,** 357–366.

Rosenbaum, J.F., Fava, M., Nierenberg, A.A. *et al.* (1995) Treatment-resistant mood disorders. In: *Treatment of Psychiatric Disorders* (ed. G. O. Gabbard), 2nd edn, Vol. 1, pp. 1275–1283. American Psychiatric Press, Washington, DC.

Rosenthal, N.E., Sack, D.A. & Gillin, J.C. *et al.* (1984) Seasonal affective disorder: a description of the syndrome and preliminary findings with light therapy. *Archives of General Psychiatry,* **41,** 72–80.

Rothschild, A.J. (1996) Management of psychotic, treatment-resistant depression. *Psychiatric Clinics of North America,* **19** (2), 237–252.

Rothschild, A.J., Samson, J.A., Bessette, M.P. & Carter-Campbell, J.T. (1993) Efficacy of the combination of fluoxetine and perphenazine in the treatment of psychotic depression. *Journal of Clinical Psychiatry,* **54,** 338–342.

455

Royal College of Psychiatrists (1995) *The ECT Handbook*. Royal College of Psychiatrists. London.

Sachs, G.S. (1996) Treatment-resistant bipolar depression. *Psychiatric Clinics of North America*, **19**, 215–236.

Sackeim, H.A., Decina, P., Canzler, M. *et al.* (1987) Effects of electrode placement on the efficacy of titrated low-dose ECT. *American Journal of Psychiatry*, **144**, 1449–1455.

Sackeim, D.G., Prudic, J. & Devanand, D.P. (1990) Treatment of medication-resistant depression with electroconvulsive therapy. In: *American Psychiatric Press Review of Psychiatry*, Vol. 9 (eds A. Tasman, S. M. Goldfiner & C. Kaufman), pp. 91–115. American Psychiatric Press, Washington, DC.

Salzman, C. (1995) Medication compliance in the elderly. *Journal of Clinical Psychiatry*, **56** (Suppl. 1), 18–23.

Sato, T., Sakado, K. & Sato, S. (1993) Is there any specific personality disorder or personality disorder cluster that measures short-term treatment outcome of major depression? *Acta Psychiatrica Scandinavica*, **88**, 342–349.

Schweizer, E., Rickels, K., Amsterdam, J.D. *et al.* (1990) What constitutes an adequate antidepressant trial for fluoxetine? *Journal of Clinical Psychiatry*, **51**, 8–11.

Scott, J. (1988) Cognitive therapy with depressed inpatients. In: *Developments in Cognitive Psychotherapy* (eds P. Tower & W. Dryden), pp. 177–189. Sage Publications, London.

Scott, J., Cole, A. & Eccleston, D. (1991) Dealing with persisting abnormalities of mood. *International Review of Psychiatry*, **3**, 19–33.

Seth, R., Jennings, A.L., Bindman, J., Phillips, J. & Bergman, K. (1992) Combination treatment with noradrenaline and serotonin reuptake inhibitors in resistant depression. *British Journal of Psychiatry*, **161**, 562–565.

Shea, M.T., Pilkonis, P.A., Beckham, E. *et al.* (1990) Personality disorders and treatment outcome in the NIMH treatment of depression collaborative research program. *American Journal of Psychiatry*, **147**, 711–718.

Shea, M.T., Widiger, T.A. & Klein, M.H. (1992) Comorbidity of personality disorders and depression: Implications for treatment. *Journal of Consulting and Clinical Psychology*, **60**, 857–868.

Slutsher, L., Hoesly, F.C., Miller, L., Williams, P., Watson, J.C. & Flemming, D.W. (1990) Eosinophilia-myalgia syndrome associated with exposure to tryptophan from a single manufacturer. *Journal of the American Medical Association*, **264**, 213–217.

Spiker, D.G., Stein, J. & Rich, C.L. (1985) Delusional depression and electroconvulsive therapy: One year later. *Convulsive Therapy*, **1**, 167–172.

Sternbach, H. (1991) The Serotonin Syndrome. *American Journal of Psychiatry*, **148**, 705–713.

Stoudemire, A., Hill, C.D., Morris, R. *et al.* (1991) Cognitive outcome following tricyclic and electroconvulsive treatment of major depression in the elderly. *American Journal of Psychiatry*, **148**, 1336–1340.

Teasdale, J.D. & Barnard, P.J. (1993) *Affect, Cognition and Change: Remodelling Depressive Thought*, Lawrence Erlbaum, Hove.

Terman, J.S., Terman, M., Schlager, D. *et al.* (1990) Efficacy of brief, intense light exposure for treatment of winter depression. *Psychopharmacology Bulletin*, **26**, 3–11.

Terman, M., Williams, J.B.W. & Terman, J.S. (1992) Light therapy for winter depression. In: *Innovations in Clinical Practice: A Source Book*, Vol. 10 (eds P. Keller & S. R. Heyman), pp. 179–221. Professional Resources Executive, Florida.

Thase, M.E. (1996) The role of Axis II comorbidity in the management of patients with treatment resistant depression. *Psychiatric Clinics of North America*, **19**, 287–310.

Thase, M.E., Mallinger, A.G., McKnight, D. *et al.* (1992) Treatment of imipramine-resistant recurrent depression. IV: A double-blind crossover study of tranycypromine for anergic bipolar depression. *American Journal of Psychiatry*, **149**, 195–198.

Thase, M.E. & Rush, A.J. (1995) Treatment-resistant depression. In: *Psychopharmacology: The Fourth Generation of Progress* (eds F. E. Bloom & D. J. Kupfer), pp. 1081–1097. Raven Press, New York.

Vaughn, C.E. & Leff, J.P. (1976) The influence of family and social factors on the course of psychiatric illness. *British Journal of Psychiatry*, **129**, 125–137.

Wehr, T.A. & Goodwin, F.K. (1987) Can antidepressants cause mania and worsen the course of affective illness? *American Journal of Psychiatry*, **144**, 1403–1411.

Weilburg, J.B., Rosenbaum, J.F., Biderman, J., Sachs, G.S., Pollack, M.H. & Kelly, K. (1989) Fluoxetine added to non-MAOI antidepressants converts non-responders to responders: a preliminary report. *Journal of Clinical Psychiatry*, **50**, 447–449.

Weilburg, J.B., Rosenbaum, J.F. & Meltzer-Brody, S. *et al.* (1991) Tricyclic augmentation of fluoxetine. *Annals of Clinical Psychiatry*, **3**, 209–213.

Whisman, M.A., Miller, I.W., Norman, W.H. &

Keitner, G.I. (1991) Cognitive therapy with depressed inpatients: specific effects on dysfunctional cognitions. *Journal of Consulting and Clinical Psychology,* **59**, 282–288.

Wilcox, D.R., Gilan, R. & Hare, E.H. (1965) Do psychiatric outpatients take their drugs? *British Medical Journal,* **2**, 790–792.

Wood, M.J. & Rubinstein, M. (1990) An atypical responder to clozapine (letter). *American Journal of Psychiatry,* **147**, 369.

Young, A.H. & Cowen, P.J. (1994) Antidepressant drugs. In: *Side-effects of Drugs Annual 17* (eds J. K. Aronson & C. J. Van Boxtell), pp. 14–24. Elsevier, Amsterdam.

Index

Index